To Lawrence J. T.
(at last I am able to
return the compliment)
with best wishes,

Bill Campbell.

Rahway, N.J.
July, 1983.

Trichinella
and Trichinosis

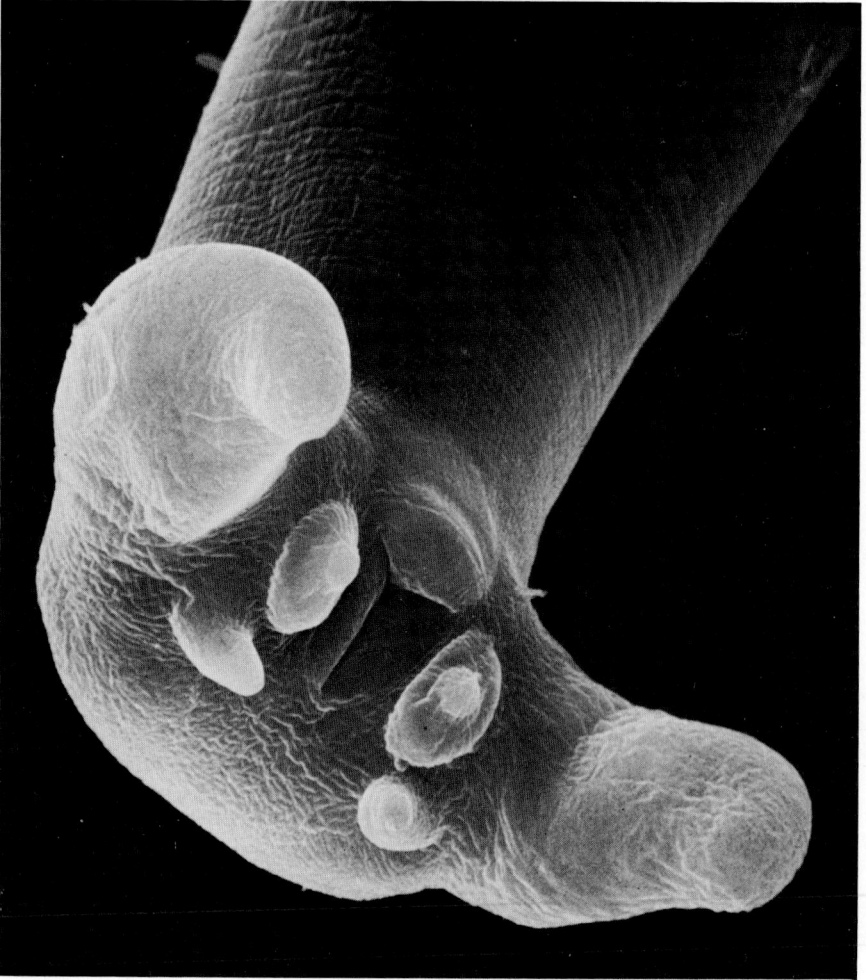

Trichinella spiralis

Posterior end of male worm (*T. spiralis nativa*) by scanning electron microscopy. Courtesy of Drs. J. R. Lichtenfels and K. D. Murrell, U.S. Department of Agriculture.

Trichinella and Trichinosis

Edited by

William C. Campbell

Merck Institute for Therapeutic Research
Rahway, New Jersey

Plenum Press • New York and London

Library of Congress Cataloging in Publication Data

Main entry under title:

Trichinella and trichinosis.

Bibliography: p.
Includes index.
1. Trichinosis. 2. Trichinella spiralis. I. Campbell, William C. (William Cecil),
1930–   . [DNLM: 1. Trichinella. 2. Trichinosis. WC 855 T8225]
RC186.T815T73 1983   616.9'654   83-2390
ISBN 0-306-41140-7

© 1983 Plenum Press, New York
A Division of Plenum Publishing Corporation
233 Spring Street, New York, N. Y. 10013

Printed in the United States of America

DEDICATED

To Dr. J. Desmond Smyth, who kindled a parasitological fire; to Dr. Arlie C. Todd, who fanned the flames; to Dr. Ashton C. Cuckler, chemotherapist *par excellence,* who suggested testing a drug against *Trichinella* and thereby induced an addiction to the affairs of that worm; to the late Dr. S. Emanuel Gould and Dr. Zbigniew Kozar, whose encouragement kept the addiction from waning; to S.J.C. and the late R.J.C., who made it all possible; and to Mary, Jenifer, Peter, and Betsy, who make it all worthwhile.

Contributors

Lyndia Slayton Blair
Merck Institute for Therapeutic Research
Rahway, New Jersey 07065

Graham A. Bullick
Department of Physiology and Cell Biology
University of Texas Medical School at Houston
Houston, Texas 77025

William C. Campbell
Merck Institute for Therapeutic Research
Rahway, New Jersey 07065

Gilbert A. Castro
Department of Physiology and Cell Biology
University of Texas Medical School at Houston
Houston, Texas 77025

David A. Denham
London School of Hygiene and Tropical Medicine
London WC1E 7HT, England

Dickson D. Despommier
Division of Tropical Medicine
School of Public Health
Columbia University
New York, New York 10032

Terry A. Dick
Department of Zoology
University of Manitoba
Winnipeg, Manitoba, Canada R3T 2N2

Anneke Elgersma
Rijks Instituut Voor de Volksgezondheid
3720 BA Bilthoven, The Netherlands

Charles W. Kim
State University of New York at Stony Brook
Stony Brook, Long Island, New York 11794

Jack C. Leighty
Dunkirk, Maryland 20754

Inger Ljungström
Department of Parasitology
National Bacteriological Laboratory
S-105 21 Stockholm, Sweden

Zbigniew S. Pawłowski
Clinic of Parasitic and Tropical Diseases
Medical Academy of Poznan
Poznan, Poland
and
Parasitic Diseases Programme
World Health Organization
Geneva 27, Switzerland

E. Joost Ruitenberg
Rijks Instituut Voor de Volksgezondheid
3720 BA Bilthoven, The Netherlands

David S. Silberstein
Department of Microbiology
Columbia University
New York, New York 10032

George L. Stewart
Laboratory of Parasitology
Department of Biology
University of Texas
Arlington, Texas 76019

Frans van Knapen
Rijks Instituut Voor de Volksgezondheid
3720 BA Bilthoven, The Netherlands

Derek Wakelin
Department of Zoology
University of Nottingham
Nottingham, England

Norman F. Weatherly
Department of Parasitology and Laboratory Practice
School of Public Health
University of North Carolina
Chapel Hill, North Carolina 27514

William J. Zimmermann
Veterinary Medical Research Institute
Iowa State University
Ames, Iowa 50011

Preface

As the modern outpouring of biological information continues at ever-increasing pace, two kinds of reviews are needed to keep the torrent in manageable form. The one assumes a working knowledge of the field in question and tries to bring the reader up to date by reporting and assessing the recent developments. The other attempts to assimilate the recent developments into a coherent restatement of the whole subject. This book falls in the latter category.

Trichinella spiralis infection has been in the medical and biological limelight for more than a century, and interest in it continues unabated—as evidenced by what Norman Stoll called the "perennially exuberant" research on trichinosis. The infection seems to offer something for almost everyone. For the physician, it offers a patient with painful and sometimes fatal disease; for the public-health official, a threat to the commonweal; for the experimental biologist, a life cycle that is unique yet easily and rapidly maintained in the laboratory; for the field ecologist, a symbiont with an affinity for an extraordinary range of wildlife species; for the pork producer, a poorer profit; for the cook, a culinary constraint; and for the diner, a dietary danger. Yet, despite this breadth of interest, and the cascade of new data, the only comprehensive books on the subject in English are those of S.E. Gould, published in 1945 and 1970. Although his work on trichinosis was virtually an avocation, Dr. Gould's passion for the subject enabled him to produce landmark treatises. His 1970 volume, *Trichinosis in Man and Animals,* with contributions from many authors, remains a treasure-house of information. But the past dozen years have brought major new findings in all aspects of trichinosis, and it is time for another stock-taking. This volume offers a fresh synthesis of old and new information, and it is hoped that the work will serve as a succinct yet comprehensive source of information on *Trichinella* as parasite and pathogen.

The use of the term *trichinosis,* rather than *trichinellosis,* will dismay some readers. Adoption of *trichinellosis* would have been baffling to others. It can be argued that as *Trichinella* was gradually becoming accepted as the correct name for the nematode genus *Trichina,* so *trichinosis* should have become superseded by *trichinellosis.* But *trichinosis* had already spread from the technical language to the vernacular, and, as in the case of *malaria* and *coccidiosis,* a new lexicon was not needed to clarify what was already perfectly clear to the scientist and layman alike. (In 1911, Ambrose Bierce's *The Devil's Dictionary* contained the entry: Trichinosis, n. The pig's reply to proponents of porcophagy.) We have two defensible words for disease caused by *Trichinella,* and with some misgiving we have chosen to stick with the one that is shorter and more venerable.

W.C.C.

Acknowledgments

The Editor is greatly indebted to the contributing authors for their fine cooperation. He especially thanks Dr. D.D. Despommier, Ms. L.S. Blair, Dr. D.A. Denham, and Dr. C.W. Kim for their wise and generous counsel throughout the planning and execution of the volume. Thanks are extended to Mrs. June Wood for typing several portions of the text, and to Mr. K. Jensen and Mr. L. Goldes of Plenum Press for their expert production of the book.

Contents

CHAPTER 3

Biology

DICKSON D. DESPOMMIER

CHAPTER 4

Biochemistry

GEORGE L. STEWART

CHAPTER 5

Anatomical Pathology
NORMAN F. WEATHERLY

CHAPTER 6

Pathophysiology of the Gastrointestinal Phase
GILBERT A. CASTRO and GRAHAM R. BULLICK

CHAPTER 10

Chemotherapy
WILLIAM C. CAMPBELL and DAVID A. DENHAM

CHAPTER 11

Clinical Aspects in Man
ZBIGNIEW S. PAWŁOWSKI

CHAPTER 12

Immunodiagnosis in Man
INGER LJUNGSTRÖM

CHAPTER 13

Epidemiology I: Modes of Transmission
WILLIAM C. CAMPBELL

CHAPTER 14

Epidemiology II: Geographic Distribution and Prevalence
CHARLES W. KIM

CHAPTER 15

Control I: Public-Health Aspects (with Special Reference to the United States)

JACK C. LEIGHTY

CHAPTER 16

Control II: Surveillance in Swine and Other Animals by Muscle Examination
WILLIAM J. ZIMMERMANN

CHAPTER 17

Control III: Surveillance in Swine by Immunodiagnostic Methods
E. JOOST RUITENBERG, FRANS VAN KNAPEN, and ANNEKE ELGERSMA

APPENDIX 1

Synopsis of Morphology
DICKSON D. DESPOMMIER and WILLIAM C. CAMPBELL

APPENDIX 2

Laboratory Techniques
LYNDIA SLAYTON BLAIR

Historical Introduction

WILLIAM C. CAMPBELL

1. PROLOGUE: GHOSTS OF CHRISTMAS PAST AND CHRISTMAS PRESENT

On a farm in Germany, Christmas 1859 meant the usual preparation of festival meats, but for a young servant woman who prepared them, the season did not bring the usual festivity. She fell ill, suffering not only from fatigue, dizziness, and fever, but also from excruciating pain in her muscles. When the new year of 1860 was barely two weeks old, she was brought to the hospital in Dresden. The diagnosis was typhoid fever, or typhus abdominalis.

It was duly entered in the books, but it was not a confident diagnosis. The woman's pain was more severe than would be expected in typhoid; she lay curled up, unable to make a movement without agony. There had been no crop of pink spots on her skin, and her spleen was not enlarged. Nevertheless, the hospital pathologist, Friedrich Albert von Zenker, thought it was typhoid, and his opinion prevailed. Unlike most pathologists of that time and place, Zenker did not confine his activities to the autopsy room. He was in the hospital wards every day, conferring with the clinicians, and this case of suspected typhoid, now unmistakably moribund, was of interest to him precisely because of the unusual muscle tenderness. In other typhoid cases, Zenker had observed hyaline necrosis in postmortem sections of muscle. The present case might provide further evidence of a link between typhoid and the degeneration of muscle tissue. Just 15 days after her

---

WILLIAM C. CAMPBELL • Merck Institute for Therapeutic Research, Rahway, New Jersey 07065.

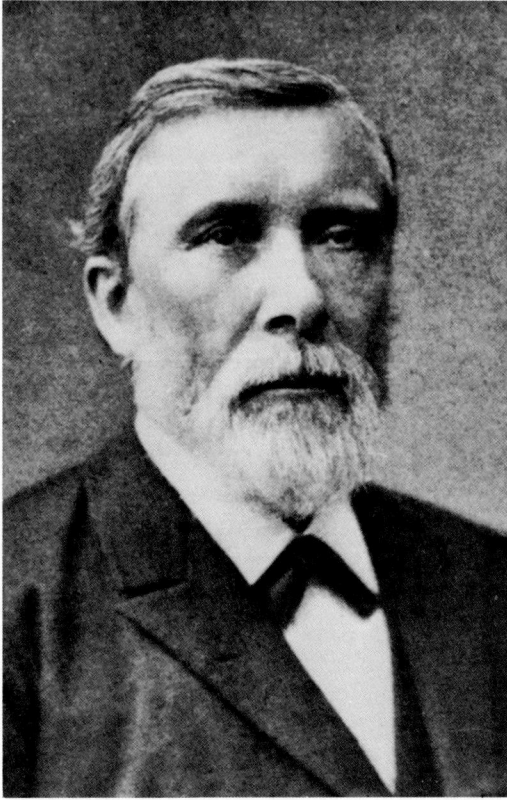

Friedrich Zenker

admission to the hospital, the young woman died. The official post-mortem examination was scheduled for the following day, but Zenker needed to examine a specimen of muscle before autolysis could distort his findings, and so, only a few hours after the patient died, he removed a sliver of muscle from her arm, crushed it, and examined it under the microscope. He was in for a surprise.

What Zenker saw was worms—dozens of minute worms wriggling in that tiny fragment of muscle tissue. He examined other pieces of skeletal muscle, and in every piece he found worms. So far as we know, no one had ever before seen quite that sight, yet Zenker knew at once what the worms were. He and many other observers had seen these worms or "trichinae" in cadavers, but each worm had been enclosed in a capsule within the muscle tissue and seemed to be doing no harm. In Zenker's case, the worms were moving vigorously in the muscle tissue,

and because they were so numerous and so widely distributed throughout the body, it seemed virtually certain that they were responsible for
the pain that had been so prominent a feature of the case. The thought
was inescapable: these worms were not only harmful but could even be
lethal. The first clinical case of trichinosis ever recognized was also the
first known fatal case.

A doctor in Postville, Iowa, does not expect to see a single clinical
case of trichinosis in his lifetime. Such infections as may occur in the
local populace are likely to be too light to arouse suspicion of trichinosis.
Yet in 1975, just four days after Christmas, a Postville doctor diagnosed
trichinosis in three patients. On the very same day, a doctor in Waterloo,
Iowa, diagnosed two cases of trichinosis—a man and his wife who had
relatives in Postville. The Postville connection turned out to be significant and to involve a particular batch of sausage. This was no ordinary
sausage; it was a venison delicacy prepared to celebrate the end of the
hunting season, and smoked over a wood fire for a couple of days.
There was no danger in that, for herbivorous animals are not normally
sources of trichinosis. But although meat from more than 100 deer had been
used, it apparently was not enough and some ground pork had
been mixed in with the venison. The result was a big batch of sausages,
a big barbecue party, many savory Christmas presents—and many cases
of trichinosis. Once the five cases had been diagnosed on December
29th, it was discovered that practically everyone who had eaten sausage
at the barbecue party had become infected. The sausage gifts had been
distributed far and wide, carrying the infective larvae with them. In all,
67 people had acquired trichinosis, but the infections were not especially
severe and there had been no fatalities (Centers for Disease Control,
1976).

The first of these episodes marks the beginning of trichinosis as a
known disease; the other gives a glimpse of trichinosis more than a
century later. The history of trichinosis is more than the history of such
episodes; it is the history of many biological discoveries, including the
first unraveling of a nematode life cycle, and it is the history of several
significant medical and sociological developments.

2. A WORM DISCOVERED (1835)

We know a good deal more about the discovery of *Trichinella spiralis*
than about the antiquity of the disease it causes. We do not know when
or where the infection first became common in man. We do not know
whether or not it was a factor in the Mosaic proscription of pork

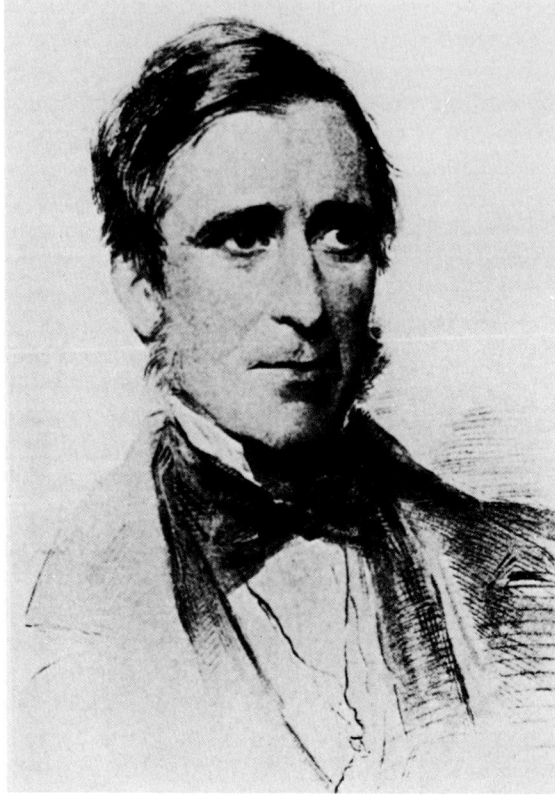

James Paget

consumption. The distinction of having been the earliest known case of *Trichinella* infection (known retrospectively, that is) belongs to a young Egyptian weaver named Makht. He lived near the River Nile about 1200 B. C.; but we did not know about his infection until 1974, at which time an intercostal muscle of his mummified body was found to contain a cyst that appeared on histological examination to be that of *Trichinella spiralis* (Millet *et al.*, 1980).

So far as we can tell, *Trichinella spiralis* was first seen on Monday, February 2, 1835, being seen on that day by James Paget, a first-year medical student, at St. Bartholomew's hospital, London. While participating in a routine *post mortem* dissection, Paget saw small white specks in the flesh of the cadaver; and having first studied them with a hand-lens, he resolved to examine them more closely with a microscope. Because the Hospital did not have a microscope, Paget went to the

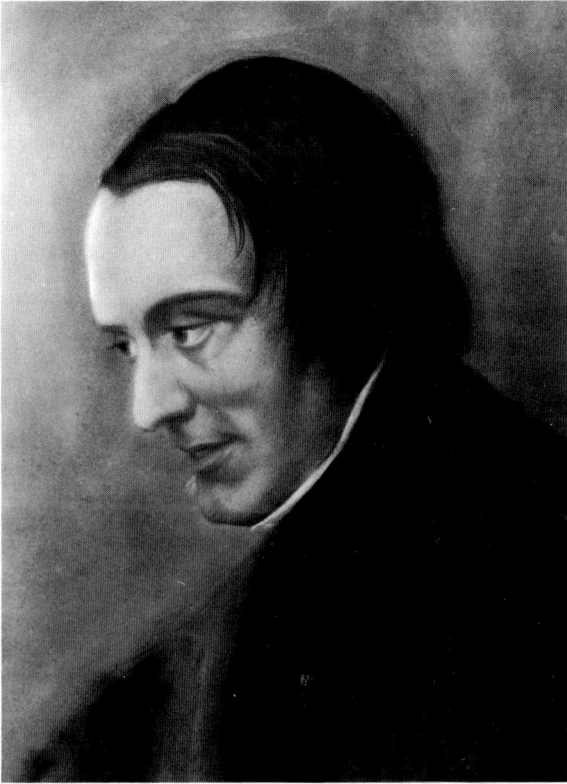

Richard Owen

Zoology Department of the British Museum. Because the Zoology Department did not have a microscope, the head of the Department took Paget to the Botany Department. Because the head of that Department was Robert Brown, the great microscopist, Paget finally got to look at his specimens through a microscope. (Brown, on being asked on that occasion if he knew anything about parasitic worms, is said to have replied "no, thank God".) Paget made some crude sketches of the cysts and the worms within, and reported his findings to the student's club of the Hospital on February 6th. He prepared a report for publication, but abandoned it in favor of a description written by Richard Owen and based on worm specimens from the same cadaver. (The specimens had been sent to Owen by Wormald, who recognized their parasitic nature either on the basis of an earlier surmise that such objects were cysticerci or, according to Paget, on the basis of the observations that Paget had just made.) The available evidence suggests that Paget and Owen made a deal in which Paget would settle for an acknowledgement of priority in Owen's paper, while Owen would provide the zoological expertise and professional clout necessary to assure early publication in a reputable journal (Campbell, 1979). Paget was not only Owen's junior in his standing at the Hospital and in English medical and scientific circles, but also lacked ready access to a microscope of high resolution. Owen (1835) promptly published a formal description of the parasite as a new species, naming it *Trichina spiralis*; and, as was his nature, he gave Paget only minimal credit for the discovery. In 1895, and again in 1896, Railliet proposed changing the name of the worm to *Trichinella* because the name *Trichina* had been applied in 1830 to a genus of fly (Gould, 1945). The new became universally accepted.

The speckled appearance of muscle in *Trichinella* infection had undoubtedly been seen many times before Paget's observation, and claims for an earlier discovery of trichinosis have been made on that basis. Even at St. Bartholomew's Hospital, Paget's contemporary, Thomas Wormald, had encountered grainy objects of similar appearance in the course of his dissections. The observation of a speck, however, is not the observation of a worm. Furthermore we generally cannot be sure, even in retrospect, that the objects seen were in fact *Trichinella* cysts. The case of Mr. Peacock, of Guy's Hospital, London, is an exception. In 1828, Peacock observed at autopsy a speckling of the muscles associated with the larynx. He made a dry preparation of the specimen for the hospital museum, and in the following year this specimen was listed in Hodgkin's Catalogue of the Museum as "No. 1361A. The Sterno-Hyoideus Muscle, speckled with numerous minute bony points". Years later, after the discovery of *Trichinella*, microscopic examination of the specimen revealed the presence of the worm, and the 1858 edition of the Catalogue reflected this new appreciation of Peacock's piece of speckled flesh. Thus 1828 is the year of the earliest known observation of the cysts of *T. spiralis* in human flesh—or the flesh of any species. This finding does not, however, alter the priority of Paget and Owen in the discovery and documentation of the worm. Peacock did not publish his observation, and did not even suspect that his "bony points" were anything but just that (Wilks, 1889).

Another physician, Friedrich Tiedemann, had seen similar objects in human flesh 7 years earlier; and his observation, moreover, was recorded in the literature (Froriep's Notizen, 1822; see Blumer, 1939). Like Peacock, Tiedemann had apparently not suspected the parasitic nature of the "stony concretions"; and although he had them chemically analyzed by his colleague Gmelin, he does not seem to have examined them microscopically. Leuckart doubted that the objects were *Trichinella* cysts because they were reported to be twice as big as one would expect such cysts to be. It is hard, however, to imagine what else they might have been. Thus, Tiedemann predates Peacock with respect to the observation of what were probably *Trichinella* cysts, but Peacock made the first observation of what were unequivocally *Trichinella* cysts.

It is generally agreed that John Hilton was the first to postulate the parastitic nature of the specks observed in human muscle. Hilton encountered speckled muscle in the dissecting room at Guy's Hospital, where he was Demonstrator of Anatomy. He examined the objects with a microscope but could not discern any internal structure. Perhaps the cysts were more calcified than were those examined by Paget approximately 2 years later. On some such slender ground must Hilton have forfeited the claim to be discoverer of one of man's most fabled parasites. Certainly it was not lack of curiosity—although Paget was later to boast of "observing" the objects where others merely "saw" them. Indeed Hilton was almost certainly the first person to attempt experimental infection of animals with *Trichinella*. Unfortunately he implanted the infected flesh subcutaneously in his rabbits; had he administered it orally, he might well have changed the course of trichinosis history. Hilton related that Addison (another luminary of Guy's Hospital) tried to culture the mysterious particles *in vitro*; but his experiment, for a variety of reasons, was unproductive (Hilton, 1833).

There are two rather mysterious aspects of Hilton's contribution. His postulation of the parasitic nature of the cysts resides entirely in the title of his article on the subject (Hilton, 1833). The title states that the speckled appearance of muscle was "probably" due to "the formation of very small cysticerci", but the text contains no suggestion of parasitism. Hilton was, of course, quite wrong in suggesting a cestode rather than a nematode parasite; but his mistake is understandable, since the cysts would indeed have resembled miniature versions of the objects that were later to be identified as tapeworm larvae. Secondly, Hodgkin, who was in a position to know, recorded that Hilton submitted his article to the Medical-Chirurgical Society on January 22, 1833 and that "the paper was read but the publication suppressed by the Council" (Wilks, 1889). This is difficult to understand since Hilton's article was in fact published in February 1833. Perhaps the Council of the Society objected to the cysticercus proposition as unsupported speculation, and were willing to approve the manuscript if that part were to be deleted. In that case, retention of the reference to cysticerci in the final portion of Hilton's title may actually have been inadvertent.

It is possible that *Trichinella* larvae were seen, and extracted from their cysts, by Henry Wood in October 1834 (Wood, 1835). His report, however, was ambiguous, and he cannot be assigned priority in the discovery of the worm (Campbell, 1979).

3. A NEMATODE LIFE CYCLE DISCOVERED (1835–1860)

Following the observations of Paget and Owen, the essentials of the morphology of *Trichinella spiralis* were described by several workers, including Farre (1835), Bischoff (1840), and Luschka (1851), and attention turned to the question of whither this new parasite went and from whence it came. Two early observations were made, each a potential revelation but each apparently failing to contribute significantly to the actual elucidation of the life cycle. In Philadelphia, in 1846, Leidy found the parasite in a piece of pork that he was having for dinner. That should have suggested something about the mode of transmission, but Leidy fell afoul of scientific authority. Deising decreed, without benefit of seeing Leidy's specimen, that it must be a different species, and almost everyone, including Leidy, apparently suspended his imaginative powers. It was not so, however, with the irrepressible Kuchenmeister, who did not fail to point out that the presence of *Trichinella* in pork suggested the infection of man by ingestion of pork, but he failed to make others pay attention. H.B. Ward called Leidy's observation "the most significant discovery among those of the many investigators who contributed to working out the life history"—but the evidence for such a claim is tenuous. Ward had earlier pointed out that the German investigators had utterly failed to grasp the import of Leidy's discovery (Ward, 1923), but subsequently reported that Virchow had acknowledged, in conversation, his indebtedness to Leidy (Ward, 1930). The second neglected observation was made in Germany. In Göttingen, Herbst was in the habit of dissecting various animals and feeding their remains to his pet badger. In November 1850, the badger itself came to the dissection table, and its muscles were found to be heavily infected with *Trichinella*. Portions of the flesh were fed to three young puppies, and several months later all of them were shown to have heavily infected muscles (Herbst, 1851). This was the first experimental evidence that the ingestion of trichinous meat would result in trichinosis. Herbst's report of 1851 should thus have been seminal, but was largely ignored (Foster, 1965).

A major turning point in the investigation of the life history of *Trichinella* was the realization in the 1840s that the worm as then known was an immature form, with Dujardin of France and von Siebold of Germany suggesting that it was the progeny of a nematode already known in the adult form (Reinhard, 1958). Later, Kuchenmeister, fresh from his success in demonstrating that a cysticercus becomes a tapeworm, went further. On the basis of excellent microscopical work, he recognized similarities between *Trichinella* and *Trichuris* and in 1855 recommended an attempt to translate the one into the other. (For Kuchenmeister, the significance of Leidy's observation was that man might become infected with whipworm by eating trichinous pork.) In 1859, his challenge was taken up by Rudolph Leuckart, the great zoologist of Giessen.

Leuckart had already begun to try to solve the *Trichinella* mystery. In 1857, he had given infected flesh to mice, and 3 days later he had found that the ingested worms had not only come out of their cysts into the gut of the mice, but also had already become much bigger than they had been when encysted in the muscle of their former host. We now know that such worms are not only bigger but also sexually mature, but they are still only a millimeter or two long, and it did not occur to Leuckart that worms so small could in fact be adults. Leuckart then decided to try the suggestion made by Kuchenmeister, but before he got started on the project, another eminent German scientist got into the act.

In July 1859, Rudolph Virchow happened on a hospital cadaver that was riddled with *Trichinella* larvae. It was a perfect source of experimental material, but Virchow was just about to leave on a trip to Norway, and the only experimental animal available was a rather sick dog. He fed it some of the infected muscle, and in a few days the dog was dead. This was one of those precious single animals that seem to mock our modern dependence on statistically significant numbers of test animals. In the intestine of that one wretched dog, Virchow found innumerable tiny nematodes that he recognized as adult worms. This was a breathtaking discovery. It was the very point that Leuckart had missed two years previously, when he failed to recognize the sexual maturity of the worms in his test mice. It was more than that. Virchow did not know whether these animals represented a new species, but he knew that they were not *Trichuris*, so his discovery also refuted Kuchenmeister's hypothesis that *Trichinella* was larval *Trichuris*—the very thing that Leuckart was just about to test. Virchow, realizing the significance of his discovery, dashed off a letter to the Paris Academy of Sciences, but his handwriting was so bad that it took two months for one of President Claude Bernard's assistants to decipher the letter and translate it into French. In the meantime, Leuckart made his move. He

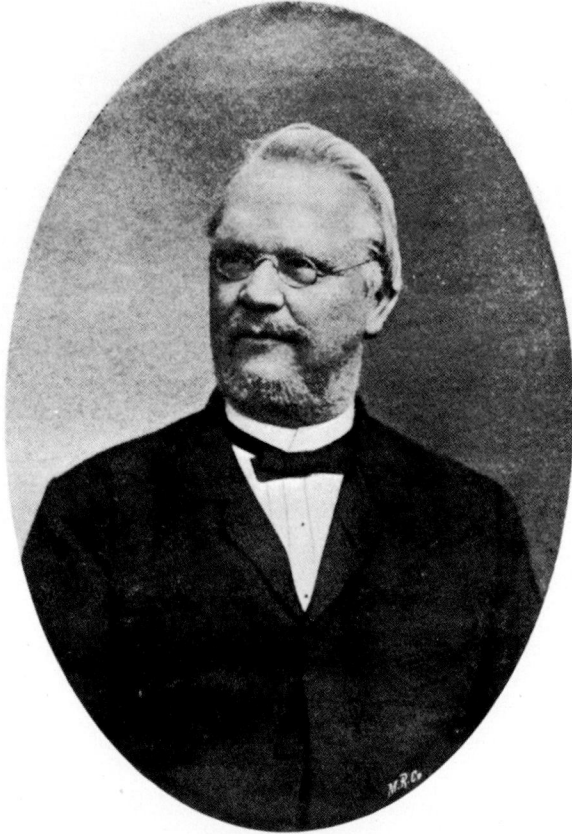

Rudolf Leuckart

gave *Trichinella*-infected muscle to a young pig. When he killed the pig 4 weeks later, he found a few dozen *Trichuris* (estimated roughly as 30–40) and took that as suggestive evidence that *Trichinella* did indeed become *Trichuris*. Although he recognized the limitation of the experiment, Leuckart, like Virchow, wanted his finding recorded with the speed and prestige that only the Paris Academy could offer. He wrote to Professor van Beneden in Belgium, asking him to present the new information at the next academy meeting. Without even waiting for the next meeting, van Beneden had the gist of Leuckart's report inserted in the printed record issued in September (van Beneden, 1859).

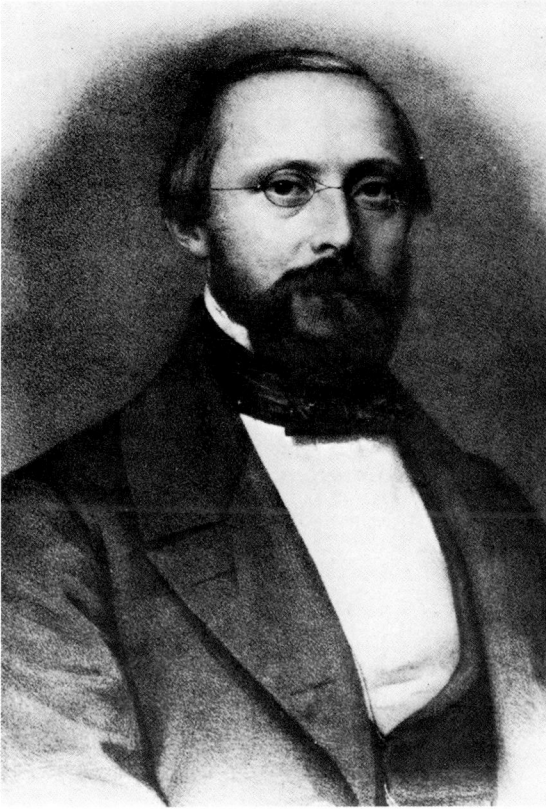

Rudolf Virchow

Unhappily, Leuckart's original *"dutzenden"* had been misread as *"du-izend,"* and Leuckart, like Virchow, paid a penalty for his imperfect penmanship. One might expect to find "dozens" of *Trichuris* in a naturally infected pig, but one would not expect to find a "thousand." Thus, Leuckart's report appeared to be a much stronger confirmation of Kuchenmeister's hypothesis than Leuckart would have wished to claim. Virchow's paper on the maturation of *Trichinella* finally appeared in November 1859 (Virchow, 1859). That month was, for another reason, a very special moment in the history of biological literature, but it might be supposed that Leuckart's immediate concern was not the appearance of Darwin's *magnum opus* but rather the appearance of Virchow's clear contradiction of Leuckart's pronouncement in support of the hypothesis that *Trichinella* becomes *Trichuris*. Leuckart's first reaction was that Virchow could not be right, but further experiments convinced him that Virchow could not be wrong (Leuckart, 1860).

It was in the month following the publication of Virchow's paper that illness befell the young woman whose case was used to introduce this chapter and who became the first person known to die of trichinosis. Zenker, the pathologist in that case, made a magnificent contribution to our knowledge of trichinosis, but his role is generally understated. His contributions, even in his lifetime, were not as widely appreciated as those of Leuckart—a matter about which Zenker was understandably unhappy (Becker and Schmidt, 1975). Zenker concluded that the innumerable unencapsulated larvae had caused the illness and death of the young woman, thereby making a discovery that Osler called the most important helminthological contribution of the 19th century. Althaus (1864) called it "no doubt the most important medical event of the last few years." Zenker, two weeks later, also examined mucus from the intestinal wall of the late patient and found adult worms, including gravid females. There is conflicting testimony as to whether this examination was prompted by knowledge of Virchow's work, but the important thing is that he realized that the intestinal adults were the progenitors of the larvae in the muscle. Zenker made good use of the young woman's musculature. Some of it he gave to a dog, some he gave to Virchow (not in the same sense), and some he gave to Leuckart. Virchow in turn gave some of the muscle tissue to a rabbit, while Leuckart fed his to a dog and to a pig. All these feedings resulted in successful infection (although Zenker also fed some other dogs in which he failed to demonstrate infection). As a result of these experiments, the three German workers were able to settle the basic points of the life cycle of *Trichinella spiralis*, including the mating of adults in the gut, the deposition of larvae by gravid female worms, the probable transport of the progeny to the muscles via the lymphatics, and the penetration of individual muscle cells, with destruction of the contractile elements and the formation of the so-called capsule from the sarcolemma. (At the risk of gross oversimplification, it could be said that it was Virchow who recognized the worm's early maturation in the gut and found larvae in mesenteric lymph nodes and inside muscle fibers; it was Zenker who found unencapsulated larvae in human musculature and recognized their pathogenicity, found the adult worms in human intestines, and suggested dissemination of their progeny via the lymphatics; and it was Leuckart who found embryos and larvae in the uterus of the adult female and obtained much of the supporting experimental data.)

It would be quite wrong, of course, to give the impression that these studies answered all questions or that they were universally accepted. Many details were missing, and many details remained controversial for many years. Hertwig (1895), in summarizing some points of dispute, related that Askenasy and Cerfontaine rejected the view that the adult females shed their larvae in the intestinal lumen and held that the worms penetrate the mucosa and submucosa to deposit their progeny. Actually, Cerfontaine (1895) believed that larviposition occurred both in the lumen and in the tissue, but considered only the latter to be of medical importance. The question was left more or less open (with some inclination toward the Askenasy–Cerfontaine position) until it was made meaningless by the recent discovery that the adults live in the mucosal tissue and not in the lumen of the crypts (see Chapter 3). The preponderance of female worms in the intestinal population was noted by Claus (1860) during experiments on rabbits and guinea pigs.

From his study of 1859, Leuckart concluded that the newborn *Trichinella* larvae reached the musculature by migrating through connective tissue. Zenker believed that they were transported by blood, perhaps reaching it via lymph (as suggested by Virchow's finding larvae in mesenteric lymph nodes), and this position was supported by the experimental work of Askenasy (Hertwig, 1895) and Cerfontaine (1895). Hertwig does not mention this as an item of controversy in the latter part of the 19th century, and perhaps the concept of vascular dissemination had already gained ascendancy. In any case, Leuckart's connective-tissue theory was eventually discredited and, after being revived briefly in modern times (see Madsen, 1974), was given the *coup de grace* by Harley and Gallichio (1971). An unfortunate *sequela* of Leuckart's teaching is that the period in which the larvae are distributed throughout the musculature is still often referred to as the "migratory phase." The term "dissemination phase" would seem more appropriate for a process that is probably a passive humoral transportation.

Some of the early workers (including Owen himself) had concluded that the *Trichinella* capsule was merely an organized exudate of host tissue. Knox (1836), among others, disagreed, and Bischoff said that Owen's position was "definitely contradicted" by the double walls of the cyst and that the capsule "is without a doubt an essential and intergral part of the worm" (translation from Bischoff, 1840). On the other hand, Dalton (1864) postulated that the capsule represented a dilation and thickening of a blood vessel of the musculature at a point where a larva had come to rest. According to Hertwig (1895), several workers (Robin,

Chalet, Chatin, Cerfontaine) contended that the capsules were formed in the connective tissue of the musculature rather than in the actual muscle fibers. Hertwig was one of many authors who confirmed the penetration of individual muscle fibers, with ensuing multiplication of nuclei and loss of striation in the vicinity of the parasite. For the next century, however, the capsule was regarded as a noncellular product of a defunct muscle fiber rather than as a transformed cell. The concepts of the infected cell as a "nurse cell" and of *Trichinella* as an *intracellular* parasite in both enteral and parenteral phases are of recent origin, and the reader is referred to Chapter 3 for further information. (In this context, it is of interest that Owen actually referred to the infected host tissue, not as necrotic, but as "morbidly altered.")

The young woman who died of trichinosis in Dresden in January 1860 provided the opportunity for Zenker to make another major breakthrough. To appreciate its significance, we must remember that despite the rapidly increasing knowledge of the biology of the parasite, its mode of transmission to man was unknown (Leuckart had become convinced that man must acquire the infection from dogs). Feeding experiments had shown that muscle-dwelling "trichinae" became gut-dwelling adults. The worms in the gut of Zenker's patient suggested that she had eaten flesh containing trichinae. He recalled that she had worked on a farm, that she had fallen ill at Christmas time, that pigs were traditionally slaughtered for the Christmas celebration, and that trichinae had been observed in the flesh of pigs (Zenker, 1860). (Zenker does not say whether he had in mind the very recent feeding experiment in pigs or Leidy's neglected earlier observation.)

Making a Sunday journey of some 80 preautomobile miles to the farm (near Plauen) where the young woman had worked, Zenker learned from the proprietor that the entire staff, including the proprietor himself, had been ill in January. Of particular importance, however, was the nature of the illness in two cases. The farm manager's wife had been severely ill with what had been thought to be typhoid fever (typhus abdominalis), but had recovered. The man who had butchered the pigs for the Christmas festivities had become ill soon afterward. In January, he developed fever (profuse sweating) and muscular pain so severe that he had been confined to bed for at least three weeks, barely able to move his legs, arms, or neck. Butchers were in the habit of eating raw meat at slaughter time.

Some remnants of the butcher's handiwork were still to be found at the farm. They included ham and sausage from a pig killed on December 21. Zenker's microscopic examination of the ham was reminiscent of his examination of his late patient. In the first fragment of meat, and every subsequent fragment, he found a multitude of larvae. He found them in the sausage, too. For Zenker, there could no longer be any doubt: his patient had acquired lethal trichinosis by eating infected pork, and the butcher and the manager's wife had probably acquired the same disease from the same source. Zenker had broken the mystery of the transmission of trichinosis.

4. FROM ZOOLOGICAL CURIOSITY TO LETHAL PATHOGEN (1860–1900)

In the quarter century that elapsed between the discovery of *Trichinella* in 1835 and the discovery of its pathogenicity in 1860, the infection was observed quite frequently in cadavers. Its potential for harm was by no means overlooked. Wood (1835) for example suspected that his patient's "acute rheumatism" was due to the parasite; but in the absence of clear-cut evidence of pathogenicity, the parasite was regarded by most clinicians as a curiosity and a plaything that allowed anatomists to indulge their impractical fondness for microscopy. At the same time, discovery of the parasite was evidence of a careful autopsy, and the finding was sufficiently uncommon to permit the anatomist to publish it. Indeed, the finding of *Trichinella* acquired a considerable *cachet*, and clinicians were known to quarrel over which of them should publish a description of the larvae in a cadaver that they had examined together (Becker and Schmidt, 1975).

Many reports of infection came from Germany, but it was clear almost from the beginning that the parasite was not confined to Europe. Bowditch and Hall discovered the worm in a cadaver in the United States in 1842. Their patient had evidently had a heavy infection, but its clinical significance was obscured by concomitant cancer. A detailed microscopic examination of the worms was being made when news of Owen's description reached them (Bowditch, 1842).

We have seen in the prologue to this chapter that the pathogenicity of *Trichinella* was demonstrated by Zenker in 1860. Equivocable cases may have been observed by others, but Zenker's was a landmark case, leaving little doubt that *T. spiralis* could be a pathogen—and a lethal one at that. It is probable that small numbers of unrecognized clinical cases had occurred in Germany and elsewhere prior to 1860. Indeed, because trichinosis is so difficult to diagnose, small numbers of unrecognized cases undoubtedly continued to occur, along with those that were increasingly becoming diagnosed as the nature of the disease became more widely known. An important feature in the recognition of the disease was the ability to diagnose it in the living patient. Parasitological diagnosis first became feasible in 1862, when Friedreich of Heidelberg (following a suggestion of Kuchenmeister) removed a piece of biceps muscle from a patient and found *Trichinella* larvae in it. Eosinophilia, one of the most consistently useful clinical signs of trichinosis, was not discovered until 1896, when T.R. Brown, who was then a medical student at Johns Hopkins University, found that a trichinosis patient had an eosinophilia of 68% (Brown, 1897). It was an unprecedented elevation in the number of eosinophils in peripheral blood, and Brown's observation became a major contribution to the diagnosis of trichinosis.

Once clinical trichinosis had been recognized, it was observed again and again. It was reported in the United States by Dalton (1864) and in Great Britain by Dickinson (1871). It was a new status symbol, and Cobbold (1872) became indignant on hearing a claim that clinical trichinosis had been seen in Ireland earlier than in England. There was, however, no disputing Germany's unenviable claim to a near monopoly on severe outbreaks. In the 30 years following Zenker's discovery of the pathogenicity of *Trichinella*, 14,817 cases were reported in Germany (Kozar, 1970), with several outbreaks involving more than 100 cases. Large outbreaks probably did not occur at that time in other countries of western Europe, for it is likely that at least some of them would have been identified as trichinosis. Whether large outbreaks occurred prior to 1860 is, of course, unknown. Glazier (1881) called attention to many historic epidemics that might have been trichinosis, but definite conclusions on the matter cannot be drawn.

It was the great outbreaks in Germany that gave *T. spiralis* worldwide notoriety. Between 1860 and 1880, there were 513 deaths out of 8491 cases, giving a mortality rate of 6% (Lehmensick, 1970), but such national statistics obscure the tragedy of the towns. In Hettstädt in 1863, there was an outbreak involving 158 cases, with 28 deaths, a mortality rate of 18% (Foster, 1965). The outbreak was apparently occasioned by the consumption of pork dishes in connection with several concurrent festivities including a celebration of the 50th anniversary of the Battle of Leipzig (and the fatalities included one aged survivor of that battle). The new biopsy method of diagnosis was employed in this outbreak, which was also notable in that the consumption of raw or smoked sausage was seen to be more hazardous than the consumption of roast pork. This not only illustrated the obvious prophylactic value of cooking pork products, but also called attention to the role of ethnic dietary preferences in determining the geographic distribution of clinical trichinosis. In 1865, there occurred in Hedersleden the most severe outbreak of trichinosis to be recorded for many years. Heder-sleden was little more than a village, having some 2100 inhabitants—of whom 337 became ill and 101 died, giving a mortality rate of 30%. Outbreaks occurred in Corbach, Hanover, Bremen, Dresden, Plauen, Anahalt, Eisleden, Jena, Leipzig, Strassfurt, and Weimar. In Linden, there were 21 fatalities out of 400 cases (Billings, 1884). In Plauen, there were 3 deaths out of 30 cases; in Calbe, 8 deaths out of 38 cases; in Bourg, 11 deaths out of 50 cases (Hun, 1869). It is hardly surprising that these events impressed upon the public, and upon the medical profession, the urgent need for control measures.

Contrasting with these large outbreaks is an "outbreak" consisting of only three cases and with considerable doubt as to the diagnosis. The episode warrants a mention only because it involves the possible solution of a riddle that was once the subject of the most intense speculation. In 1897, the Swedish explorer Andrée set off in a hydrogen-filled balloon in an attempt to drift over the North Pole. The expedition was a failure, but (like Scott's ill-fated expedition to the other pole) achieved greater renown that most successes. Andrée and his two companions perished as they trudged southward from the site of their crash landing. Discovery of their bodies and diaries in 1930 solved the mystery of their disappearance, but generated a new mystery concerning the cause of death. Food, extra clothing, and cooking oil were found at their final campsite. A couple of decades later, the illnesses recorded in the Andrée diaries were recognized as suggestive of trichinosis, and *Trichinella* larvae were found in the preserved flesh of two polar bears that had been shot by members of the expedition and used for food (Sundman, 1970). The signs and symptoms described in the English translation of the Andrée diaries (Andrée et al., 1930) may be consistent with a diagnosis of trichinosis, but they also leave room for doubt. The explorers did resort to eating raw bear meat; it is highly probable that they suffered from trichinosis, and it is quite possible that the disease was a factor in their failure to survive.

Trichinosis continues to be among the hazards of Arctic exploration (Ozeretskovskaya and Uspensky, 1957) and of Arctic life in general (see Chapters 13 and 14). Inevitably, the modern outbreaks in native Arctic people have led to speculation about possible outbreaks of historical interest. Our awareness of trichinosis in the Arctic dates from the 1930s and 1940s, but as long ago as 1919, the great Arctic explorer Stefánsson concluded that it "seems likely" that certain outbreaks of disease in the Arctic were in fact trichinosis (Stefánsson, 1919). No such caution restrained the pen of a writer of our own time. Citing an ancient prohibition on the eating of the narwhal and the white whale, Arvy

(1979) declared that "what is certain is that trichinosis existed in the Arctic by the middle of the 13th Century. . . ."

5. CONSEQUENCES (POLITICS AND PARASITES)

The new disease, and especially the German outbreaks of the 1860s, clearly showed the need for some sort of action to prevent such disasters. The police could hardly be expected to arrest the culprit, although newspaper cartoonists might wistfully suggest otherwise (Fig. 1). The consumer could not be required to cook all pork products, so the key to successful control was seen to lie in providing the consumer with pork that was safe to eat even if uncooked. In Magdeburg, the danger of raw pork was publicized and the law against selling unwholesome meat was made to include trichinous meat. That was not enough; to prevent trichinosis and not merely punish butchers for outbreaks of the disease, meat would have to be examined microscopically for "trichinae"—would have to be subjected to "trichinoscopy." Thus began a long campaign to inspect the pigs that were slaughtered in the German and Prussian states (Fig. 2). Mandatory inspection was introduced in the Duchy of Brunswick in 1863, with medical inspectors using a hand lens for initial screening and a microscope (100 magnifications) for the carcasses of unhealthy pigs. Better methods, requiring microscopy of

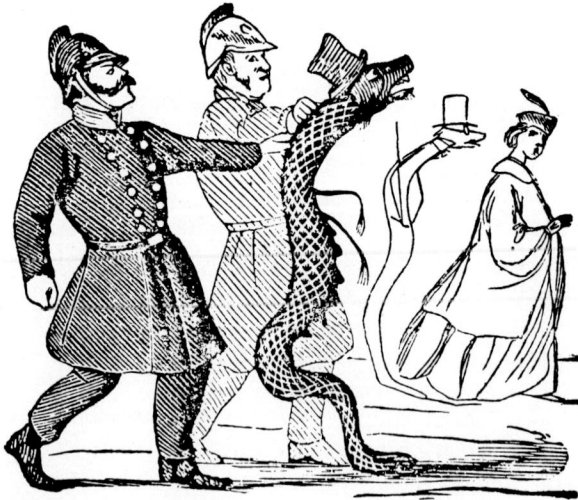

FIGURE 1. An old Danish cartoon envisioning the arrest of a trichina by the police.

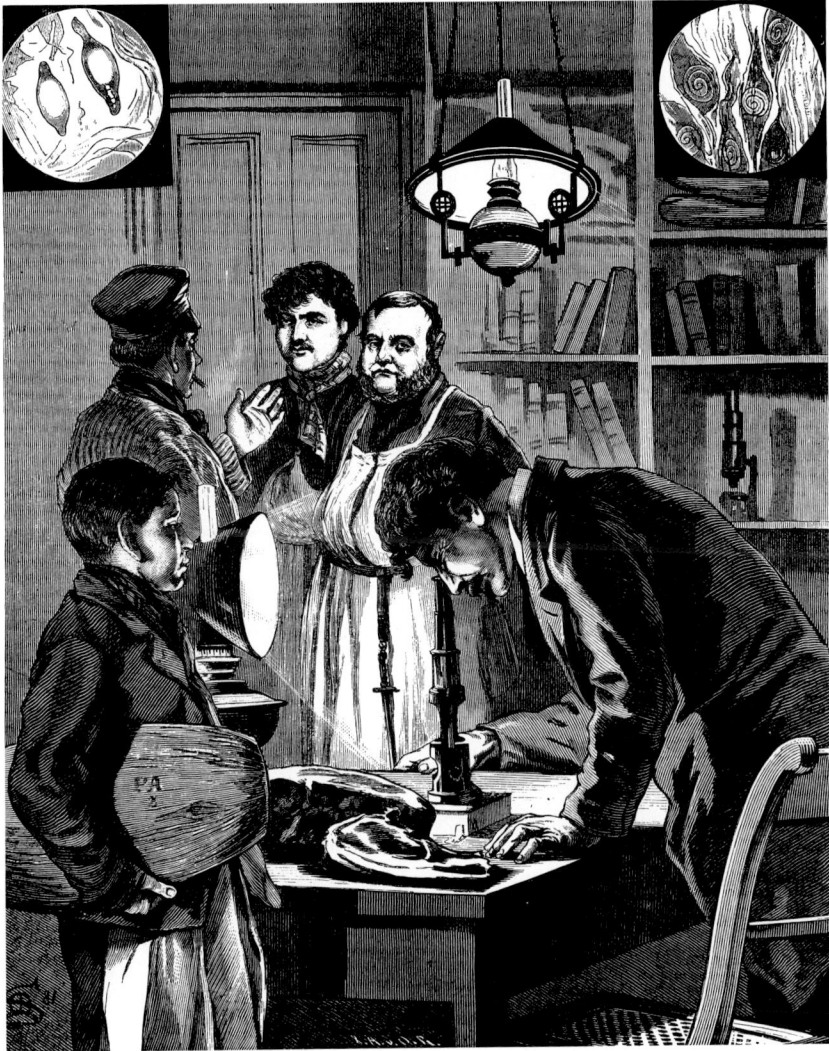

FIGURE 2. Early trichinoscopy in Germany. Butchers bring their pork to the inspector's office. From a newspaper of 1881. Granger Collection, New York.

all carcasses, were soon adopted by other local governments. In some cities, butchers banded together to carry out inspection and protect their financial and legal interests. For example, a small fraction of the selling price might go into a fund, so that any butcher who found an infected pig could be reimbursed for the loss of that carcass—and receive a congratulatory bonus as well (Hun, 1869). One butcher was jailed for a month for violating local regulations, and a physician–inspector was jailed for six months for failing to examine some pork that had caused cases of trichinosis (Glazier, 1881).

Virchow, already at the height of his professional and political power, was the natural leader of the public-health campaign. Education and trichinoscopy were his weapons. (In another context, Virchow is said to have used *Trichinella* almost literally as a weapon. Being a bluntly outspoken member of parliament, he was challenged to a duel by Bismarck, and is reported to have ignored the challenge. There is, however, an apochryphal variant of the story, in which Virchow proposed fighting the duel with a pair of sausages, one of which would contain trichinous pork. Each contestant would eat one sausage, and Bismarck would have the privilege of first choice. Bismarck allegedly declined the proposal, so Germany did not forfeit either its medical or its political *numero uno*.) The public-health campaign generated an astonishing amount of antagonism and disbelief. A skeptical veterinarian earned a footnote in the history books by allowing himself to be coerced into eating a piece of infected sausage, with painful, though not fatal, consequence (Blumer, 1939). Largely overlooked, however, is the case of a Berliner who did not believe that these little worms could be harmful and ate heavily infected sausage to prove it; he died for his unbelief (Billings, 1884). Despite this opposition, the practice of trichinoscopy spread through Prussia and the German states. The numerous local regulations were eventually standardized and applied uniformly throughout Germany in 1937 (Lehmensick, 1970).

By the end of the 19th century, the trichinoscopy of slaughtered swine had become common in Germany and in much of western Europe—but not in the United States. There are several reasons for this difference in approach. The United States had not experienced outbreaks of trichinosis, and therefore the pressure to take action regardless of difficulty or cost was less acute than in the case of Germany. Two more positive reasons are often cited for the reluctance of the United States to adopt trichinoscopy. First, the cost was considered prohibitive, especially since it would have been logistically very difficult to carry it out in the United States, with its widely scattered slaughter-houses and very high slaughter rate. Second, failure to find larvae in a small piece of muscle did not mean that the carcass was *Trichinella*-free, and therefore a stamp of approval would give a false sense of security. The weakness of that argument lies in the fact that the heavily infected carcasses, the most dangerous ones, would be detected, while those that slipped through the inspection would pose only minor threats to the public health. The historical studies of Gignilliat (1961) and Cassedey

(1971), however, suggest that there may have been another, less definable reason—a historical background that would hardly have predisposed the United States to the adoption of trichinoscopy.

In the period 1879–1888, several countries banned the importation of pork from the United States. Partial or total embargoes were imposed in 1879 by Italy, Portugal, and Greece; in 1880 by Spain and Germany (chopped pork only); in 1881 by France, Austria-Hungary, Turkey, and Romania; in 1883 by Germany (all pork products); and in 1888 by Denmark. In contrast, Britain, by far the largest importer of American pork (60% of it went to Britain and only 10% to Germany), did not exclude American pork. It was claimed then, and is still alleged by many modern authors, that the European embargoes were imposed because there was no mandatory inspection of pork for *Trichinella* in the United States, despite a high prevalence of the parasite in American swine, but the situation was not that simple.

In the 1880s, the United States had just become the world's leading exporter of pork. The European pork producers were being commercially overwhelmed, and the fact that American pork, unlike their own, was not inspected for *Trichinella* provided the perfect excuse for blocking its importation. The embargo was an especially powerful economic weapon because it could be justified on medical grounds. Since the danger of eating trichinous pork was undisputed, it may seem cynical to question the motivation for the pork embargo, but there is abundant evidence that the action was largely a matter of economic warfare. Powerful trade lobbies were involved on both the European and American sides. Further, opposing political factions within France and Germany traded accusations as to whether a pork embargo was a sanitary necessity or a commercial gimmick designed to protect the wealthy entrepreneurs while depriving the poorer people of the only meat they could afford. The United States government came under a variety of pressures. Some pork producers and many top government officials favored introduction of an American trichinoscopic inspection; other producers wanted to promote exports by reduction of tariffs against European imports; the meat packers, not wanting to foot the bill for pork inspection, demanded retaliation through the imposition of special duties on imports. The U.S. Department of Agriculture, unsure of its authority but goaded toward pork inspection by the outspoken German-trained veterinary pathologist Billings, of Nebraska, procrastinated for several years. Finally, in 1890, President Benjamin Harrison approved a bill for the introduction of trichinoscopy of export pork, accompanied by a far-from-veiled threat of retaliation against European imports. The inspection legislation was completed in 1891 (it was technically extended to apply to interstate shipments of pork

within the United States, but this provision was never put into effect)
and was duly instituted in three packing plants in Chicago (Fig. 3).
Thus the inspection system in the United States, while technically similar
to those in Europe (Fig. 4) differed in that it offered no protection to
the populace of the country in which the inspection was done. As a
further inducement to the lifting of the German embargo, the United
States removed its duty on imported German sugar and promised not
to reimpose it. Germany lifted its ban, and throughout Europe, the
doors were reopened to American pork.

Some doors were not opened wide; France replaced its ban with a
high tariff, so importation of American pork did not regain its previous
level. Germany, on the other hand, was importing more American pork
by 1895 than it had imported before the embargo. That did not please
the German meat interests, whose representatives charged that the
American pork inspection was unreliable, that the inspectors were too
few and too susceptible to bribery, and that inspected pork was in fact
causing cases of trichinosis in Germany. This did not please the Bureau
of Animal Industry (the responsible agency of the U.S. Department of
Agriculture), but did give the German regional authorities a reason for
passing local laws requiring that American pork had to be reinspected
when it reached Germany—thereby ensuring that it would become

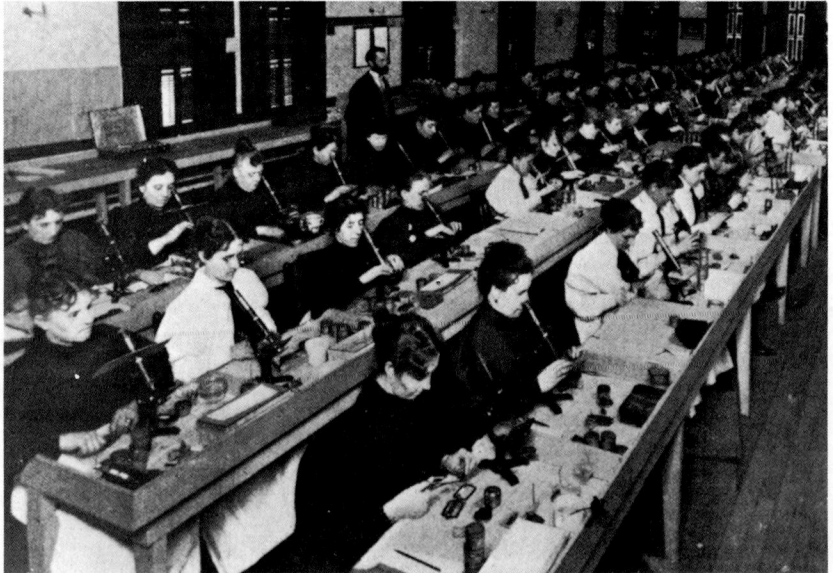

FIGURE 3. Trichinoscopy in the United States. Inspection of export pork at a meat-packing plant in Chicago, 1896.

more expensive. D.E. Salmon, Chief of the Bureau of Animal Industry, was exasperated by those German scientists who took part in this affair, describing them as "critical, bumptious, arrogant, narrow-minded individuals who have made themselves offensive by their effusive and unscrupulous efforts to convince the world that our inspection is a farce, and our science a delusion. . . ." (Cassedy, 1971). The U.S. Secretary of Agriculture was exasperated, too, and threatened to require the certification of German wine for chemical purity, on the ground that "certified American meats are as wholesome as foreign wines." Even the U.S. Ambassador to Germany was exasperated. These events of the late 1890s coincided with the eve of the Spanish-American War, but in Berlin the problem was pork. The embattled ambassador had an idea; he asked Washington for a scientific attaché to help straighten out the mess in a scientifically reputable manner.

The attaché who was attached to the embassy in Berlin in 1898 was well qualified for the job. He was Charles Wardell Stiles, later to gain a place in medical history for his work on hookworm disease. He was a trained scientist and a natural diplomat. He had already studied in Germany, and that eased his *entrée* into German scientific circles. And he must have known a thing or two about trichinosis, because he had earned his doctorate under none other than Leuckart. Stiles was immensely successful in investigating the problem in every region and at every level. He proposed that the United States forgo the small market for uncured pork and sausage and ship only pork and sausage that had been both cured and inspected by trichinoscopy. He clamped down on the cheating that went on at numerous border points and that allowed uninspected pork into Germany. He got endorsements of the United States inspection system from influential German scientists, including Virchow himself. He accumulated evidence to show that it was the German inspection system, not the American, that was unsound. Cases of trichinosis were shown, by German records, to have been due to pork inspected in Germany. Stiles pointed out that German inspectors were, by and large, part-time workers—often butchers or other tradesmen with clumsy hands and poor equipment, and so little skill in microscopy that dirty lenses (even missing lenses!) were likely to go unnoticed. American inspectors, on the other hand, were women [Fig. 3 (the solitary male is presumably the supervisor!)] with dexterous fingers and superior microscopic equipment, especially modified for rapid examination of compressed slivers of pork. Naturally, Stiles's investigations were not welcome in all quarters, and the victories gained for the United States position were not easily won. Worst of all, the outcome was something of a Pyrrhic victory. The German import regulations were changed in keeping with the new scientific evidence,

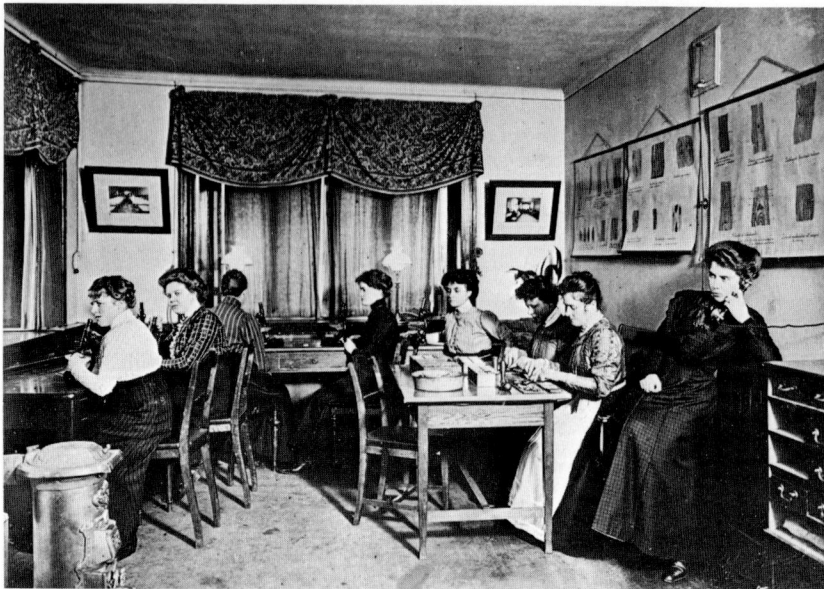

FIGURE 4. Trichinoscopy in Sweden. Women inspecting pork for trichinosis in Stockholm in 1911. The right-hand picture on the facing wall is a photograph of a similar scene, in the same room, in 1901.

but they remained protectionist. The United States exporters were afforded but little relief, and in 1906, the inspection of export pork for trichinosis was abandoned in the United States—15 years (and some 8.25 million pigs and more than 123,000 *T. spiralis* infections) after it had begun. It was revived briefly in 1964 (Gould, 1970), but again it applied only to pork destined for consumption outside the United States.

Perhaps a more significant aspect of the United States–German pork dispute was the effect it had on the prospect of trichinosis inspection in the United States. The United States authorities were not favorably impressed with what we would now call the cost–benefit ratio of the endeavor. [Many factors affect that mysterious ratio, but it may be noted in passing that in 1893 the trichinoscopy of exported pork cost the United States government $172,367, or 0.83 cent per pound of pork. In the following year, the operation was on a larger scale, and the cost was reduced to 0.16 cent per pound of pork (Salmon, 1895)] The German inspection effort involved some 100,000 inspectors (Prussia alone having about 26,000 inspectors, a body of men the size of the U.S. Army) and a cost that exceeded the entire operating expenses of the U.S. Department of Agriculture. Added to this was the consideration that more than half the cases of trichinosis that occurred in Germany after the introduction of trichinoscopy were attributable to pork that had passed inspection. The United States authorities, moreover, undoubtedly developed a degree of emotional antipathy toward trichinoscopy as a result of the prolonged squabble. In any case, the United States government rejected trichinoscopy as a measure for the protection of its citizens, a position it has maintained to the present day. The U.S. Department of Agriculture, however, has maintained an active interest in the development of improved methods of detecting *Trichinella* in swine.

Although the United States experts opted to rely on other approaches to the control of trichinosis, there is no denying the effectiveness of the German control campaign, which relied so heavily on trichinoscopy. Factors such as public education cannot be separated from the overall effect, but the fact remains that the incidence of *Trichinella* in German swine started to decline with the introduction of trichinoscopy and fell steadily until the incidence became extremely low. The incidence of *Trichinella* in swine in the United States in 1970 was higher than in Germany in 1870 (even when the figures are adjusted for the different methods of detection). The fact also remains that in the latter part of the last century, human trichinosis cases in Germany were reported at a rate of about 450 per year; in most years since World War II, West Germany has not had a single reported case of trichinosis and has enjoyed trichinosis-free periods as long as 17 years (Lehmensick, 1970). In the United States, there has not been a single trichinosis-free year since World War II; indeed, there has been an annual average of 250 reported cases for the period 1947–1970 and an average of 135 cases for the decade 1971–1980.

6. THE RECENT PAST

As the story of trichinosis takes us closer to the present day, so it takes us closer to the events and information described in the ensuing chapters. This review will not preempt those accounts, but it seems appropriate to call attention to a few miscellaneous developments that bridge the gap between the *fin de siècle* furor over trichinosis and today's rather detached approach to the problem.

A thesis published in Paris in 1921 deserves mention. Robert Ducas, a medical student working under the direction of the eminent parasitologist Emile Brumpt, undertook a series of experiments on trichinosis.

The contents of his thesis (Ducas, 1921) are mostly forgotten, but Ducas showed, among other things, that rats infected with *Trichinella spiralis* became markedly immune to subsequent infection. *Aprés Ducas le deluge!* The flood of papers that have since been published on immunity to trichinosis attests not only to the significance of the disease, but also to the appeal of rodent trichinosis as a convenient laboratory model for the study of immune responses. The findings of Ducas were confirmed and extended by McCoy (1931), whose reports stimulated much interest in the subject.

In the United States, the 1930s were marked by major public-health activities relating to *Trichinella*. Maurice Hall assembled a vast amount of information on the prevalence and epidemiology of trichinosis and indulged in hard-hitting but academically sound advocacy of public-health measures (Hall, 1937, 1938). It was not glamorous work, and not the stuff of history, but Hall in the United States, and his public-health counterparts in other lands, contributed mightily to our understanding of the infection.

In the 1930s and 1940s, many surveys were undertaken to assess the prevalence of *Trichinella* in the human population of the United States, and these have been tabulated by Zimmermann (1970). In one nationwide survey, examination of tissues from more than 5300 cadavers led to the celebrated conclusion that 16% of the population was infected (Wright *et al.*, 1944). In a particularly thorough investigation in Michigan, Gould (1943) found an infection rate of 26% in more than 900 cadavers of persons aged 50 years or more. These were shocking figures, even though most of the infections had apparently been light. Stoll (1947) estimated that the United States had three times more trichinosis than all the rest of the world combined. It must have been figures of this sort that gave rise to such pleasant fancies as the island where the cannibals' cookbook carried a footnote to the effect that American missionaries should be boiled a half-hour extra. The surveys of Wright and others provided an important yardstick, against which later prevalence rates could be measured. Modern surveys, especially that of Zimmermann *et al.* (1973), have provided evidence of a marked decline in trichinosis incidence as compared to that of the 1930s. The prevalence of *Trichinella* larvae in the population at large is now estimated at about 4%, and while that figure is low in comparison to the past, it remains high in comparison to other parts of the world (see Chapter 14).

As in the case of human infection, the prevalence of trichinosis in swine in the United States has declined in recent years. Probably the most significant event in this context is not directly concerned with *Trichinella*. In 1952, the viral agent of vesicular exanthema of swine spread across the continent from west to east. To combat the disease, and staunch the financial loss, laws were quickly passed to prohibit the feeding of uncooked garbage to swine. These measures, and similar regulations for the control of hog cholera, undoubtedly were responsible for a significant interruption of the "domestic cycle" of *Trichinella* transmission. Nevertheless, the prevalence of *Trichinella* in swine is sufficient to provide many millions of infective meals every year (Zimmermann *et al.*, 1973), and were it not for the widespread freezing and cooking of pork products, the number of human cases in the United States would be very much higher.

We have seen that the really devastating outbreaks of trichinosis occurred in 19th-century Germany. Numerically, however, the biggest known clinical outbreak occurred in 1945, and occurred not in Germany but in Northern Ireland. The date is significant. In that year, scattered concentrations of German people were to be found in many parts of Europe, where their status as prisoners of war was associated with a high degree of dietary uniformity. There were about 1200 prisoners in the camp in Northern Ireland when illness struck early in May 1945 (Day *et al.*, 1946). In one hut, all 27 prisoners were affected. On one day, 113 new cases were reported. By the end of the month, there were 705 cases, and no further cases were reported. Most were mild cases, but 88 were sufficiently severe to require hospitalization. One patient died as a result of a clot in a cerebral artery, but it was not known whether this was related to the *Trichinella* infection. The prisoners were in the habit of eating raw sausages, and the regularity of prison life made it possible to attribute the infection to locally produced pork sausages served on a particular evening about one month prior to the peak of the outbreak. Sausages from the same batch had been served to the 250 soldiers guarding the prison. There were, however, no cases of trichinosis among the guards, who (being British) preferred their sausages well cooked. If diagnoses based solely on serological and hematological findings are included in the reckoning, then the outbreak at Mosin, Poland in 1960, with 1122 persons affected, would be the largest known outbreak of *Trichinella* infection (Kozar, 1970).

Taxonomically, *Trichinella spiralis* has long been regarded as an "only child," but now there is a sibling rival to enliven the family (Trichinellidae) circle. Named *pseudospiralis*, though its spiral seems genuine enough, it does not induce encapsulation in the host muscle, and its discovery by Garkavi (1972) is a landmark in the recent history of the subject.

As in other branches of science, students of trichinosis have tended to bind together, forming multivalent linkages that have contributed to the widespread sharing of information. National conferences were held in the United States in 1952 and 1954 and in Rumania in 1958. From a Hungarian parasitological conference in 1958, plans emerged for the formation of an International Commission on Trichinellosis. This organization, sponsored by the Polish Parasitological Society, has organized or sponsored a series of international conferences on trichinosis and has arranged for the publication of a series of special issues of the Polish journal *Wiadomosci Parazytologiczne* devoted entirely to trichinosis affairs. These issues, and the published proceedings of the conferences, provide a record not only of laboratory research, but also of epidemiological and public-health aspects of trichinosis. While many individuals played important roles in organizing these activities, the leadership of Zbigniew Kozar in Poland and Emanuel Gould in the United States was of particular significance.

The innumerable contributions made in recent years to our knowledge of the genus *Trichinella* are the substance of the rest of this book. They are the substance of future histories, for it seems safe to say that the complete history of trichinosis will not be written in the foreseeable future. *Trichinella spiralis* is destined to remain with us, both in nature and in the laboratory. It is not an endangered species.

ACKNOWLEDGMENTS. For a fuller appreciation of the personalities of Zenker and Leuckart, the author is indebted to the work of Becker and Schmidt (1975). The account of diplomatic and trade difficulties associated with pork inspection relies heavily on the work of Gignilliat (1961) and Cassedey (1971). The portrait of Owen is reproduced by permission of the President and Council of The Royal College of Surgeons of England. Figure 1 is reproduced by courtesy of Dr. I. Katić. Figure 4 is reproduced from the collections of the Royal Veterinary College Library, now in the Ultana Library, Uppsala, Sweden, by courtesy of Dr. P. Räf.

REFERENCES

Althaus, J. 1864, On trichina disease: Its prevention and cure, *Med. Times Gaz.* **1**:362–364.
Andrée, S.A., Strindberg, N., and Kraenkel, K., 1930, *Andrée's Story* (translated by E. Adams-Ray), Viking Press, New York.
Arvy, L., 1979, Trichinosis in cetaceans, *Invest. Cetacea* **10**:325–330.
Becker, V., and Schmidt, H., 1975, *Die Entdeckungsgeschichte der Trichinen und der Trichinosis*, Springer-Verlag, Berlin.
Billings, F.S., 1884, *The Relation of Animal Diseases to the Public Health, and Their Prevention*, Appleton, New York, pp. 2–41.

Bischoff, T.L., 1840, Ein Fall von *Trichina spiralis*, *Med. Ann.* **6**:232–250.

Blumer, G., 1939, Some remarks on the early history of trichinosis, *Yale J. Biol. Med.* **11**:581–588.

Bowditch, H.I., 1842, *Trichina spiralis*, *Boston Med. Surg. J.* **26**:117–128.

Brown, T.R., 1897, Studies in trichinosis, *Bull. Johns Hopkins Hosp.* **8**:79–81.

Campbell, W.C., 1979, History of trichinosis: Paget, Owen and the discovery of *Trichinella spiralis*, *Bull. Hist. Med.* **53**:520–552.

Cassedey, J.H., 1971, Applied microscopy and American pork diplomacy: Charles Wardell Stiles in Germany 1898–1899, *Isis* **62**:5–20.

Center for Disease Control, 1976, Trichinosis surveillance: Annual summary, 1975, United States Department of Health, Education and Welfare, Atlanta, Georgia, p. 9.

Cerfontaine, P., 1895, Contribution à l'étude de la trichinose, *Arch. Biol.* **13**:125–145.

Claus, C., 1860, Fütterungsversuche mit Trichina spiralis, *Würzburger Naturwissenschaftliche Zeitschrift* **1**:155–157.

Cobbold, T.S., 1872, *Worms: A Series of Lectures on Practical Helminthology*, Lindsay, Philadelphia, pp. 121–127.

Dalton, J.C., 1864, Observations on *Trichina spiralis*, *Trans. N.Y. Acad. Med.* **3**:1–18.

Day, C.L. Wood, E.A., and Lane, W.F., 1946, Observations on an outbreak of trichinosis among German prisoners of war, *J. R. Army Med. Corps* **86**:58–63.

Dickinson, W.L., 1871, Three cases of trichiniasis after eating home-fed pork, *Br. Med. J.* **1**:446.

Ducas, R., 1921, L'immunité dans la trichinose, Thesis, Faculty of Medicine of Paris, Jouve, Paris, 47 pp.

Farre, A., 1836, Observations on the *Trichina spiralis*, *London Med. Gaz.*, pp. 382–387.

Foster, W.D., 1965, *A History of Parasitology*, Livingstone, Edinburgh, pp. 68–79.

Garkavi, B.L., 1972, Species of *Trichinella* from wild carnivores, *Veterinariya (Moscow)* **49**:90–101.

Gignilliat, J.L., 1961, Pigs, politics and protection: The European boycott of American pork, 1879–1891, *Agric. Hist.* **35**:3–12.

Glazier, W.C.W., 1881, Report on trichinae and trichinosis, Government Printing Office, Washington, D.C., 212 pp.

Gould, S.E., 1943, Immunological reactions in subclinical trichinosis, *Am. J. Hyg.* **37**:1–18.

Gould, S.E., 1945, *Trichinosis*, Charles C. Thomas, Springfield, Illinois, 358 pp.

Gould, S.E., 1970, *Trichinosis in Man and Animals*, Charles C. Thomas, Springfield, Illinois, 540 pp.

Hall, M.C., 1937, Studies on trichinosis, *Public Health Rep.* **52**:539–551 and 873–886.

Hall, M.C., 1938, Studies on trichinosis, *Public Health Rep.* **53**:1472–1486.

Harley, J.P., and Gallichio, V., 1971, *Trichinella spiralis*: Migration of larvae in the rat, *Exp. Parasitol.* **30**:11–21.

Herbst, M., 1851, Experiments on the transmission of intestinal worms, *Q. J. Microsc. Sci.* **1**:209–211.

Hertwig, R., 1895, Gesellschaft für Morphologie und Physiologie zu München: Officielles Protokoll, *Muenchen. Med. Wochenschr.* **42**:504–505.

Hilton, J., 1833, Notes of a peculiar appearance observed in human muscle, probably depending upon the formation of very small cysticerci, *London Med. Gaz.*, **11**:605.

Hun, E.R., 1869, *Trichina spiralis*, *Trans. N.Y. State Med. Soc.* **1869**:157–172.

Knox, 1836, Remarks on the lately discovered microscopic entozoa, infesting the muscles of the human body, *Edinburgh Med. Surg. J.* **46**:89–94.

Kozar, Z., 1970, Trichinosis in Europe, in: *Trichinosis in Man and Animals* (S.E. Gould, ed.), Charles C. Thomas, Springfield, Illinois, pp. 423–436.

Lehmensick, R., 1970, Inspection of pork and control of trichinosis in Germany, in: *Trichinosis in Man and Animals* (S.E. Gould, ed.), Charles C. Thomas, Springfield, Illinois, pp. 437–448.

Leuckart, R., 1860, On the mature condition of *Trichina spiralis, Q. J. Microsc. Sci.* **8:**168–171.

Luschka, H., 1851, Zur Naturgeschichte der *Trichinella spiralis, Z. Wiss. Zool.* **3:**69–80.

Madsen, H., 1974, The principles of the epidemiology of trichinelliasis with a new view on the life cycle, in: *Trichinellosis* (C.W. Kim, ed.), Intext Educational Publishers, New York, pp. 615–638.

McCoy, O.R., 1931, Immunity of rats of reinfection with *Trichinella spiralis, Am. J. Hyg.* **14:**484–494.

Millet, N.B., Hart, G.D., Reyman, T.A., Zimmermann, M.R., and Lewin, P.K., 1980, ROM I: Mummification for the common people, in: *Mummies, Disease and Ancient Cultures* (A. Cockburn and E. Cockburn, eds.), Cambridge University Press, Cambridge, pp. 71–84.

Owen, R., 1835, Description of a microscopic entozoon infesting the muscles of the human body, *Trans. Zool. Soc. London* **1:**315–323.

Ozeretskovskaya, N.N., and Uspensky, S.M., 1959, Group infection by trichinellosis from meat of polar bear in the Soviet Arctic (in Russian), *Med. Parazitol.* **26:**152–159.

Reinhard, E.G., 1958, Landmarks of parasitology, II. Demonstration of the life cycle and pathogenicity of the spiral threadworm, *Exp. Parasitol.* **7:**108–123.

Salmon, D.E., 1895, The Federal Meat Inspection Yearbook of the U.S. Department of Agriculture for 1894, Government Printing Office, Washington, D.C., pp. 67–80.

Steele, J.H., 1970, Epidemiology and control of trichinosis, in: *Trichinosis in Man and Animals* (S.E. Gould, ed.), Charles C. Thomas, Springfield, Illinois, pp. 493–512.

Stefánsson, V., 1919, The Stefánsson–Anderson Arctic Expedition of the American Museum, *Anthropol. Pap. Am. Mus. Nat. Hist.* **14:**445–457.

Stoll, N.R., 1947, This wormy world, *J. Parasitol.* **33:**1–18.

Sundman, P.O., 1970, Introduction, in: *The Flight of the Eagle*, Pantheon Books, New York, pp. 1–8.

Van Beneden, P.J., 1859, Observations relatives à la reproduction de divers zoophytes et à la transformation du *Trichina spiralis* en *Trichocephalus, C. R. Acad. Sci.* **49:**452–453.

Virchow, R., 1859, Recherches sur le développement du *Trichina spiralis, C. R. Acad. Sci.* **49:**660–662.

Ward, H.B., 1923, The founder of American parasitology, Joseph Leidy, *J. Parasitol.* **10:**1–21.

Ward, H.B., 1930, The discovery of the trichina, *J. Am. Med. Assoc.* **95:**1988.

Wilks, S., 1889, Lectures of Pathological Anatomy, 3rd Edition, Longman's and Co., London. p. 101–102.

Wood, H., 1835, Observations on the *Trichina spiralis, London Med. Gaz.* **16:**190–191.

Wright, W.H., Jacobs, L., and Walton, A.C., 1944, Studies in trichinosis XVI, *Public Health Rep.* **59:**669–681.

Zenker, F.A., 1860, Ueber die Trichinen-krankheit des Menschen, *Virchows Arch. Pathol. Anat.* **18:**561–572.

Zimmermann, W.J., 1970, Trichinosis in the United States, in: *Trichinosis in Man and Animals* (S.E. Gould, ed.), Charles C. Thomas, Springfield, Illinois, pp. 378–400.

Zimmermann, W.J., Steele, J.H., and Kagan, I.G., 1973, Trichiniasis in the U.S. population, 1966–70, *Health Serv. Rep.* **88:**606–623.

2

Species, and Infraspecific Variation

TERRY A. DICK

1. HISTORICAL PERSPECTIVE

Until relatively recently, there was only one species of *Trichinella*, described as *T. spiralis* (Owen, 1835) Railliet, 1895. A number of new species have been described in the past decade, namely, *T. nativa* (Britov and Boev, 1972), *T. nelsoni* (Britov and Boev, 1972),and *T. pseudospiralis* Garkavi, 1972. Other workers studied differences among isolates of *Trichinella* and considered the isolates to be geographic strains or varieties (Nelson *et al.*, 1961; Nelson and Forrester, 1962; Nelson and Mukundi, 1963; Kozar and Kozar, 1965). The term "isolate" is used here to define a number of individuals from a population isolated at a particular place and time and then propagated by serial passages through experimental hosts. The controversy over whether "new" forms of *Trichinella* are varieties, strains, sibling species, subspecies, or species persists, and adding to this controversy is the lack of clear-cut morphological differences.

A brief review of the taxonomy and morphology of *T. spiralis* is necessary prior to discussions on the speciation question.

Trichinella is the only known genus of the family Trichinellidae Ward, 1907, belonging to the superfamily Trichuroidea, order Anoplida, class Aphasmidia, and phylum Nemathelminthes. Subfamily

TERRY A. DICK • Department of Zoology, University of Manitoba, Winnipeg, Manitoba, Canada R3T 2N2.

diagnosis: Trichinellinae Ransom, 1911. Male with spicule and copulatory sheath absent. Female ovoviviparous with spherical egg surrounded with a delicate membrane and without a true eggshell; vulva in esophageal region. Adult worms in the intestine of mammals and larvae in the muscle. *Type-genus*: *Trichinella* Railliet, 1895. *Type-species*: *Trichina spiralis* (Owen, 1835). Synonyms: *T. affinis* Dies, 1851; *T. canis* Kraemer, 1853; *T. circumflexa* Polonio, 1860; *T. pseudalius* Dengler, 1863; *Pseudalius trichina* Davaine, 1863. Specific diagnosis:* body of nearly uniform diameter throughout, becoming slightly thicker posteriorly. The small head has a simple mouth opening into a distinct tubular portion of the esophagus, which in turn is surrounded by a chain of single cells characteristic of the superfamily. These cells and esophogeal tube extend approximately half the length of the body. At the posterior end of the esophagus are two cells associated with the esophageal–intestinal region. Following the esophagus is the thin-walled intestine, flask-shaped at its origin. The intestine terminates in the rectum, a muscular tube lined with chitin. In sexually mature males, the rectum is longer and its musculature thicker. Anus is terminal in both sexes. *Male*: 1.4–1.6 mm long by 40 μm thick. The single testis originates in the posterior portion of the body and extends anteriorly to about the posterior end of esophagus; here it turns back and becomes the vesicula seminalis, which terminates at the anal aperture to form a cloaca. This terminal portion of the vesicula and the cloaca can be protruded in copulation. Two conical projections 10 μm long are situated on each side of the cloaca. These are bent toward the ventral side and probably serve to hold the female *in copulo*. Between these lie four papillae, the anterior pair hemispherical, the posterior pair conical. *Female*: 3–4 mm long by 60 μm thick. The single ovary begins in the posterior end of the body, extends anteriorly for a short distance, and transforms into the uterus. The uterus transforms into the vagina near the posterior end of the esophagus, and as such extends forward to the vulva, which is on the ventral side near the middle of the esophagus and about one fifth of the body length from the anterior end. Eggs are subspherical and are 30–40 μm in diameter with a very delicate vitelline membrane, but no true eggshell. Embryos develop in the uterus and escape from the surrounding membrane. Embryos are 100–160 μm long by 9 μm thick, the anterior end being the thicker.

While general morphological characteristics were adequate to describe a single species in the genus *Trichinella*, it is more difficult to define morphologically the four species that have now been proposed.

* Taken from Hall (1916) and York and Maplestone (1969).

TABLE 1
Characteristics of Proposed *Trichinella* Species [a]

Length (mm)	Other	*T. spiralis*	*T. nativa*	*T. nelsoni*	*T. pseudospiralis*
Adult male	—	1.0 ——————————— 1.8			0.6–0.9
Adult female	—	1.3 ——————————— 3.7			1.26–2.10
Larvae	—	0.617 ————————— 1.004			0.620–0.766
Capsule (length/width)	—	1.7–2.3	1.2–1.5	1.3–2.2	
	Infectivity index	141	37	54	—

[a] From Boev *et al.* (1979).

Boev *et al.* (1979) reviewed the species of *Trichinella* and based their conclusions mostly on criteria in Table 1. Other observations made by Boev *et al.* (1979) included the smaller size of *T. pseudospiralis* (one fourth to one third smaller than the other species) and absence of a cyst. The external surface of *T. spiralis* is translucent and white, while *T. nativa* has an opaque or "matte" surface. Boev *et al.* (1979) noted that the cuticle of each species differed and that *T. nativa* is more resistant to low temperatures than the other species, while *T. nelsoni* is more resistant to high temperatures. They also reported different clinical manifestations of *T. nelsoni*, *T. spiralis*, and *T. nativa*. Their strongest evidence for the existence of distinct species was the failure of all four isolates to interbreed. Only in the case of crosses between *T. spiralis* and *T. nelsoni* were hybrids produced, but these hybrids did not propagate because males were sterile.

2. A WORKING DEFINITION OF SPECIES

To deal with the speciation question in the genus *Trichinella*, an understanding of a species is necessary. Dobzhansky (1970) defined species as "the largest and most inclusive reproductive community of sexual and cross-fertilizing individuals which share a common gene pool." Most contemporary biologists define a species as a genetically distinctive group of natural populations that share a common gene pool but are reproductively isolated from all other such groups. Species are usually separated on the basis of fairly obvious anatomical, behavioral, or physiological characters, and systematists usually rely on these in determining a species. The final criterion is always reproduction—whether or not there is actual or potential gene flow. Since isolates of *Trichinella* have very few clear-cut morphological differences, reproductive isolation is one of the main characteristics to be considered. It should be noted, however, that while it is easy to give a definition of species, Scudder (1974) is quite correct in stating that no single precise and objective definition of a species is universally acceptable and applicable.

It is well known that within the geographic range of a species, variation occurs, probably reflecting differences in the selection pressures operating on populations as a result of environmental differences. Since *Trichinella* is found in homeothermic animals, environmental pressure may be largely restricted to hosts or groups of hosts in a given geographic area. Perhaps resistance to freezing in those isolates recovered from holarctic regions may be an additional selective factor.

How then does speciation occur if all species originate from one population at some point in time? Most biologists believe that in the vast majority of cases (excluding speciation by polyploidy), the initiating factor in speciation is geographic separation. At first, the only reproductive isolation will be geographic isolation by physical separation, and the separated populations will still be potentially capable of interbreeding. Therefore, according to the modern concept of species, they will still belong to the same species. Eventually, they may become so different genetically that there would be no effective gene flow between them even if they were to come into contact. When this point in divergence has been reached, two populations are considered to be two separate species.

As two populations diverge, they accumulate differences that will lead to development of intrinsic isolating mechanisms. These mechanisms encompass biological characteristics that prevent two populations from sharing a common area or from interbreeding effectively if they again occur in the same location. In other words, speciation is initiated when through external barriers the two populations become entirely allopatric or occupy different ranges. Speciation is not completed until the two populations have evolved isolating mechanisms that will keep them allopatric or that will keep their gene pools separate even when they are sympatric or have the same range. These isolating mechanisms could be the same or different for allopatric or sympatric species. Dobzhansky *et al.* (1977) classified reproductive isolating mechanisms as premating (prezygotic) and postmating (zygotic). The former impede or prevent hybridization of members of different populations, and hence the production of hybrid zygotes. The latter reduce the viability or fertility of hybrids that have arisen. Prezygotic isolating barriers are: (1) ecological or habitat isolations, which occur when species occupy different habitat (biotypes) in the same territory; (2) seasonal or temporal isolation, which is found between populations in which members reach sexual maturity at different times, usually at different seasons of the year; (3) ethological or sexual isolation, which is a result of weakening, or absence, of sexual attraction between females and males of different species; (4) mechanical isolation, which comes about because of different sizes or shapes of the genitalia, making copulation and sperm transfer difficult or impossible; (5) gametic isolation, which results from female and male gametes failing to attract each other, or from spermatozoa of one species being inviable in the sexual ducts of another species. Postmating or zygotic isolating mechanisms are as follows: (1) hybrid inviability, which eliminates many or all hybrid individuals before they reach sexual maturity; (2) hybrid sterility, which disrupts the process of gamete formation in the hybrids, so that they fail to produce functioning sex cells; and (3) hybrid breakdown, which reduces the viability or fertility in the progeny of hybrids, i.e., in F_2 or in back-cross generations.

There are no examples where all the prezygotic or zygotic isolating mechanisms described above occur between two species. Usually, there are two or more isolating mechanisms that reinforce separation. In the short run, however, it is immaterial whether species are kept separate by ecological, ethological, or hybrid-sterility barriers. Reproductive isolation is not an all-or-none phenomenon, but is rather one of degree. For example, a hybrid may be wholly sterile, or it may have its fertility reduced below that of the parental stock.

The question of hybrid inviability, sterility, and breakdown is a complex one. A hybrid zygote may be aborted soon after its formation or during any stage of the life cycle. Hybrid individuals may be less competitive in a given environment, but there are also well-documented examples of somatic hybrid vigor. Sterility is due to problems in germ-cell formation, a good example being the failure of some or all chromosomes to pair properly at meiosis.

Partial or complete fertility in one or both sexes does occur in some interspecific hybrids. However, hybrid breakdown may occur in the second or back-cross generations. In summary, then, crosses between species almost always result in less viable offspring, but if hybrids are produced they either break down in the subsequent hybrid generations, or, in back-crosses of these hybrids to parental stock, males are usually sterile. Thus, reproductive isolation is maintained and the two breeding stocks would be considered bona fide species.

3. TERMINOLOGY

Lines of isolates of *Trichinella* have been described as strains and races by Rappaport (1943a,b), Nelson and Mukundi (1963), Kozar and Kozar (1965), Nelson *et al.* (1966), Schad *et al.* (1967), Kruger *et al.* (1969), Ozeretskovskaya *et al.* (1970), Pawlowski and Rauhut (1971), Britov and Boev (1972), Bessonov *et al.* (1975), Siddiqi and Meerovitch (1976a,b), Machnicka (1979), and Stoll *et al.* (1979) and as varieties by Britov and Smirnova (1966),Pereverzeva (1966), Grétillat and Vassiliades (1968), Britov (1969, 1971), Ozerestskovskaya *et al.* (1969), Pereverzeva *et al.* (1971a,b, 1974), Komandarev *et al.* (1975), Belozerov (1976), Mutafova and Komandarev (1976), Komandarev and Mihov (1977), Dick and Belosevic (1978), Belosevic and Dick (1979, 1980a,b), and Dick and Chadee (1981). Some workers have referred to lines of *Trichinella* as geographic isolates (Sukhdeo and Meerovitch, 1977, 1979, 1980; Dick and Chadee, 1981). Some of the aforementioned workers have also referred to isolates of *Trichinella* as distinct species (Britov, 1975, 1977a, 1980; Garkavi, 1976; Komandarev *et al.*, 1975; Tomasovicova, 1975; Komandarev and Mihov, 1977; Barus *et al.*, 1979; Boev *et al.*, 1979). Finally, Boev *et al.* (1979), in a review of the genus, concluded that *T. nativa*, *T. nelsoni*, and *T. pseudospiralis* were sibling species of *T. spiralis*.

The term "variety" or "strain" lacks precision, but is often used to define geographic races of wild species. Races and subspecies may be "incipient species," but this does not imply that every race will some day become a separate species, only that some of them may do so if genetic divergence proceeds far enough. A subspecies or race may be defined as a group of natural populations within a species that differ genetically but are not reproductively isolated. Turesson (1922) proposed the term "ecotype" for local populations of plant species arising as a result of the genotypical response to particular kinds of habitats. Some ecological geneticists have used the term ecotype for what could otherwise be called races or subspecies. An even more controversial term is that of "semispecies" proposed by Mayr (1970) and defined as "showing some of the characteristics of species and some of subspecies." Grant (1971) defined semispecies as "populations that are neither good races nor good species but are connected by a reduced amount of interbreeding and gene flow." In other words, semispecies are borderline situations between races and species. On the other hand, Dobzhansky (1970) described species that are isolated reproductively but differ only in some apparently minor and not easily visible details or are identical in outward appearance as sibling species.

TABLE 2
Designation of North American *Trichinella* Isolates

Host	Latitude	Longitude	Year established
Pig	43°00′N	81°00′W	1952
Pig	44°00′N	63°00′W	1980
Polar bear	58°00′N	95°00′W	1976
(*Ursus maritimus*)			
Wolverine	55°00′N	100°00′W	1979
(*Gulo gulo*)			
Marten	56°00′N	99°00′W	1980
(*Martes americana*)			
Arctic fox	69°15′N	105°00′W	1980[1,2,3,4a]
(*Alopex lagopus*)			

[a] Four isolates from same host species and geographic area.

Trichinella isolates from various sources are impossible to identify by inspection of one individual, and because of the difficulties in identification, it seems appropriate at this time to designate any population of *Trichinella* recovered from a given host as a geographic isolate. Classification as a geographic isolate as used here makes no assumptions as to systematic position, but merely indicates the location from which the particular isolate was recovered. Dick and Chadee (1981) and Chadee and Dick (1982a) have designated North American isolates of *Trichinella* by including in the name the host species, latitude, longitude, and the year in which the parasite was recovered (Table 2).

4. DISTRIBUTION OF ISOLATES

The distribution of *Trichinella* species and isolates is known for a number of geographic locations. Figure 1 outlines the locations of those *Trichinella* for which there is some information on biological characteristics, some of it being derived from interbreeding experiments. The main geographic areas include Africa, England, India, Europe, North America, and the U.S.S.R.

Based on the work of Boev *et al.* (1979), the geographic distribution of the species of *Trichinella* has been outlined as follows: *T. spiralis* is associated with domestic pigs and primarily restricted to those parts of the world where pigs are widely used as food. According to Boev *et al.* (1979), the *Trichinella* recovered from wild pigs is the same species, but information on biological characteristics and reproductive isolation is

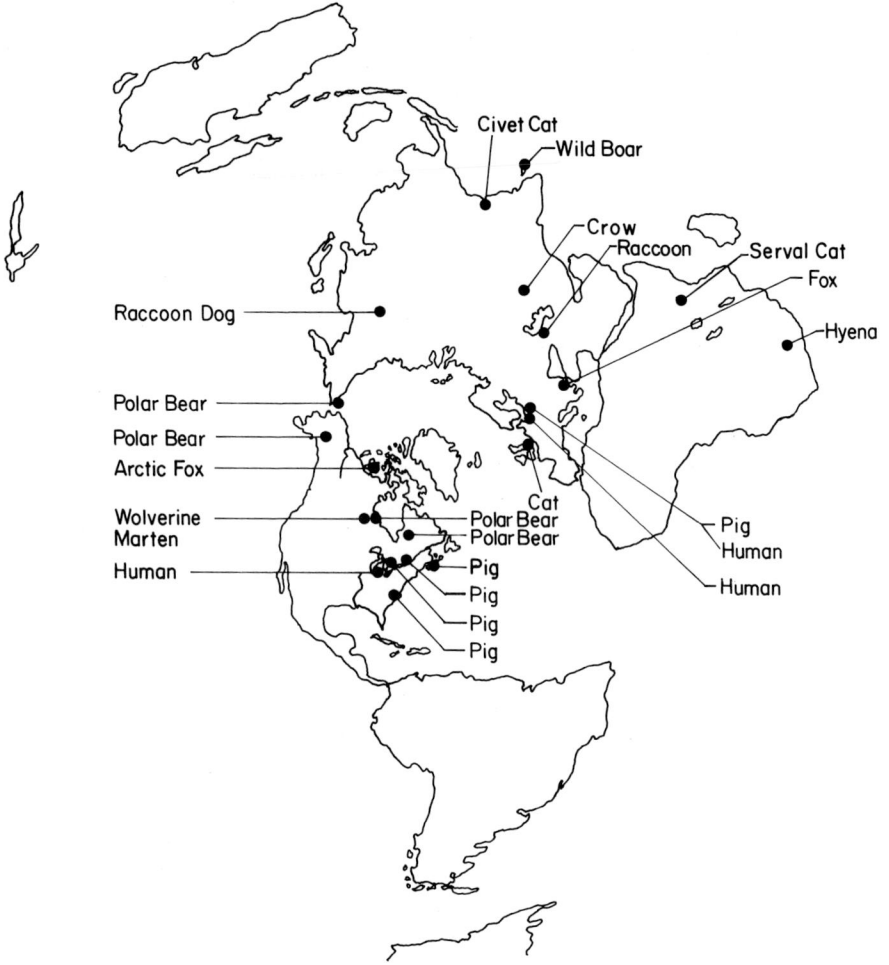

FIGURE 1. Distribution of isolates of *Trichinella* for which some information on their biology is available.

lacking. The geographic distribution of *T. pseudospiralis* is not well known, although it has been reported from the Caucasus of the U.S.S.R. and more recently from Chokpak in the headland of the Talassk mountain range of Tein-Shan by Shaikenov (1980). Boev *et al.* (1979) suggest that a small *Trichinella* discovered in India may also be *T. pseudospiralis*. Observations by Rausch *et al.* (1956), Zimmerman and

Hubbard (1969), and Wheeldon (personal communication) indicate that a form of *Trichinella* occurs in birds from North America. Boev *et al.* (1979) stated that *T. nativa* is typically a northern species and is characteristic of circumpolar regions of Asia, North America, and Europe (Boev *et al.*, 1979; Sukhdeo and Meerovitch, 1977). Boev *et al.* (1979) also suggested that the southern limit of its range is about the 40th parallel. *Trichinella nelsoni* is considered to be the "southern" species of *Trichinella* by Boev *et al.* (1979) and is found in Africa (Nelson and Mukundi, 1963; Kruger *et al.*, 1969), in Europe south of the Ukraine (Britov, 1971), in Estonia and Sweden (Boev *et al.*, unpublished), in Bulgaria (Komandarev *et al.*, 1975), in Switzerland (Shaikenov *et al.*, 1977), in Spain (Boev *et al.*, 1978), in middle Asia (Boev *et al.*, 1975), and in southern Kazakhstan (Boev *et al.*, unpublished). *Trichinella nativa* and *T. nelsoni* are reported to occur as sympatric species in Tajikistan and Estonia (Boev *et al.*, 1979). This is the first such report on sympatric speciation in *Trichinella*.

The general distribution of *Trichinella* in North America is reasonably well documented (Cameron, 1970; Rausch, 1970; Zimmerman, 1970), but distribution of species or isolates is far from clear. Sukhdeo and Meerovitch (1977) concluded that the north-temperate, tropical, and arctic isolates of *Trichinella* most likely correspond to the three species of *Trichinella*: *T. spiralis*, *T. nelsoni*, and *T. nativa*. There is no question that there is an arctic form of *Trichinella* in North America, since this is well documented in studies by Read and Schiller (1969), Arakawa and Todd (1971), Dick and Belosevic (1978), Belosevic and Dick (1979, 1980a,b), Dick and Chadee (1981), and Chadee and Dick (1982a,b). The southern limit of this arctic isolate of *Trichinella* appears to be about the 50°N latitude (Dick and Chadee, 1981), but more information is required on isolates of North America, particularly those north and south of the 40th parallel. Two isolates from near the 40th parallel from pigs have been studied by Dick and co-workers and were found to have similar characteristics, which differed from the characteristics of arctic isolates. More work needs to be done on isolates from wild animals from this region and from the southern part of the United States and Mexico before a clear picture of distribution emerges. Also, it is quite possible that infections in wild animals in the Rocky Mountains may represent a southern extension of the range of *Trichinella* having characteristics of arctic *Trichinella*. Biological characterization of *Trichinella* isolates from animals inhabiting the Rocky Mountain range and wild pigs in the southern United States would be most helpful in revealing patterns of distribution of *Trichinella* in North America.

5. CRITERIA FOR SPECIES AND ISOLATES

The criteria usually employed to define isolates and species of *Trichinella* include morphology of larvae and adults, particularly length and width (Schad *et al.*, 1967; Arakawa and Todd, 1971; Garkavi, 1972; Sukhdeo and Meerovitch, 1977; Boev *et al.*, 1979; Belosevic and Dick, 1979, 1980a), shape of cyst (Boev *et al.*, 1979), and pathogenicity or virulence (Kozar and Kozar, 1965). The most common characteristic used to date is that of reproductive potential as defined by larvae per gram of host tissue following infection with a given inoculum (Nelson and Mukundi, 1963; Kozar and Kozar, 1965; Kruger *et al.*, 1969; Arakawa and Todd, 1971; Pawlowski and Rauhut, 1971; Pereverzeva *et al.*, 1974; Bessonov *et al.*, 1975; Tomasovicova, 1975; Garkavi, 1976; Siddiqi and Meerovitch, 1976a,b; Schad *et al.*, 1967). Another method employs interbreeding techniques between species or isolates (Britov, 1971, 1975, 1977a; Bessonov *et al.*, 1975; Komandarev *et al.*, 1975; Sukhdeo and Meerovitch, 1977; Belosevic and Dick, 1980a). Larval production is greatly influenced by the species of experimental host used (see Section 5.5), and interbreeding experiments have generated considerable controversy concerning methodology and interpretation (see Section 5.1).

Until recently, no detailed profile for any one isolate was available. In an effort to standardize and define in detail the biological characteristics of isolates, the following approach was taken in our laboratory. Assessment was made of these parameters:

1. Capacity to interbreed with *T. spiralis* (standard domestic pig isolate and other isolates).
2. Morphological measurements of adults (these measurements included length and width of male and female worms and length of uterus of female).
3. Morphological measurements of larvae, including total length and width; lengths of gonad, intestine, stichosome, and rectum; and postgonad distance in males and females.
4. Intestinal distribution as determined by the median location of each population of *Trichinella* in the small intestine: that point of the intestine from which 50% of the worms were anterior and 50% of the worms were posterior. It was assumed that worms in each 5% (1/20th) of the intestine were evenly distributed.
5. *In vitro* release of newborn larvae by 7-day-old females over a 24-hr period.
6. Longevity of worms during the intestinal phase.

7. Virulence in different hosts.
8. Reproductive-capacity index (RC1), defined as (number of muscle larvae recovered/number of larvae in inoculum) and determined 40 days postinfection.
9. Longevity of muscle larvae, as evidenced by lack of infiltration or calcification or both of worms in the muscle.
10. Behavior patterns, especially with respect to sexual attraction.
11. Sensitivity to the drug thiabendazole.

These characteristics were based on a constant inoculum (400 larvae/mouse) and a standard outbred genetic strain of mouse host.

5.1. Genetic Criteria

The emphasis on genetic aspects of *Trichinella* has been on chromosome number and breeding potential between isolates or species or both. Penkova and Romanenko (1973) examined spermatogenesis and ovogenesis of *T. spiralis* Owen, 1835 var. *domestica*; *T. spiralis* Owen, 1835 var. *nativa*; and *T. pseudospiralis* Garkavi, 1972. Bessonov *et al.* (1975) assessed the karyotypes of *T. nativa*, *T. spiralis*, and *T. pseudospiralis*, and Mutafova and Komandarev (1976) studied the karyotype of a laboratory strain of *Trichinella* that was identified as *T. nelsoni*. Penkova and Romanenko (1973) found that chromosome number and shape were similar for all *Trichinella* studied and that the diploid number of chromosomes in females was six and in males five. Bessonov *et al.* (1975) found that *T. spiralis*, *T. nativa*, and *T. pseudospiralis* could not be differentiated by their karyotypes. They reported that the diploid complement of chromosomes of the female in the metaphase consisted of one pair of acrocentric, one pair of submetacentric, and one pair of metacentric chromosomes. Males had in their mitotically dividing spermatogonia five rodlike chromosomes including two large acrocentric, two small submetacentric, and one metacentric chromosome. Mutafova and Komandarev (1976) found that in *T. nelsoni*, the second largest, slightly submetacentric chromosome in males was univalent and therefore the sex chromosome. There were differences in the length of chromosomes and mean chromosome centromere index. Major differences were noted between the first chromosome pair and the rest.

Centromere index determination revealed that each pair of chromosomes differed in location of centromere. Mutafova and Komandarev (1976) noted a faintly stained zone at the end of the short arm of the first pair of chromosomes and suggested that this may be an indication that these chromosomes bear a satellite. Mutafova and Komandarev (1976) also reported that their results do not agree with those of Geller and Gridasova (1974), who reported that the largest chromosome pair is acrocentric. Mutafova and Komandarev (1976) found the largest chromosome pair to be almost submetacentric and not the longest acrocentric chromosome as reported by Geller and co-workers. Mutafova and Komandarev (1976) concluded that these differences may be species-specific.

While there is some controversy in interpretation of karyotypes, it is in breeding experiments that the greatest differences have been reported. Some of these differences appear to be related to methodology, but most are probably related to the isolates studied. Reproductive isolation is of fundamental importance in the designation of species (see Section 2). The problem with breeding in *Trichinella* is the uncertainty as to whether a negative result with one breeding pair is clearcut evidence of reproductive isolation, and on the other hand whether multiple-pair breeding is error-free. Most of the work on breeding has been carried out by Britov and co-workers, Meerovitch and co-workers, and Dick and co-workers. The method of breeding varies among laboratories. Britov (1977a), Komandarev *et al.* (1975), Sukhdeo and Meerovitch (1977), and Shaikenov (1980) infect experimental hosts with a stomach tube. Belosevic and Dick (1980a) preferred to use surgical transplantation, since rates of infection appeared to be higher. Use of single or multiple breeding pairs also differs among laboratories. Britov (1971) discussed methods for cross-infections including single and multiple pairs. The criteria for sexing *Trichinella* larvae are of critical importance for breeding experiments and were defined as follows by Belosevic and Dick (1980a): *Male*: distance of 60–70 μm from posterior pole of gonad to the end of the worm, rectum length about 50 μm, blunt anterior pole of gonad, intestine crossing the gonad from ventral (convex) to dorsal (concave) surface, intestinal blub lying ventral to the gonad. *Female*: distance of 30–40 μm from posterior pole of gonad to the end of the worm, rectum length about 25–30 μm, pointed anterior pole of gonad, intestine always on the dorsal side, intestinal bulb lying dorsal to the gonad. Britov (1977b) points out the danger of multiple-pair breeding because of problems in sexing and rightly points out morphological anomalies that make it difficult to sex some *Trichinella* larvae. These include males and females with double crossovers of the intestine from concave to convex and back to the concave surface. Britov (1977b) also noted that males were found with the intestinal bulb midway between concave and convex surfaces (his Type IV males) and not unlike the characteristic of his Type I females. These same morphological forms have been observed in our laboratory, but are not used for breeding experiments. The greatest chance of error exists with the Type IV males and Type I females if care in selection is not rigorous. In breeding experiments, only those males should be chosen that have the intestinal bulb close to the convex surface, distinct crossover from convex to the concave surface, gonad rounded at the anterior end, long rectum, and no vaginal plate [a series of large cells at the site of the future vaginal opening (see Villella, 1966)]. In the case of females, only those worms should be chosen that have the intestinal bulb close to the concave surface and the intestine continuing close to this surface to the rectum. The vaginal plate should be present, and the rectum should be short. Most critical is that the ovary must be sharply pointed at its anterior end and this point must be close to the convex surface, and the beginnings of the cells forming the uterus should be evident. In other words, the ovary should be pointed and appear to extend slightly anterior to the posterior end of the stichosome and be close to the convex surface. Using these criteria, over 300 larvae have been sexed and transplanted into the mouse duodenum and recovered 5 days later to assess sexing accuracy. Transplants of 5, 10, or 20 males or females have been made, but no sexing errors occurred. Mice were also transplanted with groups of 5, 10, or 20 males or females and examined on day 30–40 postinfection for the presence of muscle larvae. Over 400 larvae have been assessed for sexing accuracy by this method, but no muscle larvae were found, indicating that none of the infections had been bisexual.

Britov (1971), using both single and multiple pairs in his breeding experiments, found that there was genetic isolation of two *Trichinella* varieties: *T. spiralis* var. *domestica* and *T. spiralis* var. *nativa*. Using multiple-pair breeding trials only, Britov (1977a) defined the genetic relationship among *T. pseudospiralis*, *T. spiralis*, *T. nativa*, and *T. nelsoni* and concluded that the degree of closeness was as follows and in decreasing order: *T. nelsoni* and *T. spiralis*; *T. nelsoni* and *T. nativa*, and *T. nativa* and *T. pseudospiralis*. The remotest relationship was between *T. spiralis* and *T. nativa*. When the females of a younger species (see Section 7) were fertilized by males of an older species, hybridization was always more successful than when the sexual combination of *Trichinella* species was reversed. Britov (1977a) found in a cross between *T. nelsoni* and *T. spiralis* that 18 of 29 mice produced hybrid larvae, but fewer larvae were produced, and hybrid males were sterile while females were fertile. Back-crosses of hybrid females to *T. spiralis* males produced larvae, but they were not infective. Mice receiving hybrid larvae only did not harbor worms in the muscle, indicating that there was hybrid breakdown. Reproductive isolation between single breeding pairs of a laboratory strain and *T. spiralis*, *T. nativa*, and *T. pseudospiralis* and between a fox isolate and *T. spiralis*, *T. nativa*, and *T. psuedospiralis* was reported by Komandarev *et al.* (1975). Sukhdeo and Meerovitch (1977) found that there was complete reproductive isolation between arctic and north-temperate and tropical isolates and partial reproductive isolation between the north-temperate and tropical isolates, such that the tropical females could not be fertilized by north-temperate males or by north-temperate–tropical hybrid males. Shaikenov (1980), using one breeding pair per experimental trial,found that a newly isolated *Trichinella* species from *Corvus frugilegus* did not breed with *T. spiralis*, *T. nativa*, or *T. nelsoni*, but did breed with the previously isolated *T. pseudospiralis*. Bessonov *et al.* (1975) conducted breeding experiments using single pairs of worms and various combinations of male and female *T. spiralis*, *T. nativa*, and *T. pseudospiralis* and concluded that there was insufficient evidence to consider *T. nativa* and *T. spiralis* separate species. They did find, however, that *T. pseudospiralis* was reproductively isolated from *T. spiralis* and *T. nativa*.

Recent work by Belosevic and Dick (1980a) and Dick and Chadee (1982b) raises new questions concerning gene flow among the various isolates of *Trichinella*. Isolates from a polar bear and a wolverine interbreed readily with each other in both single- and multiple-pair breeding trials and with the pig isolate of *Trichinella* in multiple-pair breeding experiments. However, although large numbers of single-pair breeding trials have been carried out between *T. spiralis* var. *pseudospiralis* and the wolverine and polar bear isolates, no offspring were produced. In multiple-pair crosses between *T. spiralis* var. *pseudospiralis* and the wolverine isolate, offspring were produced, and the RCI (see Section 5.5) was 1.76. Two subsequent generations in the same strain of mice produced RCIs of 2.18 and 0.33. The RCIs for *T. spiralis* var. *pseudospiralis* and the wolverine and polar bear isolates in the same strain of mice were 22, 22, and 42, respectively. A cross between *T. spiralis* var. *pseudospiralis* and the polar bear isolate produced an RCI of 0.52 in mice. Subsequent generations had an RCI of 0.92 in mice, but when transferred to hamsters, the RCI increased until it reached a value of 211 by generation seven. The same hybrid passed through hamsters and then to mice gave an RCI of 10.51 at generation nine. All hybrids of *T. spiralis* var. *pseudospiralis* lacked cysts in the muscle stage of the life cycle. The points to note from these hybrids are: (1) their infectivity was low initially, usually lower than either of the parent stock; (2) their infectivity increased in subsequent generations; (3) their RCIs were influenced by the host species; and (4) there was no hybrid breakdown. Finally, back-crosses indicated that hybrids were viable when crossed to parental stock. On the other hand crosses between *T. spiralis* from pigs and *T. spiralis* var. *pseudospiralis* have not produced any offspring, even when multiple breeding pairs were used. Certainly, in North America, there is the potential for gene flow between isolates from polar bear and wolverine and between these two isolates and *T. spiralis* and *T. spiralis* var. *pseudospiralis*. It is also clear that experimental hosts can have a remarkable effect on the infectivity levels of these hybrids.

5.2. Morphological Criteria

In Section 1, the general description and morphology of the species were given. This section will deal with morphological differences based on isolates or species, or both, and the influence of host on worm size. Tables 3 and 4 list measurements of those adult *Trichinella* that have been studied, and Tables 5 and 6 list measurements of larvae. According to Boev *et al.* (1979), adult *T. pseudospiralis* is smaller than *T. spiralis*, with males ranging from 0.62 to 1.026 mm in length and females ranging from 1.26 to 2.038 mm. The size range for *T. spiralis* isolated from pigs varies from 1.13 to 2.2 mm in length for males and 1.54 to 3.35 mm for females. It is interesting to note that Railliet (1895 cited in Hall, 1916) recorded measurements of 1.2–2.2 mm in length for males and 3.5–4.4 mm for females. the arctic isolates of *Trichinella* are considerably smaller in size, ranging in length for males from 0.97 to 1.22 mm and for females from 1.49 to 2.15 mm. The effect of passaging and host species on worm size was shown by Schad *et al.* (1967), who observed a decrease in size of worms for strains isolated from civet cats and pigs. Similarly, Chadee and Dick (unpublished) observed a decline in size with passages through outbred Swiss Webster mice. Length and width measurements do not appear to be good criteria for separating isolates or species of *Trichinella*. On the other hand, Bessonov *et al.* (1978) compiled differences between *T. pseudospiralis* and *T. spiralis*; the number of stichocytes appeared to be somewhat different, although there was overlap with respect to males but not females. Two recent studies (Barus *et al.*, 1979; Hulinska and Saikenov, 1980), using scanning electron microscopy, evaluated the speciation problem in *Trichinella*. Barus *et al.* (1979) concluded that *T. spiralis*, *T. nelsoni*, and *T. nativa* had differences in the morphology of the copulatory appendages (pseudobursa) and that this contributed to their reproductive isolation. Hulinska and Saikenov (1980) found differences in the shape of the lateral processes of the pseudobursa, the position of cloaca opening, and the shape of the second pair of cloacal papillae at the level of the pore, but not in line with the first pair of papillae. Hulinska and Saikenov (1980) are conservative in their interpretation and concluded

TABLE 3
Measurements of *Trichinella* Adult Males

Authority	Location	Designation	Width (mm)	Length (mm)			Pseudo-bursa	Esoph-agus	Sticho-some	Distance between anal papillae	Number of stichocytes
				Total	Sticho-some	Esoph-agus					
Arakawa and Todd (1971)	Arctic	Strain from polar bear	0.032	1.10	—	—	—	—	—	—	—
	Arctic	Strain—Alaskan dog	0.032	1.10	—	—	—	—	—	—	—
	North Carolina	Strain—pig	0.032	1.13	—	—	—	—	—	—	—
Schad *et al.* (1967)	Michigan	Strain—human	0.033	1.14	—	—	—	—	—	—	—
	India	Strain—civet cats	—	0.99[a]	—	—	—	—	—	—	—
				1.23[b]	—	—	—	—	—	—	—
	Canada	Strain—pig	—	1.58[a]	—	—	—	—	—	—	—
				1.26[c]	—	—	—	—	—	—	—
Sukhdeo and Meerovitch (1977)	Canada	Isolate—*T. spiralis* (pig)	—	1.22 ± 0.001	—	—	—	—	—	—	—
		Isolate—*T. nativa?* (polar bear)	—	0.97 ± 0.001	—	—	—	—	—	—	—
		Isolate—*T. nelsoni?* (serval cat)	—	1.14 ± 0.001	—	—	—	—	—	—	—
Belosevic and Dick (1979)	Canada	*T. spiralis*—pig	0.033 ± 0.003	1.21 ± 0.10	—	—	—	—	—	—	—
		Isolate—polar bear	0.029 ± 0.004	1.22 ± 0.09	—	—	—	—	—	—	—

Reference	Country	Isolate							
Chadee and Dick (unpublished)	Canada	Isolate—wolverine	0.031 ± 0.022	1.16 ± 0.080[d]	0.44 ± 0.042	0.13 ± 0.023	—	—	—
			0.032 ± 0.002	1.10 ± 0.092[e]	0.40 ± 0.038	1.13 ± 0.021			
Garkavi and Gineev (1976)	U.S.S.R.	T. pseudospiralis (raccoon)	0.027–0.035	0.62–0.9	0.27–0.35	0.1–0.16	—	—	—
Bessonov et al. (1975)	U.S.S.R.	T. pseudospiralis—raccoon (from Garkavi, 1972)	0.027–0.035	0.62–0.9	0.27–0.35	—	—	—	49–54
Shaikenov (1980)	U.S.S.R.	T. pseudospiralis from crow	0.025–0.032	0.873–1.026	0.34–0.41	0.135–0.172	—	—	—
Barus et al. (1979)	—	Trichinella sp.	—	—	—	—	0.012–0.014	0.009–0.010	—
		T. spiralis					0.017–0.020	0.006–0.007 0.009–0.012	—
		T.nelsoni					0.18 0.19	0.008 0.012–0.014	—

[a] Generation 4. [b] Generation 9. [c] Generation 5. [d] Generation 3. [e] Generation 10.

TABLE 4
Measurements of *Trichinella* Adult Females

Authority	Location	Designation	Width (mm)	Length (mm)					Distance from vulva to anterior end	Number of stichocytes
				Total	Stichosome	Esophagus	Uterus	Ovary		
Arakawa and Todd (1971)	Arctic	Strain from polar bear	0.032	1.54	—	—	—	—	—	—
	Arctic	Strain—Alaskan dog	0.030	1.49	—	—	—	—	—	—
	North Carolina	Strain—pig	0.031	1.54	—	—	—	—	—	—
	Michigan	Strain—human	0.032	1.54	—	—	—	—	—	—
Schad et al. (1967)	India	Strain—civet cats	—	2.04[a]	—	—	—	—	—	—
				2.24[b]	—	—	—	—	—	—
	Canada	Strain—pig	—	3.35[a]	—	—	—	—	—	—
				2.35[c]	—	—	—	—	—	—
Sukhdeo and Meerovitch (1977)	Canada	Isolate—*T. spiralis* (pig)	—	2.65 ± 0.003	—	—	1.86 ± 0.036	—	—	—
		Isolate—*T. nativa?* (polar bear)	—	1.93 ± 0.002	—	—	1.20 ± 0.34	—	—	—
		Isolate—*T. nelsoni?* (serval cat)	—	2.17 ± 0.003	—	—	1.42 ± 0.031	—	—	—

Reference	Country	Species/isolate								
Belosevic and Dick (1979)	Canada	T. spiralis—pig	0.038 ± 0.003	2.19 ± 0.24	—	—	1.36 ± 0.20	—	—	—
		Isolate—polar bear	0.038 ± 0.005	2.12 ± 0.26	—	—	1.26 ± 0.19	—	—	—
Chadee and Dick (unpublished)	Canada	Isolate—wolverine	0.035 ± 0.003	2.15 ± 0.20[d]	0.47 ± 0.067	0.15 ± 0.027	1.31 ± 0.15	0.20 ± 0.052	—	—
			0.036 ± 0.004	1.87 ± 0.18[e]	0.41 ± 0.034	0.14 ± 0.022	1.24 ± 0.15	0.17 ± 0.036	—	—
Garkavi and Gineev (1976)	U.S.S.R.	T. pseudospiralis (raccoon)	0.029– 0.035	1.26– 2.10	0.32– 0.40	0.12– 0.19	—	—	0.35– 0.40	—
Bessonov et al. (1975)	U.S.S.R.	T. pseudospiralis— raccoon (from Garkavi, 1972)	0.029– 0.035	1.26– 2.10	0.32– 0.4	—	—	—	0.35– 0.4	39–42
Shaikenov (1980)	U.S.S.R.	T. pseudospiralis from crow	0.35– 0.38	1.34– 2.038	0.324– 0.416	0.14– 0.18	0.707– 1.242	0.140– 0.23	—	—
Barus et al. (1979)	—	Trichinella sp.	—	—	—	—	—	—	—	—
		T. spiralis	—	—	—	—	—	—	—	—
		T. nelsoni	—	—	—	—	—	—	—	—

[a] Generation 4. [b] Generation 9. [c] Generation 5. [d] Generation 3. [e] Generation 10.

TABLE 5
Measurements of *Trichinella* Male Larvae

Authority	Designation	Length (mm)						Postgonad distance (mm)
		Width	Total	Gonad	Intestine	Sticho some	Rectum	
Belosevic and Dick (1980b)	*T. spiralis*—pig	0.029 ± 0.002	1.009 ± 0.071[a]	0.259 ± 0.037	0.319 ± 0.041	0.683 ± 0.070	0.056 ± 0.005	0.003 ± 0.005
		0.029 ± 0.002	1.010 ± 0.061[b]	0.258 ± 0.032	0.325 ± 0.036	0.683 ± 0.061	0.054 ± 0.007	0.064 ± 0.006
	Isolate—polar bear	0.033 ± 0.005	0.857 ± 0.064[a]	0.262 ± 0.029	0.307 ± 0.028	0.547 ± 0.052	0.048 ± 0.007	0.054 ± 0.007
		0.029 ± 0.002	0.974 ± 0.065[b]	0.272 ± 0.032	0.328 ± 0.031	0.637 ± 0.068	0.053 ± 0.008	0.061 ± 0.008
Chadee and Dick (unpublished)	Isolate—wolverine	0.028 ± 0.002	0.740 ± 0.073[c]	0.194 ± 0.021	0.220 ± 0.024	0.391 ± 0.043	0.028 ± 0.006	0.038 ± 0.005
		0.031 ± 0.002	0.762 ± 0.056[d]	0.192 ± 0.015	0.212 ± 0.019	0.339 ± 0.038	0.035 ± 0.005	0.045 ± 0.005
Garkavi (1972)	*T. pseudospiralis*	0.03– 0.04	0.65– 0.85[e]	—	—	—	—	—
Raillet (1895), from Hall (1916)	*T. spiralis*	0.03	0.8– 1.0[e]	—	—	—	—	—

[a] Generations 1–5.   [b] Generations 6–12.   [c] Generation 3.   [d] Gereration 10.   [e] Sex of larvae not stated.

TABLE 6
Measurements of *Trichinella* Female Larvae

Authority	Designation	Width	Length (mm)					Vaginal primoidium	Post-gonad distance (mm)
			Total	Gonad	Intestine	Sticho-some	Rectum		
Belsoevic and Dick (1980b)	T. spiralis—pig	0.029 ± 0.003	1.030 ± 0.053[a]	0.291 ± 0.030	0.315 ± 0.027	0.712 ± 0.047	0.025 ± 0.004	—	0.033 ± 0.005
		0.032 ± 0.003	1.043 ± 0.048[b]	0.309 ± 0.033	0.339 ± 0.034	0.700 ± 0.051	0.026 ± 0.003	—	0.035 ± 0.004
	Isolate—polar bear	0.029 ± 0.003	0.876 ± 0.065[a]	0.281 ± 0.035	0.299 ± 0.033	0.579 ± 0.054	0.021 ± 0.003	—	0.027 ± 0.004
		0.029 ± 0.003	0.999 ± 0.060[b]	0.299 ± 0.041[b]	0.321 ± 0.039	0.681 ± 0.061	0.023 ± 0.003	—	0.030 ± 0.004
Chadee and Dick (unpublished)	Isolate—wolverine	0.028 ± 0.003	0.799 ± 0.086[c]	0.224 ± 0.032	0.238 ± 0.035	0.448 ± 0.044	0.010 ± 0.003	0.292 ± 0.028	0.015 ± 0.003
		0.038 ± 0.002	0.833 ± 0.071[d]	0.236 ± 0.026	0.244 ± 0.028	0.456 ± 0.042	0.010 ± 0.003	0.298 ± 0.025	0.016 ± 0.035

[a] Generations 1–5. [b] Generations 6–12. [c] Generation 3. [d] Generation 10.

that the differences in the configuration of the pseudobursa of the males of *T. spiralis*, *T. nativa*, *T. nelsoni*, and *T. pseudospiralis* were not sufficient to warrant separation as independent species. Dick (unpublished) examined the male genitalia of *T. spiralis* var. *pseudospiralis* and *T. spiralis* from pig isolate, but also felt that differences were not pronounced enough to support species separation on morphological grounds.

Larval morphology is well understood with respect to differentiating between male and female larvae for breeding experiments (Villella, 1966; Britov, 1977a,b; Belosevic and Dick, 1980a). There is, however, considerably less known about the general morphology of larvae (Tables 5 and 6) and the influence of rapid passage on the morphology of both male and female larvae. In the case of two isolates (polar bear and wolverine), both were found to increase in size with passaging through outbred Swiss Webster mice.

In contrast, adults of the wolverine isolate showed a slight decline with passaging (Tables 3 and 4). To date, we have no detailed morphological study of selected isolates of *Trichinella* throughout its distribution. What is needed now is a thorough morphological study, including scanning electron microscopy, to determine whether there are substantial and significant differences among the various forms of *Trichinella*.

5.3. Biochemical and Immunological Criteria

The biochemical and immunological characteristics of isolates and species of *Trichinella* are incompletely understood. Ozeretskovskaya *et al.* (1970) worked with strains of *Trichinella* isolated from polar bear, man, and pig. Larvae of all three strains, when subjected to differential disk electrophoresis on polyacrylamide gels, had identical numbers of protein bands (16). Differences in staining intensities of the bands were noted among the isolates, and a characteristic feature of the protein extract from the polar bear isolate was a distinct separation of the fractions of the α_2-globulins. Ermolin and Efremov (1974), examining somatic extracts of *T. spiralis* and *T. pseudospiralis*, were unable to find any differences using techniques of immunodiffusion, immunoelectrophoresis, and disk electrophoresis in polyacrylamide gels. An analysis of blood serum fractions by Ozeretskovskaya *et al.* (1970) over the course of infection of "arctic" and "laboratory" strains revealed that the polar bear isolate or arctic strain in white mice caused less hypoproteinemia in the earlier stage of the disease and less hypergammaglobulinemia in the later stages than the "laboratory" strain. They concluded that the arctic strain of *Trichinella* had a lower immunogenicity than other strains. Work by Penkova (1974) using an *in vitro* microprecipitation test and cross-absorption of antisera against *T. spiralis* and *T. pseudospiralis* found the isolates to be serologically identical. *Trichinella pseudospiralis* appeared to be more immunogenic as indicated by higher titers of precipitating antibodies. Belozerov (1976) used the indirect immunofluorescent test to test for serological differences among *T. spiralis*, *T. nativa*, and *T. pseudospiralis*, but was unable to show clear-cut differences. Bessonov *et al.* (1978), using an *in vitro* microprecipitation test, found that *T. spiralis* and *T. nativa* had practically the same number of precipitates, 173–178 and 256–272, after 18 and 36 hr. In anti-*T. pseudospiralis* sera, microprecipitation was more marked (226–286 and 350–359 precipitates on *T. spiralis* and *T. nativa* larvae after 18 and 36 hr incubation and 399–483 on *T. pseudospiralis*). Bessonov *et al.* (1978) concluded that *T. pseudospiralis* was more immunogenic than *T. nativa* and *T. spiralis*. Sukhdeo and Meerovitch (1979) examined the antigenic characteristics of arctic, north-temperate, and tropical insolates of *Trichinella* using homologous and heterologous hyperimmune rabbit antisera and two-dimensional immunoelectrophoresis. Arctic and north-temperate isolates yielded 27 components and the tropical isolate 28. Heterologous combinations between the arctic and north-temperate isolates suggested a sharing of 19–20 antigens, between arctic and tropical isolates a sharing of 21 antigens, and between the tropical and north-temperate isolates a sharing of 24–25. The arctic isolate differed from both the north-temperate and the tropical isolate by 6–7 antigens, while the tropical and north-temperate isolates differed by 3 antigens. Sukhdeo and Meerovitch (1979) suggested that only *T. nativa* should be considered a different species, while *T. spiralis* and *T. nelsoni* may represent subspecies. Other work by Belosevic and Dick (unpublished) comparing the amino acid composition of an arctic isolate from a polar bear and *T. spiralis* from a pig (Table 7) showed some minor differences in amino acid composition, but no striking difference in levels of a specific amino acid. In summary, neither biochemical nor immunological methods have shown consistent differences between isolates or species.

5.4. Sensitivity to Drug Treatment

Very little is known about the comparative sensitivity of various isolate of *Trichinella* to drugs. Kociecka (1971) emphasized the importance of *T. spiralis* strains and suggested that differences in strain sensitivity to thiabendazole may contribute to differences in experimental results. In the treatment of trichinellosis, Ozeretskovskaya *et al.* (1970) noted that thiabendazole is less active on muscle stages of

TABLE 7
Amino Acid Composition of Muscle Larvae of *Trichinella spiralis* and an
Isolate from Polar Bear Recovered from Crl:COBS CFW(SW) Mice at Day
40 Postinfection

Amino acid	Pig isolate		Polar bear isolate	
	Average (nmoles/ml)[a]	Relative number (arginine = 1)	Average (nmoles/ml)[a]	Relative number (arginine = 1)
Cysteic acid	14.04	0.06	39.88	0.36
Aspartic acid	638.00	2.68	310.50	2.82
Threonine	260.90	1.10	141.40	1.28
Serine	307.00	1.29	158.60	1.44
Glutamic acid	565.70	2.38	284.90	2.58
Proline	266.10	1.12	139.00	1.26
Glycine	383.50	1.61	219.20	1.99
Alanine	483.30	2.03	244.00	2.21
Valine	288.20	1.21	171.40	1.55
Methionine	84.36	0.35	19.11	0.17
Isoleucine	244.70	1.03	137.60	1.25
Leucine	401.00	1.69	222.30	2.02
Norleucine	48.69	—	30.00	—
Tyrosine	186.80	0.79	78.01	0.71
Phenylalanine	187.30	0.79	100.20	1.00
Histidine	128.60	0.54	68.50	0.62
Lysine	388.20	1.61	205.30	1.86
Ammonia	1263.00	—	601.50	—
Arginine	237.70	1.00	110.36	1.00

[a] Average of two trials.

synanthropic (pig) strains of *Trichinella* than on arctic strains and suggested that this is related to difficulty of the drug in penetrating the fibrous capsule. On the other hand, Spaldonova *et al.* (1978), working with *T. pseudospiralis*, were unable to show significant differences in efficacy of the benzimidazole anthelmintics, including thiabendazole. This was interesting, since *T. pseudospiralis* is not encysted.

Studies by Chadee *et al.* (1983), working with three isolates of *Trichinella* (polar bear, wolverine, and pig) and *T. spiralis* var. *pseudospiralis* using the drug thiabendazole [(2-(4'-thiazolyl) benzimidazole) Merck and Co. Inc.], found substantial differences among these forms of *Trichinella*. Outbred male white mice [Crl:COBS CD-1 (1CR)] were used throughout the study. The drug was incorporated in pelleted feed at concentrations of 0.03–0.06% and tested against the intestinal stage on days 2–7 of infection; against migrating and preencystment larvae

(0.03–0.1%) on days 4–20 postinfection, for convenience here termed "migratory phase"; against the early muscle phase (0.03–0.5%) on Days 20–40; and against the later muscle phase (0.03–0.1%) on days 40–60. Efficacy was determined by measuring the *in vitro* release of newborn larvae by female worms or the number of larvae recovered from muscle 40 and 60 days postinfection. During the intestinal stage, chemosterilization was obtained with 0.05% thiabendazole for the pig isolate and *T. spiralis* var. *pseudospiralis* and with 0.03% for the polar bear and wolverine isolates. Drug treatment during the "migratory phase" at sustained low dosages (0.03–0.1%) was effective in reducing the muscle larvae, and efficacy was similar for all the *Trichinella* isolates. Efficacy during early and late muscle stages varied among isolates. Low drug dosages (0.03–0.15%) were ineffective against *T. spiralis* var. *pseudospiralis*, but a higher dosage (0.5%) was highly effective against all the *Trichinella* isolates. *Trichinella* sensitivity varied, the most susceptible at high dosage (0.5%) being the polar bear and wolverine isolates, with 99% efficacy, and *T. spiralis* var. *pseudospiralis*, with 100% efficacy. Thiabendazole in the case of the pig isolate was only 74% effective. For all isolates, larvae recovered from mice treated at high and low dosages were not infective when introduced to mice. Sustained low thiabendazole treatment (0.1%) from 40 to 60 days postinfection was effective in reducing the number of muscle larvae of the polar bear and wolverine isolates. Differences in drug sensitivity among isolates cannot be separated from the biology of the isolates. For example, the sensitivity to thiabendazole as measured by reduction in the number of larvae recovered from the muscle is related to the length of the intestinal phase and time of treatment; the shorter the intestinal phase, the lower the number of larvae recovered, particularly when drug treatment is of a fixed duration.

There is little doubt that drug sensitivity varies among isolates of *Trichinella*, but the unresolved question is whether these differences are more pronounced in relatively "new" isolates as opposed to isolates that have long been passaged in experimental hosts, particularly mice and rats. A fresh pig isolate should be evaluated to determine its sensitivity to drugs and then compared to current laboratory isolates.

5.5. Effect of Host on Reproductive-Capacity Index

It has been known for some time that infectivity of isolates or species, or both, of *Trichinella* is influenced by host, particularly the experimental host. Table 8 outlines infection levels of *Trichinella* as reported in a few selected papers. These papers were chosen because

TABLE 8
Infection Levels of *Trichinella* in Selected Hosts

Authority	Source	Location	Number of larvae inoculated	Experimental host	Larvae/gram
Nelson and Mukundi (1963)	Human	Kenya	219–408	Rat (Nairobi)	10–20
	Cat	London	219–408	Rat (Nairobi)	2,402–4,805
	Human	Kenya	2,500	Pig (Landrace)	1.6
	Cat	London	2,500	Pig (Landrace)	205.5
Nelson *et al.* (1966)	Serval cat	Kenya	100	Rat	3
			100	Mouse	37
			100	Hamster	1
			200	Guinea pig	83
			200	Rabbit	13
	Polar bear	Alaska	100	Rat	0
			100	Mouse	168
			100	Hamster	93
			200	Guinea pig	133
			200	Rabbit	15
	Cat	England	100	Rat	181
			100	Mouse	186
			100	Hamster	188
			200	Guinea pig	268
			200	Rabbit	108

				6,000–24,000		4.7–21.0
Kruger et al. (1969)		Hyena	South Africa	6,000–24,000	Pig	4.7–21.0
Kozar and Kozar (1965)		Baboon	Kenya	15,000	Rat	26–2,162
				500	Mouse	1,474
		Pig	Poland	500	Mouse	2,732
		Human	Poland	500	Mouse	2,276
Siddiqi and Meerovitch (1976b)		Rat from pig	Canada	3,000	Rat (albino)	7,822
				3,000	Rat (hooded)	6,342
				640	Mouse	6,343
		Baboon	Kenya	3,000	Rat (albino)	842
				3,000	Rat (hooded)	54
				640	Mouse	2,000
		Polar bear	Alaska	3,000	Rat (albino)	25
				3,000	Rat (hooded)	57
				640	Mouse	1,335
Garkavi (1976)	T. spiralis		—	500	Rat	300
				200	Hamster	28.3
	T. pseudospiralis		—	500	Rat	49
				200	Hamster	213
	T. nelsoni		—	500	Rat	5.5
				400	Hamster	7
	T. nativa		—	500	Rat	0
				200	Hamster	16

the Alaskan and Kenyan strains in several of the studies came from the same source. *Trichinella nelsoni*, as far as is known, originated from the Kenya isolate. It is clear from these papers that experimental design varies among research groups, and in some cases the infective dose is an approximation (Table 8). The history of isolates is difficult to follow, since they are not always maintained within one genetic line of a particular host and in some cases not even within the same species of host. For example, by 1963, the Kenyan strain had been passaged as follows: several cat (*Felis serval*), mongoose (*Myonax sanguineus*), monkeys (*Cercopithecus aethiops*), and baboons (*Papio doguera*). The current host of the Kenyan strain may be mouse or guinea pig, depending on the particular laboratory. This probably accounts for its increased infectivity to mice in some laboratories. Kozar and Kozar (1965) pointed out that a change of host is likely to affect the infectivity of an isolate. Similar observations were made by Zimoroi (1964), who found that in the initial passage of *T. spiralis* strains from wolves, foxes, genets, and martens through mice and guinea pigs, there was a reduced infectivity, but in subsequent generations, these strains were almost equal to a pig strain maintained in guinea pigs. Arakawa and Todd (1971) also showed that an arctic isolate, initially infecting mice at very low levels, was much more infective after several passages through mice and suggested an increased adaptability of the arctic isolate. There is also evidence that the host can suppress infection levels of an isolate and influence the level of infection in subsequent infections. Dick and Chadee (1981), working with the pig, polar bear, and wolverine isolates, obtained the following results: RCIs in Crl COBS CFW(SW) mice were 152, 72, and 22 (an average of 10 generations), for pig, polar bear, and wolverine isolates, respectively. When transferred to raccoons, the indices were 10.59, 10.87, and 43.87, for pig, polar bear, and wolverine isolates. When the polar bear isolate, with an RCI of 10.87 in raccoons, was passaged from raccoon to the original strain of mice, the RCIs were 26.89, 29.77, and 52.97 for generations one, two, and three. It is apparent that even though the host (raccoon) influence was operating for one generation only, it had a dramatic influence on reproductive capacity for at least three generations. Similarly, as reported in Section 5.1, hybrids are influenced by the host, and a period of adaptation to a new host may be necessary. It is likely that prolonged passage in a given host will eventually stabilize the RCI of a given isolate.

RCIs are relatively stable for a given isolate. For example, the mean RCI for the polar bear isolate over 15 generations was 63.45 ± 19.34, and the range of values was 40.67–100.63 (Belosevic and Dick, 1979). The mean RCI for *T. spiralis* from pigs for 11 generations was 151.27

± 27.30, with a range of 124.14–201.25. Similarly, the mean RCI of the wolverine isolate for 10 generations was 22.23 ± 10.43, with a range of 7.21–39.22 (Chadee and Dick, unpublished). These values are significantly different and are therefore reliable characteristics for these isolates.

Results for isolates maintained in Crl COBS CFW(SW) mice are presented in Table 9. It is clear that isolates treated in the same way behave quite differently in different hosts; the pig isolate has a high RCI in rats, while the RCIs of the polar bear and wolverine isolates are quite low. This is a characteristic reported for most wild isolates, including the Kenyan strain. Of considerable interest is the behavior of all three isolates in a wild-type host, such as *Peromyscus*, where differences become less pronounced. The influence of host genetics becomes obvious when the RCI (31) of the wolverine isolate in *Mus* is compared to the RCI (11) for a cross of a wild-type *Mus* to a laboratory strain of *Mus* [Crl COBS CFW(SW)] and this RCI in turn is compared to the RCI (17) for a cross between *Mus* × COBS mice and parental COBS mice. The effects are even more complex when we compare RCIs in hosts to the release of larvae *in vitro* by 7-day-old females from the same host. Using the wolverine isolate as an example, we find that

TABLE 9
Reproductive-Capacity Indices of *Trichinella* Isolates from Various Hosts

	Isolate		
Host[a]	*T. spiralis* (pig)[b]	Polar bear[b]	Wolverine[c]
Crl COBS CFW (SW) mice (outbred)	151	63	22
AHF:(SW) mice (outbred)	139	45	—
CD-1 mice (outbred)	94[c]	44[c]	43
Sec-J mice (inbred)	94	29	32
Sprague–Dawley rats (outbred)	204	7	3
Hamster (*Mesocricetus auratus*)	—	203[d]	270
Peromyscus maniculatus	33	19	10
Cleithrionomys gapperi	33	52	—
Microtus pennsylvanicus	75	64	—
Mus musculus (wild-type)	—	—	30.72
Hybrid *Mus* × Crl:COBS	—	—	10.65
Hybrid *Mus*–Crl × Crl:COBS	—	—	16.50

[a] Infection dose 400 except for rats (2000) and hamsters (500).
[b] Data taken from Belosevic and Dick (1979).
[c] Chadee and Dick (unpublished).
[d] Data from Dick and Belosevic (1978) plus unpublished data.

the RCI in rats is 3, in Crl COBS CFW(SW) mice is 22, and in *Mus* is 31, but the *in vitro* larval release per female per 24 hr in rats is 29, in Crl COBS is 30, and in *Mus* is 28. Clearly, then, differences in RCIs reflect more subtle aspects of the biology of an isolate as it interacts with the host immune system. Not only do these isolates have stable and reproducible characteristics within a host, but also, within an isolate, we see different characteristics in different hosts. The interaction of isolates of *Trichinella* and host species is extremely complex under laboratory conditions, and we can expect to find the same complexity under natural conditions.

5.6. Other Biological Characteristics

This section deals with variation in cyst morphology, resistance to freezing, virulence of isolates, intestinal distribution, *in vitro* larval release by 7-day-old females over a 24-hr period, duration of the intestinal stage, and viability of muscle larvae.

Some investigators have compared the cyst morphology of isolates or species or both, and Boev *et al.* (1979) have given a succinct review. Using a length-to-width ratio, or form index, they found that the index of *T. spiralis* is 1.7–2.3, that of *T. nativa* is 1.2–1.5, and that of *T. nelsoni* is 1.8–2.2. The shape and size of the cyst are influenced by the host, and this has been observed in wild carnivores as well as experimental hosts (Dick, unpublished). The reliability of cyst morphology as a biological characteristic needs further evaluation in a number of different hosts.

The importance of resistance to freezing by arctic isolates has become apparent from observations by Brandly and Rausch (1950), Clark *et al.* (1972), Dick and Belosevic (1978), Dick and Chadee (1981), Dies (1980), and Boev *et al.* (1979). Infective larvae have been recovered from wolf muscle frozen for 18 months at $-10°C$ (Dies, 1980), from polar bear muscle frozen for 12 months at $-15°C$ (Dick and Belosevic, 1978), and from arctic fox frozen at $-15°C$ for 14 months (Chadee and Dick, 1982a). Eaton (1979) reported that Ozeretskovskaya recovered living *Trichinella* larvae from polar bear meat frozen for more than 2 years. Boev *et al.* (1979) stated that *T. nativa* is a dozen times more resistant to low temperature in comparison with other species, while *T. nelsoni* is more resistant to high temperatures. There appear to be conflicting observations on temperature resistance of *T. nelsoni*, since Shaikenov (1980) stated that *T. pseudospiralis* died at -12 to $-17°C$ after 3 days, while *T. nelsoni* and *T. nativa* remained alive for more than 6 months. It would be interesting to know whether these results were obtained from experimental hosts or from wild carinvores, since Dick and Belosevic (1978) were unable to maintain freezing resistance of the polar bear isolate in laboratory mice. Recently raccoons have been experimentally infected with an arctic fox isolate and the carcasses frozen. Larvae recovered up to 270 days postfreezing were infective to laboratory mice.

Virulence of *Trichinella* isolates has been reported in a number of studies (Culbertson and Kaplan, 1938; McCoy, 1931; Rappaport, 1943a; Kozar and Kozar, 1965; Belosevic and Dick, 1979; Dick and Chadee, 1981), and results are outlined in Table 10. Again, it becomes obvious that comparisons are difficult, since different strains of host and parasite were used. Strains of *Trichinella* from pigs and humans did not appear to have different levels of virulence. On the other hand, strains isolated from wild animals varied considerably. The polar bear isolate was the most virulent in mice, with the Kenyan strain being less virulent and the wolverine isolate the least virulent. This is interesting, since the polar bear and wolverine isolates are definitely arctic isolates, yet these observations suggest that high virulence may not be a characteristic of all arctic isolates. Britov (1980) reported that every species of *Trichinella* has its own microbial symbionts that are transferred transovarially.

TABLE 10
Virulence of *Trichinella* Isolates

Authority	Designation	Number of larvae	Host	Remarks
Glaser (1920)[a]	*T. spiralis*	1,200[b]	Mice	Fatal
Trawinski (1935)[a]	*T. spiralis*	>150–200[b]	Rats	90% of population dead in 10–15 days
Culbertson and Kaplan (1938)	*T. spiralis*	300[b]	Mice	69.1% died within a month
McCoy (1931)	*T. spiralis*	40[c]	Rats	Lethal in 12–35 days
		70[c]	Rats	Lethal in 2–7 days
Rappaport (1943a)	Strain B—human	50–60[c]	Mice	Majority died; no
	Strain W—pig	50–60[c]	Mice	difference among
	Strain Y—human	50–60[c]	Mice	strains
Kozar and Kozar (1965)	Strain—human	2,000[b]	Mice	20 of 20 died
	Strain—pig	2,000[b]	Mice	20 of 20 died
	Strain—Kenyan	2,000[b]	Mice	6 of 20 died
	Strain—pig	15,000[b]	Rats	10 of 10 died
	Strain—Kenyan	15,000[b]	Rats	1 of 10 died
Dick and Chadee (1981)	Strain—pig	2,400[b]	Mice	50% dead on day 8
	Strain—polar bear	1,700[b]	Mice	50% dead on day 9
	Strain—wolverine	2,800[b]	Mice	50% dead on day 4

[a] From Rappaport (1943a). [b] Total number of larvae in inoculum. [c] Infection dose (larva/g of host).

Perhaps different microorganisms affect the virulence of *Trichinella* isolates.

Comparisons of intestinal distribution in different isolates of *Trichinella* are limited to work by Pawlowski and Rauhut (1971), Belosevic and Dick (1979), Sukhdeo and Meerovitch (1980), and Chadee and Dick (1982b). Pawlowski and Rauhut (1971)found that intestinal distribution of an old strain of *Trichinella* isolated from pigs differed significantly from the distribution of another pig strain and a strain isolated from humans. It should be noted that their old strain was maintained in experimental hosts (rats) for a number of years and that its distribution is similar to the distribution of a pig isolate of *Trichinella* in rats reported by Dick and Silver (1980). Work by Belosevic and Dick (1979) showed that worm position (defined as an averaged median value for a point on the length of the intestine at which 50% of worms were anterior and 50% of worms were posterior to that point) in the same strain of mouse for *T. spiralis* pig and polar bear isolates was 17 and 24, respectively. Similarly, Chadee and Dick (unpublished) showed that worm position for the wolverine isolate was 24 in the same strain of mice, but distribution was statistically different in other host strains and species. On the other hand, Sukhdeo and Meerovitch (1980) found that the adults of Alaska, Canada, and Kenya isolates occupied similar sites along the intestine. Intestinal position may be a quantifiable biological characteristic for some isolates if the same experimental host is used.

In vitro larval release by female worms over a 24-hr period, measured on day 7 postinfection, differs among the pig, polar bear, and wolverine isolates. *In vitro* larvae release on day 7 for the pig isolate was 56, for the polar bear isolate 21 (Belosevic and Dick, 1979), and for the wolverine isolate 31 (Dick and Chadee, 1981). Whether or not significant differences in larval release will persist among isolates, or groups of isolates, can be clarified only when data on other isolates are available.

Duration of the intestinal stage is influenced by host and strain of *Trichinella*. Chadee *et al.* (1983) found that worm longevity in CD-1 outbred white mice was 16 days for the pig isolate, 11 days for the polar bear isolate and *T. spiralis* var. *pseudospiralis*, and 12 days for the wolverine isolate. Intestinal longevity in Crl COBS CFW(SW) mice was 17 days for the pig isolate, 15 days for the polar bear isolate (Belosevic and Dick, 1979), and 12 days for the wolverine isolate (Chadee and Dick, 1982b). Adults of the three strains of *Trichinella* studied by Pawlowski and Rauhut (1971)disappeared from the intestine by day 14. Ozeretskovskaya *et al.* (1970) reported that the prepatent period of arctic trichinosis is long, but it is not known whether the intestinal stage in man is extended.

The viability of muscle-dwelling larvae in experimental hosts varies among isolates. Boev *et al.* (1979) stated that larvae of *T. nativa* in man, swine, and rats decayed in large numbers. Work by Belosevic and Dick (1980a) showed that survival of the polar bear isolate in mice was considerably lower than for the pig isolate. On the other hand, Chadee and Dick (1982b) found that the wolverine isolate had a much higher survival rate in the same period of time (600 days). Differences in cellular infiltration of cysts and/or calcification are evident when one examines wild carnivore muscle. In some individuals, a high level of infiltration and calcification is apparent, and in others no evidence of calcification is noted. Usually, these differences are attributed to age of infection, and that is probably the correct interpretation for some of the animals. It is also possible that we are observing, in some samples at least, the end result of the host–parasite interaction of isolates differing in virulence or immunogenicity.

6. *TRICHINELLA SPIRALIS* var. *PSEUDOSPIRALIS*—AN ENIGMA

The conservative approach is taken here in classifying the *pseudospiralis* isolate as *T. spiralis* var. *pseudospiralis*, since there is evidence for some gene flow between it and other isolates of *Trichinella*, particularly in North America (see Section 5.1). There is no question that this isolate differs from other *Trichinella* isolates by its infectivity to birds, its smaller size, and the lack of a cyst in the muscle stage of its life cycle. Other morphological features are less convincing as good species characteristics, but scanning electron microscopy by Barus *et al.* (1979) and Hulinska and Saikenov (1980) suggests that there may be differences in size of the pseudobursa and the position and shape of anal papillae (see Section 5.2). Evidence for distinct biochemical and immunogenic properties of *T. spiralis* var. *pseudospiralis* differs among workers (see Section 5.3) and at this point is not too convincing. While the muscle-phase of *T. spiralis* var. *pseudospiralis* was sensitive to thiabendazole (Chadee *et al.*, 1983), the level of drug treatment did not appear to be related to lack of a cyst, since other *Trichinella* isolates were sensitive to the same drug levels. The lack of cyst appears to be a unique characteristic of *T. spiralis* var. *pseudospiralis*, but its importance to the biology of that organism is not clear. Experiments dealing with sexual attraction among *T. spiralis*, a *Trichinella* isolate from a polar bear, and *T. spiralis* var. *pseudospiralis* showed that the last was less attracted to either of the other two isolates than these isolates were to each other (Belosevic and Dick, 1980b). For this reason, Belosevic and Dick (1980b) concluded that *T. spiralis* var. *pseudospiralis* was distinct from *T. spiralis*, but were careful not to identify it as a separate species.

The distribution of *T. spiralis* var. *pseudospiralis* is not well delineated (Boev *et al.*, 1979), and there has been uncertainty over whether it was originally isolated from a raccoon, *Procyon lotor*, or a raccoon-dog, *Nycteureutes procyonoides*. It appears certain now that the original isolation of *T. spiralis* var. *pseudospiralis* was from an American raccoon (*P. lotor*)in the U.S.S.R., and most Russian literature supports this observation (Boev *et al.* 1979). Until recently, the only record of *T. spiralis* var. *pseudospiralis* in wild populations was that of Garkavi (1972). Work by Shaikenov (1980) reported *T. spiralis* var. *pseudospiralis* from two crows, *Corvus frugilegus*, out of a total of 744 birds from the order Falconiformes and family Corvidae in the headland of Tien-Shan, U.S.S.R. This finding is of considerable importance, since it is convincing evidence that *T. spiralis* var. *pseudospiralis* occurs more widely in wild populations and is not just an anomaly isolated once. It is also strong evidence to support the comments of Boev *et al.* (1979) that maintenance of *T. pseudospiralis* in nature is dependent on meat-eating birds.

7. SPECIATION IN *TRICHINELLA*

Even though there are considerable lacunae in our understanding of ecological and genetic aspects of *Trichinella*, there is much that we do know. It seems apparent that there is some geographic segregation of *Trichinella*. There are holarctic forms of *Trichinella* circulating primarily through arctic carnivores usually referred to as either arctic isolates or *T. nativa*. This type of *Trichinella* is resistant to freezing in carcasses of wild carnivores, and it has an opaque appearance or matte cuticle. Resistance to freezing is not retained in experimental animals, suggesting that if it is genetic, it is considerably influenced by the host. The arctic isolate has low infectivity in experimental rats and pigs and is less infective to mice than the temperate form isolated from pigs. There is also a temperate-to-north-temperate form primarily associated with pigs and rats, but unfortunately there is very little information on isolates recovered from carnivores, such as black bears and foxes from the temperate region. The relationship between isolates from wild pigs and domestic pigs is not clear, but these isolates are generally considered to belong to the same group or strain of *Trichinella*. The major distinguishing characteristics are high infectivity to rats, mice, and pigs and low resistance to freezing. The low freezing resistance may be more apparent than real, since there is no information on the response of temperate or north-temperate forms of *Trichinella* to freezing when in the flesh of wild carnivores. Most of the north-temperate forms have been passaged rapidly and for long periods of time in laboratory animals, usually mice and rats. Consequently, they are highly selected forms of *Trichinella* and are therefore probably furthest removed from the characteristics of a "natural" *Trichinella*. Yet this form is considered typical of what may be the only species of *Trichinella*, i.e., *T. spiralis*.

Trichinella nelsoni is considered to be a "southern" species by Boev *et al.* (1979), yet its distribution extends from Africa to as far north as Sweden and Estonia (approximately the 50th or 60th parallel). This "southern species" or "Kenya isolate" has characteristics similar to those of the holarctic form, particularly low infectivity to mice, rats, and pigs, although considerable differences were found in infectivity levels among laboratories when the same isolate was studied. The Kenya isolate has low virulence, a characteristic shared by the wolverine isolate, which by all other characteristics is considered an arctic isolate. It has been suggested that the Kenya isolate is resistant to freezing, but this is not well substantiated.

The form of *Trichinella* most different is *T. spiralis* var. *pseudospiralis* or *T. pseudospiralis*, which to date has been recovered from the Caucasus region of the U.S.S.R. and the Tien-Shan mountain region. There is increasing evidence that it is also present in birds from North America. Its major distinguishing features are lack of cyst in the muscle stage, small size, and infectivity to birds. It is generally felt that it is widely distributed in scavenging and carnivorous birds, but more studies are needed to get an adequate indication of its distribution.

There is very little detailed information on *Trichinella* morphology other than that described in the 19th and early 20th centuries. This is probably because researchers had been convinced that only one species exists in nature. What is even more surprising is that no concerted effort was made to measure normal morphological and biological variation within a species that has such a remarkable range of hosts. For example, we have no detailed comparative morphological information on arctic isolates, even though a number have been studied. Extensive information on biological characteristics is lacking, with the exception of infectivity levels in experimental hosts. It is clear now, however, that the host, natural or experimental, can have an immediate and long-lasting influence on infectivity levels. It is also well known that by following an isolate through a number of generations, biological characteristics such as reproductive capacity in a given host, intestinal distribution, *in vitro* larval release by females, virulence, longevity in intestine and muscle, and basic breeding potential appear to be stable, predictable, and statistically significant characteristics for a specific isolate. It is also known that the host can affect these characteristics to a considerable extent. There appear to be two factors involved in defining these isolates, a basic genetic component that is more or less stable and a component that is quite variable, i.e., an environmental influence, predominantly expressed via the host.

The major isolating mechanism in the process of speciation is probably geographic isolation, at least in the initial stages. It is difficult to imagine complete geographic isolation in species with such a wide range of hosts, including some of the large carnivores that move great distances. It is conceivable, however, that cycling of a *Trichinella* isolate could be localized if it utilized a relatively limited number of hosts, none of which ranges widely. Perhaps this occurs in the case of African isolates, but it would seem highly unlikely with arctic isolates or for *T. spiralis* var. *pseudospiralis* in its bird hosts. This type of selection pressure could account for differences in biological characteristics without assuming complete speciation. The implication here is that speciation, while in progress, has not as yet been completed.

Other isolating mechanisms besides geographic isolation are involved. If an isolate differs in its niche within the intestine and the time it stays in the intestine, these factors would influence the chance of its interacting with another isolate or species. It is known that the preferred site in the intestine of experimental animals varies among isolates, but there is no evidence that the site selected is sufficiently different to prevent overlap of populations of any two isolates or species. Longevity does not appear to be different enough, nor is the molting pattern sufficiently different, to make two populations asynchronous (Belosevic, Chadee, and Dick, unpublished).

The most important isolating mechanism between two populations is reproductive, either pre- or postzygotic. Little direct information is available on prezygotic isolating mechanisms, but there is some evidence that male reproductive structures differ among *T. spiralis, T. nativa, T. nelsoni,* and *T. pseudospiralis* (Barus *et al.,* 1979; Hulinska and Saikenov, 1980). Ethological evidence showed that *T. spiralis* var. *pseudospiralis* is less attracted to an isolate from polar bear and one from a pig (Belosevic and Dick, 1980b), suggesting a degree of isolation. There is also evidence that although sperm transfer occurs, embryogenesis is not initiated (Britov, 1977a), suggesting incompatibility of sperm and ovum among "species" of *Trichinella*. Reproductive isolation usually occurs by postzygotic mechanisms by which nonviable hybrids are produced. If this were true in all breeding experiments, the question of speciation in *Trichinella* would be easily solved. However, while some studies showed hybrid nonviability, other studies clearly showed hybrid viability without hybrid breakdown. The question of reproductive isolation among arctic forms or *T. nativa*, temperate-to-north-temperate forms or *T. spiralis*, African forms or *T. nelsoni*, and *T. spiralis* var. *pseudospiralis* or *T. pseudospiralis* is still not resolved. Furthermore, because a clear picture of normal variation within an isolate or species is not available, we cannot be sure even whether a hybrid was isolated. It is highly likely because of the variation in characteristics among isolates that some hybrids have already been isolated.

Breeding studies have given insight into the speciation question. *Trichinella spiralis* and *T. nelsoni* will interbreed, but their hybrids are nonviable. Arctic isolates interbreed readily. The wolverine and polar bear isolates interbreed with the pig isolate reasonably well, while the wolverine and polar bear isolate breed with *T. spiralis* var. *pseudospiralis* to a lesser degree. The pig isolate and *T. spiralis* var. *pseudospiralis* do not interbreed, but as pointed out previously, the pig isolate is modified by extensive passaging through experimental hosts, and this may account for inability to interbreed. This interpretation should be viewed with caution, since a new pig isolate in our laboratory did not breed with a new arctic fox isolate. Thus, while new isolates may in some instances be more compatible reproductively, there appear to be fundamental genetic differences among some isolates.

Do these genetic differences warrant classifying various form of *Trichinella* as distinct species? For the time being, the author does not think so. There is no doubt that there are pronounced differences such as the inability of *T. spiralis* and *T. spiralis* var. *pseudospiralis* to interbreed, but *T. spiralis* interbreeds with the arctic isolates, which in turn breed with *T. spiralis* var. *pseudospiralis*. What is even more remarkable is that *T. spiralis* var. *pseudospiralis* isolated from the U.S.S.R. interbreeds with arctic isolates from North America. There appears to be some gene flow between these and other isolates. The two exceptions are gene flow between *T. spiralis* and *T. spiralis* var. *pseudospiralis* and between *T. nelsoni* and arctic isolates, although interbreeding between *T. spiralis* and *T. nelsoni* produced nonviable hybrids. If *Trichinella* does not have several separate species, how are these differences to be explained? It is possible that we are dealing with a series of semispecies or incipient species in various stages of speciation. Most will probably disappear or become part of the normal variation of *T. spiralis*, while others such as *T. spiralis* var. *pseudospiralis* may progress to a full species designation, particularly if they stay relatively isolated geographically and utilize a bird host. The African isolates appear to have the strongest case for geographic isolation and selection pressures due to the host species involved, and they, too, may be progressing toward species status. The African isolates need to be interbred with a much wider range of isolates before reproductive isolation can be clearly stated. Taking all breeding data together and assuming that experimental work was done properly, there does not appear to be good reproductive isolation at present. There may be an inability of tropical and arctic forms to interbreed, but both of them breed with the north-temperate form. This suggests a latitudinal cline of variants or isolates with distinct characteristics that nevertheless allows some gene flow among the isolates. *Trichinella spiralis* var. *pseudospiralis*, as evidenced by breeding experiments, has affinities to arctic isolates, suggesting on the one hand a long association with arctic forms and on the other hand that its unique characteristic, lack of cyst, may be recently acquired. Other workers have suggested that *T. spiralis* var. *pseudospiralis*, because of its association with birds, may be the ancestral form of *T. spiralis*. Arctic isolates are probably the oldest form of *Trichinella* and *T. spiralis* from pigs the youngest. The African isolates may be a refugium that was derived from large carnivores isolated in Africa following glaciation, but still retained some characteristics of arctic isolates.

8. FUTURE CONSIDERATIONS

1. There is a need to define adequately the species *T. spiralis* through studies to determine its normal variation. The studies should include comparisons of morphological data, other biological characteristics, and work on geographical isolates from closely related areas in a number of individuals of the same host species and in different host species from the same area. This would determine the degree of normal variation for a specific isolate and give baseline data for comparing isolates around the world.

2. The ability of *Trichinella* isolates to resist freezing needs to be evaluated, particularly in those isolates recovered from wild animals from all regions of the world. Furthermore, information is urgently needed as to whether or not resistance to freezing is a genetic characteristic of arctic isolates only.

3. Well-defined and universally accepted standards for designating isolates are essential for future comparisons. A detailed history of each isolate should be maintained and should include number of passages, length of passages, genetic designation of experimental host, and

experimental techniques for digesting, isolating, and infecting with larvae.

4. Methods should be standardized for breeding experiments; both single and multiple breeding pairs should be used, and if a hybrid is produced, reproductive capacity should be determined and hybrid viability clearly established.

5. The population genetics of *Trichinella* needs to be studied, and the range of variability within its gene pool needs to be determined. Electrophoretic patterns of proteins from isolates should be made and compared with well-defined biological characteristics. Immunoelectrophoretic techniques have shown promise for distinguishing among African, arctic, and north-temperate forms of *Trichinella*. Electrophoresis, immunoelectrophoresis, and isoelectric focusing should be applied to isolates closely related by geography or by host species as well as to those forms considered to have greater differences.

6. More comparative work on the range of virulence possible for isolates, and sensitivity to drugs, is essential if trichinellosis is to be properly treated. Public-health officials should be aware that differences do exist, particularly with respect to infections originating from wild animals. Causes of increased virulence should be evaluated and should include immunogenic properties of isolates and their potential as carriers of pathogens.

7. Geographic distribution and biological characteristics of *Trichinella* within a region are not well defined. Considerably more information is required from South America, southern Asia, the southern United States, and Mexico. Biological characterization of isolates from the Rocky Mountain region of North America would help clarify the factors that influence the distribution of arctic isolates in North America.

8. A concerted effort to find *T. spiralis* var. *pseudospiralis* in North American animals, particularly birds, would help clarify the range of this parasite and its affinities to other forms of *Trichinella*.

9. It will become increasingly difficult to keep accurate records on geographic isolates of *Trichinella* as more are discovered and studied. Perhaps to ensure a degree of taxonomic order in the genus *Trichinella*, we should consider subspecies status, i.e., *T. spiralis spiralis*, *T. spiralis nativa*, *T. spiralis nelsoni*, and *T. spiralis pseudospiralis*. It should be noted, however, that by definition they are not "good" subspecies, since they lack distinct morphological differences.

In summary, the major tasks to be addressed in the resolution of the species problem in the genus *Trichinella* are to determine normal variation of characteristics of isolates, establish the extent of local populations or demes, and determine the degree of genetic similarity among these local populations. Finally, having determined the normal variation at the deme or local population level, we can start to apply principles of population genetics to define speciation in the genus.

REFERENCES

Arakawa, A., and Todd, A.C., 1971, Comparative development of temperate zone and arctic isolates of *Trichinella spiralis* in the white mouse, *J. Parasitol.* **57**:526–530.

Barus, V., Tenora, F., Wiger, R., Genov, T., and Komandarev, S., 1979, Scanning electron microscopic studies on males of *Trichinella* species, *Folia Parasitol.* **26**:97–101.

Belosevic, M., and Dick, T.A., 1979, *Trichinella spiralis*: Comparison of stages in host intestine with those of an arctic *Trichinella* sp., *Exp. Parasitol.* **48**:432–446.

Belosevic, M., and Dick, T.A., 1980a, *Trichinella spiralis*: Comparison with an arctic isolate, *Exp. Parasitol.* **49**:266–276.

Belosevic, M., and Dick, T.A., 1980b, Chemical attraction in the genus *Trichinella*, *J. Parasitol.* **66**:88–93.

Belozerov, S.N., 1976, Serological identification of *Trichinella* strains and species by indirect immunofluorescent test, *Gelmintol. Byull.* **18**:5–8.

Bessonov, A.S., Penkova, R.A., and Uspensky, A.V., 1975, On the independence of *Trichinella* species, *Waid. Parazytol.* **21**:561–575.

Bessonov, A.S., Penkova, R.A., and Gumenshehikova, V.P., 1978, *Trichinella pseudospiralis* Garkavi, 1972: Morphological and biological characteristics and host specificity, in: *Trichinellosis* (C.W. Kim and Z.S. Pawlowski, eds.), University Press of New England, Hanover, New Hampshire pp. 79–93.

Boev, S.N., Shaikenov, B., and Tazieva, Z., 1975, Sibling species of *Trichinella* in Kazakhstan and Middle Asia, *Second Europ. Multicol. Parasitol. Trogir.* 1–6 Sept., pp. 80–81.

Boev, S.N., Bondareva, V.I., Sokolova, I.B., Tazieva, Z.H., and Shaikenov, B., 1978, *Trichinellae* and Trichinellosis in Kazakhstan, Abstracts, Asian Congress on Parasitology, Bombay, India.

Boev, S.N., Britov, V.A., and Orlov, I.V., 1979, Species composition of Trichinellae, *Wiad. Parazytol.* **25**:495–503.

Brandly, P.J., and Rausch, R., 1950, A preliminary note on trichinosis investigations in Alaska, *Arctic* **3**:105–197.

Britov, V.A., 1969, Some differences between natural and synanthropic strains of *Trichinella*, *Wiad. Parazytol.* **15**:555–560.

Britov, V.A., 1971, Biologic methods of determining *T. spiralis* Owen, 1835 varieties, *Wiad. Parazytol.* **17**:477–480.

Britov, V.A., 1975, The importance of the identification of *Trichinella* in the prophylaxis of trichinelliasis, *Vopr. Prirodnoi Ochaguvusti Bolesni Alma-Ata.* **7**:109–112.

Britov, V.A., 1977a, Detection of the genetic relationship among nematode species of the genus *Trichinella*, *Genetika* **13**:1025–1029.

Britov, V.A., 1977b, On the technique of crossing of *Trichinella*, *Parasitologia* **11**:460–461.

Britov, V.A., 1980, The species of *Trichinella*, their specificity and their role in initiating disease in humans and animals, *Helminthologia.* **17**:63–66.

Britov, V.A., and Boev, S.N., 1972, Taxonomic rank of various strains of *Trichinella* and their circulation in nature, *Vestn. Akad. Nauk. SSSR* **28**:27–32.

Britov, V.A., and Smirnova, M.I., 1966, About *Trichinella spiralis* strains, *Wiad. Parazytol.* **12**:527–530.

Britov, V.A., Ermolin, G.A., Tarakanov, V.I., and Nikitin, T.L., 1971, Genetic isolation of two variants of *Trichinella*, *Med. Parazitol. Bolezni* **5**:515–521.

Cameron, T.W.M., 1970, Trichinosis in Canada, in: *Trichinosis in Man and Animals* (S.E. Gould, ed.), Charles C. Thomas, Springfield, Illinois, pp. 374–377.

Chadee, K., and Dick, T.A., 1982a, Designation and freezing resistance of isolates of *Trichinella spiralis* from wild carnivores, *J. Wildl. Dis.* **18**:169–173.

Chadee, K.C., and Dick, T.A., 1982b, Biological characteristics and host influence on a geographical isolate of *Trichinella* (Wolverine: 55°00′N, 100°00′W, 1979), *J. Parasitol.* **68**:451–456.

Chadee, K., Dick, T.A., and Faubert, G.M., 1983, Sensitivity of *Trichinella* sp. isolates to thiabendazole, *Can. J. Zool.* (in press).

Clark, P.S., Brownsberger, E. Saslow, A.R., Kagan, I.G. Nobel, G.R., and Maynard, J.E., 1972, Bear meat trichinosis, *Ann. Intern. Med.* **76**:951–956.

Culbertson, J.T., and Kaplan, S.S., 1938, A study upon passive immunity in experimental trichiniasis, *Parasitology* **30**:156–166.

Dick, T.A. and Belosevic, M., 1978, Observations on a *Trichinella spiralis* isolate from a polar bear, *J. Parasitol.* **64**:1143–1145.

Dick, T.A., and Chadee, K., 1981, Biological characterization of some North American isolates of *Trichinella spiralis*, in: *Trichinellosis* (C.W. Kim, E.J., Ruitenberg, and T.S. Teppema, eds.), Reedbooks, Surrey, England, pp. 23–27.

Dick, T.A., and Chadee, K., 1983, Interbreeding and gene flow in the genus *Trichinella*, *J. Parasitol.* (in press).

Dick, T.A., and Silver, B.B., 1980, Intestinal distribution of *Trichinella spiralis* in rats, *J. Parasitol.* **66**:472–477.

Dies, K., 1980, Survival of *Trichinella spiralis* larvae in deep-frozen wolf tissue, *Can. Vet. J.* **21**:38.

Dobzhansky, T., 1970, *Genetics of the Evolutionary Process*, Columbia University Press, New York.

Dobzhansky, T., Ayala, F.J., Stebbins, G.L., and Valetine, J.W., 1977, *Evolution*, W.H. Freeman, San Francisco.

Eaton, P.D.R., 1979, Trichinosis in the Arctic, *Can. Med. J.* **120**:22.

Ermolin, G.A., and Efremov, E.E., 1974, *Trichinella spiralis*: Isolation and purification of the main functional antigen from decapsulated larvae, in: *Trichinellosis* (C.W. Kim, ed.), Intext Educational Publishers, New York, pp. 187–197.

Garkavi, B.L., 1972, Species of *Trichinella* isolated from wild animals, *Veterianariya* **10**:90–91.

Garkavi, B.L., 1974, The cross immunity of superinvasion between *Trichinella spiralis* and *T. pseudospiralis* in white mice and rats, *Parasitologia* **4**:299–301.

Garkavi, B.L., 1976, Susceptibility of laboratory animals to *Trichinella* from synanthropic and natural nidi of the North Caucasus, *Parazitologia* **10**:154–157.

Garkavi, B.L., and Gineev, A.M., 1976, *Trichinella* in wild animals in northern Caucasus, *Vopr. Prirodnoi Oclyagovosti Boleznei* **8**:136–139.

Geller, E.R., and Gridasova, L.F., 1974, The karyotype and ovogenesis of *Trichinella spiralis* (Owen, 1835), *Med. Parazit. Parzit. Bolezni* **3**:324–326.

Grant, V., 1971, *Plant Speciation*, Columbia University Press, New York.

Grétillat, S., and Vassiliades, G., 1968, Réceptivés comparées du chat et du pore domestiques á la souche ouest-africaine de *Trichinella spiralis* (Owen, 1835), *C. R. Acad. Sci.* **266**:1139–1141.

Hall, M.C., 1916, Nematode parasites of mammals of the orders Rodentia, Lagomorpha, and Hyracoidea, *Proc. U.S. Natl. Mus.* **50**(213):1–258.

Hulinska, D., and Shaikenov, B., 1980, Scanning electron microscopic studies on developmental adult stages of four *Trichinella* species, *Angew. Parasitol.* **21:**150–158.

Kociecka, W., 1971, Behaviour of *Trichinella spiralis* larvae with animals treated by thiabendazole and hydrocortisone, *Wiad. Parazytol.* **17:**625–640.

Komandarev, S., and Mihov, L., 1977, On the species belongings of two *Trichinella* strains from Bulgaria, *Khelmintologiya* **3:**46–54.

Komandarev, S., Britov, V., and Mihov, L., 1975, Identification of two *Trichinella* strains from Bulgaria, *C. R. Acad. Bulg. Sci.* **28:**1541–1542.

Kozar, Z., and Kozar, M., 1965, A comparison of the infectivity and pathogenicity of *Trichinella spiralis* strains from Poland and Kenya, *J. Helminthol.* **39:**19–34.

Kruger, S.P., Collins, M.H., van Niekerk, J.W., McCully, R.M., and Basson, P.A., 1969, Experimental observations on the South African strain of *T. spiralis*, *Wiad. Parazytol.* **15:**546–554.

Machnicka, B., 1979, The problem of geographical strains of *Trichinella spiralis* and their biological properties, *Wiad. Parazytol.* **25:**197–205.

Mayr, E., 1970, *Populations, Species and Evolution*, Harvard University Press, Cambridge.

McCoy, O.R., 1931, Immunity of rats to reinfection with *Trichinella spiralis*, *Am. J. Hyg.* **14:**484–494.

Mutafova, T., and Komandarev, S., 1976, On the karyotype of a laboratory *Trichinella* strain from Bulgaria, *Z. Parasitenkd.* **48:**247–250.

Nelson, G.S., and Forrester, A.T.T., 1962, Trichinosis in Kenya, *Wiad. Parazytol.* **8:**17–28.

Nelson, G.S., and Mukundi, J., 1963, A strain of *Trichinella spiralis* from Kenya of low infectivity to rats and domestic pigs, *J. Helminthol.* **37:**329–338.

Nelson, G.S., Rickman, R., and Pester, F.R.N., 1961, Feral trichinosis in Africa, *Trans. R. Soc. Trop. Med. Hyg.* **55:**514–517.

Nelson, G.S., Blackie, E.J., and Mukundi, J., 1966, Comparative studies on geographical strains of *Trichinella spiralis*, *Trans. R. Soc. Trop. Med. Hyg.* **60:**471–480.

Ozeretskovskaya, N.N., Romanova, V.I., Alekseeva, M.I., Pereverzeva, E.V., and Uspenskii, S.M., 1969, Physiological and biochemical characteristics of natural Arctic synanthropic North Caucasian and laboratory strains of *Trichinella spiralis*, *Wiad. Parazytol.* **15:**561–570.

Ozeretskovskaya, N.N., Romanova, V.I., Alekseeva, M.I., Pereverzeva, E.V., and Uspenskii, S.M., 1970, Human trichinosis in the Soviet Arctic and the characteristics of the strain of arctic *Trichinella*, in: *Productivity And Conservation in Northern Circumpolar Lands* (W.A. Fuller and P.G. Kevan, eds.), *INNC Publ. N. Ser.* **10:**133–142.

Pawlowski, Z., and Rauhut, W., 1971, Comparative observations on three local strains of *Trichinella spiralis*, *Wiad. Parazytol.* **17:**481–486.

Penkova, R.A., 1974, Identification of *Trichinella* species by the use of microprecipitation test on live larvae, *Bull. All-Union K.I. Skryabin Inst. Helminthol.* **13:**80–85.

Penkova, R.A., and Romanenko, L.N., 1973, The investigation of *Trichinella* chromosomes, *Proc. All-Union K.I. Skryabin Inst. Helminthol.* **20:**133–142.

Pereverzeva, E.V., 1966, About strains of *Trichinella spiralis*, *Wiad. Parazytol.* **12:**531–541.

Pereverzeva, E.V., Ozeretskovskaya, N.N., Uspenski, S.M., and Veretennikova, N.L., 1971a, Studies on helminthofauna and muscle phase of trichinellosis in polar bear from Wrangel Island, *Wiad. Parazytol.* **17:**451–463.

Pereverzeva, E.V., Ozeretskovskaya, N., and Veretennikova, N.L., 1971b, Histomorphological studies of polar bear *Trichinella* strain, *Wiad. Parazytol.* **17:**465–475.

Pereverzeva, E.V., Ozeretskovskaya, N.N., and Veretennikova, N.L., 1974, On the peculiarities of the development of *Trichinella* larvae (isolated from muscles of a raccoon) in white mice, *Wiad. Parazytol.* **20:**67–80.

Rappaport, I., 1943a, A comparison of three strains of *Trichinella spiralis*. I. Pathogenicity and extent of larval development in the musculature, *Am. J. Trop. Med.* **23**:343–350.

Rappaport, I., 1943b, A comparison of three strains of *Trichinella spiralis*. II. Longevity and sex ratio of adults in the intestine and rapidity of larval development in the musculature, *Am. J. Trop. Med.* **23**:351–362.

Rausch, R.L., 1970, Trichinosis in the Arctic, in: *Trichinosis in Man and Animals* (S.E. Gould, ed.), Charles C. Thomas, Springfield, Illinois, pp. 348–373.

Rausch, R., Babero, B.B., Rausch, R.V., and Schiller, E.L., 1956, Studies on the helminth fauna of Alaska. XXVII. The occurrence of larvae of *Trichinella spiralis* in Alaskan mammals, *J. Parasitol.* **42**:259–271.

Read, C.P., and Schiller, E.L., 1969, Infectivity of *Trichinella* from the temperate and arctic zones of North America, *J. Parasitol.* **55**:72–73.

Schad, G.A., Nundy, S., Chowdhury, A.B., and Bandyopadhyay, A.K., 1967, *Trichinella spiralis* in India. II. Characteristics of a strain isolated from a civet cat in Calcutta, *Trans. R. Soc. Trop. Med. Hyg.* **61**:249–258.

Scudder, G.G.E., 1974, Species concepts and speciation, *Can. J. Zool.* **52**:1121–1134.

Shaikenov, B., 1980, Spontaneous infection of birds with *Trichinella pseudospiralis* Garkavi, 1972, *Folia Parasitol.* **27**:227–230.

Shaikenov, B., Tazieva, Z.H., and Horning, B., 1977, Zur Ätiologie der Naturherd-Trichinellose in der Schweiz, *Acta Trop.* **34**:327–350.

Siddiqi, M.N., and Meerovitch, E., 1976a, Host–parasite relationship in trichiniasis. I. Infectivity of various strains of *Trichinella spiralis* in rats, *Pak. J. Zool.* **8**:183–189.

Siddiqi, M.N., and Meerovitch, E., 1976b, Host–parasite relationship in trichiniasis. II. Infectivity of various strains of *Trichinella spiralis* in mice, guinea pigs and two strains of rats, *Pak. J. Zool.* **8**:191–197.

Spaldonova, R., Corba, J., and Tomasovicova, O., 1978, Comparison of the efficacy of different benzimidazole anthelmintics against *Trichinella spiralis* and *Trichinella pseudospiralis*, in: *Trichinellosis* (C.W. Kim and Z.S. Pawlowski, eds.), University Press of New England, Hanover, New Hampshire, pp. 437–443.

Stoll, L., Fuhr, R., and Haase, M., 1979, The biological behaviour of different *Trichinella spiralis* strains: Investigations in pigs, *Arch. Lebensmittelhyg.* **30**:13–16.

Sukhdeo, M.V.K., and Meerovitch, E., 1977, Comparison of three geographical isolates of *Trichinella*, *Can. J. Zool.* **55**:2060–2064.

Sukhdeo, M.V.K., and Meerovitch, E., 1979, A comparison of the antigenic characteristics of three geographical isolates of *Trichinella*, *Int. J. Parasitol.* **9**:571–576.

Sukhdeo, M.V.K., and Meerovitch, E., 1980, A biological explanation for the differences in infectivity of geographical isolates of *Trichinella*, *Can. J. Zool* **58**:1227–1231.

Tomasovicova, O., 1975, Poultry—a new host of *Trichinella pseudospiralis* (Garkavi, 1972), *Biologia (Bratislava)* **30**:821–826.

Turesson, G., 1922, The genotypical response of the plant species to its habitat, *Hereditas* **3**:211–350.

Villella, J.B., 1966, Morphologic criteria for distinguishing the sex of *Trichinella spiralis* larvae from muscle, *J. Parasitol.* **52**:908–910.

Yorke, W., and Maplestone, P.A., 1969, *The Nematode Parasites of Vertebrates*, Hafner, New York.

Zimmerman, W.J., 1970, Trichinosis in the United States, in: *Trichinosis in Man and Animals* (S.E. Gould, ed.), Charles C. Thomas, Springfield, Illinois, pp. 378–400.

Zimmerman, W.J., and Hubbard, E.O., 1969, Trichinosis in wildlife of Iowa, *Am. J. Epidemiol.* **90**:84–92.

Zimoroi, I., 1964, Natural outbreaks of trichinellosis in Kursk region, Thesis for candidate degree, Kursk.

3

Biology

DICKSON D. DESPOMMIER

1. INTRODUCTION

Most of the broad aspects of the life cycle of *Trichinella* were uncovered during the 50 years following its discovery and description by Paget and Owen in 1835 and are highlighted in Chapter 1, which deals with the history of this nematode. Nevertheless, many details of its enteral and parenteral life were not described until after 1960, and many have yet to be described. For instance, it is now known that *Trichinella* lives as an intracellular parasite, except for its brief life as a migratory newborn larva, making it the largest example of this type of commonly occurring organism. These findings have radically influenced thinking concerning the specific ways in which *Trichinella* derives its livelihood from the host.

Trichinella is one of the least host-specific parasites in nature. It has been shown both experimentally and through surveys on sylvatic animal populations that *Trichinella* can infect almost any mammalian species (Leuckart, 1860; McCoy, 1932; Hemmert-Halswick and Bugge 1934; Alicata, 1935; Schwartz, 1938; Roth, 1939; Sawitz, 1939; Kuitunen-Ekbaum and Webster, 1947; Larsh and Hendricks, 1949; Humes and Akers, 1952; Berezantsev, 1954; Chute and Covalt, 1960; Cameron, 1960; Nelson and Forrester, 1962; Rausch, 1962). The Chinese hamster represents the exception, being the only known nonpermissive mammalian host (Ritterson, 1959). However, even this host is susceptible to the enteral phase of the infection. It is generally agreed that other

DICKSON D. DESPOMMIER • Division of Tropical Medicine, School of Public Health, Columbia University, New York, New York 10032.

TABLE 1
***Trichinella* Life Cycle**[a]

Stage	Description	References
Enteral phase		
1. Ingestion of raw or undercooked meats containing the infective L_1 larva	This step in the infection was well described by many investigators during the 1800s and 1900s.	Herbst (1851)
2. Digestion of host tissue and release of infective L_1 larvae in the stomach	Experiments in a variety of mammalian species revealed this aspect of the life cycle.	Virchow (1859), Leuckart (1860)
3a. Entry of infective L_1 larva into its intra-multicellular niche	Scanning and transmission electron-microscopic studies revealed that the enteral phase of infection occurred within the cytoplasm of columnar cells.	Wright (1979)
3b. Four larval stages (L_1–L_4) leading to adulthood	Both light and transmission electron-microscopic studies in mice and rats showed that four molts are needed for maturation of *Trichinella* to the adult stage.	Villella (1958), Ali Khan (1966), Kozek (1971a,b)
4. Occurrence of mating within the intra-multicellular niche	Studies in mice revealed that mating occurs within the enteral niche between 30 and 40 hr after oral infection.	Gardiner (1976)

5. Production of newborn L₁ larvae	Newborn L₁ larvae are shed beginning on day 5 after entering the intramulticellular niche, and then enter the lamina propria region of the villus tissue.	Heller (1933)

Parenteral phase

6. Migration of L₁ larva to lymph, then blood-stream	Experiments involving cannulation of the thoracic duct in rats showed that up to 70% of all newborn L₁ larvae migrate to the bloodstream via the lymphatics.	Basten and Beeson (1970), Harley and Gallicchico (1971)
7. Entry of newborn L₁ larva into its intracellular niche (i.e., the striated skeletal muscle cell)	Intracellular life within the muscle cell begins by newborn L₁ larva penetrating the sarcolemmal membrane.	Despommier (1976)
8–9. Growth and development of the larva in its Nurse cell	Trichinella induces permanent alterations in its intracellular niche leading to the formation of the Nurse cell. The worm then grows and differentiates without molting into an infective L₁ larva.	Ribas-Mujal and Rivera-Pomar (1968), Stewart (1973), Despommier (1975)
10. Mature Nurse cell–infective L₁ larva complex	Growth and differentiation of Trichinella are complete within 20 days after entry of the larva into the intracellular niche.	Despommier et al. (1975)

a See Fig. 1 for diagram.

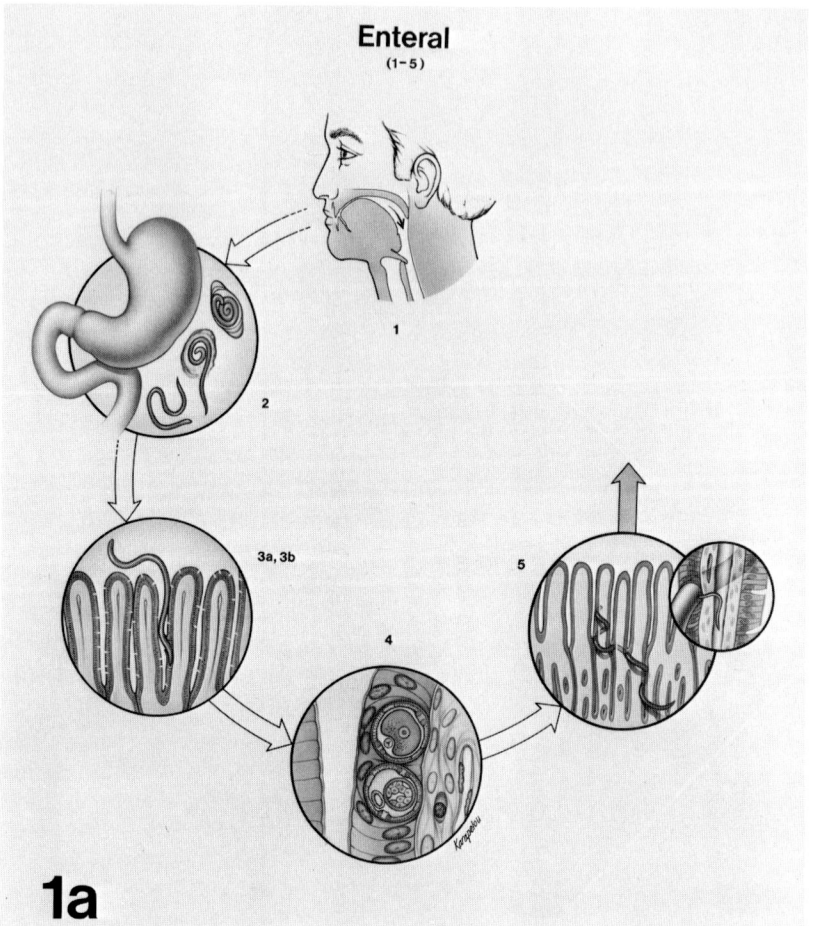

Enteral
(1-5)

1a

FIGURE 1. (1a) Enteral, (1b) parenteral *Trichinella* life cycle (see Table 1 for description).

classes of vertebrates are either refractory to infection with *Trichinella* or harbor *Trichinella* only when their body temperatures are adjusted experimentally to 35–37°C (Leuckart, 1860; Ducas, 1921; Gaugusch, 1950; Zimmermann *et al.*, 1962; Smirnov, 1963). Presented below is a detailed description of the life cycle of *Trichinella* as discerned from experimental infections in mice, rats, guinea pigs, and rabbits. A synoptic account of the morphology of the parasite may be found in Appendix 1.

The life cycle of *Trichinella* is diagrammed in Fig. 1 and described in Table 1; the numbers in brackets following the text subheads are

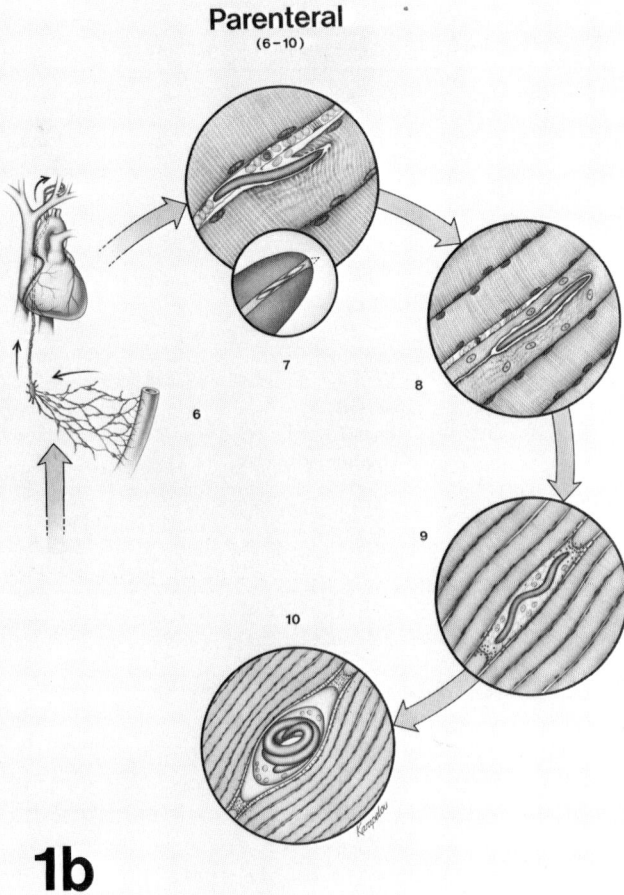

FIGURE 1. (*Continued*)

those of the life-cycle stages in Fig. 1 and Table 1. The nomenclature used for the stages of *Trichinella* throughout the discussion is given in Table 2.

2. INGESTION OF THE INFECTIVE FIRST-STAGE LARVA [1]

The infection begins when infective first-stage (L_1) larvae (Ali Khan, 1966; Kozek, 1971a) are swallowed. Prior to carefully conducted studies on the molting cycle (Villella 1958; Ali Khan, 1966; Kozek 1971a,b), investigators were not in agreement as to which larval stage

TABLE 2
Nomenclature of the Stages of *Trichinella spiralis*

Stage	Location in host	Time present during life cycle	Synonyms in the literature
Infective L$_1$ larva[a]	Enteral	0.9 hr after infection	Muscle larva, infective larva, juvenile
L$_2$ larva	Enteral	10–14 hr after infection	None
L$_3$ larva	Enteral	15–22 hr after infection	None
L$_4$ larva	Enteral	23–30 hr after infection	None
Adult	Enteral	31 hr and continuing to days, weeks, or months after infection	None
Newborn L$_1$ larva	Enteral	As long as adults are present	Prelarva, embryo, newborn larva
Migratory L$_1$ larva	Parenteral	Unknown, probably no longer than 1 day	Migratory larva
Preinfective L$_1$ larva	Parenteral	0–14 days after entering muscle cell	Muscle larva, immature juvenile
Infective L$_1$ larva[a]	Parenteral	15 days up to 30 years	Muscle larva, infective larva, juvenile

[a] These are the same larval stage.

the infective muscle larva represented. Arguments against its status as an L$_1$ larva arose because the L$_1$ undergoes both a remarkable series of developmental changes and increased growth on entering the muscle cell. It was therefore inferred that molting must also have occurred. These speculations were not substantiated by electron-microscopic studies on the muscle phase (Despommier, 1975), while four molts were identified with the enteral phase of its life, thereby placing *Trichinella* in register with most other nematode species.

3. DIGESTION OF HOST TISSUES AWAY FROM THE INFECTIVE FIRST-STAGE LARVA [2]

If muscle larvae are ingested as part of an infected meal, then infected host muscle tissue and Nurse cell must first become digested away from the parasite in the stomach for the worms to be released. It is presumed that this is accomplished by the action of acidified pepsin. This phase of the infection lasts for only minutes, and the larva does not undergo any developmental changes while in the stomach. Unfortunately, this larval stage has served as the traditional starting point in numerous *in vitro* studies involving metabolism, ecdysis, and other phenomena and probably has been selected more because of the ease of its acquisition than because of its relevance to the life cycle.

4. INTRAMULTICELLULAR ENTERAL NICHE

4.1. Entrance of the Infective First-Stage Larva [3a]

Once digestion has proceeded sufficiently to free them, the L_1 larvae rapidly enter their intracellular niche in the small intestine (Fig. 2) (Wright, 1979), doing so in as little as 10 min after being released from the muscle tissues (Despommier et al., 1978). The intracellular niche actually consists of a row of columnar epithelial cells into which the larva penetrates. Since the L_1 larva is approximately 1 mm in length by 35–38 μm in diameter, and each columnar cell measures approximately 32 μm × 8.5 μm, the worm occupies about 117 columnar cells during this early phase. Thus, it is more proper to refer to this stage of the infection as the intramulticellular stage. Surprisingly, there is no disintegration of host cells as the result of penetration by the larva; rather, the cells stretch to accommodate the nematode (Fig. 3). There is fusion of columnar-cell membranes with each other to form a syncytium (Wright, 1979), similar to that found in *Trichuris muris* infections (Lee and Wright, 1978). The mechanism or mechanisms by which the infective L_1 larva enters columnar cells are not known, since ultrastructural evidence strongly suggests that this stage does not possess a stylet (Bruce, 1970b). While the columnar epithelium of the small intestine is the natural intramulticellular niche occupied by *Trichinella*, other epithelial tissues can also become infected under experimental conditions. For instance, the pregnant rat uterus is a suitable niche, promoting growth and development of *Trichinella* to the adult stage (McCoy, 1936). Interestingly, no adult worms matured in the uteri of nonpregnant rats. Chick embryo membranes or the amniotic sac of rat embryos can also serve as a suitable environment for worm maturation (McCoy, 1936). Unfortunately, no histological evidence was presented to permit the identification of the precise location of the adult worms within these abnormal environments. In another study, a few adult male worms were recovered from diffusion chambers (0.45-μm-pore-size filters) that were first filled with infective L_1 larvae, then implanted intraperitoneally in CFW strain mice for 7 days (Despommier and Wostmann, 1968). No adult female worms developed in the diffusion chambers.

Precisely where in the small intestine the infective L_1 larva begins

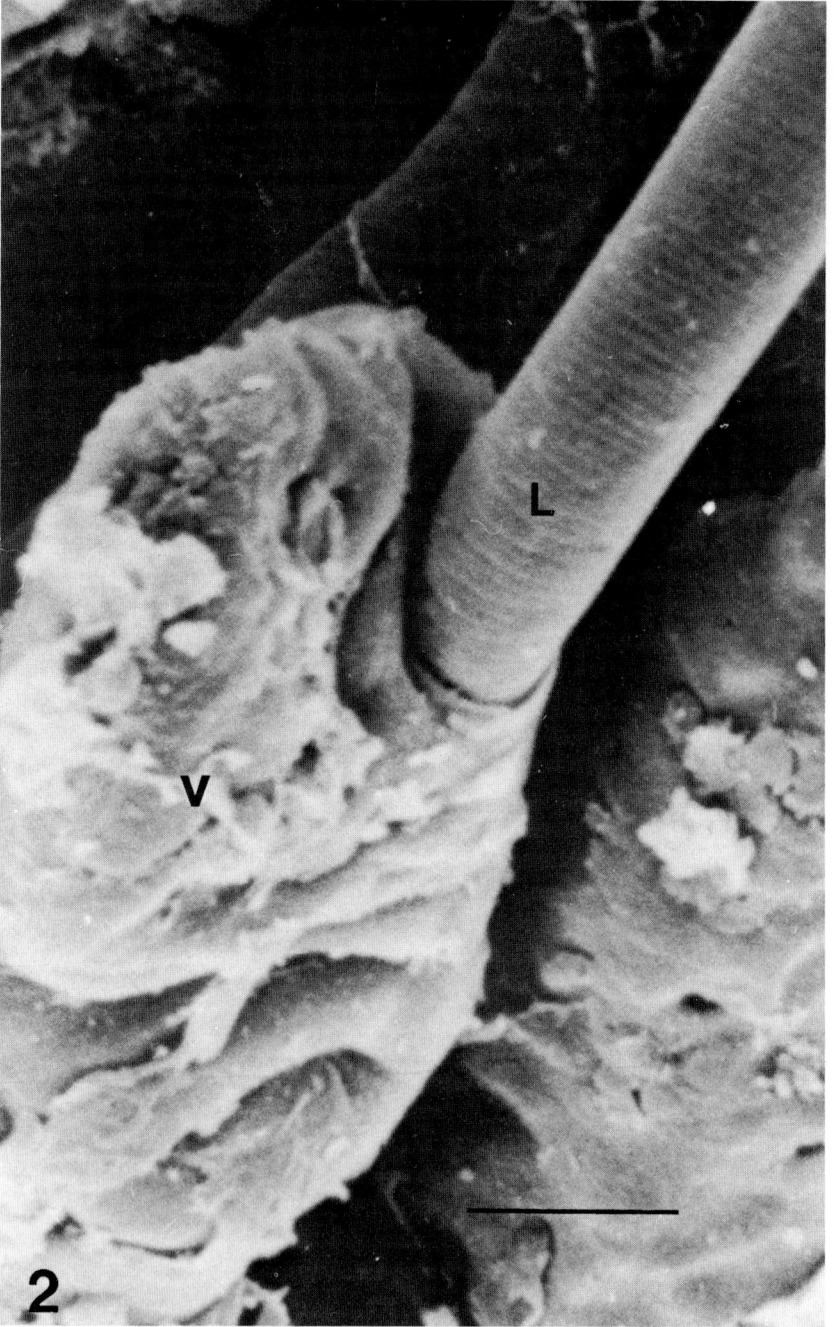

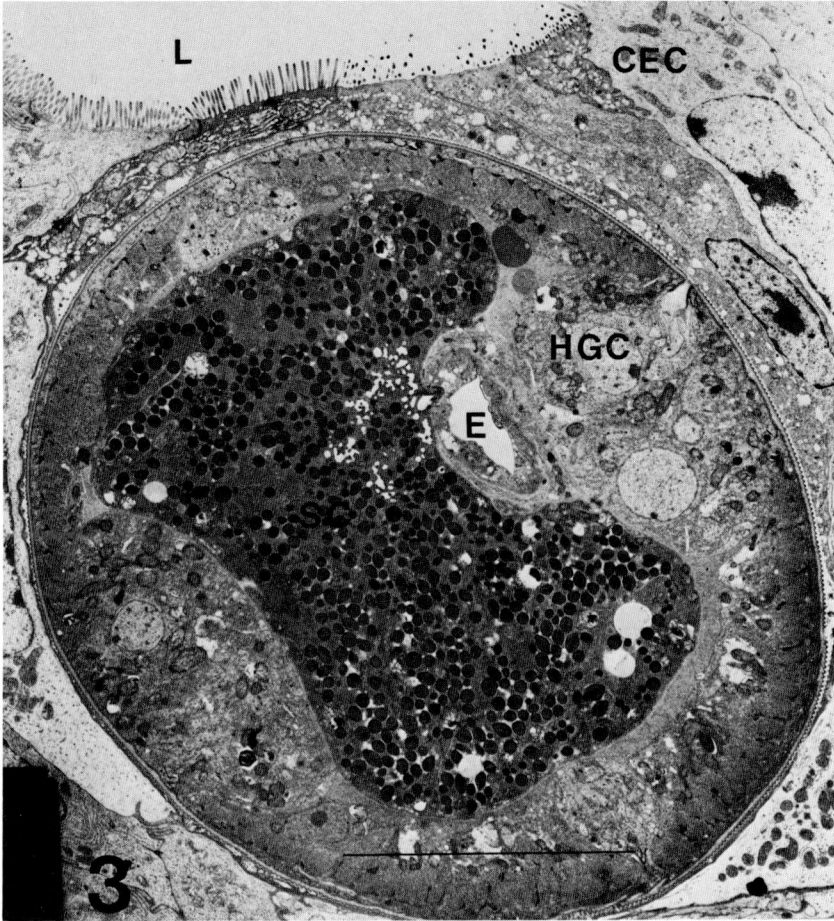

FIGURE 3. Transmission electron micrograph of the adult *Trichinella* in its intramulti-cellular niche. (E) Esophagus; (CEC) columnar epithelial cell; (SC) stichocyte; (HGC) hypodermal gland cell; (L) lumen of small intestine. Scale bar: 10 μm. Courtesy of Dr. K. A. Wright.

its enteral life (i.e., duodenum, jejunum, or ileum) has been the subject of several major investigations in which mice, rats, and guinea pigs served as hosts (Gursch, 1949; Larsh and Hendricks, 1949; Podhajecky, 1962; Campbell, 1967; Denham, 1968; Kennedy, 1976; Dick and Silver, 1980; Sukhdeo and Croll, 1981). It is generally agreed that the

←——————————————————————————————

FIGURE 2. Scanning electron micrograph of an infective L₁ larva (L) in the act of penetrating the columnar epithelium of the villus (V) in the small intestine of a mouse. Scale bar: 40 μm. Courtesy of Dr. M. Sukhdeo.

duodenum is the site in which the majority of larvae in a given dose establish. However, at least in the guinea pig and the outbred ICI or inbred agouti mouse, larvae establish more often in the jejunum and ileum (Roth, 1938; Denham, 1968). Even infections that normally establish in the duodenum can be made to settle elsewhere. For instance, if large volumes of fluid (e.g., 0.5–1.0 ml per mouse) accompany the larvae, as may be the case in experimentally induced infections, over 50% will be found further down in the small intestine, in either the jejunum or the ileum (Sukhdeo and Croll, 1981). Furthermore, if infective L_1 larvae are introduced into the jejunum or ileum, they will develop to adults and remain there (Dick and Silver, 1980).

Gut motility also plays a role in worm location. Intestine inhibited with smooth-muscle relaxants harbored a majority of worms in the anterior most portion of the duodenum (Sukhdeo and Croll, 1981). In contrast, the more active the peristalsis, the farther down in the gut tract the infective L_1 larvae established (Larsh and Hendricks, 1949; Sukhdeo and Croll, 1981).

Unisexual infections were found in different locations; female worms were distributed in the gut as in the bisexual infection, while male worms had a somewhat random distribution (Sukhdeo and Croll, 1981). The age of the host alters the site selection of the infective L_1 larvae (Larsh and Hendricks, 1949; Campbell, 1967; Dick and Silver, 1980), with worms taking up residence farther down in the gut in young mice (24–48 days old) as compared to old mice (130–140 days old).

While most mammals can serve as a host for *Trichinella*, various altered physiological states within a given host can dramatically influence the number of worms that establish themselves in the enteral niche. Newborn mice were shown to be innately resistant to an incoming infection (Bass and Olson, 1965). In contrast, studies on old mice (22 months old) have shown that they harbor more infective L_1 larvae in their muscles than their younger (4-months-old) counterparts (R. B. Crandall, 1975). However, it was not determined whether or not this differential susceptibility was due to an increased number of worms that established themselves in the gut.

Sex of the host can influence the number of infective L_1 larvae recoverable from muscle, although not always in the same way. For instance, ICI strain female mice (see Table 6) harbored more than 3 times as many infective L_1 larvae (241,000) as did their male counterparts (63,400) (Denham and Martinez, 1970). In contrast, female hooded rats had fewer infective L_1 larvae than males (Manku and Hamilton, 1972). In neither of those studies was it determined which stage of the infection was affected by this host characteristic.

In one instance, the diet of the host was shown to influence the establishment of an incoming infection. Rats fed a diet designed to induce protein–calorie malnutrition were more susceptible to infection than well-nourished controls (Saowakontha, 1975). Hyperalimentation of rats 2 days prior to infection resulted in fewer adult worms recovered at day 7 (Castro *et al.*, 1974). However, it was not determined how many infective L_1 larvae became established at the beginning of the infection (i.e., on day 1 or 2).

The intestinal flora plays a role in the establishment of a primary infection (Stefanski and Przyjalkowski, 1964). Germ-free mice showed an irregular pattern regarding the take of infection and, regardless of the sex or age of mice, invariably harbored fewer adults at day 5 than conventional controls (Przyjalkowski and Golinska, 1976). More larvae became established in the small intestine if germ-free mice were first colonized by enteric bacterial species such as *Escherichia coli, Bacillus mesentericus, B. subtilis,* or *Pseudomonas aeruginosa,* thereby converting them to gnotobionts (Przyjalkowski, 1968; Przyjalkowski and Wescott, 1969). Interpretation of these data must, however, await further work on the physiological and biochemical requirements for infection in the enteral niche by the L_1 larva, since many changes are brought about in the gut during conventionalization of germ-free hosts.

Adrenalectomy prior to infection decreased the number of infective L_1 larvae that took up residence in the gut, as evaluated on day 3 of infection. The effects of adrenalectomy were reversed by pretreatment of adrenalectomized mice with hydrocortisone, corticosterone, and prednisone (Pawlowski, 1967a,b). It does not seem likely that host immune effects would be exerted against the infection during the first 3 days, since acquired resistance usually takes 6–7 days to develop in a primary infection. Therefore, it is probable that some other host factor or factors were affected by adrenalectomy, which in turn influenced the number of larvae that established. The fact that at least some larvae in the adrenalectomized host proceeded to adulthood suggests a differential response of the parasite to this altered host state, and perhaps indicates that not all infective L_1 larvae have the same ability to infect, even when they are all derived from hosts that harbor a fully developed complement of "infective" L_1 larvae.

Body temperature exerts a strong influence on the establishment of the enteral infection. In one study, outbred mice maintained at 8–10°C throughout the infection harbored significantly fewer *Trichinella* adults at day 5 than did controls that were maintained at 36°C (Lightner and Ulmer, 1974). The difference in larval infectivity between the two temperature groups was even more striking when inbred Swiss mice served as the host. Fewer infective L_1 larvae became established in hibernating hamsters than in their nonhibernating counterparts (Chute, 1961). Bats became infected when maintained at 30–34°C, and a few adult worms were recovered at days 7 and 12 after infection. However, only two adult worms developed in one hibernating bat out of 50 (Chute and Covalt, 1960). It is well established that serum glucose levels are reduced during hibernation and thus may also have influenced the establishment of worms. However, serum glucose levels may also become reduced during the first week of the enteral phase in nonhibernating hosts (Pawlowski, 1967c; Castro *et al.*, 1967; Stewart, 1978). It might therefore be reasonable to presume that lower than normal levels of glucose prior to infection do not affect the number of larvae that go on to complete their life cycle in the enteral niche. The decline in serum glucose is thought to reflect the fact that *Trichinella* induces a malabsorption of glucose during the enteral phase (Castro *et al.*, 1967).

Rarely is the entire dose of infective L_1 larvae accounted for as adult worms, even in the most permissive hosts. Error in counting is obviously a major factor, but there is often a larger difference between the number of worms recovered and the number given than can be explained by methodological procedures alone. Damage to larvae during isolation by peptic digestion may also account for a small proportion of the loss. The factors that determine this crucial parasite characteristic have not been systematically investigated.

4.2. Molting and Development [3b]

Once in its enteral niche, four molts ensue in rapid succession, taking a total of about 30 hr. The rapidity of the molting cycle of *Trichinella* is truly remarkable. The selective pressures that have been brought to bear on this aspect of the worm's biology have obviously favored those individuals that could accomplish their molting within this brief time span. It is likely that a large component of the environment that was responsible for this adaptation was the host's immune system, a topic that is discussed in depth in Chapter 8.

Table 3 contains data derived from three major studies on the molt cycle. While minor discrepancies exist among these studies regarding the time of each molt for each sex of worm, all present incontrovertible evidence that four molts occur in the small intestine and that adult worms are produced as early as 24 hr after oral infection. If the molting times shown in Table 3 are averaged for each stage, then both sexes appear to develop at about the same rate. However, for each individual study, the molting times of the sexes may indeed be different. Such differences need to be explained in terms of the strain of host and parasite before their biological significance can be assessed.

TABLE 3
Molting Cycle for Male and Female Worms

Molt	Female				Male			
	Ali Khan (1966)	Kozek (1971a)	Villella (1958)	$\bar{X}^a$	Ali Khan (1966)	Kozek (1971a)	Villella (1958)	$\bar{X}^a$
$L_1 \to L_2$	12 hr	10 hr	6 hr	8 hr	10 hr	9 hr	12 hr	10 hr
$L_2 \to L_3$	19 hr	15 hr	12 hr	12 hr	17 hr	13 hr	18 hr	16 hr
$L_3 \to L_4$	26 hr	21 hr	18 hr	22 hr	24 hr	18 hr	24 hr	22 hr
$L_4 \to$ adult	36 hr	28 hr	24 hr	29 hr	29 hr	25 hr	30 hr	28 hr

[a] Mean hour of molt to nearer hour.

Molting most likely occurs in the intramulticellular niche (Wright, 1979). Investigations on site selection by the infective L_1 larva (Despommier et al., 1978; Wright, 1979) or the adult (Gardiner, 1976) presented no morphological evidence for discarded cuticles in columnar epithelial tissues. Unfortunately, in all in vivo studies so far conducted on molting, worms were removed from the host before being examined. However, it is possible that if molting does occur within the cytoplasm of epithelial cells, cuticles become compressed and hence inapparent.

There have been many in vitro attempts to study and influence the molting of Trichinella (Weller, 1943; Kim, 1961, 1962; Meerovitch, 1962, 1965a,b; Tarakanov, 1963, 1964, 1970; Tarakanov and Krasnova, 1971; Thomas, 1965; Berntzen, 1965; Hitcho and Thorson, 1971; Sakamoto, 1979). All the aforecited studies began with pepsin–HCl-isolated infective L_1 larvae, a transient stage of the infection that is biologically equivalent to that found in the stomach. In all but two of these attempts, it was found that under a variety of culture conditions, infective L_1 larvae underwent multiple cuticle formation without apolysis. In many cases, the larvae eventually died. The two successful studies (Berntzen, 1965; Sakamoto, 1979) presented evidence indicating that cuticle formation and four complete molts from L_1 to adult occurred if infective L_1 larvae were first exposed to pancreatin and trypsin after they were isolated from host muscle tissue by pepsin–HCl digestion. In addition, pancreatin- and trypsin-treated larvae were allowed to crawl through fine-mesh stocking material, an apparently necessary prerequisite to achieving their first molt. The two conditions closely mimicked the in vivo situation the worm encounters when it enters the small intestine.

Hence, molting in Trichinella, at least from L_1 to L_2, seems to be analogous to that seen in other animals, particularly snakes, in which old skins must be removed in two stages, namely, by snagging them on

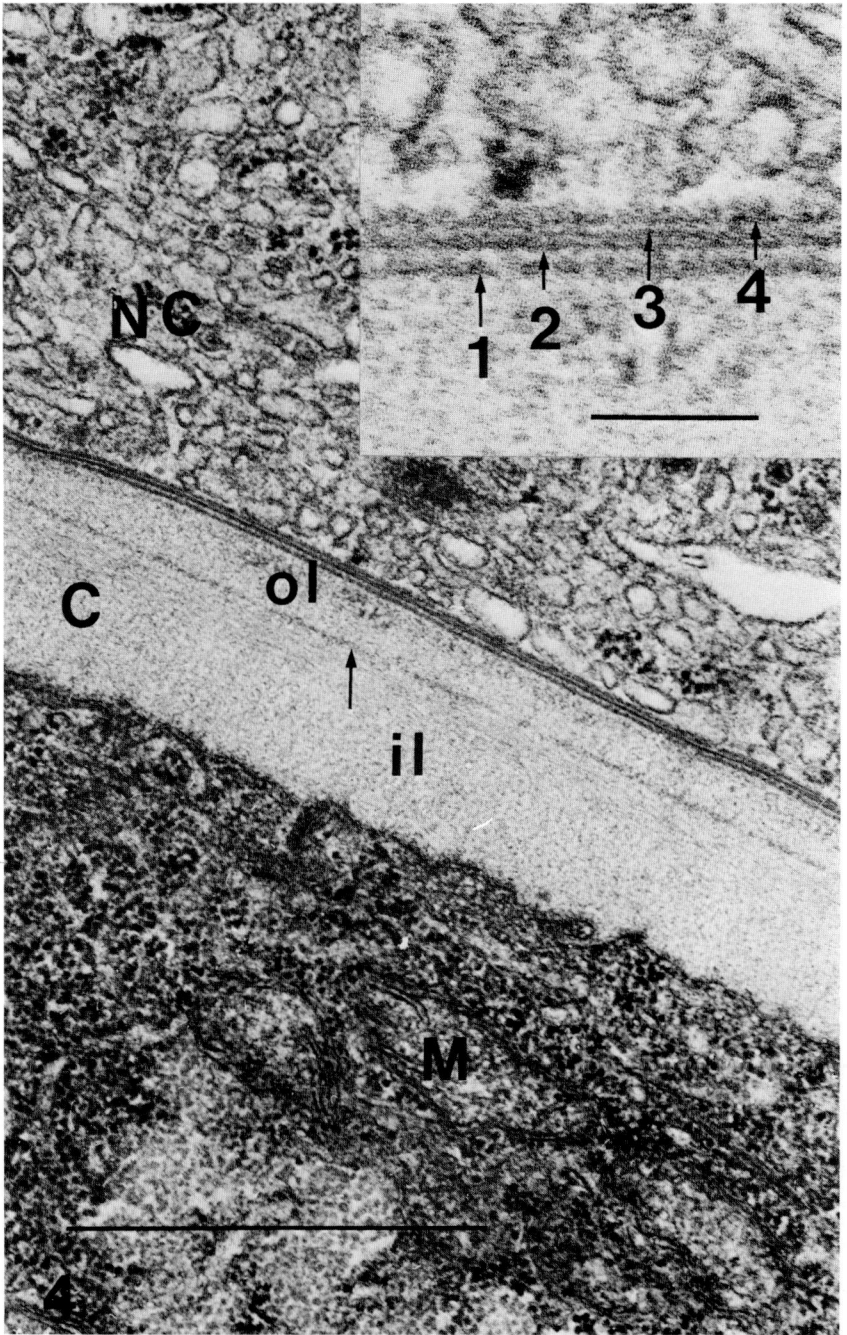

inanimate objects, then literally crawling out of them. Similarly, *Trichinella* may need a physical barrier against which to rub in order to remove a portion or all of its outer cuticular layers [i.e., layers 3 and 4 (see Figs. 4 and 5a). The microvillus cell surface could serve this purpose. *In vitro*, ecdysis from L_2 through to the adult stage apparently proceeded without additional outside physical aid. Despite these two apparent successes in culturing *Trichinella*, the mechanism or mechanisms that control molting cannot yet be examined in as much detail as they have been, for instance, in *Phocanema decipiens*, or in certain free-living nematodes such as *Caenorhabditis elegans*. This is due primarily to the fact that no simple *in vitro* culture system exists for *Trichinella* in which growth constituents and other nutritional components, which may play a role in ecdysis, can easily be manipulated. In retrospect, it is also now apparent that those investigators who employed the pepsin-isolated infective L_1 larva for studies on metabolism (Stannard *et al.*, 1938; von Brand *et al.*, 1952; Stoner and Hankes, 1955; Castro and Fairbairn, 1969) inadvertently selected an inappropriate stage of the infection to work with, since, as already pointed out, *Trichinella* does all its molting and growth after reaching the small intestine.

Trichinella does not significantly increase in width over these 30 hr, which most likely reflects the high degree of selection imposed by its intramulticellular environment. Worms of greater width would probably not be accommodated within the cytoplasm of columnar epithelial cells and therefore would be selected against. In contrast, increases in worm length can easily be tolerated. Thus, the adult female grows significantly in length following the last molt, increasing over 1.5 times for 30 hr to day 5, occupying about 415–425 columnar cells. Male growth is less substantial, increasing only 20–30% during those 4 days.

Although worm growth is not one of the main features of the molting cycle, *Trichinella* undergoes extensive morphogenesis during this time, maturing into adult male and female worms. Every major tissue is remodeled, including cuticle, hypodermal gland cell, muscle, nerve, genital primordium, gut tract, and stichosome. A hallmark of its development is its almost complete utilization of glycogen stores (Ferguson and Castro, 1973). It would be interesting to investigate how much glycogen is ultimately converted into various worm tissues in

←

FIGURE 4. Transmission electron micrograph of the cuticle (C) of the infective L_1 larva of *Trichinella*. The cuticle consists of an outer layer (ol), an inner layer (il), and an electron-dense layer (↑). (N) Nurse cell; (M) mitochondria. Scale bar: 5 μm. *Inset:* High magnification shows the four layers (arrows 1, 2, 3, and 4) associated with the Nurse cell–parasite interface. Scale bar: 0.5 μm.

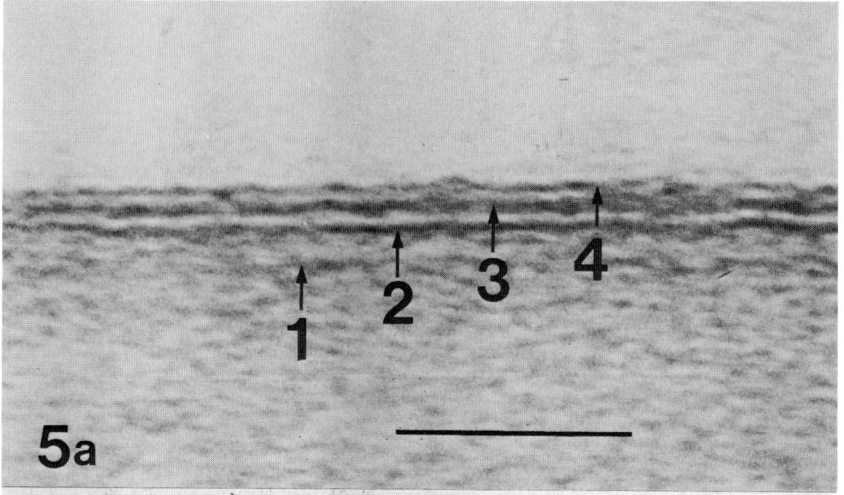

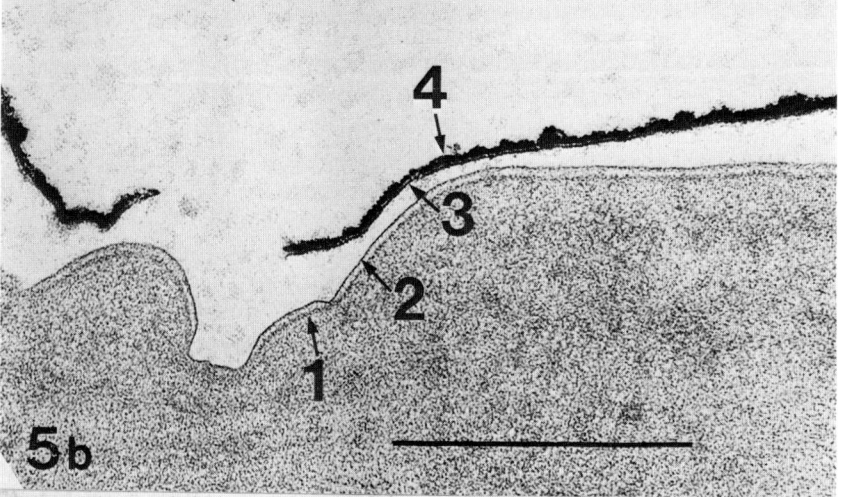

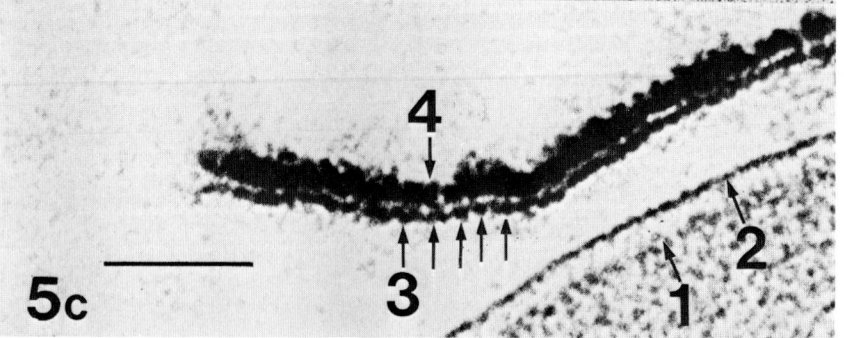

relation to how much host-derived precursors are needed by the worm in this complex process.

The cuticle of the infective L_1 larva (Fig. 4) is composed of two major regions separated by an electron-dense zone (Beckett and Booth-royd, 1961; Despommier et al., 1967; Ribas-Mujal and Rivera-Pomar, 1968; Bruce, 1970a; Kozek, 1971b; Purkerson and Despommier, 1974). As already alluded to, two thin, membranelike layers (i.e., 3 and 4) surround the outermost region of the cuticle, while two others (layers 1 and 2) lie just beneath them. These four structures were originally described as three layers (Beckett and Boothroyd, 1961), but the micrographs failed to resolve layers 3 and 4. Layers 3 and 4 are found only on the surface of the cuticle of the infective L_1 larva. Ribas-Mujal and Rivera-Pomar (1968) first described them in the parenteral phase and proposed that both were host-derived structures, forming a rather large physiologically active space for the worm while in its Nurse cell. They further suggested that the true outer surface of the cuticle was actually layer 2. However, other investigators were able to demonstrate that with proper fixation and slow dehydration through an extensively graded series of ethanol, layers 3 and 4 were never anatomically separated from the worm's surface (Purkerson and Despommier, 1974). Hence, it is likely that if there is a physiological space between the parasite and the infected host cell, it is nanometers, not micrometers, wide. Layers 3 and 4 survive host digestion in the stomach and are closely associated with the cuticular surface (Fig. 5a), even after treat-ment for 1 hr in 1% pepsin–1% concentrated HCl (Despommier et al., 1967). Unpublished results from the author's laboratory have shown that alpha chymotrypsin or papain did not cause ultrastructural damage to either layer 3 or 4. In contrast, trypsin (0.25% at 37°C for 1 hr at pH 8.2) digested a significant portion of layer 4 and induced a thickening and "beading" of layer 3 (Fig. 5b and 5c). Numerous breaks also occurred in layers 3 and 4 when pepsin-isolated infective L_1 larvae were agitated gently under the conditions described above. Wright

←——

FIGURE 5. (5a) Transmission electron micrograph of the infective L_1 larva after isolation from host tissue by pepsin–HCl digestion. Layers 3 and 4 remain closely associated with the cuticular surface (i.e., layer 2). Scale bar: 0.5 μm. (5b) Transmission electron micrograph of the cuticular surface of the pepsin–HCl-isolated infective L_1 larva following a 1-hr digestion in 0.25% trypsin at pH 8.2. Layers 3 and 4 have undergone partial digestion. Furthermore, they have become broken at various points and are no longer closely associated with the cuticular surface. Scale bar: 2 μm. (5c) High-magnification view of a portion of cuticle seen in (5b). Layer 3 appears to be degraded at regular intervals (arrows), whereas layer 4 has become thicker as the result of exposure to trypsin digestion. Scale bar: 0.5 μm.

(personal communication) observed that layer 4 was not present *in situ* in some worms 3 hr after oral infection, and Kozek (1971b) showed that layer 4 was no longer present at 6 hr after oral infection. However, the precise fate of layers 3 and 4 throughout the first hours of the enteral phase was not systematically investigated in any of these experiments. The surface of the infective L_1 larva is antigenic (Sulzer, 1965; Despommier *et al.*, 1967; M.J. Brzosko and Gancarz, 1969; Novoselska, 1974; Mackenzie *et al.*, 1978), and antibodies are formed during the infection that adhere specifically to layer 4 (Despommier *et al.*, 1967). More attention will be given to the antigenity of the cuticular surface of all stages in Chapter 9.

Throughout the molt cycle, the cuticle changes in structure (Kozek 1971b), and resembles the cuticle of the adult (Fig. 6) as early as the second molt.

The hypodermal gland cell is an unusual structure (Fig. 7) of unknown function found in the family Trichuridae as well as in other families of free-living nematodes (Wright and Hope, 1968). This cell periodically interrupts the surface of the cuticle, and its ultrastructure in the adult has been described by Bruce (1970a). In the adult, this

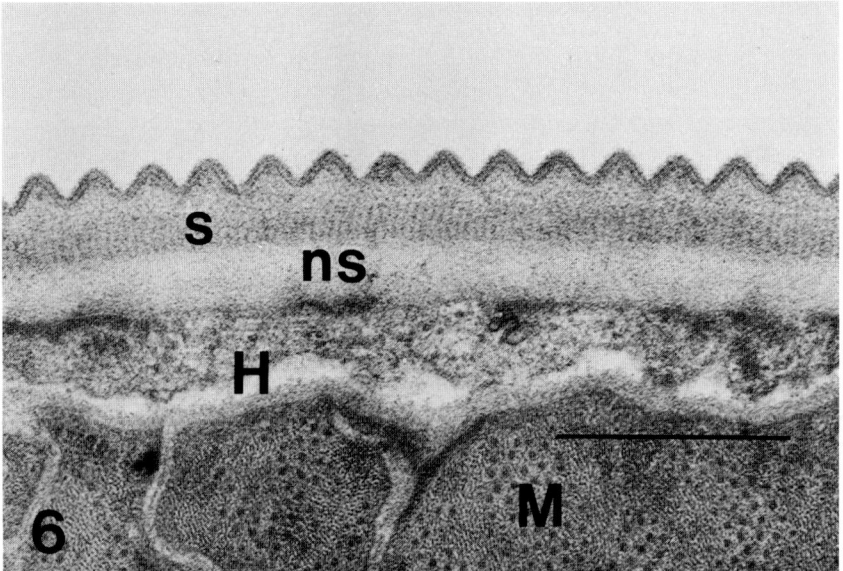

FIGURE 6. Transmission electron micrograph of the cuticle of the adult. The outer surface is bounded by two layers, while the matrix is composed of a striated (s) and a nonstriated (ns) layer. (M) Muscle; (H) hypodermis. Scale bar: 2 μm.

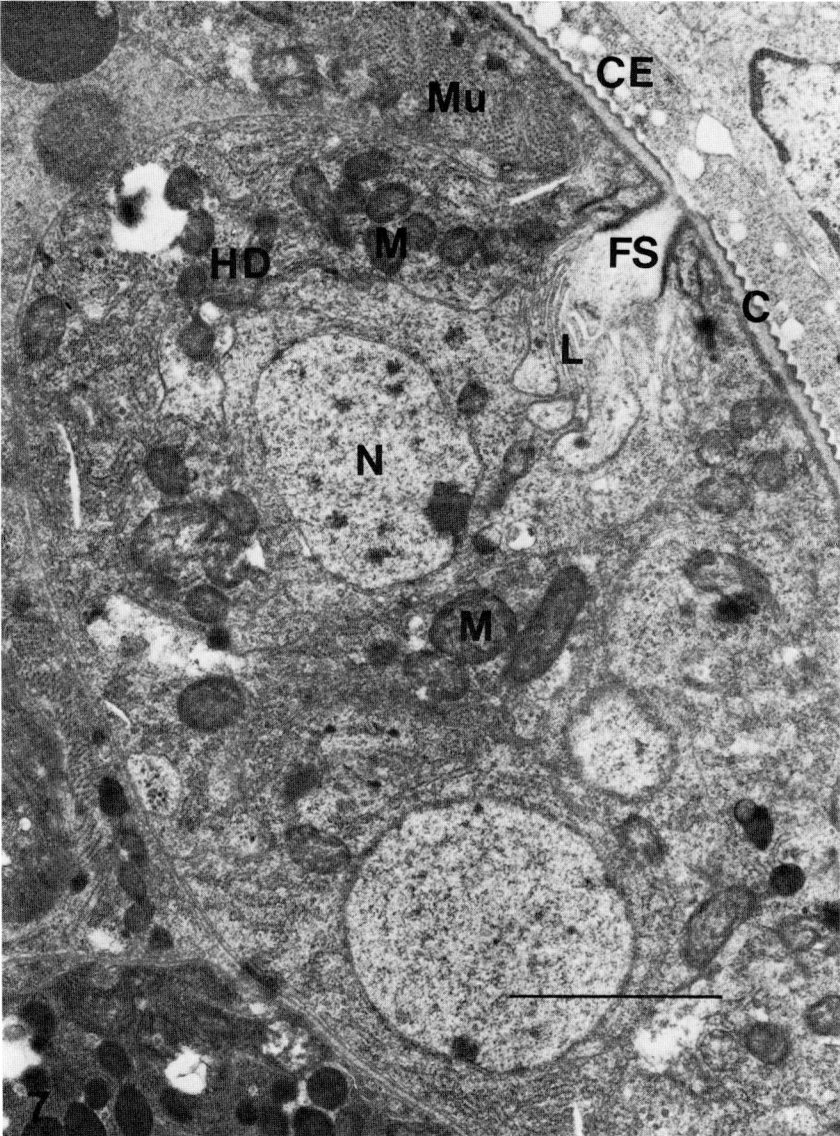

FIGURE 7. Transmission electon micrograph of the hypodermal gland cell (HD) of the adult worm. (N) Nucleus; (L) lamellae; (M) mitochondria; (C) cuticle; (Mu) muscle; (FS) fine strands; (CE) columnar epithelial cell. Scale bar: 2 μm. Courtesy of Dr. K.A. Wright.

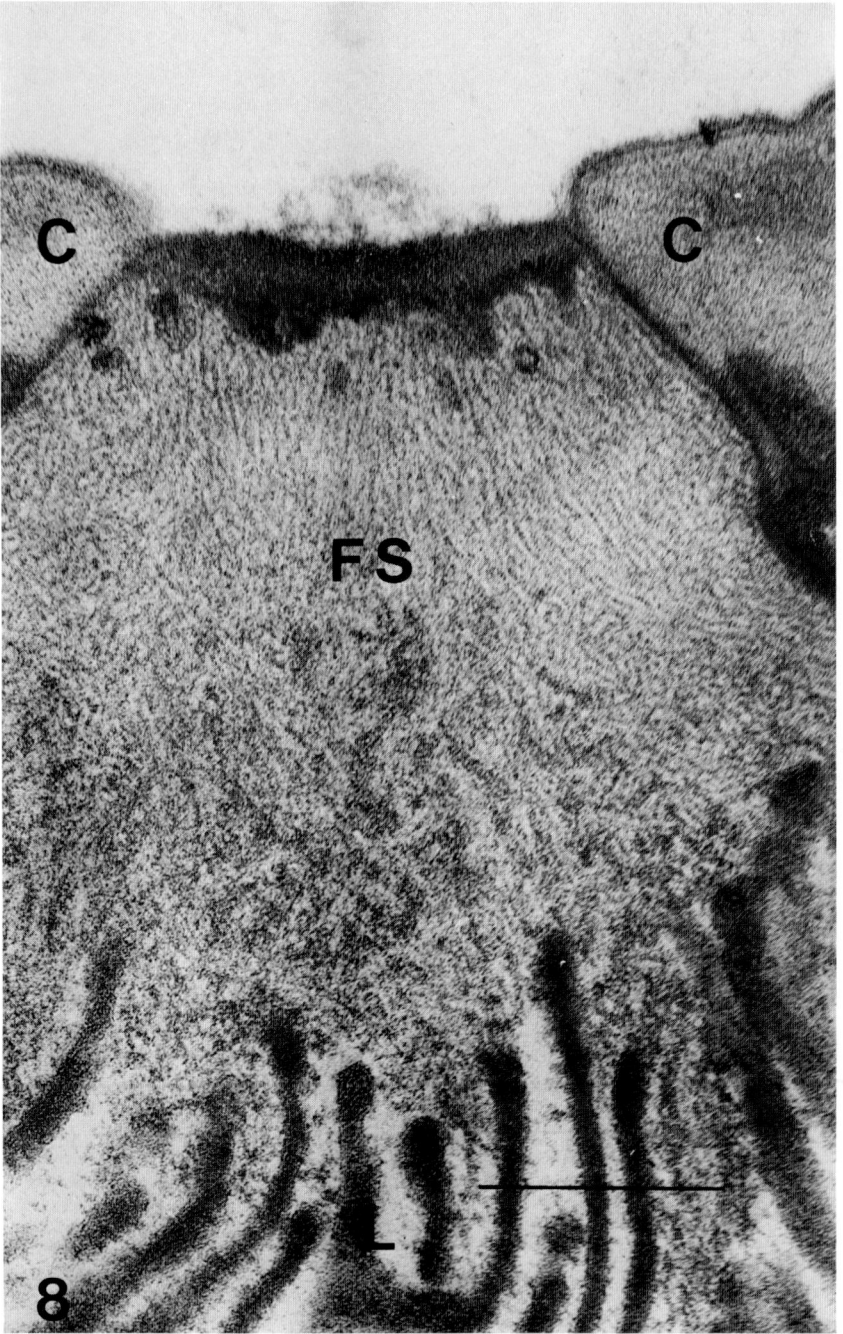

subcuticular cell forms four rows, two dorsal and two ventral, that run for most of the length of the body, totaling some 200–300 cells. Its pore is positively stained by the argentaffine reaction (Richels 1955), according to the method of Lison (1936). The infective L_1 larva does not possess this cell, but all other stages (i.e., L_2 to adult) of the enteral infection do (Bruce, 1970a). In another study, the same investigator showed that newborn L_1 larvae do not have hypodermal gland cells. Some atypical cells interpreted as being hypodermal gland cells were seen in 9- to 10-day-old preinfective L_1 larvae (Bruce, 1974). However, it is doubtful that they were indeed gland cells, since they failed to communicate through the cuticular surface.

The extracellular content of the cell in the adult worm forms a plug of fibrous material (Fig. 8) and is most likely secreted into its lumen, since this material was present in newly formed gland cells lying beneath the surface of the old cuticle during the time of molting (Wright, personal communication). In the preinfective L_1 larva, the fibrous material was shown to be susceptible to pepsin–HCl digestion (Bruce, 1974). It was therefore reasoned that this cell type might not occur in the infective L_1 larva, since this later stage must traverse the stomach prior to entering the columnar epithelium of the small intestine. The fact that 24 to 28-hr-old larvae (i.e., L_4 larvae) do not establish an infection when given orally (Katz, 1960) gives some support for this supposition. In contrast, it is known that the adult worm can survive and reproduce after passing through the stomach (Katz, 1960; Matoff, 1961, 1963). These results could reflect differences in the maturation of the hypodermal gland cell, but it is obvious that more information is needed regarding the structure and function of this interesting cell before this question can be resolved.

While the function of the hypodermal gland cell remains unknown, any consideration of its role in the worm's biology must take into account the niche in which the enteral stages live. The intramulticellular environment of the adult worm brings it into direct contact with naked host cytoplasm (Wright, 1979). Ultrastructurally, the architecture of hypodermal gland cell suggests a high degree of metabolic activity associated with its convoluted membranous inner cavity.

The musculature of the larval and adult stage of *Trichinella* consists of somatic and esophageal muscles, as well as muscles that are associated with the reproductive tract. The somatic musculature of the L_1 larva is

←───

FIGURE 8. Transmission electron micrograph of the fine-strand portion of a hypodermal gland cell. Note the denser appearance of the outer surface of the fine strands (FS). (L) Lamellae; (C) cuticle. Scale bar: 1 μm.

composed of a single row of cells lying just beneath the hypodermis (Figs. 9 and 10) and extends the length of the worm. The general pattern is maintained throughout its life cycle (Fig. 11). From the little evidence available in the literature on the structure of its somatic musculature, it can be stated that *Trichinella* does not differ significantly from nematodes that exhibit a meromyarian type of arrangement (Hope, 1969). Hence, each somatic muscle cell consists of a contractile portion lying closest to the hypodermis, while the cell body contains glycogen, mitochondria, and the nucleus. If *Trichinella* muscle is typical, then one would predict that the somatic muscle cells fuse together at various points along them, thereby creating a syncytium. However, the concept of fused muscle cells may apply only to nematodes that exhibit poly-myarian somatic musculature. Similarly, they would be expected to send out cytoplasmic processes that would connect to one of four nerve cords, thereby completing the myoneural junction typical of other nematodes (Debell, 1965). These observations have yet to be made on the somatic musculature of *Trichinella*.

The somatic musculature undergoes some change during molting. The muscle cells of the L_1 larva remain similar in overall structure to adult muscle cells except that adult muscle cells are more elongated and numerous (Richels, 1955) and contain less glycogen than those of the infective L_1 larva (Bruce, 1970a; Ferguson and Castro, 1973). Glycogen reserves of the larva become rapidly depleted while it develops to an adult worm, decreasing from approximately 15% dry weight as infective L_1 larva to only about 1% dry weight as an adult (Ferguson and Castro, 1973). It is therefore tempting to speculate that the energy available for muscular contraction may shift from endogenous to exogenous sources during morphogenesis.

The worm is motile and exhibits typical snakelike movement in all its stages except the pepsin-isolated infective L_1 larva, which repeatedly coils and uncoils (Fig. 12). Motility can be directional, since all enteral stages (i.e., L_1 to adult) are able to migrate toward a heat source when placed into differentially warmed 0.85% NaCl (Despommier, 1973). The relevance of such heat-seeking behavior to its life cycle has yet to be demonstrated, however.

The capillary esophagus is surrounded by a small amount of muscle tissue (Fig. 13), while the anus also has muscle associated with it. The physiology and biochemistry of the muscle system of *Trichinella* are in need of much research, since nothing is known of either.

One of the least-studied aspects of the biology of *Trichinella* has been its nervous system. No investigations aimed solely at describing its physiology have been described, and only a few fragmented reports

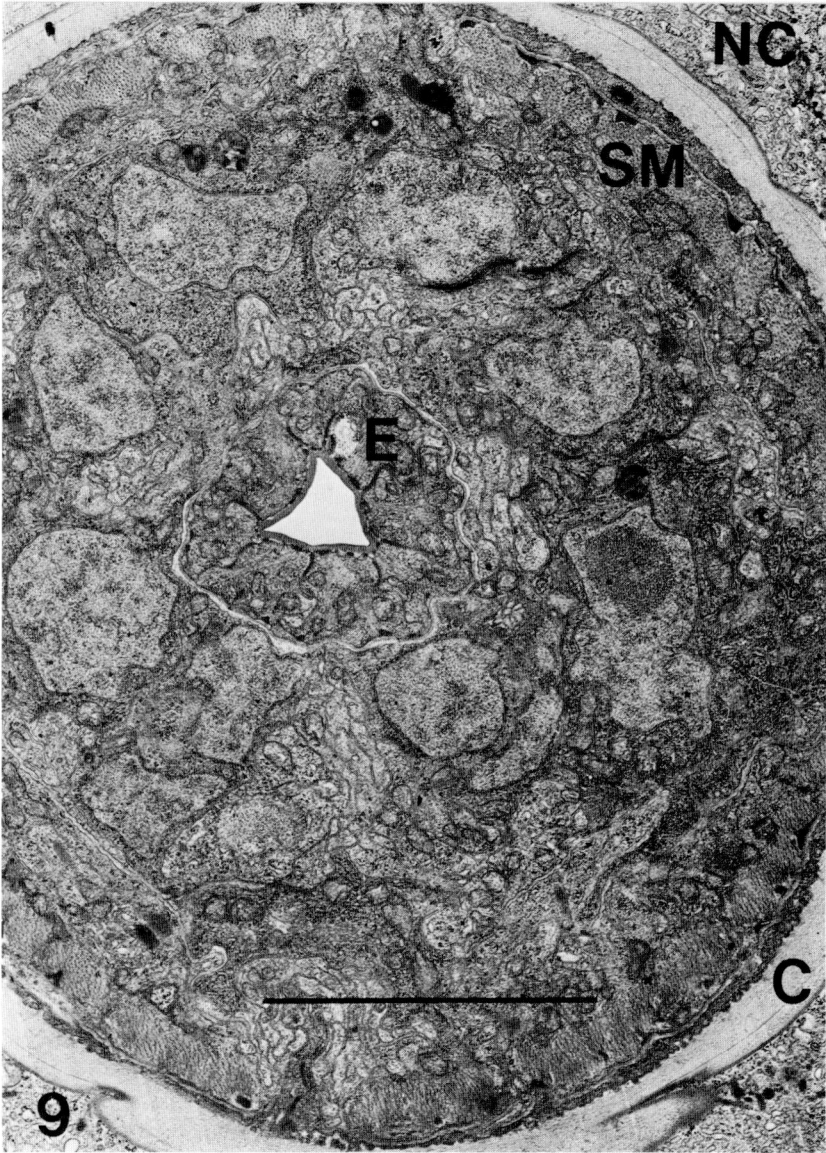

FIGURE 9. Transmission electron micrograph of the infective L₁ larva *in situ*. The somatic musculature (SM) consists of a single row of muscle cells that lie just beneath the hypodermis. (NC) Nurse cell; (C) cuticle; (E) esophagus. Scale bar: 10 μm.

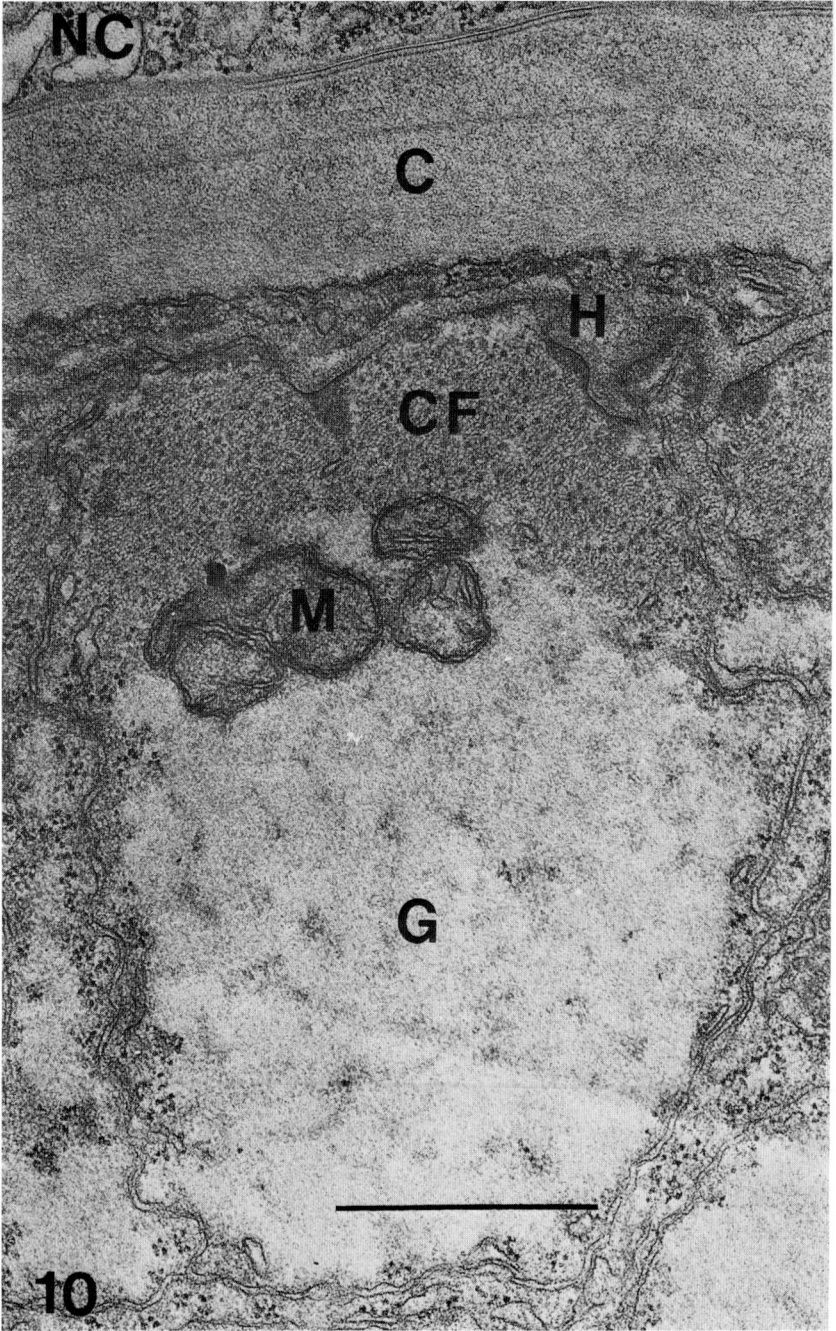

can be found dealing with its anatomy (Richels, 1955; Ramisz, 1965; Shanta and Meerovitch, 1967; Bruce, 1970b). This is particularly regrettable, since so much useful information on the structural and functional aspects of nematode behavior has already been gleaned from experiments on free-living nematodes in recent years (Zuckerman, 1980).

The nervous system of the L_1 larva is basically the same as that of the adult, consisting of a cephalic nerve ring that gives rise to four main nerve cords: two lateral, one dorsal, and one ventral. Nothing is known about the number of ganglia in the L_1 larva, but the adult worm possesses six in its anterior end (Richels, 1955). Each somatic muscle cell is presumably innervated as previously described. The neurotransmitter system may involve acetylcholine, since acetylcholinesterase has been histochemically demonstrated in nervous tissues of the adult (Ramisz, 1965). There are no obvious sensory papillae at either end of the worm, regardless of its stage of development. However, modified hypodermal gland cells in the anterior region of the adult suggest a sensory function, since dendritic processes leading into the gland cell have been observed (McLaren, 1976).

Behavioral studies are scant, but as already mentioned, all enteric-phase stages can detect and respond to a heat gradient by migrating toward the highest tempertaure (Despommier, 1973). These data prove that *Trichinella* possesses thermal receptors that are integrated with its musculature, probably by the cephalic nerve ring. Interestingly, adults of *Trichinella* removed from the immune host are not able to react as well to a thermal gradient as are worms derived from nonimmune hosts (Despommier, unpublished data), a phenomenon common to other species of nematodes as well (McCue and Thorson, 1965). It is probable that *Trichinella* also perceives its presence in the small intestine by receptors, but specifically which host stimuli are received and processed by the infective L_1 larva remains undiscovered. In this regard, the phenomenon of rapid expulsion [see Chapter 8 (Section 2.3)] may be a useful host response with which to explore the physiology of initiation of infection in the gut (McCoy, 1940), since the great majority of worms are unable to establish themselves in the enteral niche under this special host-induced environment.

The ability of adults of either sex to detect an individual of the opposite sex gives evidence for chemoreceptors sensitive to pheromones

←───

FIGURE 10. Transmission electron micrograph of a single somatic muscle cell of the infective L_1 larva. The cell is composed of contractile filaments (CF), mitochondria (M), and glycogen (G). (H) Hypodermis; (C) cuticle; (NC) Nurse cell. Scale bar: 2 μm.

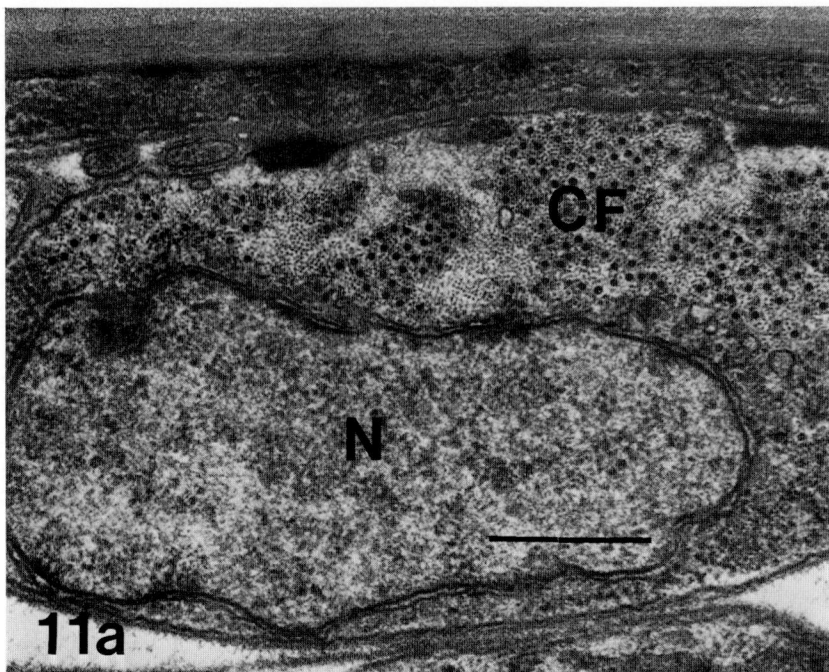

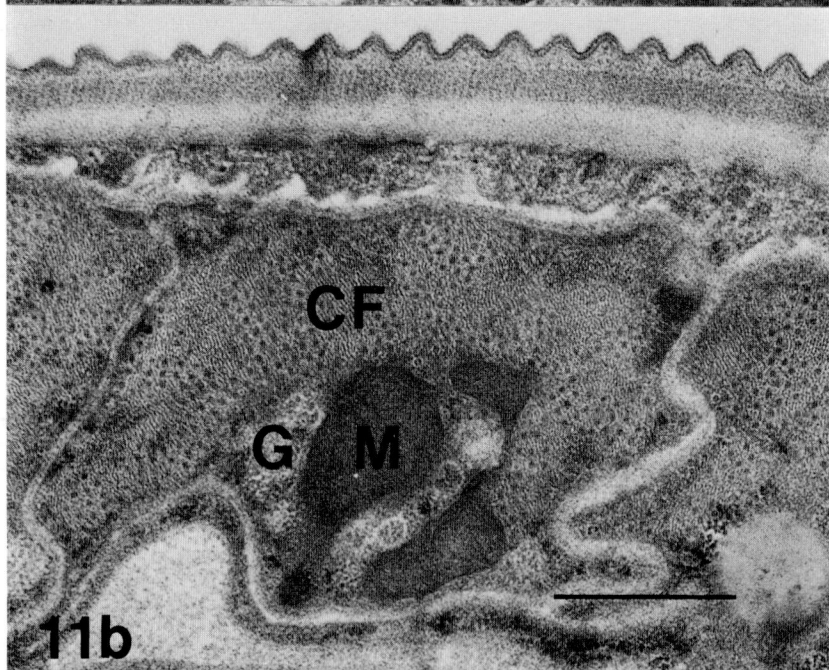

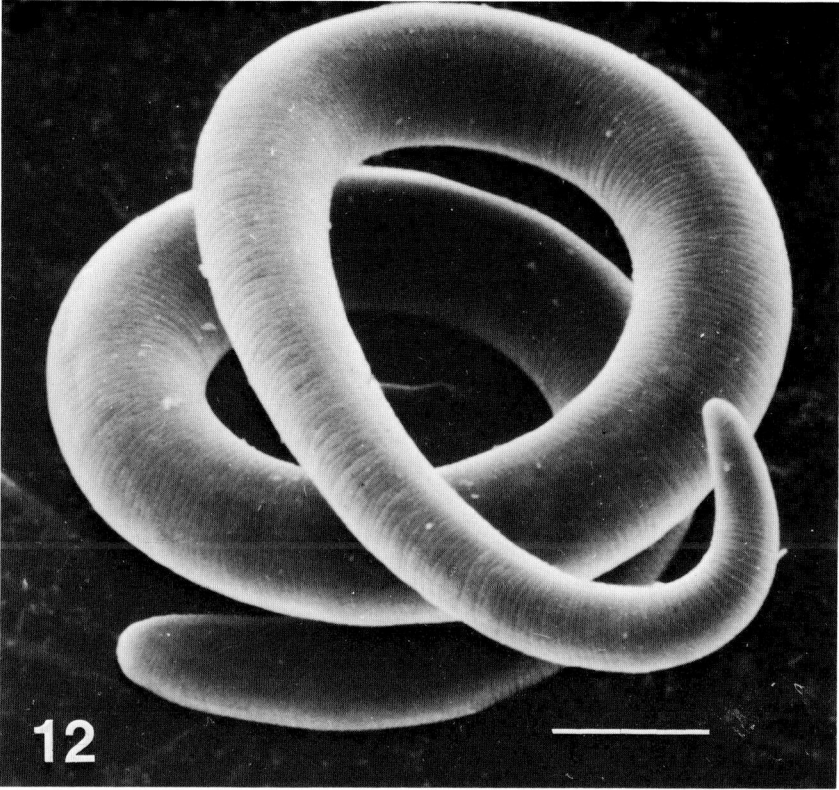

FIGURE 12. Scanning electron micrograph of a pepsin–HCl-isolated infective L_1 larva. Worms thus isolated exhibit coiling and uncoiling behavior. Scale bar: 40 μm. Courtesy of Dr. J. Burnham.

(Bonner and Egtes, 1967) and is dealt with more thoroughly in Section 5. Finally, experiments conducted *in vitro* with the newborn L_1 larva strongly suggest that this stage is able to perceive and respond to various electrical stimuli (Hughes and Harley, 1977).

It is obvious from this brief discussion that the nervous system of *Trichinella* plays a vital role throughout its life, and it is hoped that

←——————————————————————————

FIGURE 11. Transmission electron micrographs of the somatic musculature of the adult worm. (11a) The nucleus (N) and contractile filaments (CF) are prominent features in this view. Scale bar: 2 μm. Courtesy of Dr. K.A. Wright. (11b) Each muscle cell is composed of contractile filaments (CF), mitochondria (M), and glycogen (G). Note that the somatic muscle cell of the adult contains less glycogen than that of the infective L_1 larva (see Fig. 13). Scale bar: 2 μm.

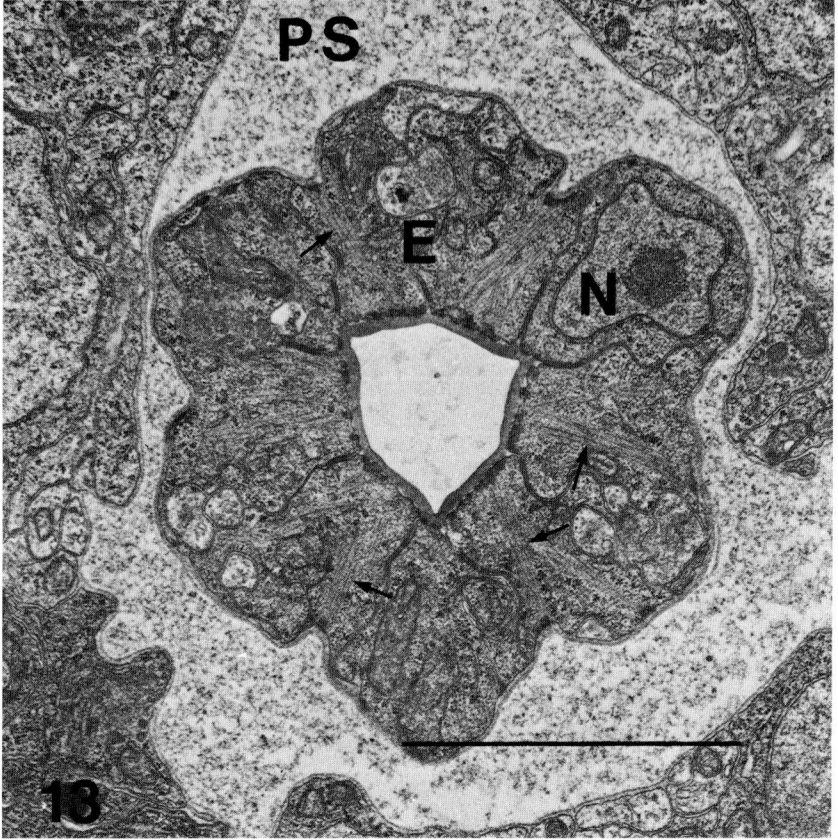

FIGURE 13. Transmission electron micrograph of the esophagus (E) of an infective L_1 larva. The musculature (arrows) of the esophagus consists primarily of radiate muscle fibers that attach to the inner membrane bordering the cuticular lining. (N) Nucleus; (PS) pseudocoelom. Scale bar: 5 μm.

more experimentation will be conducted in the future on this important aspect of *Trichinella* biology.

The organs of reproduction are partially undifferentiated in the infective L_1 larva, but mature rapidly during its 30 hr of morphogenesis (Wu and Kingscote, 1957; Villella, 1958; Berntzen, 1965; Ali Khan, 1966; Shanta and Meerovitch, 1967; Kozek, 1971a, 1975). Nonetheless, male and female infective L_1 larvae can be distinguished from each other, as shown in Table 4 (Hemmert-Halswick and Bugge, 1934; Villella, 1966; Ali Khan, 1966; Kozek, 1975; Sukhdeo and Meerovitch, 1977). The advanced state of sexual development exhibited by the infective L_1 larva is unique among nematodes. The selective pressures that have resulted in this high degree of maturation are probably inexorably linked to its need for rapid development in the gut following oral infection.

The most striking external changes in morphology occur during male worm development. The copulatory appendages and their associated structures are present as early as the L_2 larva (Fig. 14). Structures associated with the copulatory appendages, namely, the two sets of smaller accessory papillae, can be seen in outline below the cuticle of the L_3 larva (Fig. 15), but are fully developed only in the adult (Fig. 16). The purpose or purposes to which these accessory papillae are put during mating is not known, since the actual act of mating has not been observed. It is presumed that the copulatory bell (Fig. 17) is inserted inside the vulva of the female, and perhaps the papillae help to position the male just prior to this event.

Sperm production occurs shortly before or immediately following the last molt, since spermatozoa have been observed in the vas deferens at the time of the last molt (Wu, 1955a; Ali Khan, 1966; Kozek, 1971a). In the female, the single ovary and oviduct develop progressively throughout the molt cycle.

All enteral and parenteral stages of *Trichinella* possess a complete intestinal tract. The intestinal tract remains largely unaltered throughout the molting cycle. Three regions can be distinguished morphologically, namely, the esophagus, the midgut, and the hindgut. Both the esophagus (Fig. 18) and the hindgut are lined with an extension of cuticle (Beckett and Boothroyd, 1961; Bruce, 1966, 1970b; Despommier *et al.*, 1967; Backwinkel and Themann, 1972). It has been stated that both the adult and newborn L_1 larva possess a stylet in the anteriormost

TABLE 4
Sexual Characteristics of the Male and Female Infective L_1 Larva

Characteristic	Male	Female	References
Intestinal tract	Crosses over genital primordium	Always dorsal to genital primordium	Villella (1966)
Intestinal bulb	Ventral to genital primordium	Dorsal to genital primordium	Sukhdeo and Meerovitch (1977)
Genital primordium	Anterior pole blunted	Anterior pole pointed	Sukhdeo and Meerovitch (1977)
Length of rectum	50 μm	25 μm	Ali Khan (1966), Kozek (1975)

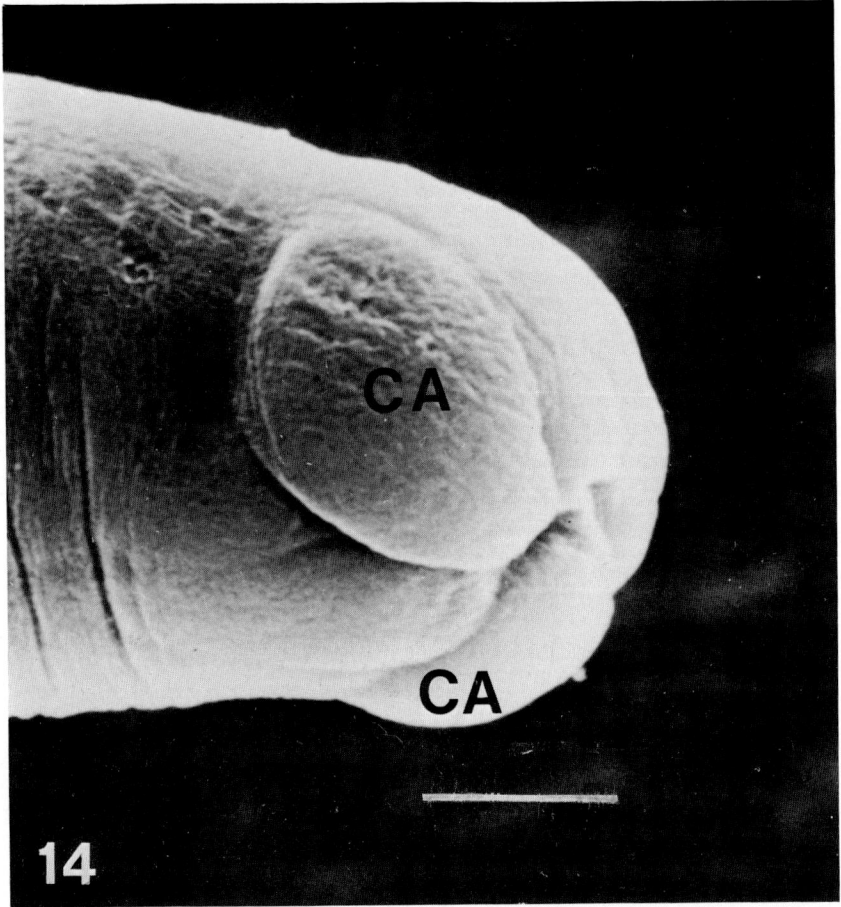

FIGURE 14. Scanning electron micrograph of a 13-hr-old male L_2 larva. The copulatory appendages (CA) are visible. No accessory papillae can be seen. Scale bar: 5 μm. Courtesy of Dr. J. Burnham.

region of the esophagus (van Someren, 1939) that is presumably used to gain entrance into cells. While some convincing morphological evidence (Fig. 19) exists regarding the occurrence of a stylet in the newborn L_1 larva, photographic data clearly showing a stylet in the adult worm have not been presented. Furthermore, as previously stated, no stylet was observed in the infective L_1 larva (Bruce, 1970b).

The midgut is lined with columnar epithelium, with each cell possessing microvilli (Fig. 20), suggesting that they function to absorb nutrients (Beckett and Boothroyd, 1960; Bruce, 1966; Despommier *et al.*, 1967). However, no *in vitro* or *in vivo* study has yet demonstrated the absorptive capacity of the intestinal tract of *Trichinella* at any time during or after its molting cycle in the gut. Indeed, many *in vitro* studies on the infective L_1 larva and adult have shown just the opposite, namely, that the intestinal tract is capable of secretion (Campbell, 1955; Chipman, 1957; Jackson, 1959; Mills and Kent, 1965; Despommier and Müller, 1970, 1976). Jackson (1959) showed that infective L_1 larvae that were incubated in media containing fluorescin-labeled normal immunoglobulin did not ingest the tagged host protein. In contrast, immu-

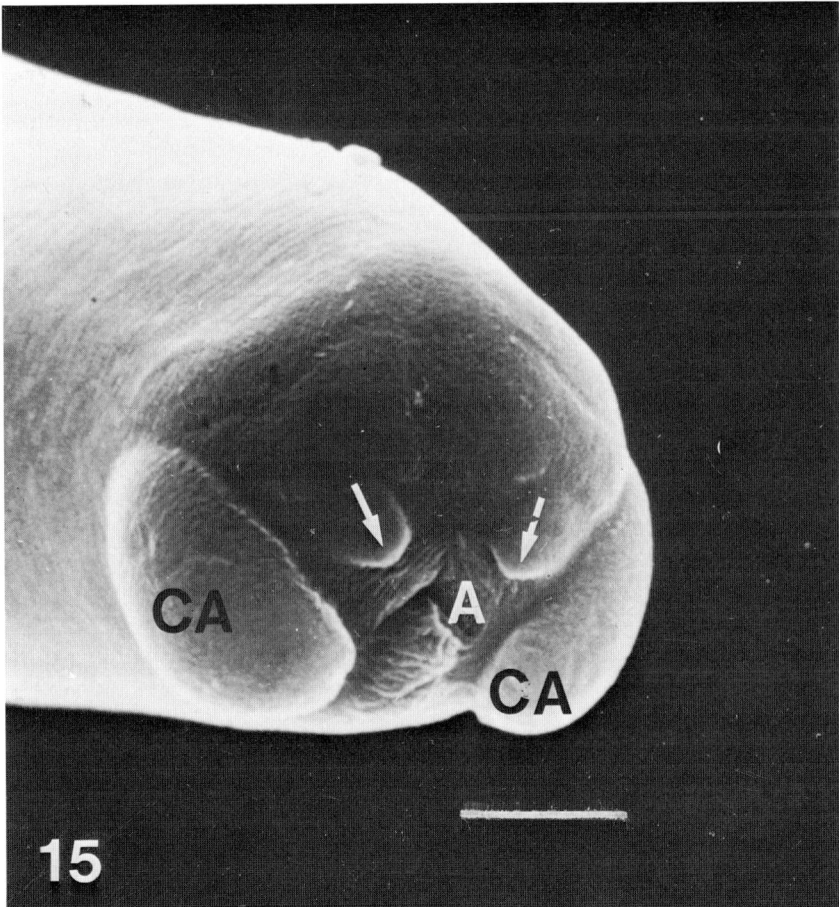

FIGURE 15. Scanning electron micrograph of a 17-hr-old L_3 male larva. The copulatory appendages (CA) and two accessory papillae (arrows) are now both visible. The cloaca (A) can also be seen. Scale bar: 5 μm. Courtesy of Dr. J. Burnham.

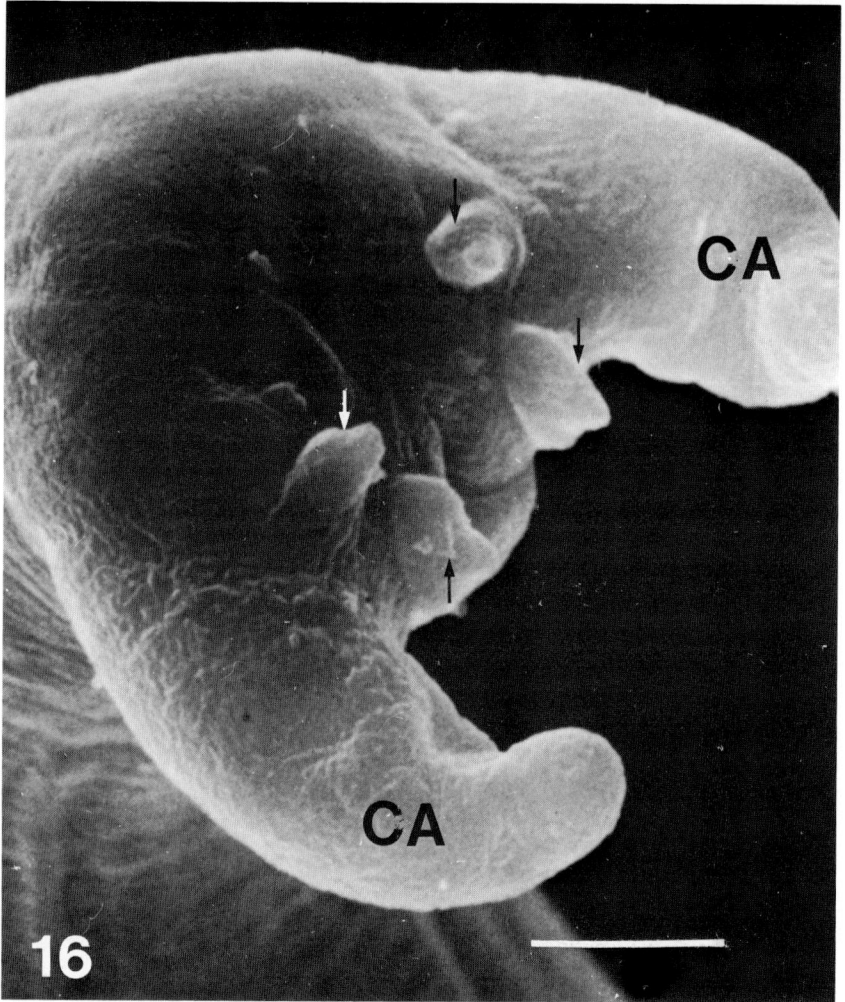

FIGURE 16. Scanning electron micrograph of a mature male adult worm. The copulatory appendages (CA) and all four accessory papillae (arrows) are now fully developed. Scale bar: 5 μm. Courtesy of Dr. J. Burnham.

noprecipitates developed at the oral and anal orifices of infective L_1 larvae incubated in antibodies directed against the whole infection. When infective L_1 larvae were incubated in a maintenance medium containing ferritin particles (Despommier *et al.*, 1967), no ferritin was ever observed within the gut tract of the worm.

Little is known concerning the nutritional requirements of adult

Trichinella, and nothing is known about its mechanism of feeding. Since the adult contains only small amounts of glycogen (Ferguson and Castro, 1973), it is reasonable to assume that its energy requirements are met either by food that the host ingests or by the substance of the host itself. In this regard, Castro *et al.* (1976) have shown that hyper-alimentation of rats did not affect the life of the worm when this procedure was initiated from day 2 through day 7 of infection. It seems unlikely that so much has been learned in recent years concerning its immunology and epidemiology, yet nothing has been discerned about the basic life-sustaining process of feeding, but that is the case. When its nutritional needs and mechanism of nutrient recruitment are finally elucidated, a much clearer picture will be formed as to the parasitic nature of this nematode.

The stichosome (Fig. 21) consists of a row of 50–55 discoid cells (Chitwood, 1930; Chitwood and Chitwood, 1950; Richels, 1955; Wu, 1955b; Villella, 1970) called stichocytes and occupies the anterior half of the infective L_1 larva. The structure and function of this organ have

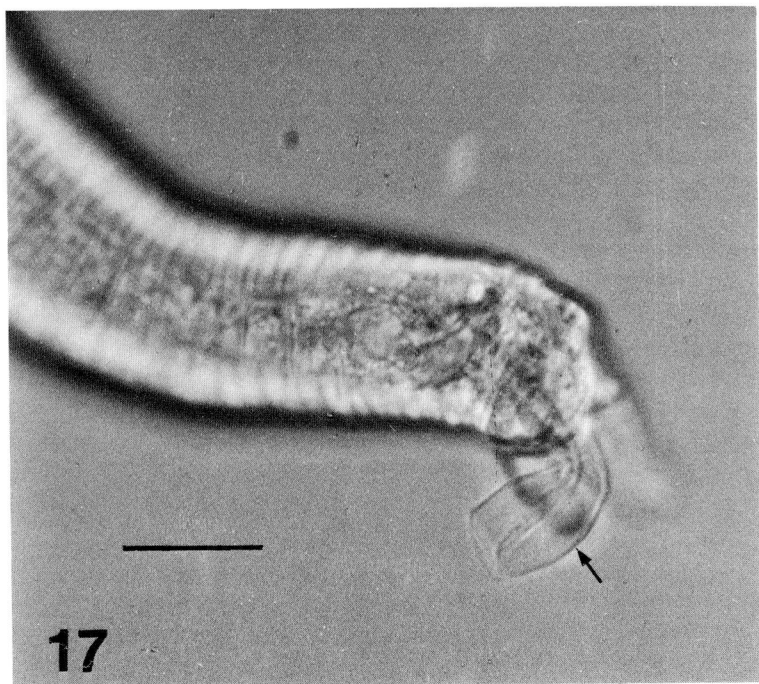

FIGURE 17. Fully extended copulatory bell (arrow) of the mature male adult. Scale bar: 20 μm. Courtesy of Dr. J. Burnham.

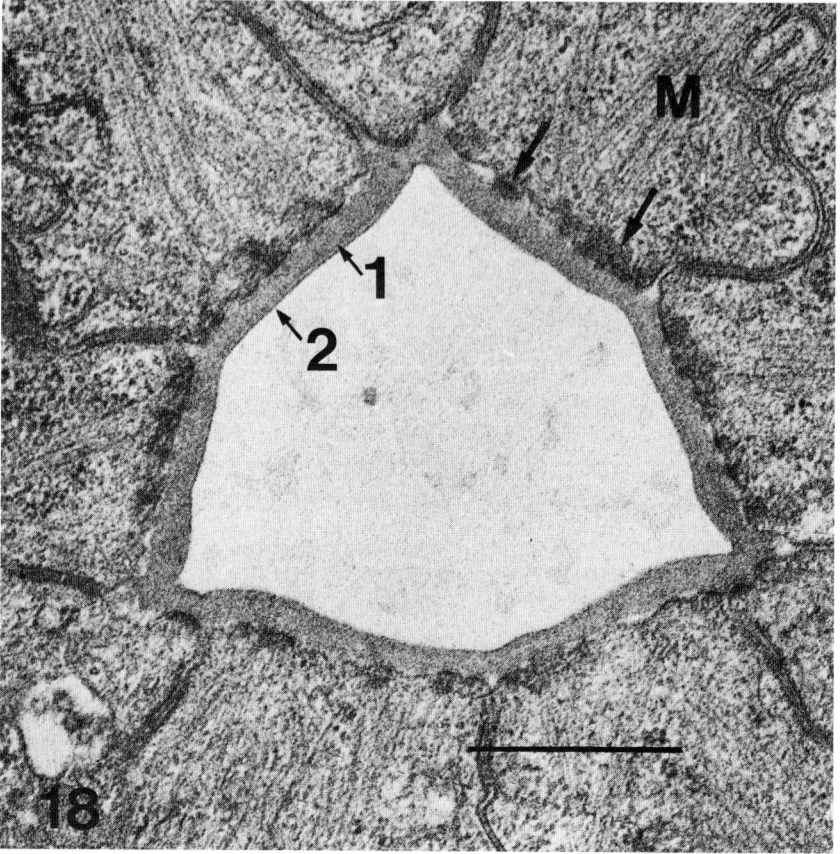

FIGURE 18. Transmission electron micrograph of the esophagus of an infective L_1 larva. The cuticular lining has two layers (1, 2) contiguous with layers 1 and 2 of the outer cuticle (see Fig. 4 and 5). Note the musculature (M) and its points of attachment (arrows) to the membrane on the inner surface of the cuticular lining. Scale bar: 1 μm.

been investigated, and its cells have been shown to possess secretory granules, the contents of which are antigenic (Campbell, 1955; Jackson, 1959; Mills and Kent, 1965; W. Brzosko *et al.*, 1965; Despommier and Müller, 1970, 1976; Kozek and Crandall, 1974).

There are two kinds of stichocytes in the infective L_1 larva: beta-granule-containing cells (Figs. 22 and 23) and alpha-granule-containing cells (Figs. 24 and 25), both of which have been described in some ultrastructural detail (Despommier and Müller, 1976). These two cell types secrete the contents of their granules during the molt cycle, with almost all the granules being absent from the stichocyte by the 30th hour of infection (Despommier, 1974). The contents of each granule empty into the canaliculi and from there pass into the duct that communicates with the lumen of the esophagus (Figs. 26 and 27) (Bruce, 1970a; Despommier, 1974). The antigenicity of the granule contents is discussed in detail in Chapter 9. The function and precise site of action

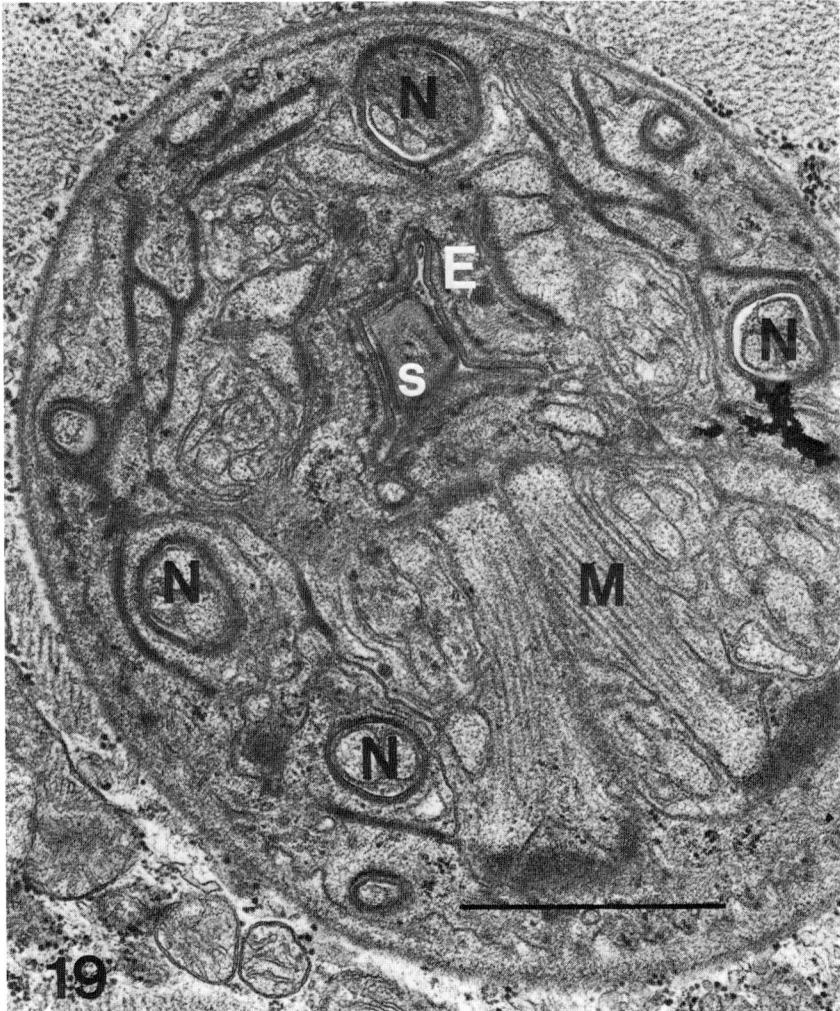

FIGURE 19. Transmission electron micrograph of a migratory L_1 larva fixed and sectioned 1 hr after penetrating a striated skeletal muscle cell. The esophagus (E) and stylet (s) are clearly visible. Note the well-developed musculature (M), which presumably is used to move the stylet in and out. Various portions of nerve (N) are also seen in this view. Scale bar: 1 μm.

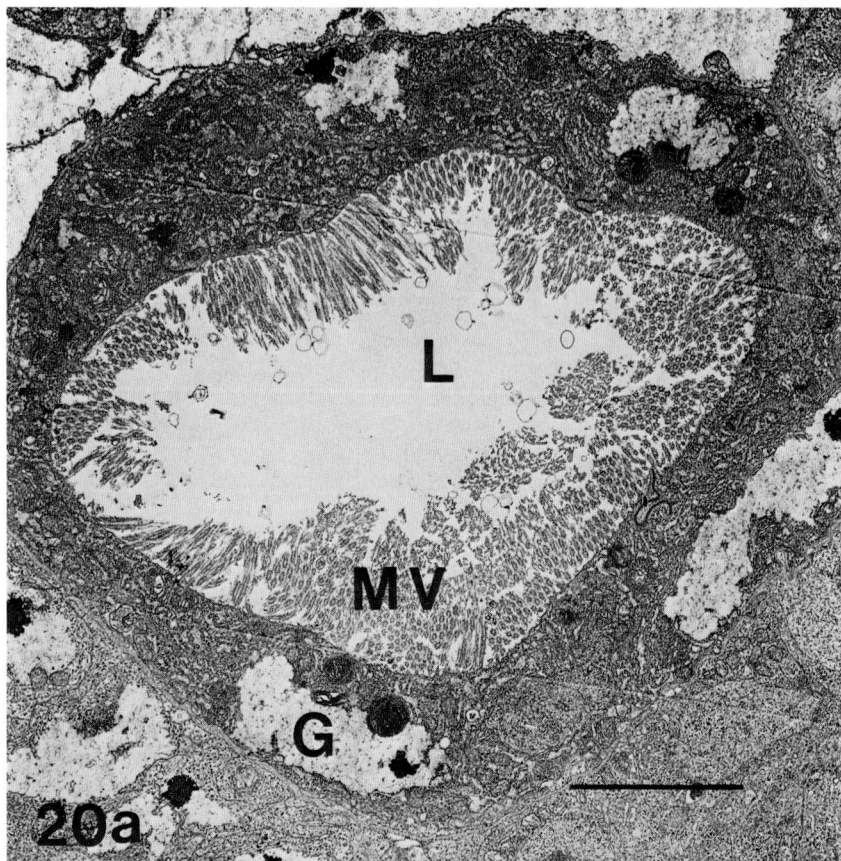

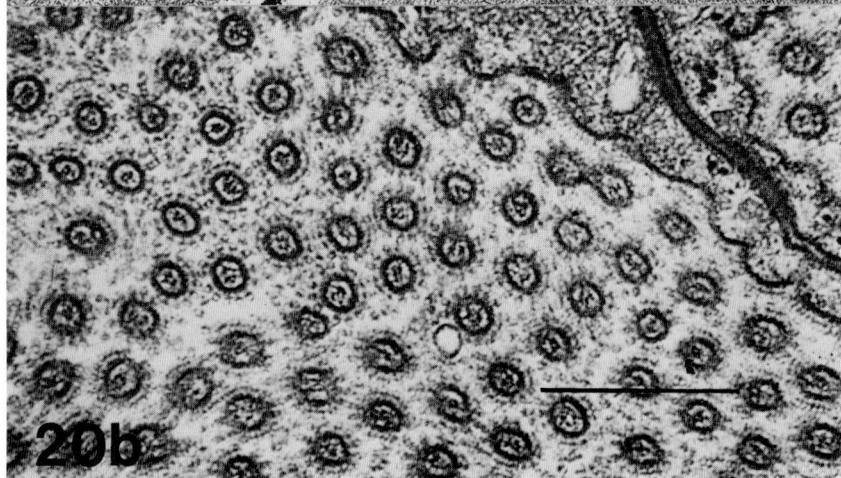

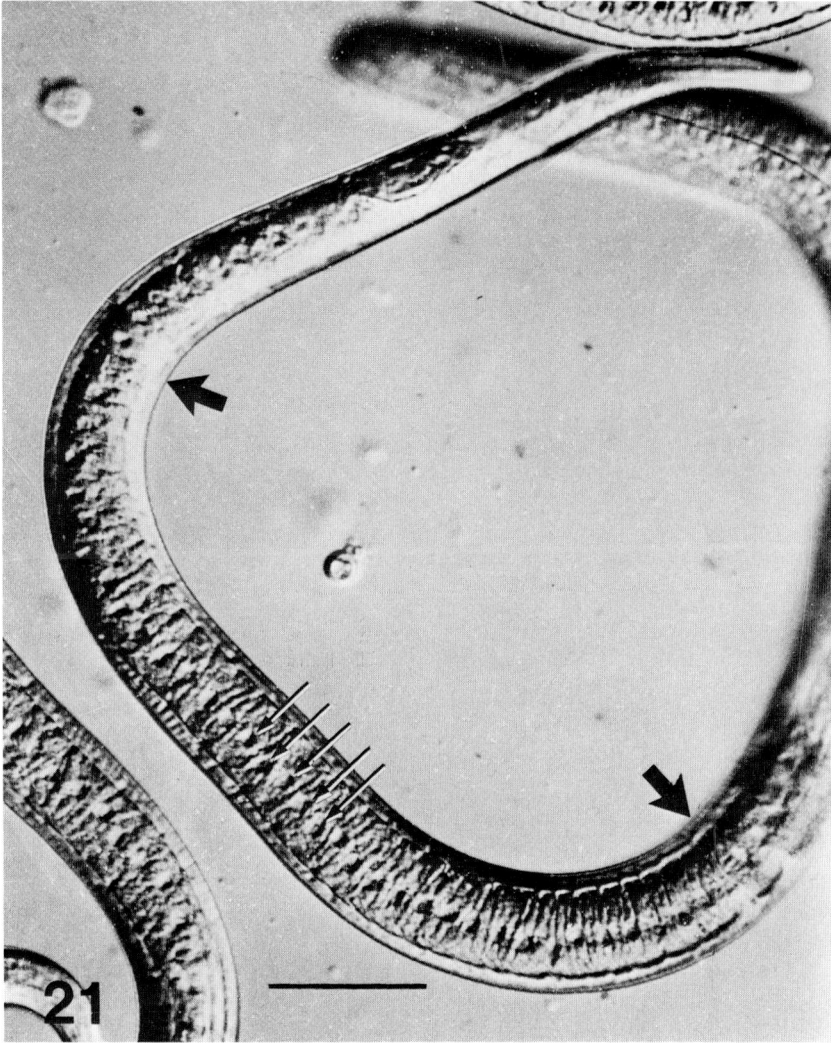

FIGURE 21. Stichosome region of the infective L_1 larva. The large arrows delineate its beginning and end. Each stichosome contains about 50–55 stichocytes (arrows). Nomarski interference microscopy. Scale bar: 50 μm.

FIGURE 20. (20a) Transmission electron micrograph of the midgut of an infective L_1 larva. The microvilli (MV) are seen in both cross and longitudinal section. (G) Glycogen; (L) lumen. Scale bar: 2 μm. (20b) Transmission electron micrograph of microvilli in the midgut of an infective L_1 larva. Scale bar: 0.3 μm.

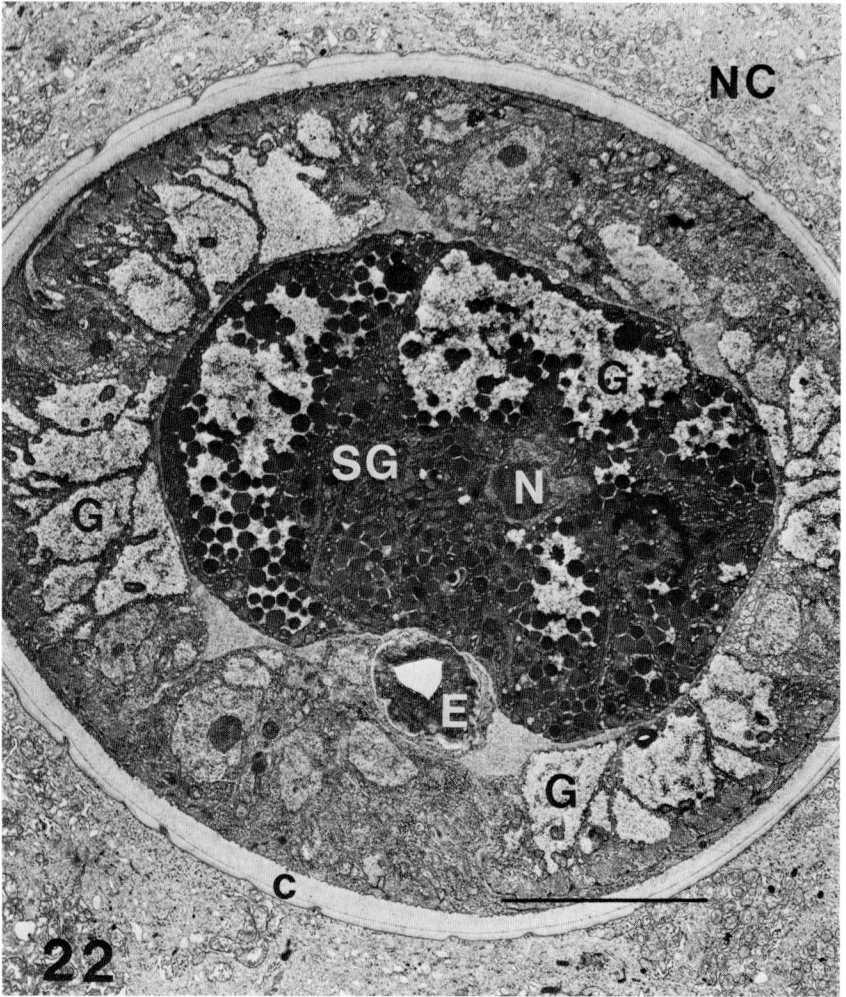

FIGURE 22. Transmission electron micrograph of a beta-secretory-granule (SG)-containing stichocyte from an infective L₁ larva. (E) Esophagus; (G) glycogen; (N) nucleus; (C) cuticle, (NC) Nurse cell. Scale bar: 8 μm.

--→

FIGURE 23. Transmission electron micrograph of a portion of a beta-granule-containing stichocyte from an infective L₁ larva. The secretory granules (SG) are embedded in glycogen (G). Mitochondria (M) and rough endoplasmic reticulum (rer) are present in abundance. Scale bar: 1 μm.

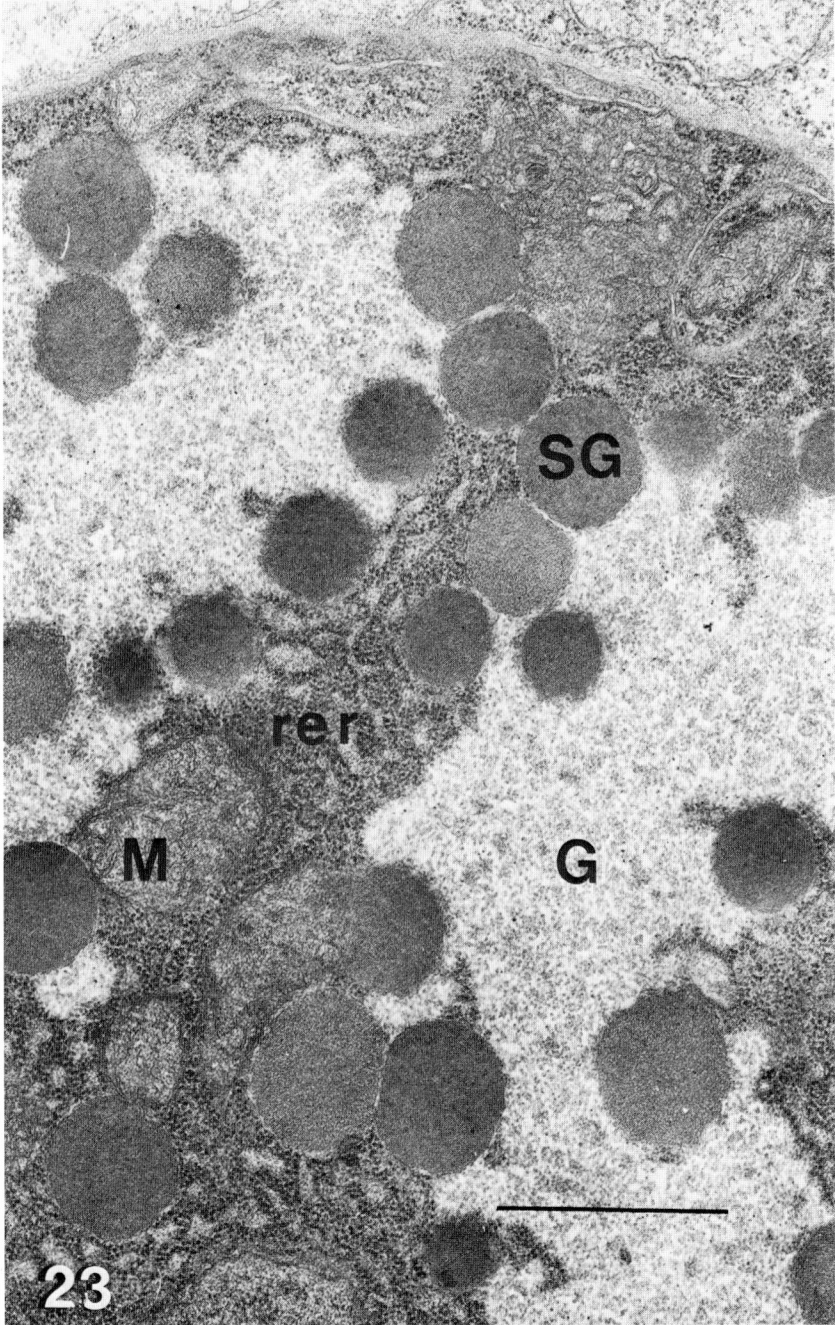

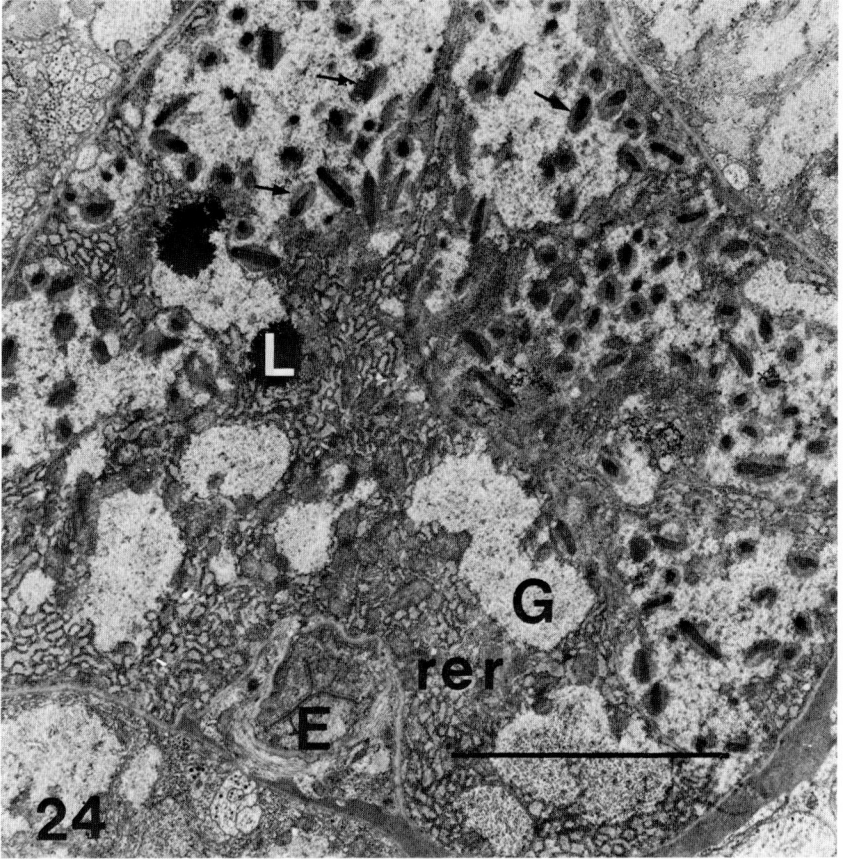

FIGURE 24. Transmission electron micrograph of an alpha-secretory-granule-containing stichocyte from an infective L_1 larva. Arrows indicate granules. The nucleus is not seen in this section. (G) Glycogen; (rer) rough endoplasmic reticulum; (L) lipid droplet; (E) esophagus. Scale bar: 10 μm.

of these secretions in the host are still not known, but broad speculations have been offered (Despommier, 1974; Despommier and Müller 1976), since the immune responses directed against them have such profound influences on the outcome of the infection (Despommier, 1977). These speculations included the possibility that they might be enzymes. The

———→

FIGURE 25. Transmission electron micrograph of a portion of alpha-granule-containing cytoplasm from the stichocyte of an infective L_1 larva. The alpha granules contain a dense core (c) and are bounded by a single unit membrane (arrow). Glycogen (G) and rough endoplasmic reticulum (rer) are also typically found in this cell type. Scale bar: 1 μm.

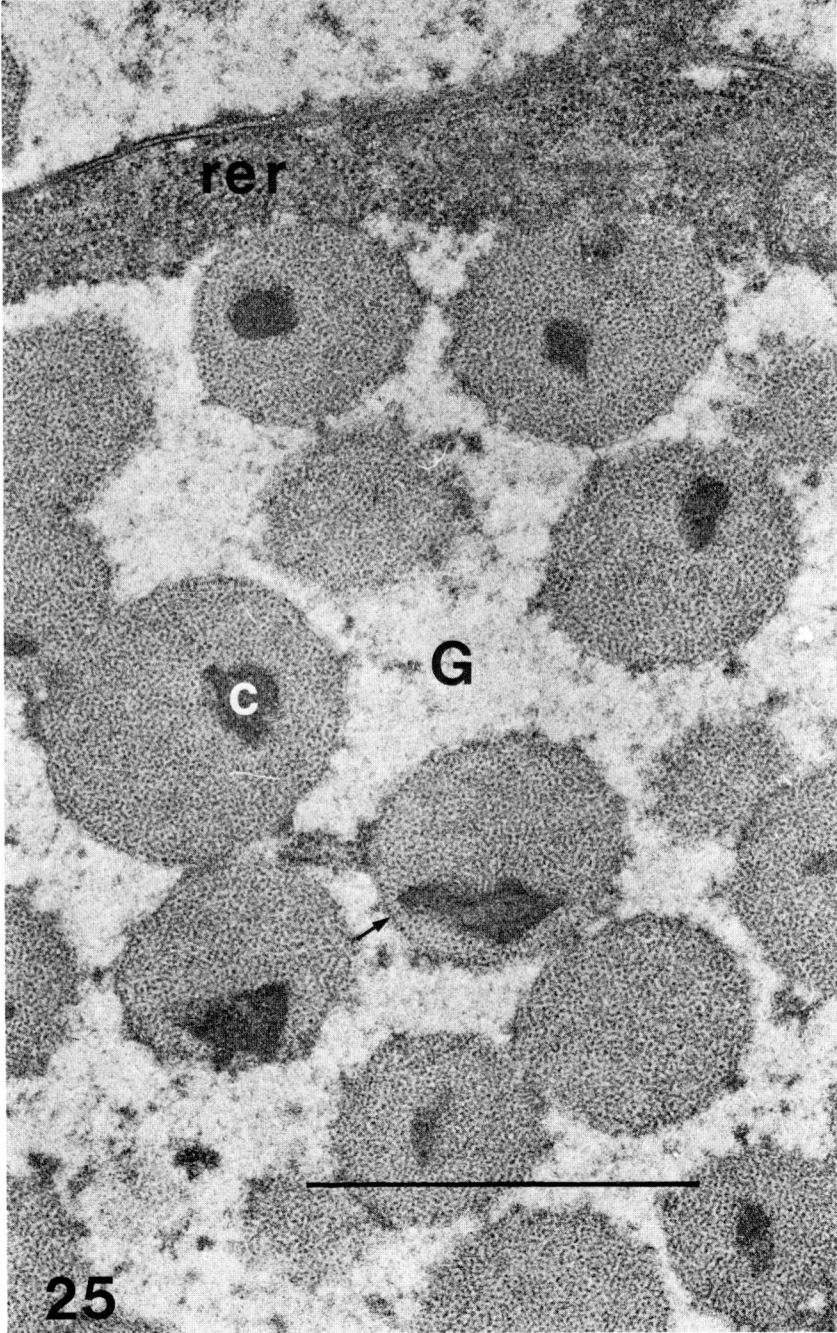

rer

c

G

25

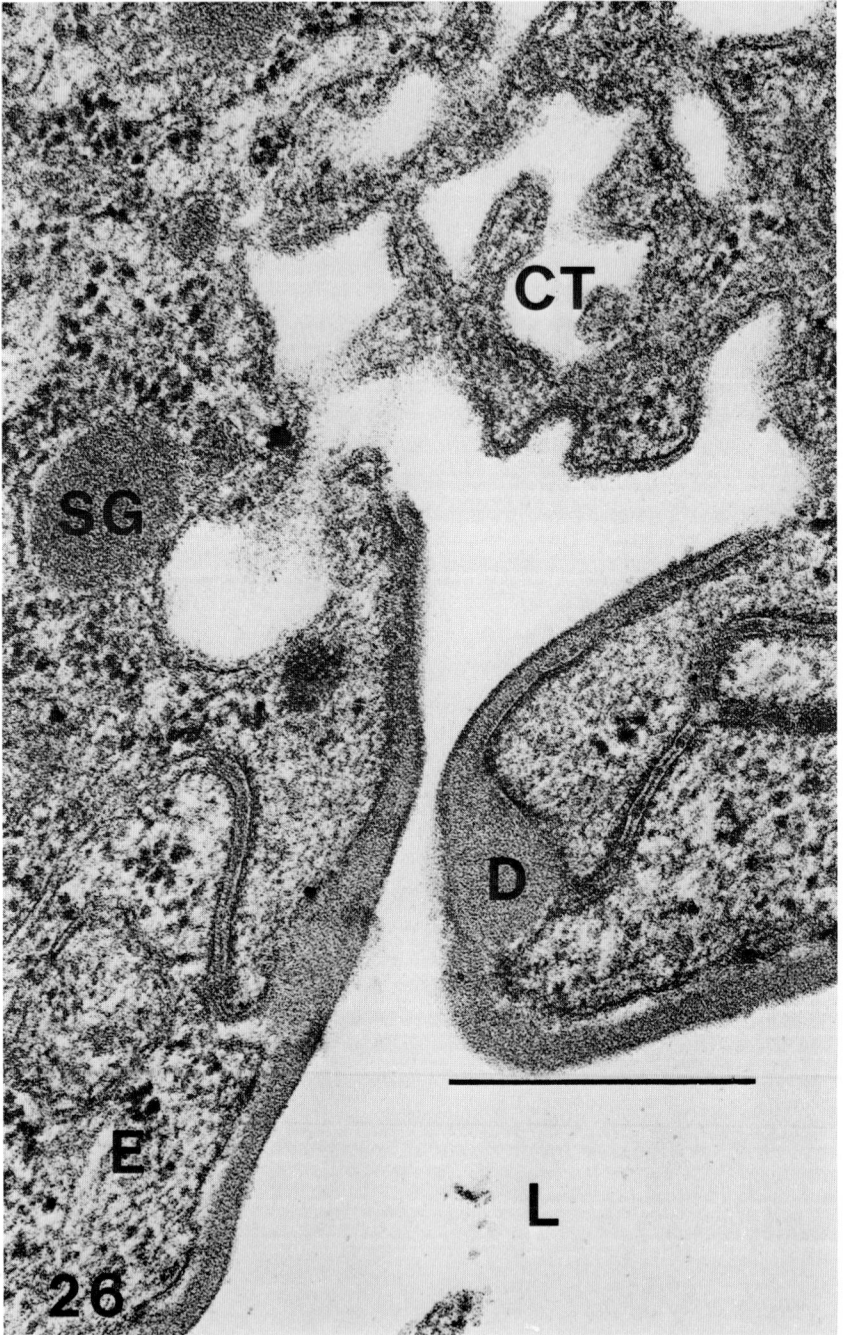

fact that host immune responses that act against these secretions are reversible by transplanting worms from immune animals to nonimmune recipients (Bell *et al.*, 1979) argues in favor of their functioning outside the worm. While no enzymatic activities have yet been ascribed to any particular fraction of the secretions obtained from any stage of *Trichinella*, this statement merely reflects the paucity of data concerning them, rather than summarizes an extensive series of negative experiments.

The stichocyte of the adult (Fig. 28) differs significantly from that of the infective L_1 larva, although their number (see Figs. 3 and 29) remains the same throughout the molt cycle (Richels, 1955). Shortly after the fourth molt, the stichocyte cells of the adult reorganize, now being devoid of both secretory granules and glycogen (Despommier, 1974). Stichocyte mitochondria elongate and increase in number. In addition, much rough endoplasmic reticulum exists throughout the cytoplasm of the stichocyte, particularly in the peripheral region of the cell. The duct (Fig. 30) remains open both to the canalicular tree on the cell side and to the lumen of the esophagus on the intestine side. At 48 hr after infection, secretory granules can once again be observed within its cytoplasm. These new granules are of a more irregular shape and are somewhat larger than those found in the infective L_1 larva. Furthermore, throughout adult life, the cytoplasm does not become empty of secretory granules, despite evidence that they are being secreted (Chipman, 1957). Therefore, it is probable that the stichosome functions continuously in the adult, in contrast to its apparent stage-specific function in the preadult worm. No recent work has been done on the chemistry or immunology of the adult secretions. Therefore, until each secreted protein has been isolated and purified from both the adult and infective L_1 larva, no useful speculation can be offered as to their respective roles in the worm's biology.

4.3. Mating [4]

Immediately following sexual maturity, mating occurs (Hemmert-Halswick and Bugge, 1934; Wu and Kingscote, 1957; Ali Khan, 1966; Kozek, 1971a; Gardiner, 1976), presumably within the intramulticellular niche. Sperm have been observed in mature female worms as early as

←

FIGURE 26. Transmission electron micrograph of the region of the duct (D) that connects the canalicular tree (CT) with the lumen (L) of the eosphagus (E). Note the thickening of cuticle within the duct and its extension into the distal portion of the canalicular tree. A beta secretory granule (SG) can be seen in the leftmost portion of the cell. Scale bar: 1 μm.

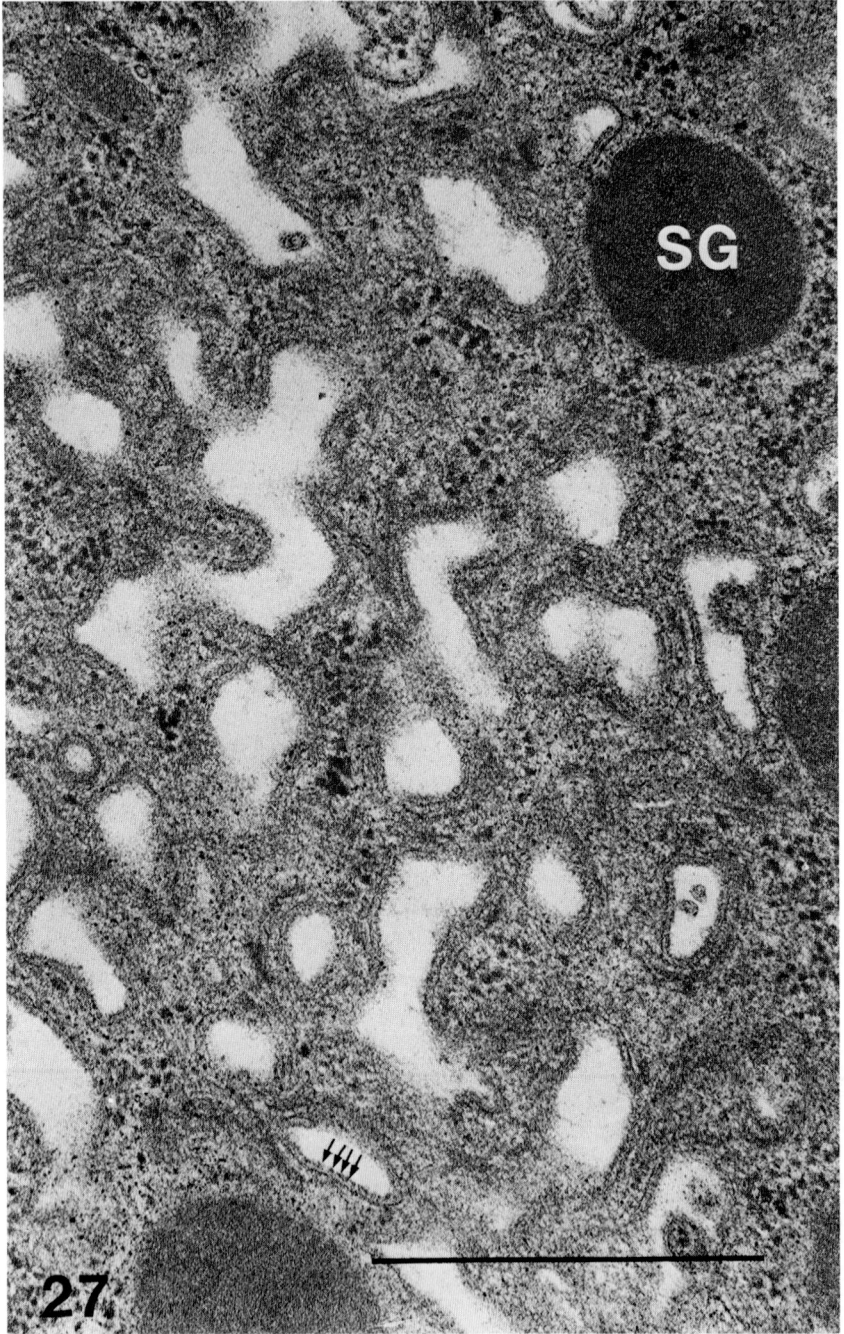

30 hr after infection (Kozek, 1971a; Gardiner, 1976), but usually females are not inseminated until 37–40 hr after infection (Wu and Kingscote, 1957; Ali Khan, 1966).

The solitary telogonic ovary of the female is located in the hindmost region and produces eggs from the epithelium lining that organ. The haploid number of chromosomes in the egg is three, while somatic cells possess six (Penkova and Romanenko, 1973; Bessonov et al., 1976). However, nothing is yet known about meiosis in either sex. Oogenesis occurs at the interface of the ovary and its lumen. The flattened cells nearest the lumen round up and increase in size, eventually becoming cuboidal (Wu, 1955a). The free-floating ova are irregular in size, measuring about 25 μm in diameter, and possess a large centrally placed nucleus.

As Wu (1955a) pointed out, spermatogenesis in *Trichinella* is unusual, taking place along the epithelial lumen of the single testis. The nonflagellated sperm are produced from the irregularly shaped columnar cells and pass into the lumen of the testis. From there, they enter the vas deferens, eventually to reside in the seminal vesicle. During copulation, the sperm pass into the female through the copulatory bell and can then be found throughout the seminal receptacle. The number of chromosomes in the sperm is either two or three, while the somatic cells have five. Therefore, sex of the offspring is determined by the male.

Numerous experiments have established that in the gut, just prior to the time of insemination, the ratio of females to males is about 1.5–2:1 (Boyd and Huston, 1954; Podhajecky, 1963; Denham, 1968) and remains that way up to the time in the infection when immune expulsion of adults begins (Rappaport, 1943; Gursch, 1949; Campbell and Cuckler, 1966). These data suggest either that there is differential survival of female zygotes or that a mechanism similar to meiotic drive is in operation. However, before mating can occur, it is obvious that adult worms of each sex must first come into contact. How this is accomplished has been the subject of several studies. If a host receives a randomly selected pair of infective L_1 larvae, in some instances, a complete infection is established, with worms eventually being found in the muscle (Doerr and Menzl, 1933; Matoff, 1935; Wolffhugel, 1938; Chirasak, 1971; Mikhail and Soliman, 1978). Furthermore, when a

←───

FIGURE 27. Transmission electron micrograph of a portion of the canalicular tree of a beta-granule-containing stichocyte from an infective L_1 larva. The lining of each lumen within the tree has small regularly arranged granules (arrows). (SG) Beta secretory granule. Scale bar: 1 μm.

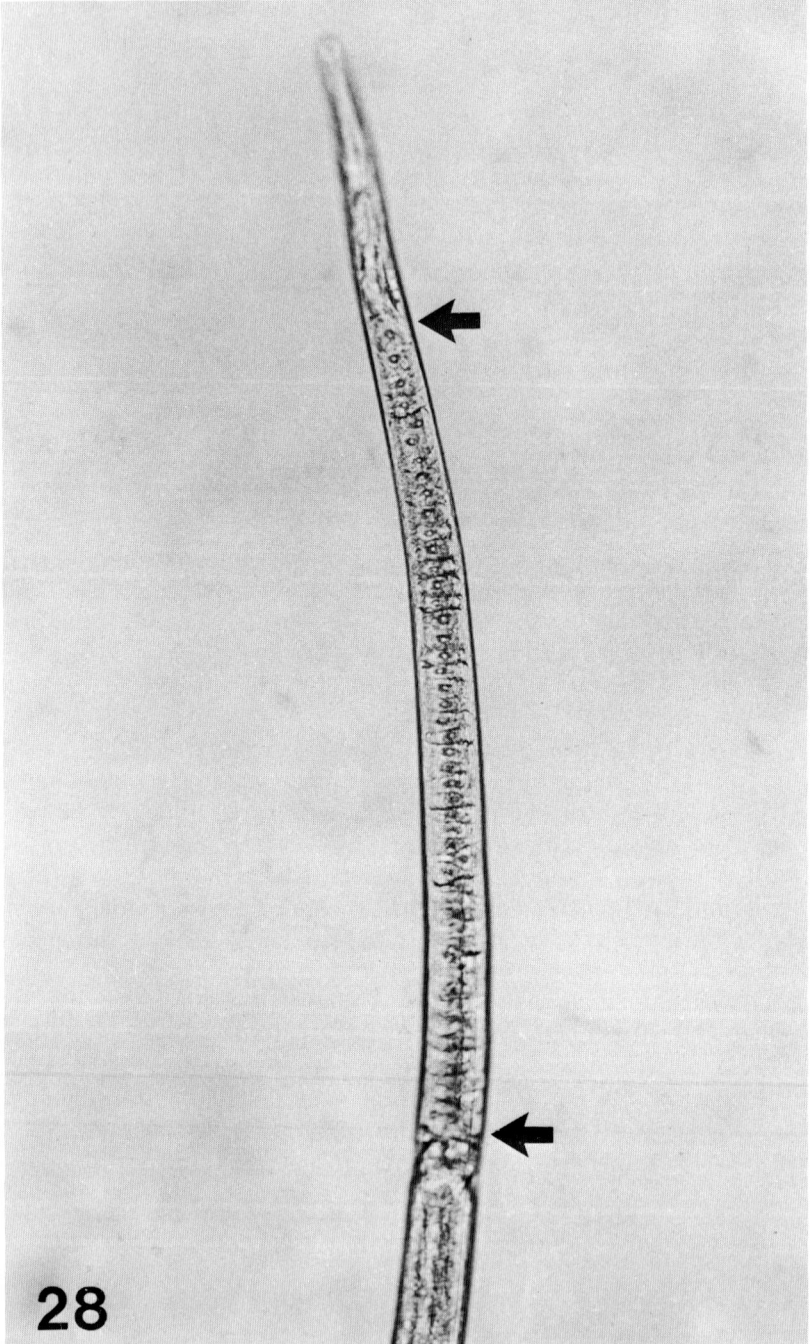

28

single unsexed infective L_1 larva was given orally to a mouse, followed by another infective L_1 larva 4 days later, 9% of all mice developed a complete infection (Campbell and Yakstis, 1969). In order for just a few worms to succeed in mating within the apparent vastness of the enteral niche, an attraction pheromone system must be operative. *In vitro* experiments have been carried out to investigate this possibility. In one study, it was found that female worms attracted male worms, and attracted them more strongly than males attracted females (Bonner and Etges, 1967). In addition, the study showed that females neither attracted nor repelled other females. However, males clearly repelled other males. Belosevic and Dick (1980) obtained similar results with regard to heterosexual attraction; females of *Trichinella* attracted males, but the reciprocal experiment was not done. In addition, they showed that males repelled each other, thereby confirming earlier findings (Bonner and Etges, 1967). However, when females were tested, they too repelled each other in the migration chamber. The reason for this last difference between the two studies was not clear from the data presented in either work.

In vivo studies using monosexual infections gave results that supported the findings that females neither attracted nor repelled each other, while males repelled each other (Sukhdeo and Croll, 1981). In these experiments, it was clearly shown that females become distributed in the anterior region of the small intestine in a pattern indistinguishable from that of a natural infection. However, infections with only males showed a nonaggregated distribution, the males being found in almost equal numbers in both the anterior and posterior regions of the small intestine. Therefore, it appears as though the males of *Trichinella* exhibit territorial behavior. The selective advantage of a system consisting of an attractant and a repellent is obvious, since mating success would then be maximized.

During infection, it is commonly observed that all females become fertilized. Since, as already mentioned, the sex ratio of females to males is about 2:1, for all females to become inseminated, each male must mate, on the average, two times (i.e., males do not die after mating). The attractant–repellent system of pheromones would favor the mating success of this sex ratio, and it is probable that the female attractant overrides the signals from the male repellent. To date, there is no information regarding the chemical nature of the female pheromone, but studies with heterologous isolates of *Trichinella* (i.e., *T. spiralis* var.

FIGURE 28. Stichosome of the adult worm. The arrows delineate the stichosome. Nomarski interference microscopy. Courtesy of Mr. Eric Gravé.

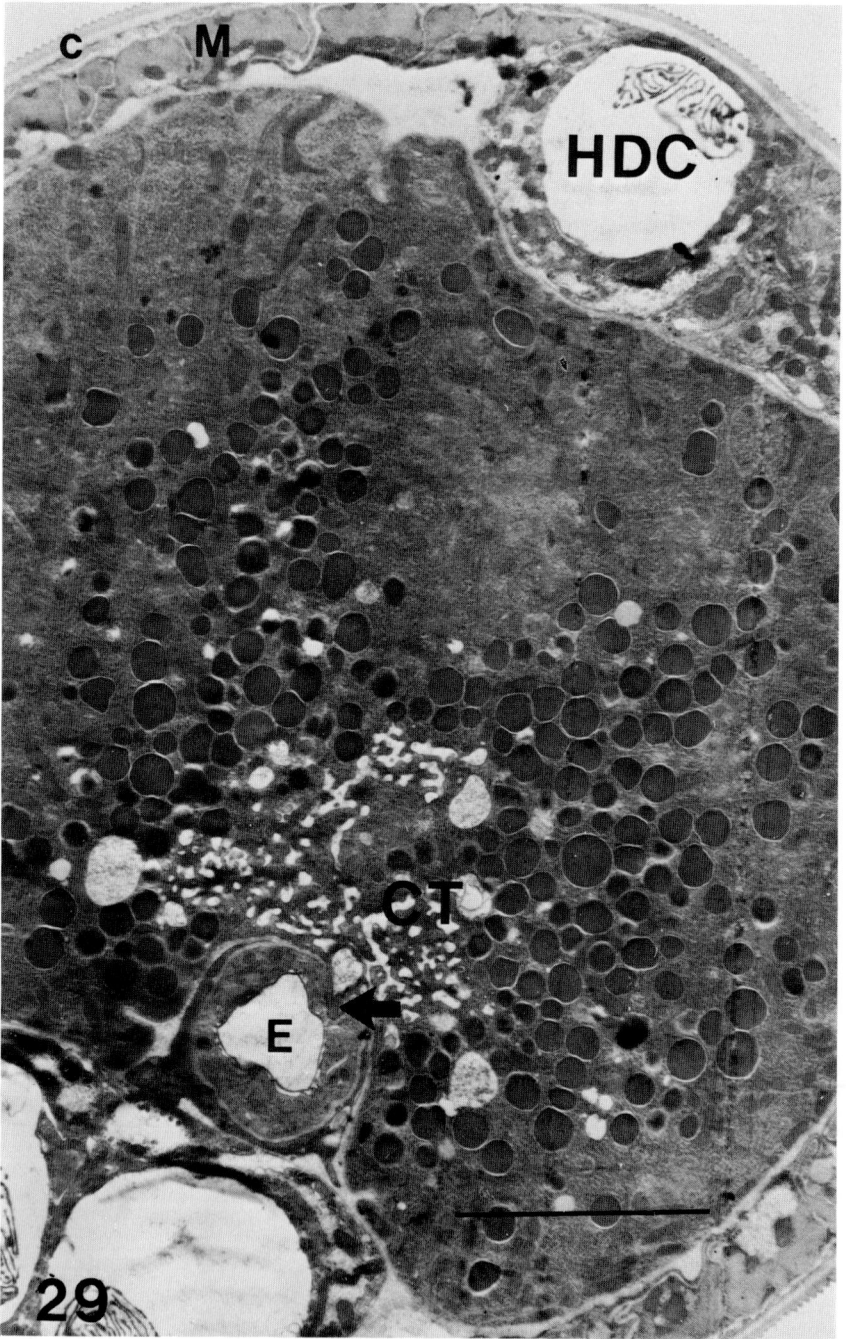

pseudospiralis and an arctic strain of *Trichinella*) indicated that males of all strains tested detect and respond to the same pheromone (Belosevic and Dick, 1980). A major unanswered question regarding this pheromone system is where and when the males come into contact with it. Since it is now established that both sexes live within the intramulticellular niche and have been observed there during the time of mating (i.e., 30 hr after infection), theories regarding the ways in which the males detect and respond to the female pheromone must take this fact into account. Another unanswered question raised by this system is how the males who have encountered one female know to leave her after mating and to seek another mate. It is possible that the pheromone is not produced by females that have recently mated.

With regard to the act of mating itself, the positioning of two adult worms within a common host-cell cytoplasm does not seem possible given the dimensions of host columnar cells. It is more probable, therefore, that both worms occupy adjacent rows of cells when engaged in sexual contact, and that is consistent with what has been observed (Gardiner, 1976).

The length of time that the enteral infection lasts appears to be largely under the control of the immune system of the host and is discussed in detail in Chapter 8. It should be pointed out, however, that the maximum life-span of adult *Trichinella* has never been determined. The longest-lived adult worms were recovered from athymic nude mice and were 83 days old (Ruitenberg *et al.*, 1977), although over 80% were gone by day 40, and nearly 95% had egressed from the small intestine by day 65. The experiment would have been extended to a longer observation period, but all mice died by the 83rd day. Regrettably, adult counts in athymic (*nu/nu*) mice were not carried out at earlier time points, which would have permitted calculation of the mean life-span of the adult worm (i.e., the time in the infection at which 50% of the adults were no longer present in the small intestine). It is probable that adult worms produced newborn L_1 larvae throughout the infection period (i.e., all 83 days), as judged by the large numbers of infective L_1 larvae recovered from the musculature of *nu/nu* mice at day 40 (170,400) and day 50 (175,700).

←——

FIGURE 29. Transmission electron micrograph of a stichocyte of an adult worm. Another stichocyte cell of an adult, *in situ*, is seen in Fig. 3. The secretory granules are irregularly shaped and occupy the central region of cytoplasm. In addition, the canalicular tree (CT), duct (arrow), and esophagus (E) are filled with precipitated material presumably derived from the contents of the granules. Hypodermal gland cell (HDC), musculature (M), and cuticle (c) can also be seen in this view. Scale bar: 5 μm.

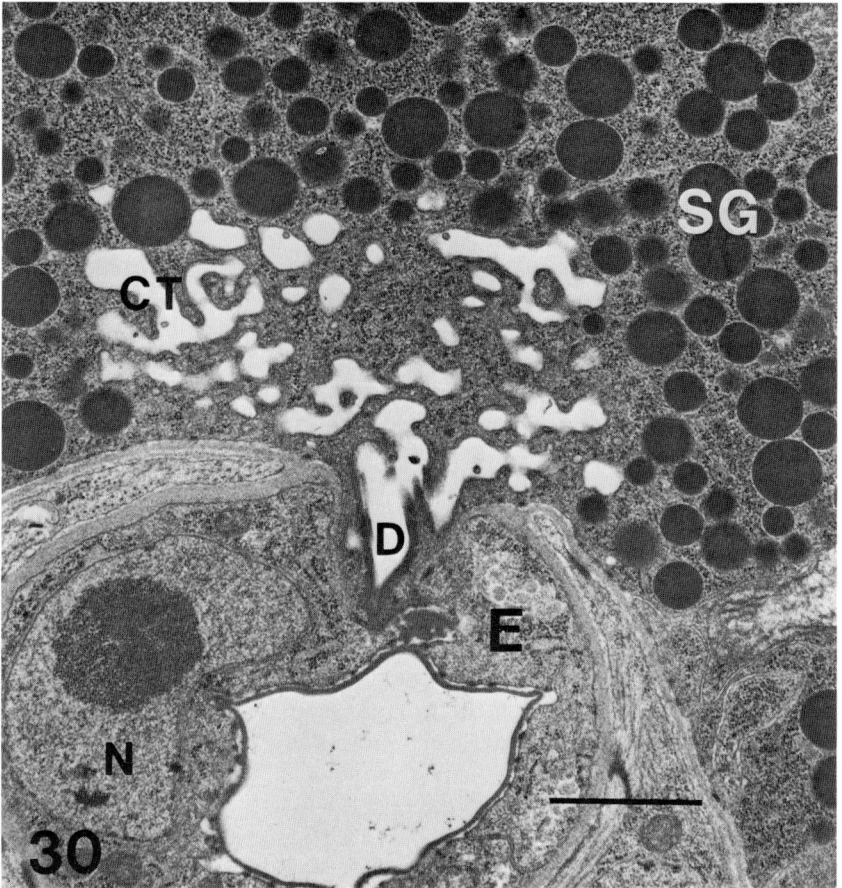

FIGURE 30. Transmission electron micrograph of the duct region of a stichocyte from an adult worm. The duct (D), canalicular tree (CT), secretory granules (SG), nucleus (N), and esophagus (E) are seen in this view. Scale bar: 1 μm. Courtesy of Dr. K.A. Wright.

4.4. Fecundity [5]

Fertilization of ova occurs at the junction of the ovary and seminal receptacle (Wu, 1955a), signaling the production of newborn L_1 larvae. As previously stated, insemination occurs at about 30 hr following oral infection. Embryogenesis takes about 90 hr, because the first newborn L_1 larvae are not shed until day 5 after infection (Denham and Martinez, 1970; Harley and Gallicchico, 1971).

Following fertilization, the egg develops through typical embryological stages (i.e., blastule, gastrula) and finally into a recognizable larva

(Berntzen, 1965). The report that *Trichinella* molts once within the vitelline membrane (Berntzen, 1965) has not been confirmed, and such a molt seems unlikely, since, as already detailed, the worm undergoes four typical molts in the intestine. The embryology of *Trichinella* has not been thoroughly studied, although some morphological data exist (Berntzen, 1965). Nothing is known about the physiological or biochemical features of intrauterine development.

The larvae (Fig. 31) are born live, passing through the vulva (i.e., birth pore or genital pore). The fecundity of single worms has been investigated, as well as the total number of infective L_1 larvae produced during an infection. Table 5 shows data from several carefully conducted experiments in which the fecundity of single female worms was determined. As can be seen, widely different results were obtained and most likely reflect host differences, as well as possible parasite strain variation.

The number of infective L_1 larvae recovered at day 30 or later from a given infection has been used by many investigators as an index of the overall success of the infection in a given host. Counts of infective L_1 larvae recovered from various inbred strains of mice are listed in Table 6, and are representative of the variation noted for other species of host as well. This kind of determination has limited value in that differences between hosts in the number of infective L_1 larvae recovered do not allow the investigator to identify the phase of the infection that is different. The possibilities for differences include: (1) number of adult worms that become established in the host; (2) total number of newborn L_1 larvae produced per female; (3) longevity of adults in the intramulticellular enteral niche; (4) survival of newborn L_1 larvae during migration; and (5) successful establishment and growth of infective L_1 larvae in the intracellular parenteral niche. Furthermore, total counts of infective L_1 larvae reveal nothing concerning daily total production of infective L_1 larvae. In this regard, two different experimental designs

TABLE 5
Production of Infective L_1 Larvae by Single Female Worms

Host species	Number of infective L_1 larvae recovered	Reference
Rat	1100	Nolf (1937)
Rat	345	Edney *et al.* (1953)
Rat	200	Wolffhugel (1938)
Mouse	1600	W. C. Campbell and Yakstis (1969)
Mouse	1660	Chirasak (1971)

TABLE 6
Relationship between Defined Strains[a] of Mice and Number of Infective L_1 Larvae Recovered from the Musculature

Host	Mean number of infective L_1 larvae given orally	Number of infective L_1 larvae recovered from the musculature[b]	Reference
B_{10} LP *nu/nu*	300	176,700	Ruitenberg *et al.* (1977)
SJL	200	44,200	Rivera-Ortiz and Nussenzweig (1976)
AKR	200	25,200	Rivera-Ortiz and Nussenzweig (1976)
LAF_1	200	13,200	Rivera-Ortiz and Nussenzweig (1976)
DBA/1	200	8,500	Rivera-Ortiz and Nussenzweig (1976)
ICI female	400	241,000	Denham and Martinez (1970)
ICI male	400	63,400	
NIH	400	18,600	Wakelin (1980)
SWR	400	36,300	Wakelin (1980)
B_{10}	400	65,100	Wakelin (1980)
B_{10} B_r	400	83,000	Wakelin (1980)
B_{10} D_2	400	49,000	Wakelin (1980)
T.O.	300	50,000	James and Denham (1975)
Biozzi strain	50	9,700	Perrudet-Badoux *et al.* (1975, 1978)
F 24–26	200	32,000	
(High responder)	300	19,000	
Biozzi strain	50	20,300	Perrudet-Badoux *et al.* (1975, 1978)
F 24–26	200	34,000	
(Low responder)	300	30,000	
C_3HeB/FeJ	150	42,000	Wassom *et al.* (1979)
CBA/J	150	33,000	Wassom *et al.* (1979)
RF/J	150	25,000	Wassom *et al.* (1979)
AKR/J	150	23,000	Wassom *et al.* (1979)
C58/J	150	22,000	Wassom *et al.* (1979)
DBA/J	150	20,000	Wassom *et al.* (1979)
SWR/J	150	16,000	Wassom *et al.* (1979)
BUB/Bn J	150	15,000	Wassom *et al.* (1979)
A/J	100	1,699	Tanner (1978)
C57B1/6	100	2,800	Tanner (1978)
BALB/c	100	1,100	Tanner (1978)
AKR	100	1,400	Tanner (1978)
DBA/1	100	2,700	Tanner (1978)
SJL	100	2,500	Tanner (1978)
LAF/J	100	3,500	Tanner (1978)
A/J X C57B1/6	100	3,300	Tanner (1978)
BN	200	36,400	Stephanski and Kozar (1969)
R III	200	67,000	Stephanski and Kozar (1969)
BALB	200	88,200	Stephanski and Kozar (1969)
C_3H	200	103,200	Stephanski and Kozar (1969)

[a] Most of the strains of mice listed are inbred. However, in some instances, this information was not stated in the text; therefore, the term "defined strains" was chosen.

[b] The time at which each experiment was ended after oral infection varied; 30 or 35 days was the most common time of termination.

have been employed. In the first instance, the drug methyridine (Janitschke, 1962) was used to limit each day's infection by eliminating the adults in the host without affecting the L_1 larvae already produced by them (Denham and Martinez, 1970). Different groups of male mice, all of which were infected on the same day, were given drug on day 5, 6, 8, 10, 12, 17, or 21 after infection. Counts of infective L_1 larvae were made on all groups of mice at day 35 after infection. Maximum numbers of infective L_1 larvae were produced on day 7 of the infection. However,

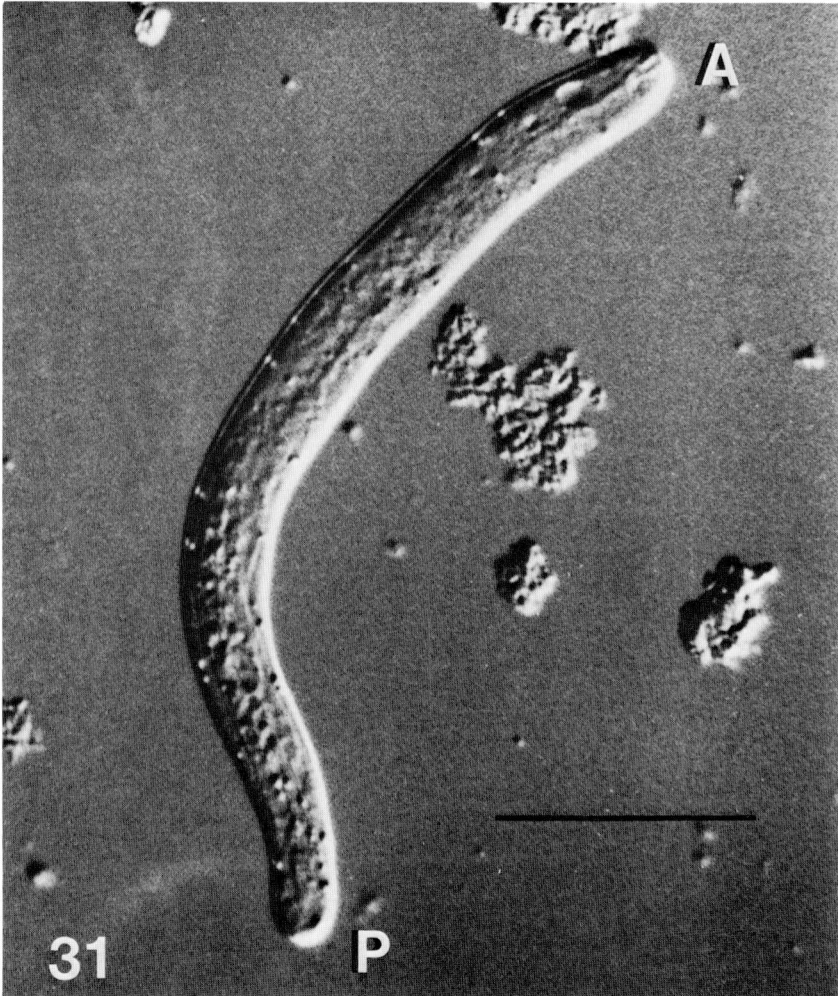

FIGURE 31. Newborn larva. (A) Anterior; (P) posterior. Nomarski interference microscopy. Scale bar: 20 μm.

in this instance, only those newborn L_1 larvae that successfully developed in the musculature were counted. A second approach employed cannulation of the thoracic duct of infected rats from days 4 to 15 after infection, with subsequent enumeration of migratory L_1 larvae in 24-hr samples of lymph (Harley and Gallicchico, 1971). Day 9 was the day on which most migratory L_1 larvae were recovered (Table 7). The total number of migratory L_1 larvae collected in lymph between days 4 and 15 of infection (142,270) represented over 60% of the total infective L_1 larvae produced (225,000). While much was learned concerning the kinetics of daily total production of migratory L_1 larvae, these data did not indicate whether all migratory L_1 larvae recovered by cannulation were capable of completing the life cycle, since their infectivity was not measured.

To determine rates of production of newborn L_1 larvae per female, an *in vitro* system was devised whereby individual adult female worms were allowed to shed newborn L_1 larvae for 24 hr (Despommier *et al.*, 1977). Enumeration of newborn L_1 larvae shed *in vitro* was carried out on various days after a primary infection in CFW (random-bred) mice. In addition, the total number of adult female worms present on days 7, 9, and 11 was also determined. When the total number of newborn L_1 larvae produced per day *in vitro* was multiplied times the total

TABLE 7
Number of Migratory L_1 Larvae Produced
Each Day as Ascertained from Cannulation
of the Thoracic Duct[a]

Day of collection of lymph after infection	Mean number of migratory L_1 larvae recovered per rat[b]
4	0
5	0
6	3,090
7	10,040
8	22,126
9	53,261
10	23,277
11	18,490
12	8,453
13	3,490
14	43
15	0

[a] After Harley and Gallicchico (1971).
[b] Each rat received 3000 infective L_1 larvae via the oral route.

TABLE 8

Relationship between the Number of Newborn L₁ Larvae Shed *in Vitro* and the Number of Infective L₁ Larvae Recovered at Day 30[a]

Day after infection	Number of newborn L_1 larvae shed per female	Number of females	Total number of newborn L_1 larvae produced	Number of infective L_1 larvae recovered from the musculature
5	10^b	111	1,110	—
6	130	111[c]	14,430[c]	—
7	125	111	13,870	—
8	65	89[c]	5,785[c]	—
9	38	68	2,585	—
10	20	35[c]	700[c]	—
11	0	3	0	—
		TOTAL:	38,480	39,000

[a] Derived from Despommier *et al.* (1977).
[b] Estimated from another experiment in that same series.   [c] Interpolated.

number of females present, then added together for each day of the infection, the total number (38,480) of newborn L_1 larvae produced *in vitro* was within 2% of the actual number (39,000) of infective L_1 larvae recovered at day 30 after infection (Table 8). These data strongly suggest that the *in vitro* shedding of newborn L_1 larvae can be used to predict the overall success of the infection, at least for CFW mice. Variation in shed rate among individual worms for any given day was low, but shed rate did vary from day to day, and was correlated with the development of host immunity.

Experiments in which various host and *in vitro* conditions were systematically altered were conducted by Stewart *et al.* (1980) to further define the *in vitro* shed-rate assay for adult worm fecundity. No differences in shed rates were noted between single females and groups of females or between individual females incubated together with male worms. However, adult females derived from the ileum or jejunum shed fewer newborn L_1 larvae than did those from the duodenum. Temperature also affected shed rate, with fewer newborn L_1 larvae being shed at temperatures that were above or below 37°C. Finally, female worms from heavy infections (500 or more per mouse) shed fewer worms than those adults derived from mice infected with low numbers (125 or 250). These later findings correlate well with earlier *in vivo* studies on superinfections and fecundity (Tanner, 1968; Chirasak, 1971). In the earlier studies, it was clearly shown that fewer infective L_1 larvae per female worm were produced in heavy infections.

5. INTRACELLULAR PARENTERAL NICHE

5.1. Migration of the First-Stage Larva to the Niche [6]

Besides a brief stay in the stomach by the infective L_1 larva at the time of initial infection, the only other time point at which *Trichinella* is not within cells is during its migration to the muscle cell. The route in the host that *Trichinella* takes to reach its intracellular parenteral niche has been investigated by many researchers (Cerfontaine, 1895; Askanazy, 1895; Graham, 1897; Staubli, 1905; Mauss and Otto, 1942; Berntzen, 1965; Nelson *et al.*, 1966; Basten and Beeson, 1970; Harley and Gallicchio, 1971). The most convincing evidence regarding its route through the body comes from two studies on rats in which the thoracic duct was cannulated during infection. In the first study, newborn larvae were recovered in large numbers between days 6 and 7 after oral inoculation (Baston and Beeson, 1970). However, this was an incidental finding, since the purpose of the experiments was to collect lymphocytes, not worms. When the lymph collected from infected donors on the aforementioned days was injected intravenously into recipients, as many as 50,000 infective L_1 larvae were recovered from the musculature at day 30 after injection.

A more systematic study employed infected rats that were cannulated from days 4 to 15 following oral infection with 3000 infective L_1 larvae (Harley and Gallicchio, 1971). In addition, these investigators attempted to collect migratory L_1 larvae from blood, abdominal fluid, and various tissues including lung, liver, and kidneys.

As mentioned in Section 6, the results of this study showed that over 60% of all migratory L_1 larvae were collected in lymph, with the rest being found in various organs, especially the liver and lung. Moreover, on day 9 after infection, the number of larvae in lymph was 97% of the total number recovered on that day, and clearly suggested that this was the dominant route of migration used by *Trichinella* to get from the enteral to the parenteral niche (Table 9). The results also showed that this stage of the infection did not spend any appreciable amount of time in the bloodstream, since few migrating L_1 larvae were ever recovered from blood, regardless of the time in the infection period at which the collection was made. However, studies aimed at determining exactly how long the migratory L_1 larva spends in the host prior to penetrating a cell, be it striated muscle or other, has yet to be determined.

From what is now known, it is probable that the migratory L_1 larva first enters the lamina propria of the villus. That is accomplished by

TABLE 9
Number of Migratory L_1 Larvae Recovered
from Rats at Day 9^a after Oral Infection[b]

Tissue	Number of migratory L_1	Percentage of L_1 larvae
Abdominal cavity	80	0.1
Blood[c]	132	0.2
Kidney	269	0.5
Liver	380	0.7
Lung	458	0.8
Lymph[d]	53,261	97.7
	54,580	100

[a] Day of maximum number of migratory L_1 found in most tissues examined from days 4 to 15.
[b] Derived from Harley and Gallicchico (1971).
[c] The assumption is made that each rat had an average total blood volume of 11 ml.
[d] Collected over a 24-hr period.

the aid of its stylet. Once there, it penetrates the lymphatic vessel and, less frequently perhaps, the capillary. Those larvae that reach the lymphatic vessel arrive in the general circulation by way of the thoracic duct. Whether this is accomplished by a passive or an active process on the part of the parasite is not known.

Evidence derived from experiments in which attempts were made to infect rats by various routes with newborn L_1 larvae collected *in vitro* supports the view that migration occurs primarily through the blood-stream once the migrating L_1 larvae enter the thoracic duct (Dennis *et al.*, 1970). In these studies, it was clearly demonstrated that injecting newborn L_1 larvae by the intravenous route produced infections in the musculature equal to 80% of the initial dose. In contrast, less than 10% of the larvae succeeded in infecting muscle if they were injected subcutaneously, intraperitoneally, or intradermally. Other investigators have confirmed that the intravenous route gives high yields of infections in the muscles (Ruitenberg and Steerenberg, 1976; James and Denham, 1975; James *et al.*, 1977; Perrudet-Badoux and Binaghi, 1978).

Before *Trichinella* enters the muscle cell (Fig. 32), it must first locate the cell. Numerous studies have conclusively shown that only the striated skeletal muscle cell is a suitable intracellular niche for the continued development of *Trichinella*. However, transient infections of cells in various organs, including heart muscle (Dunlap and Weller, 1933), brain tissue (Most and Abeles, 1937; Schope, 1949), retina and choroid of the eye (Schoop *et al.*, 1961), and liver (Mauss and Otto, 1942) have

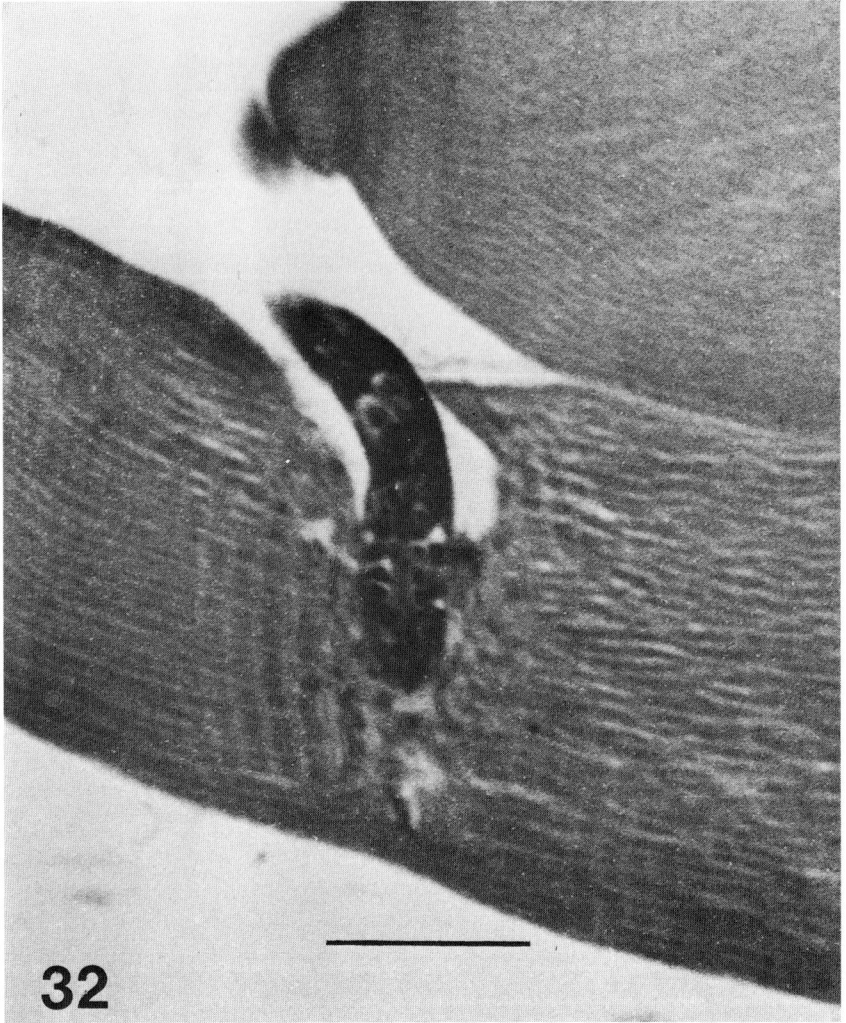

FIGURE 32. Migratory L_1 larva penetrating a striated skeletal muscle cell. Scale bar: 20 μm.

been reported. Indeed, it is precisely this indiscriminate behavior during migration that results in much of the disease in the human infection with this pathogen. Migrating L_1 larvae have also been commonly observed in blood (Staubli, 1905; Harley and Gallicchico, 1971), cerebrospinal fluid (van Cott and Lintz, 1914), less frequently in mother's milk (Denham, 1966), and of course of lymph (Basten and Beeson,

1970; Harley and Gallicchico, 1971). Apparently, *Trichinella* does not cross the placenta (Augustine, 1934; Denham, 1966). From these observations, it can be concluded that *Trichinella* is not selective in its penchant for penetrating host cells. Nonetheless, the vast majority of L_1 larvae end up in striated skeletal muscle cells, a cell type that comprises some 40% of the total weight of the soft tissues of most mammalian species. If other cell types are routinely entered by the migrating L_1 larvae, then *Trichinella* must also be able to exit from them and continue to seek out its natural habitat. Unfortunately, to date, no *in vitro* system using living cells has been developed for studying this important aspect of *Trichinella's* life cycle.

However, some *in vitro* studies have been carried out in migration chambers using newborn L_1 larvae to gain insight into their ability to move toward various chemical and galvanic stimuli designed to simulate some of the conditions that might be expected to occur next to striated skeletal muscle cells (Hughes and Harley, 1977). It was shown that worms had a positive taxis toward a 120-mV stimulus and were repelled by a 90-mV stimulus. In addition, worms were attracted to the negative pole of the 120-mV stimulus. *Trichinella* was repelled by a concentration gradient of KCl, while gradients of phosphocreatine and glycogen had no effects on its migration. These data support the concept that once *Trichinella* comes close to a striated skeletal muscle cell, it is first attracted to the cell, and then rapidly initiates its penetration into the cell after emerging from the capillary.

As previously stated, it is likely that *Trichinella* enters its intracellular parenteral niche by the aid of its stylet. However, penetration mechanisms involving enzymes have not yet been ruled out. Studies in which newborn L_1 larvae were injected directly into muscle bundles showed that penetration had occurred as early as 10 min after injection (Despommier *et al.*, 1975). However, as already mentioned, the rapidity with which *Trichinella* enters its parenteral niche has yet to be determined under natural migratory conditions.

Studies have been done to determine which striated skeletal muscles are most frequently infected, and the relative number of infective L_1 larvae in each, in both naturally occurring and experimentally induced infections in a variety of mammalian hosts, including pig (Thornbury, 1897; Olsen *et al.*, 1964), mouse (Barriga, 1978; Stewart and Charniga, 1980), rat (Leonard and Beahm, 1941; Oliver, 1961), and man (Forrester *et al.*, 1961). In general, the pattern that emerges from these studies supports the commonly held view that muscles that are the most active throughout the wake–sleep cycle of the host (i.e., diaphragm and masseter) harbor the highest percentage of the infective L_1 larvae from a given infection. However, the correlation between muscle activity and relative number of infective L_1 larvae is less striking for muscles that are not known to have a high level of metabolic activity. Thus, in the mouse, the abdominal muscles harbored the fewest worms, while significantly more *Trichinella* were recovered from the pectoralis group (Stewart and Charniga, 1980). A more consistent correlation existed between the physical location of the muscle (i.e., cranial to the caudal margin of the rib cage vs. caudal to the rib cage) and the percentage of *Trichinella* recovered, the higher percentage of larvae being found in the former group (Stewart and Charniga, 1980). If the migrating L_1 larvae are passively carried to the muscles by the general circulation, then the amount of vascularization for a given muscle should determine the resulting number of infective L_1 larvae, providing that no tropism is operative. The results of Hughes and Harley (1977), on the other hand, suggest that the frequency of muscle contractions, and hence the negative 120-mV potential attendant contraction, should greatly influence the resulting number of larvae present in them.

5.2. Entrance of the Migratory First-Stage Larva [7]

Many aspects of the life cycle already discussed are peculiar to *Trichinella*. Its degree of differentiation and growth as an L_1 larva in the muscle cell, now to be described, serves further to exemplify the uniqueness of its biology. The site of penetration shows signs of disruption consistent with the view that entry into the muscle cell is largely a mechanical process (Fig. 32). Immediately after pentrating the muscle fiber, the larva migrates just under its surface, coming to rest several worm-lengths away from its point of entry.

The worm, now termed the preinfective L_1 larva, begins a protracted period of postembryonic growth and development without molting (Wu, 1955b; Ali Khan, 1966; Villella, 1970; Kozek, 1971a,b; Despommier, 1974; Despommier *et al.*, 1975). The growth of *Trichinella* during its parenteral life has been studied extensively using infections initiated orally with infective L_1 larvae (Richels, 1955; Wu, 1955b; Berntzen, 1965; Ali Khan, 1966; Villella, 1970; Kozek, 1971a,b; Stewart, 1973). With this approach, newborn L_1 larvae begin life within the parenteral niche at various times, and consequently their further development is nonsynchronous. Therefore, studies on the growth of the larva or its organs have usually been carried out on the largest or most developed worms that could be found on a given day of the infection. Biological variation in any worm-growth parameter is a valid assumption for any cohort of larvae, but no such variation could be measured under the foregoing scheme, representing a major disadvantage to this approach.

Nonetheless, much basic information regarding the morphology of postembryonic development has been gleaned from these nonsynchronous infections. Stewart (1973) used drug-abbreviated infections, limiting the age difference between the oldest and youngest larvae to 6 days, thereby reducing, but not eliminating, the variation in the age of the worms being assayed. The approximate age of the larvae in nonsynchronous infections can be estimated by subtracting 5 or 6 days from the "days after infection" age. This will result in an error of between 24 and 48 hr in the calculation of the age of the worm. Hence, the real age of the larva will be referred to from now on when data from these studies are discussed.

Synchronous growth of larvae was achieved by injection of newborn L_1 larvae directly into muscle tissue (Despommier et al., 1975), thereby permitting a detailed study of the kinetic aspects of its growth, which included the concept of variation (Fig. 33) and, by serendipity, led to the observation of a migratory L_1 larva penetrating a muscle cell (Despommier, 1977). In this study, it was found that the volume of

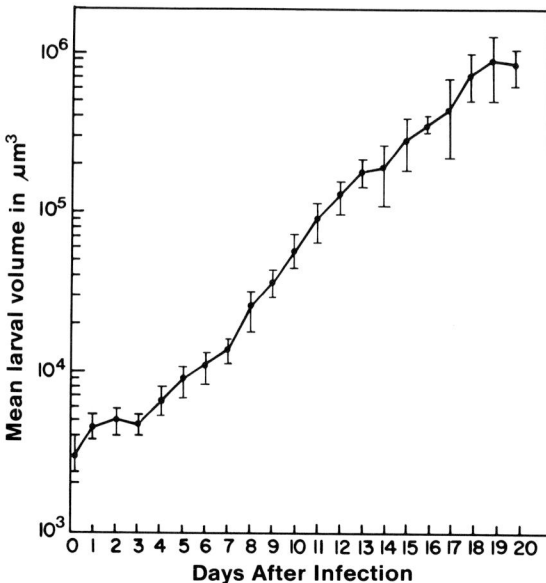

FIGURE 33. Growth curve of the larva in its intracellular niche. The worm increases its volume by about 39% per day beginning on day 4 and ending on day 19 after entering the muscle cell.

Trichinella increased exponentially beginning on day 4 after entry of the larva into its intracellular niche and continued until day 19. Within the first 24 hr of its parenteral phase, the worm doubled its original volume, but did not increase further until day 4. This cessation of worm growth was also noted in nonsynchronous infections (Wu, 1955b). During this early phase of its intracellular life, the larva was associated with non-membrane-bound host cytoplasm (Despommier, 1975). The pause in its growth cycle on days 2 and 3 occurred at a time when its intracellular niche was undergoing radical rearrangement of both a physiological and a biochemical nature (Stewart, 1973; Stewart and Read, 1972, 1973a,b, 1974; Maier and Zaiman, 1966; Farris and Harley, 1977). Structural changes associated with these host-cell alterations strongly correlate to the loss of muscle-cell characteristics and the acquisition of Nurse-cell characteristics (Faaske and Themann, 1961; Ribas-Mujal and Rivera-Pomar, 1968; Backwinkel and Themann, 1972; Despommier, 1975). It is most likely that these host-cell changes were necessary before worm growth could resume. Regrettably, there have been no biochemical studies that deal with this aspect of its parenteral life. The biochemical changes in the host striated muscle cell that occur during the parenteral phase are dealt with in Chapter 7.

5.3. Growth and Development [8–9]

Trichinella grows and differentiates maximally between days 4 and 20 after penetrating the muscle cell, as determined from synchronous (Despommier *et al.*, 1975) and nonsynchronous infections (Richels, 1955; Wu, 1955a; Villella, 1970). The only major organ that develops fully during this time is the stichosome (Richels, 1955; Wu, 1955b; Ali Khan, 1966; Bruce, 1974; Despommier, 1975; Despommier and Müller, 1976). The genital primordium remains primitive throughout this phase, although, as already stated, it does undergo some sexual differentiation. The cuticle thickens progressively throughout this period, but does not undergo further differentiation.

The number of stichocytes in the stichosome increases from about 19 or 20 on day 1 of intracellular life (Richels, 1955) to about 50–55 at day 20 (Richels, 1955; Wu, 1955b; Villella, 1970; Despommier and Müller, 1976). Maximum increase in stichocyte numbers occurs on days 6–10 after intracellular infection (Richels, 1955; Wu, 1955b).

The stichocytes differentiate into cells containing either alpha-granules or beta-granules. The alpha-granule cells occupy the last third of the stichosome and number about 10–15, while the beta-granule cells constitute the rest of the stichosome, numbering some 35–40

(Despommier and Müller, 1976). Mature alpha-granule stichocytes contain about 2000 granules, while beta-granule stichocytes contain about 3000 granules.

Ultrastructural studies are in conflict as to the time of onset of secretory-granule formation (Bruce, 1974; Despommier, 1974; Despommier and Müller, 1976). Synchronous infections initiated with newborn L_1 larvae have shown that no granules of either type are present in the stichocytes until day 14 after intracellular infection. Since the granules contain antigens (Jackson, 1959; M.J. Brzosko and Gancarz, 1969; Despommier and Müller, 1976), the antigenicity of the cell can be examined for time of onset of antigen synthesis and granulogenesis by immunohistochemical techniques. Antigenicity of the stichocyte was first noted in 14-day-old larvae, as detected by the horseradish-peroxidase-labeled-antibody method (E.A. Zimmerman *et al.*, 1973). Crandall and Kozek (1974) used fluorescin-labeled antibodies on frozen sections of tissue infected with nonsynchronously growing larvae and detected antigenicity in the stichocytes of 9- and 11-day-old preinfective L_1 larvae, but not in younger worms (4 and 6 days old). In these studies, the stichocytes remained antigenic in all older worms tested. The use of frozen, nonfixed tissue, rather than deparaffinized sections of fixed worms, most likely accounted for the difference between these two studies with regard to the time of onset of stichocyte antigenicity, because any soluble antigens not incorporated within granules would have leached out during the handling procedures associated with the perioxidase-labeled-antibody technique. These studies strongly suggest that antigen synthesis begins on about day 9 or 10 after penetration, while granulogenesis occurs later, around day 14. Since Bruce (1974) did not include experiments on antigenicity of the stichocyte, his results cannot be compared with the findings cited above.

The stichocyte of the preinfective and infective L_1 larva possesses a fully formed canalicular tree and duct, but probably does not secrete significant amounts of cell product during the parenteral phase. Rather, this row of cells is stage-specific and is functional for *Trichinella* during the first 30 hr of life in its enteral niche, as previously outlined. However, there is some evidence that a brief period of secretion of antigens specific to the stichocyte occurs just prior to granulogenesis (Crandall and Kozek, 1974), resulting in the stimulation of antibodies against them. In this regard, it has been shown that intravenous infection initiated with newborn L_1 larvae results in both a viable muscle infection and a high degree of protection (Despommier, 1971; James and Denham, 1974), suggesting that the protection-inducing antigens identified with the stichosome (Despommier and Müller, 1976; Despommier and Laccetti, 1981) were indeed secreted into the host. Morphological evidence in support of this view is derived from ultrastructural studies that showed that the rough endoplasmic reticulum, canaliculi, duct, and esophagus were filled with precipitated material during the period just prior to granulogenesis (i.e., days 10–13). No such material was observed in any of these locations after completion of granulogenesis on day 16.

Immunity induced by *Trichinella* while in its parenteral niche would have selective advantage for that cohort of worms and its host, since humoral antibodies and other protective immune responses could not reach them (Crandall and Kozek, 1974), and would serve to protect its host from future potentially lethal *Trichinella* infections that it might encounter. The time at which *Trichinella* becomes infective for another host during its intracellular life has been the subject of many early studies in which nonsynchronous infections were used. Villella (1970) reviewed this literature and concluded that the time during muscle development at which *Trichinella* can go on to complete the enteral phase of its life cycle in another host varies from day 17 to day 21 after oral infection. This is equivalent to a worm age of 12–16 days and signals the maturation point of the infective L_1 larva. Some larvae were infective on day 14 of a synchronous infection, and most were infective by day 16 (Despommier, unpublished observation). It is therefore tempting to speculate that infectivity is dependent on the presence of secretory granules in the stichocytes. From other considerations, this would at least seem plausible, since the contents of the granules appear to be needed for essential (albeit unknown) worm functions. It is interesting to note that while infectivity is achieved by *Trichinella* by day 16, the worm does not stop growing until day 20, increasing its volume about 2.4 times.

As mentioned, the preinfective L_1 larva lives within naked host cytoplasm, but sometime between days 10 and 14 after infection, layers 3 and 4 can be observed for the first time (Fig. 34), surrounding the cuticle (Despommier, 1975). It is not known whether these two layers are actually typical membranes, or from whence they are derived (i.e., host or parasite). The layers remain closely associated with the cuticular surface throughout the rest of the life of the larva (Beckett and Boothroyd, 1961; Ribas-Mujal and Rivera-Pomar, 1968; Purkerson and Despommier, 1974; Despommier, 1975). No views have been published of the oral or anal orifice of *Trichinella* showing the ultrastructural relationship of this area of the worm to the cytoplasm of the Nurse cell. Thus, it is possible that these regions of the worm remain exposed to naked host cytoplasm after layers 3 and 4 are formed. This point

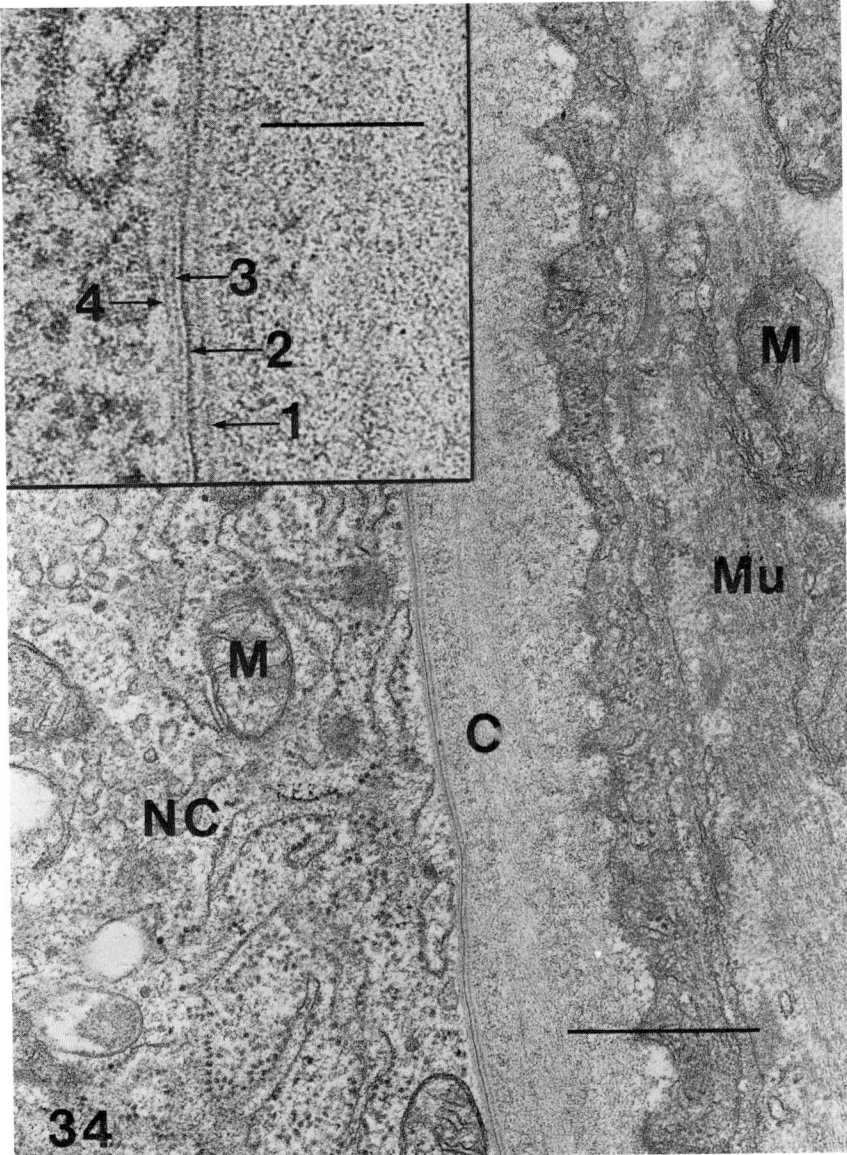

FIGURE 34. Transmission electron micrograph of a 14-day-old larva in its Nurse cell (NC). The four layers (arrows 1, 2, 3, and 4 of inset) are associated with the Nurse cell–parasite interface. Layers 1 and 2 are cuticular (see also Figs. 4 and 5). The precise origins of layers 3 and 4 have not yet been determined. (M) Mitochondria; (C) cuticle; (Mu) muscle. Scale bars: figure 2 μm; inset: 0.5 μm.

becomes critical in discussing nutrient recruitment by the infective L_1 larva. If layers 3 and 4 completely surround the worm, then any exogenous nutrient must traverse the modified sarcolemma of the nurse cell, pass through its whorls of smooth membranes, and finally cross layers 4 and 3, in that order. Once inside layer 3, nutrients could then enter the worm by either the oral or the transcuticular route, if such a route exists. If the oral cavity remains in contact with naked host cytoplasm, then the permutations of possible feeding mechanisms increase considerably. However, further speculation regarding nutrient recruitment is unlikely to be useful until more ultrastructural data on this aspect have been presented. Furthermore, autoradiographic studies at the electron-microscopic level regarding the route of movement of low-molecular-weight precursors for macromolecular synthesis by the worm have not yet been conducted. Such studies might also help to resolve the question of feeding mechanisms.

5.4. Mature Nurse Cell–Infective First-Stage Larva Complex [10]

Growth of the L_1 *Trichinella* larva ceases on day 20 after muscle penetration, the larva having increased its volume from day 0 to day 20 by over 270 times. The worm, fully coiled in its Nurse cell (Fig. 35), now awaits a new host in which to begin its enteral phase. The mature Nurse cell–infective L_1 larva complex can remain in a stable, infectious configuration as long as the host remains alive and does not calcify it (Pagenstecher, 1865). Calcification occurs at rates that vary not only among species of host, but also among individuals within a given species. Nurse cell–infective L_1 larva complexes have been found calcified as soon as 6 months after infection, but lethal calcification is usually not observed around Nurse cell–infective L_1 larva complexes in experimental infections of mice and rats.

While the growth of the parenteral worm is complete by day 20, the Nurse cell continues to differentiate, increasing the amount of collagen that is found in its hypertrophied glycocalyx (Ritterson, 1966; Bruce, 1970c; Stewart and Read, 1972; Teppema *et al.*, 1973; Despommier, 1975). Uptake studies, detailed in Chapter 4, also suggest that the turnover rates for many Nurse cell and parasite components are high and remain so throughout the rest of the period of muscle infection.

ACKNOWLEDGMENTS. The author thanks Drs. K. Wright, S. Holmes Giannini, R. Isenstein, and D. Silberstein, and I. Dunn and C. Kotas,

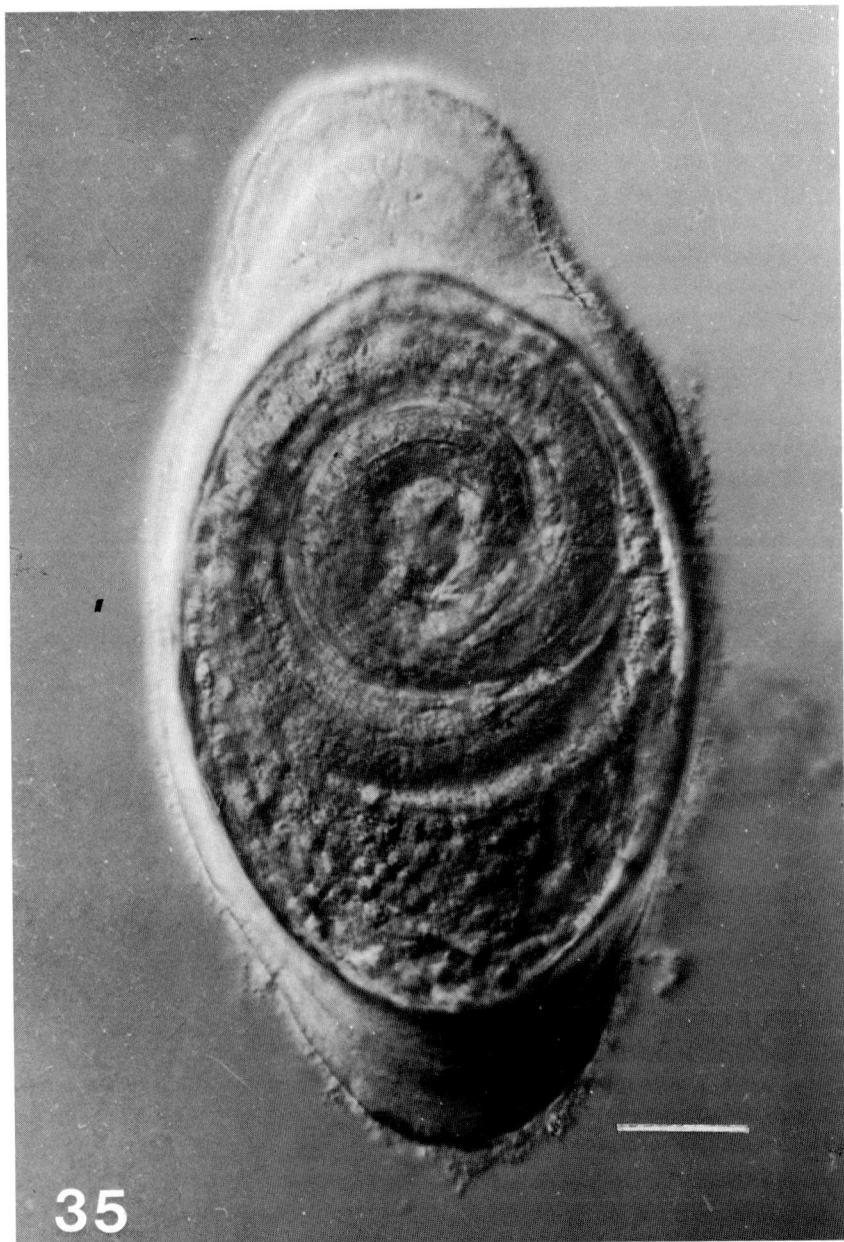

FIGURE 35. Nurse cell–infective L$_1$ larva complex. Nomarski interference microscopy. Scale bar: 50 μm. Courtesy of Mr. Eric Gravé.

for their helpful suggestions and critical review. He especially thanks Mrs. T. Terilli for typing this manuscript, and Mrs. C. Lewinter, and I gratefully acknowledge my wife, Mrs. J. Despommier, for proofreading the final version.

REFERENCES

Alicata, J.E., 1935, Infectivity of *Trichinella spiralis* after successive feedings to rabbits, *J. Parasitol.* **21:**431.

Ali Khan, Z., 1966, The post-embryonic development of *Trichinella spiralis* with special reference to ecdysis, *J. Parasitol.* **52:**248–259.

Askanazy, M., 1895, Zur Lehre von der Trichinosis, *Virchows Arch. Pathol. Anat.* **141:**42–71.

Augustine, D.L., 1934, Studies on the subject of prenatal trichinosis, *Am. J. Hyg.* **29:**115–122.

Backwinkel, K-P., and Themann, H., 1972, Elektronenmikroskopische Untersuchungen über die Pathomorphologie der Trichinellose, *Beitr. Pathol.* **146:**259–271.

Barriga, O.O., 1978, Reliability of muscle samples to estimate *Trichinella* infections in the mouse, *J. Parasitol.* **64:**954–955.

Bass, G.K., and Olson, L.J., 1965, *Trichinella spiralis* in newborn mice: Course of infection and effect on resistance to challenge, *J. Parasitol.* **51:**640–644.

Basten, A., and Beeson, P.B., 1970, Mechanisms of eosinophilia. II. Role of the lymphocyte, *J. Exp. Med.* **131:**1288–1304.

Beckett, E.B., and Boothroyd, B., 1960, The ultrastructure of the "cilia-like" processes in the mid-gut of *Trichinella spiralis* larvae, in: *Proc. Eur. Reg. Conf. on Electron Microscopy*, Vol. II, Delft, pp. 938–941,

Beckett, E.B., and Boothroyd, B., 1961, Some observations on the fine structure of the mature larva of the nematode *Trichinella spiralis*, *Ann. Trop. Med. Parasitol.* **55:**116–124.

Bell, R.D., McGregor, D.D., and Despommier, D.D., 1979, *Trichinella spiralis*: Mediation of the intestinal component of protective immunity in the rat by multiple phase-specific, antiparasitic responses, *Exp. Parasitol.* **47:**140–157.

Belosevic, M., and Dick, T.A., 1980, Chemical attraction in the genus *Trichinella*, *J. Parasitol.* **66:**88–93.

Berezantsev, Y.A., 1954, Raccoon dog as a new host of *Trichinella*, *Dokl. Akad. Nauk. SSSR* **94:**791.

Berntzen, A.K., 1965, Comparative growth and development of *Trichinella spiralis in vitro* and *in vivo* with a redescription of the life-cycle, *Exp. Parasitol.* **16:**74–106.

Bessonov, A.S., Penkova, R.A., Gumenshchickova, V.P., 1976, *Trichinella pseudospiralis* Garkavi, 1972: Morphological and biological characteristics and host specificity, in: *Trichinellosis* (C. Kim, ed.), University Press of New England, Hanover, New Hampshire, pp. 79–93.

Bonner, T.P., and Etges, F.J., 1967, Chemically mediated attraction in *Trichinella spiralis*, *Exp. Parasitol.* **21:**53–60.

Boyd, E.M., and Huston, E.J., 1954, The distribution, longevity and sex ratio of *Trichinella spiralis* in hamsters following an initial infection, *J. Parasitol.* **40:**686–690.

Bruce, R.G., 1966, The fine structure of the intestine and hind-gut of the larva of *Trichinella spiralis*, *Parasitology* **56:**359–365.

Bruce, R. G., 1970a, *Trichinella spiralis*: Fine structure of body wall with special reference to formation and molting of cuticle, *Exp. Parasitol.* **28**:499–511.

Bruce, R.G., 1970b, Structure of the esophagus of the infective juvenile and adult *Trichinella spiralis, J. Parasitol.* **56**:540–549.

Bruce, R.G., 1970c, The structure and composition of the capsule of *Trichinella spiralis* in host muscle, *Parasitology* **60**:223–227.

Bruce, R.G., 1974, Occurrence of hypodermal gland cells in the bacillary band of *Trichinella spiralis* during two phases of its life cycle, in: *Trichinellosis* (C. Kim, ed.), Intext, New York, pp. 43–49.

Brzosko, M.J., and Gancarz, Z., 1969, Immunoelectronmicroscopic studies on antibody binding to the cuticle of *Trichinella spiralis* larvae, *Wiad. Parazytol.* **15**:606–617.

Brzosko, W., Gancarz, Z., and Nowoskawski, A., 1965, Immunofluorescence in the serological diagnosis of *Trichinella spiralis* infection, *Med. Doswi. Mikrobiol.* **17**:325–332.

Cameron, T.W.M., 1960, Trichinosis in Canada, *Wiad. Parazytol.* **6**:304–321.

Campbell, C.H., 1955, The antigenic role of the excretion and secretions of *Trichinella spiralis* in the production of immunity in mice, *J. Parasitol.* **41**:483–491.

Campbell, W.C., 1967, Distribution of *Trichinella spiralis* in the small intestine of young mice, *J. Parasitol.* **53**:395–397.

Campbell, W.C., and Cuckler, A.C., 1966, Further studies on the effects of thiabendazole on trichinosis in swine, with notes on the biology of the infection, *J. Parasitol.* **52**:260–279.

Campbell, W.C., and Yakstis, J.J., 1969, Mating success and fecundity of pairs of *Trichinella* larvae administered to mice, *Wiad. Parazytol.* **15**:526–532.

Castro, G. A., and Fairbairn, D., 1969, Carbohydrates and lipids in *Trichinella spiralis* larvae and their utilization *in vitro, J. Parasitol.* **55**:51–58.

Castro, G.A., Olson, L.J., and Baker, R.D., 1967, Glucose malabsorption and intestinal histopathology in *Trichinella spiralis*-infected guinea pigs, *J. Parasitol.* **53**:595–612.

Castro, G.A., Johnson, L.R., Copeland, E.M., and Dudrick, S.J., 1974, Development of enteric parasites in parenterally fed rats, *Proc. Soc. Exp. Biol. Med.* **146**:703–706.

Castro, G.A., Johnson, L.R., Copeland, E.M., Dudrick, S.J., *et al.*, 1976, Course of infection with enteric parasites in hosts shifted from enteral to total parenteral, J. Parasitol. **62**:353–359.

Cerfontaine, P., 1895, Contribution a l'étude da la trichinose, *Arch. Biol.* **13**:125–145.

Chipman, P.B., 1957, The antigenic role of the excretions and secretions of adult *Trichinella spiralis* in the production of immunity in mice, *J. Parasitol.* **43**:593–598.

Chirasak, K., 1971, Output of larvae and life span of *Trichinella spiralis* in relation to worm burden and superinfection in the mouse, *J. Parasitol.* **57**:289–297.

Chitwood, B.G., 1930, The structure of the esophagus in the Trichuroidea, *J. Parasitol.* **17**:35–42.

Chitwood, M.D., and Chitwood, B.G., 1950, *An Introduction to Nematology*, University Park Press, Baltimore.

Chute, R.M., 1961, Infection of *Trichinella spiralis* in hibernating hamsters, *J. Parasitol.* **47**:25–29.

Chute, R.M., and Covalt, D.B., 1960, The effect of body temperature on the development of *T. spiralis* in bats, *J. Parasitol.* **46**:855–858.

Crandall, C.A., and Kozek, W., 1974, Immunogenicity of the stichosome of *Trichinella spiralis*, in: *Trichinellosis* (C. Kim, ed.), Intext, New York, pp. 231–238.

Crandall, R.B., 1975, Decreased resistance to *Trichinella spiralis* in aged mice, *J. Parasitol.* **63**:566–567.

Debell, J.T., 1965, A long look at neuromuscular junctions in nematodes, *Q. Rev. Biol.* **40**:233–251.

Denham, D.A., 1966, Infections with *Trichinella spiralis* passing from mother to filial mice pre- and post-natally, *J. Helminthol.* **40**:291–296.

Denham, D.A., 1968, Immunity to *Trichinella spiralis*. III. The longevity of the intestinal phase of the infection in mice, *J. Helminthol.* **62**:257–268.

Denham, D.A., and Martinez, A.R., 1970, Studies with methyridine and *Trichinella spiralis*. 2. The use of the drug to study the rate of larval production in mice, *J. Helminthol.* **44**:357–363.

Dennis, D., Despommier, D.D., and Davis, N., 1970, The infectivity of the newborn larva of *Trichinella spiralis* in the rat, *J. Parasitol.* **56**:974–977.

Despommier, D.D., 1971, Immunogenicity of the newborn larva of *Trichinella spiralis*, *J. Parasitol.* **57**:531–535.

Despommier, D.D., 1973, A circular thermal migration device for the rapid collection of large numbers of intestinal helminths, *J. Parasitol.* **59**:933–935.

Despommier, D.D., 1974, The stichocyte of *Trichinella spiralis* during morphogenesis in the small intestine of the rat, in: *Trichinellosis* (C. Kim, ed.), Intext, New York, pp. 239–254.

Despommier, D., 1975, Adaptive changes in muscle fibers infected with *Trichinella spiralis*, *Am. J. Pathol.* **78**:477–496.

Despommier, D., 1976, Musculature. in: *Ecological Aspects of Parasitology* (C.R. Kennedy, ed.), North-Holland, Amsterdam, pp. 270–285.

Despommier, D.D., 1977, Immunity to *Trichinella spiralis*, *Am. J. Trop. Med. Hyg.* **26**:68–75.

Despommier, D.D., and Laccetti, A., 1981, *Trichinella spiralis*: Partial characterization of antigens isolated by immuno-affinity chromatography from the large-particle fraction of the muscle larva, *J. Parasitol.* **67**:332–339.

Despommier, D.D., and Müller, M., 1970, The stichosome of *Trichinella spiralis*: Its structure and function, *J. Parasitol.* **56** (Sect. II, Part I), Second Int. Congr. Parasitol., pp. 76–77.

Despommier, D.D., and Müller, M., 1976, The stichosome and its secretion granules in the mature muscle larva of *Trichinella spiralis*, *J. Parasitol.* **62**:775–785.

Despommier, D.D., and Wostmann, B.S., 1968, Diffusion chambers for inducing immunity to *Trichinella spiralis* in mice, *Exp. Parasitol.* **23**:228–233.

Despommier, D.D., Kajima, M., and Wostmann, B.S., 1967, Ferritin-conjugated antibody studies on the larva of *Trichinella spiralis*, *J. Parasitol.* **53**:618–624.

Despommier, D.D., Aron, L., and Turgeon, L., 1975, *Trichinella spiralis*: Growth of the intracellular (muscle) larva, *Exp. Parasitol.* **37**:108–116.

Despommier, D.D., Campbell, W.C., and Blair, L., 1977, The *in vivo* and *in vitro* analysis of immunity to *Trichinella spiralis* in mice and rats, *Parasitology* **74**:109–119.

Despommier, D., Sukhdeo, M., and Meerovitch, E., 1978, *Trichinella spiralis*: Site selection by the larva during the enteral phase of the infection in mice, *Exp. Parasitol.* **44**:209–215.

Dick, T.A., and Silver, B.B., 1980, Intestinal distribution of *Trichinella spiralis* in rats, *J. Parasitol.* **66**:472–477.

Doerr, R., and Menzl, E., 1933, Studien über den Mechanismus der Trichinelleninfektion. VIII. Vergleichende Untersuchungen über die Empfanglichkiet der Ratte und des Meerschweinchens für die Infektion *per os, Zentralbl. Bakteriol. Parasitenkd. Infektionskr. Hyg. Abt. 1: Orig.* **128**:177–188.

Ducas, R., 1921, L'immunite dans la Trichinose, Thesis, Jouve et Cie, Paris, 47 pp.

Dunlap, G.L., and Weller, C.V., 1933, Pathogenesis of trichinous myocarditis, *Proc. Soc. Exp. Biol. Med.* **30**:1261–1262.

Edney, J.M., Arbogast, F., and Stepp, J., 1953, Productivity in gravid *Trichinella spiralis* (Owen, 1835) transplanted into laboratory rats, *J. Tenn. Acad. Sci.* **28**:62–68.

Faaske, E., and Themann, H., 1961, Elektronmicroskopische Befunde an der Muskelfasen nach Trichinbefall, *Virchows Arch. Pathol. Anat.* **334**:459–474.

Farris, K.N., and Harley, J.P., 1977, *Trichinella spiralis*: Alteration of gastrocnemius muscle kinetics in the mouse, *Exp. Parasitol.* **41**:11–70.

Ferguson, J.D., and Castro, G.A., 1973, Metabolism of intestinal stages of *Trichinella spiralis*, *Am. J. Physiol.* **255**:85–89.

Forrester, A.T., Nelson, G.S., and Sander, G., 1961, The first record of an outbreak of trichinosis in Africa south of the Sahara, *Trans. R. Soc. Trop. Med. Hyg.* **55**:503–513.

Gardiner, C.H., 1976, Habitat and reproductive behavior of *Trichinella spiralis*, *J. Parasitol.* **62**:865–870.

Gaugusch, Z., 1950, Studies on the infection of poikilothermic animals with *T. spiralis*, *Ann. Univ. Mariae Curie-Sklodowska Vet. Med.* **5**(Sect. DD):95–106.

Graham, J.Y., 1897, Beiträge zur Naturgeschichte der *Trichina spiralis*, Arch. Mikrosk. Anat. **50**:219–275.

Gursch, O.F., 1949, Intestinal phase of *Trichinella spiralis* (Owen 1835) Railliet, 1895, *J. Parasitol.* **35**:19–26.

Harley, J.P., and Gallicchico, V., 1971, *Trichinella spiralis*: Migration of larvae in the rat, *Exp. Parasitol.* **30**:11–12.

Heller, M., 1933, Entwickelt sich die *Trichinella spiralis* in der Darmlichtung ihres Wirtes?, *Z. Parasitenkol.* **5**:370–392.

Hemmert-Halswick, A., and Bugge, G., 1934, Trichinen und Trichinose, *Ergeb. Allg. Pathol.* **28**:313–392.

Herbst, G., 1851, Beobachtungen über *Trichina spiralis* in Betreff zu Vebertragung der Ergewudwurmer, *Nachr. Georg-August Univ. Konigl. Ges. Wiss. Goettingen* 262–264.

Hitcho, P.J., and Thorson, R.E., 1971, Possible molting and maturation controls in *Trichinella spiralis*, *J. Parasitol.* **57**:787–793.

Hope, W.D., 1969, Fine structure of the somatic muscles of the free-living marine nematode *Dentostoma californicum* Steiner and Abin 1933 (Leptosomatidae), *Proc. Helminthol. Soc. Wash.* **36**:10–29.

Hughes, W.L., and Harley, J.P., 1977, *Trichinella spiralis*: Taxes of first-stage migratory larvae, *Exp. Parasitol.* **42**:363–373.

Humes, A.G., and Akers, R.P., 1952, Vascular changes in the cheek pouch of the golden hamster during infection with *Trichinella spiralis* larvae, *Anat. Rec.* **114**:103–113.

Jackson, G.J., 1959, Fluorescent antibody studies of *Trichinella spiralis* infections, *J. Infect. Dis.* **105**:97–117.

James, E.R., and Denham, D.A., 1974, The stage specificity of the immune response to *Trichinella spiralis*, in: *Trichinellosis* (C. Kim, ed.), Intext, New York, pp. 345–351.

James, E.R., and Denham, D.A., 1975, Immunity to *Trichinella spiralis*. VI. The specificity of the immune response stimulated by the intestinal stage, *J. Helminthol.* **49**:43–47.

James, E.R., Maloney, A., and Denham, D.A., 1977, Immunity to *Trichinella spiralis*. VII. Resistance stimulated by the parenteral stages of the infection, *J. Parasitol.* **63**:720–723.

Janitschke, B., 1962, Untersuchungen an Meerschweinchen über die Wirkung von Promintic und Ruelene auf Larven von *Trichinella spiralis* und *Toxocara canis*, Dissertation, Free University, Berlin.

Katz, F.F., 1960, The oral transplantation of intestinal stages of *Trichinella spiralis, J. Parasitol.* **46**:500–504.

Kennedy, M.W., 1978, Kinetics of establishment, distribution and expulsion of the enteral phase of *Trichinella spiralis* in the NIH strain of mouse, in: *Trichinellosis* (C. Kim and Z. Pawlowski, eds.), University Press of New England, Hanover, New Hampshire, pp. 193–205.

Kim, C.W., 1961, The cultivation of *Trichinella spiralis in vitro, Am. J. Trop. Med. Hyg.* **10**:742–747.

Kim, C.W., 1962, Further study on the *in vitro* cultivation of *Trichinella spiralis, Am. J. Trop. Med. Hyg.* **11**:491–496.

Kozek, W.J., 1971a, The molting pattern in *Trichinella spiralis*. I. A light microscope study, *J. Parasitol.* **57**:1015–1028.

Kozek, W.J., 1971b, The molting pattern in *Trichinella spiralis*. II. An electron microscopy study, *J. Parasitol.* **57**:1029–1038.

Kozek, W.J., 1975, *Trichinella spiralis*: Morphological characteristics of male and female intestine-infecting larvae, *Exp. Parasitol.* **37**:380–387.

Kozek, W.J., and Crandall, C.A., 1974, Immunogenicity of the stichosome of *Trichinella spiralis* in mice, in: *Trichinellosis* (C. Kim, ed.), Intext, New York, pp. 231–237.

Kuitunen-Ekbaum, E., and Webster, D., 1947, Trichinosis in wild rats in Toronto, *Can. J. Public Health* **38**:76–78.

Larsh, J.E., Jr., and Hendricks, J.R., 1949, The probable explanation for the differences in localization of adult *Trichinella spiralis* in young and old mice, *J. Parasitol.* **35**:101–106.

Lee, T.D.G., and Wright, K.A., 1978, The morphology of the attachment and probable feeding site of the nematode, *Trichuris muris* (Shrank 1788) Hall 1916, *Can. J. Zool.* **56**:1889–1905.

Leonard, A.B., and Beahm, E.H., 1941, Studies on the distribution of *Trichinella* larvae in the albino rat, *Trans. Kans. Acad. Sci.* **44**:419–433.

Leuckart, R., 1860, *Untersuchungen über Trichina spiralis*, Winter, Leipzig, 57 pp.

Lightner, L.K., and Ulmer, M.J., 1974, *Trichinella spiralis*: Effect of environmental temperature on mice, *Exp. Parasitol.* **35**:262–265.

Lison, L., 1936, *Histochimie Animale*, Gautier-Villars, Paris.

Mackenzie, C.D., Preston, P.M., and Ogilvie, B.M., 1978, Immunological properties of the surface of parasitic nematodes, *Nature (London)* **276**:826–827.

Maier, D.M., and Zaiman, H., 1966, The development of lysosomes in rat skeletal muscle in trichinosis myositis, J. Histochem. Cytochem. **14**:396–400.

Manku, S., and Hamilton, R., 1972, The effect of sex and sex hormones on the infection of rats by *Trichinella spiralis, Can. J. Zool.* **50**:597–602.

Matoff, K., 1935, Versuche zur Feststellung der Mindestzahl von Muskeltrichinellen, welche zur Invadierung von Mäusen, Ratten, Meerschweinchen, Kaninchen und Hunden erförderlich ist, *Tierarztl. Rundsch* **41**:466–471.

Matoff, K., 1961, Further studies on muscle trichinellosis produced by infection with intestinal forms, *Z. Parasitenkd.* **20**:470–476.

Matoff, K., 1963, On the transplantation of young intestinal trichinellae, *Z. Parasitenkd.* **22**:495–513.

Mauss, E.A., and Otto, G.F., 1942, The occurrence of *Trichinella spiralis* larvae in tissues other than skeletal muscles, *J. Lab. Clin. Med.* **27**:1384–1387.

McCoy, O.R., 1932, Experimental trichiniasis infections in monkeys, *Proc. Soc. Exp. Biol. Med.* **30**:85–86.

McCoy, O.R., 1936, The development of trichinae in abnormal environments, *J. Parasitol.* **22**:54–59.

McCoy, O.R., 1940, Rapid loss of *Trichinella* larvae fed to immune rats and its bearing on the mechanisms of immunity, *Am. J. Hyg.* **32:**105–116.

McCue, J.F., and Thorson, R.E., 1965, Host effects on the migration of *Nippostrongylus brasiliensis* in a thermal gradient, *J. Parasitol.* **51:**414–417.

McLaren, D.L., 1976, Nematode sense organs, in: *Advances in Parasitology*, Vol. 14 (B. Dawes, ed.), Academic Press, New York, pp. 195–265.

Meerovitch, E., 1962, *In vitro* development of *Trichinella spiralis* larvae, *J. Parasitol. (Suppl.)* **48:**34.

Meerovitch, E., 1965a, Studies on the *in vitro* axenic development of *Trichinella spiralis*. I. Basic culture techniques, pattern of development and the effects of the gaseous phase, *Can. J. Zool.* **43:**69–79.

Meerovitch, E., 1965b, Studies on the *in vitro* axenic development of *Trichinella spiralis*. II. Preliminary experiments on the effects of farnesol, cholesterol, and an insect extract, *Can. J. Zool.* **43:**81–85.

Mikhail, E.G., and Soliman, A.A., 1978, Productivity of one pair of *Trichinella spiralis* larvae administered to rats, *J. Egypt. Soc. Parasitol.* **8:**219–226.

Mills, C.K., and Kent, N.H., 1965, Excretions and secretions of *Trichinella spiralis* and their role in immunity, *Exp. Parasitol.* **16:**300–310.

Most, H., and Abeles, M.M., 1937, Trichinosis involving the nervous system: A clinical and neuropathologic review, with report of two cases, *Arch. Neurol. Psychiatry* **37:**589–616.

Nelson, G.S., and Forrester, A.T.T., 1962, Trichinosis in Kenya, *Wiad. Parazytol.* **8:**17–28.

Nelson, G.S., Blackie, E.J., and Mukundi, S., 1966, Comparative studies of geographical strains of *Trichinella spiralis*, *Trans. R. Soc. Trop. Med. Hyg.* **60:**471–480.

Nolf, L.O., 1937, The transplantation of gravid *Trichinella spiralis*, *J. Parasitol.* **23:**574.

Novoselska, L.S., 1974, Common features between cuticle antigens of *Trichinella* larvae and hen, dog, and guinea pig muscles, *C. R. Acad. Bulg. Sci.* **27:**12–21.

Oliver, V.L., 1961, The distribution of trichinae larvae in the muscles of experimentally infected rats, Dissertation, University of Alabama, 56 pp.

Olsen, B.S., Villella, J.B., and Gould, S.E., 1964, Distribution of *Trichinella spiralis* in muscles of experimentally infected swine, *J. Parasitol.* **50:**489–495.

Pagenstecher, H.A., 1865, *Die Trichinen*, Engelmanns, Leipzig, 116 pp.

Pawlowski, Z., 1967a, Hormones of the adrenal cortex in experimental trichinellosis of rats. I. Effect of prednisone on the number of mature and larval forms, *Acta Parasitol. Pol.* **14:**163–172.

Pawlowski, Z., 1967b, Adrenal cortex hormones in intestinal trichinellosis. II. Effect of adrenalectomy, desoxycorticosterone and glucocorticoids on the course of trichinellosis in rats, *Acta Parasitol. Pol.* **15:**157–170.

Pawlowski, Z., 1967c, Adrenal cortex hormones in intestinal trichinellosis. III. Effects of adrenalectomy and hydrocortisone, insulin, alloxan and glucose treatment on elimination of *Trichinella spiralis* adult in hooded rats, *Acta Parasitol. Pol.* **15:**179–189.

Penkova, R.A., and Romanenko, L.N., 1973, Studies on *Trichinella* chromosomes, *Tr. Vses. Inst. Gel'mintol. K.I. Skryabina* **20:**133–142.

Perrudet-Badoux, A., and Binaghi, R.A., 1978, Immunity against newborn *Trichinella spiralis* larvae in previously infected mice, *J. Parasitol.* **64:**187–189.

Perrudet-Badoux, A., Binaghi, R.A., and Biozzi, G., 1975, *Trichinella* infestation in mice genetically selected for high and low antibody production, *Immunology* **29:**387–390.

Perrudet-Bodoux, A., Binaghi, R.A., and Bonssac-Aron, Y., 1978, *Trichinella spiralis* infection in mice: Mechanism of the resistance in animals genetically selected for high and low antibody production, *Immunology* **35:**519–522.

Podhajecky, K., 1962, Localization of intestinal trichinellae in the small intestine of mice in their intestinal phase, *Wiad. Parazytol.* **8:**633–636.

Podhajecky, K., 1963, Male–female ratio of *Trichinella spiralis* in various phases of infection in white mice, *Biologia* **18:**75–78.

Przyjalkowski, Z., 1968, Effect of intestinal flora and of a monoculture of *E. coli* on the development of intestinal and muscular *Trichinella spiralis* in gnotobiotic mice, *Bull. Acad. Pol. Sci. Cl. 2* **16:**433–437.

Przyjalkowski, Z.W., and Golinska, Z., 1978, Host response to intestinal infection with *Trichinella spiralis* and *Trichinella pseudospiralis* in germ-free and conventional mice, in: *Trichinellosis* (C. Kim and Z.S. Pawlowski, eds.), University Press of New England, Hanover, New Hampshire, pp. 141–150.

Przyjalkowski, Z., and Wescott, R., 1969, *Trichinella spiralis:* Establishment in gnotobiotic mice infected by *Bacillus mesentericus, B. subtilis,* and *Pseudomonas aeruginosa, Exp. Parasitol.* **25:**8–12.

Purkerson, M., and Despommier, D.D., 1974, Fine structure of the muscle phase of *Trichinella spiralis* in the mouse, in: *Trichinellosis* (C. Kim, ed.), Intext, New York, pp. 7–23.

Ramisz, A., 1965, Studies on the nervous system of nematodes by means of histochemical method for active acetycholinesterase. I. *Trichinella spiralis* and *Syphacia abvelata. Acta Parasitol. Pol.* **13:**205–214.

Rappaport, I., 1943, A comparison of three strains of *Trichinella spiralis.* II. Longevity and sex ratios of adults in the intestine and rapidity of larval development in the musculature, *Am. J. Trop. Med. Hyg.* **23:**351–362.

Rausch, R.L., 1962, Trichinellosis in the Arctic. in: Trichinellosis (Z. Kozar, ed.), Pol. Sci. Publ., Warsaw, pp. 80–86.

Ribas-Mujal, D., and Rivera-Pomar, J.M., 1968, Biological significance of the early structural alterations in skeletal muscle fibers infected by *Trichinella spiralis, Virchows Arch. A* **345:**154–168.

Richels, I., 1955, Histologische Studien zu den Problemen der Zellkonstanz: Untersuchungen zur Mikroskopischen Anatomie im Lebenszyklus von *Trichinella spiralis, Zentralbl. Bakteriol.* **163:**46–84.

Ritterson, A.L., 1959, Innate resistance of species of hamsters to *Trichinella spiralis* and its reversal by cortisone, *J. Infect. Dis.* **105:**253–266.

Ritterson, A.L., 1966, Nature of the cyst of *Trichinella spiralis, J. Parasitol.* **52:**157–161.

Rivera-Ortiz, C.I., and Nussenzweig, R., 1976, *Trichinella spiralis:* Anaphylactic antibody formation and susceptibility in strains of inbred mice, *Exp. Parasitol.* **39:**7–17.

Roth, H., 1938, On the localization of adult trichinae in the intestine, *J. Parasitol.* **24:**225–231.

Roth, H., 1939, Experimental studies on the course of trichina infection in guinea pigs. II. Natural susceptibility of the guinea pig to experimental trichina infection, *Am. J. Hyg.* **29:**(Sect. D):89–104.

Ruitenberg, E.J., and Steerenberg, P.A., 1976, Immunogenicity of the parenteral stages of *Trichinella spiralis, J. Parasitol.* **62:**164–166.

Ruitenberg, E.J., Elgersma, A., Kruizinga, W., *et al.* 1977, *Trichinella spiralis* in congenitally athymic (nude) mice: Parasitological, serological and haematological studies with observations on intestinal pathology, *Immunology* **33:**581–587.

Sakamoto, T., 1979, Development and behavior of adult and larval *Trichinella* cultured *in vitro, Mem. Fac. Agric. Kagoshima Univ.* **15**(24):107–114.

Saowakontha, S., 1975, The relationship between protein–calorie malnutrition and trichinosis. II. Immunological response in rats fed low and high protein diets, *Southeast Asian J. Trop. Med. Public Health* **6:**79–81.

Sawitz, W., 1939, *Trichinella spiralis*: Incidence of infection in man, dogs and cats in the New Orleans area as determined in postmortem examinations, *Arch. Pathol.* **28**:11–21.

Schoop, G., Lieb, W.A., and Lamina, J., 1961, Die Parasiten des Auges: Tierexperimentelle Untersuchungen über die Trichinose des Auges, *Klin. Monatsbl. Augenheilkd.* **139**:433–465.

Schope, M., 1949, Encephalitis bei der Trichinose mit Nachweis einer *Trichinella* in Gehirm, *Arch. Psychiatr. Nervenkr.* **181**:603–610.

Schwartz, B., 1938, Trichinosis in swine and its relationship to public health, *J. Am. Vet. Med. Assoc.* **92**:317–337.

Shanta, C.S., and Meerovitch, E., 1967, The life cycle of *Trichinella spiralis*. I. The intestinal phase of development, *Can. J. Zool.* **45**:1255–1260.

Smirnov, G.G., 1963, Natural modality of trichinellosis in the Arctic, *Ter. Arkh.* **42**:338–344.

Stannard, J.N., McCoy, O.R., and Latchford, W.B., 1938, Studies on the metabolism of *Trichinella spiralis* larvae, *Am. J. Hyg.* **27**:666–682.

Staubli, C., 1905, Klinische und experimentelle Untersuchungen über Trichinosis, *Verh. Kongress. Med. (Wiesbaden)* **22**:353–362.

Stefanski, W., and Przyjalkowski, Z., 1964, The influence of certain bacteria on the establishment of trichinae in the digestive tract of the mouse, *Bull. Acad. Vet. Fr.* **37**:131–135.

Stefanski, W., and Kozar, M., 1969, Degree of resistance of some mouse strains to *Trichinella spiralis* infections, *Wiad. Parazytol.* **15**:571–575.

Stewart, G.L., 1973, Studies on chemical pathology in trichinosis, Thesis, Rice University, Houston.

Stewart, G., 1978, *Trichinella spiralis*: Alterations of blood chemistry in the mouse, *Exp. Parasitol.* **45**:287–297.

Stewart, G.L., and Charniga, L.M., 1980, Distribution of *Trichinella spiralis* in muscles of the mouse, *J. Parasitol.* **66**:688–689.

Stewart, G.L., and Read, C.P., 1972, Ribonucleic acid metabolism in mouse trichinosis, *J. Parasitol.* **58**:252–256.

Stewart, G.L., and Read, C.P., 1973a, Desoxyribonucleic acid metabolism in mouse trichinosis, *J. Parasitol.* **59**:164–167.

Stewart, G.L., and Read, C.P., 1973b, Changes in RNA in mouse trichinosis, *J. Parasitol.* **59**:997–1005.

Stewart, G.L., and Read, C.P., 1974, Studies on biochemical changes in trichinosis. I. Changes in myoglobin, free creatine, phosphocreatine, and two protein fractions in mouse muscle, *J. Parasitol.* **60**:996–1000.

Stewart, G.L., Krama, G.W., Reddington, J.J., and Hamilton, M., 1980, Studies on *in vitro* larvaposition by adult *Trichinella spiralis*, *J. Parasitol.* **66**:94–99.

Stoner, R.D., and Hankes, L.V., 1955, Incorporation of C^{14}-labelled amino acids by *Trichinella spiralis* larvae, *Exp. Parasitol.* **4**:435–444.

Sukhdeo, M.V.K., and Croll, N.A., 1981, The location of parasites within their hosts: Factors affecting longitudinal distribution of *Trichinella spiralis* in the small intestine, *Int. J. Parasitol.* **11**:163–168.

Sukhdeo, M.V.K., and Meerovitch, E., 1977, Comparison of three geographical isolates of *Trichinella*, *Can. J. Zool.* **55**:2060–2064.

Sulzer, A.J., 1965, Indirect fluorescent antibody tests for parasitic diseases. I. Preparation of a stable antigen from larvae of *Trichinella spiralis*, *J. Parasitol.* **56**:717–721.

Tanner, C.E., 1968, Relationship between infecting dose, muscle parasitism, and antibody response in experimental trichinosis in rabbits, *J. Parasitol.* **54**:98–107.

Tanner, C.E., 1978, The susceptibility to *Trichinella spiralis* of inbred lines of mice differing at the H-2 histocompatibility locus, *J. Parasitol.* **64**:956–957.

Tarakanov, V.I., 1963, The *in vitro* cultivation of *Trichinella spiralis*, the agent of trichinellosis, in: *Gelminty Tcheloveka, Zhivatnykh, i Rastenii i Borba s Nimi*, Moscow, pp. 78–82.

Tarakanov, V.I., 1964, The culture of *Trichinella spiralis* larvae up to the sexually mature stage in artificial nutrient media, *Veterinariya (Moscow)* **3**:43–47.

Tarakanov, V.I., 1970, The influence of artificial nutrient media on the *in vitro* development of *Trichinella* larvae, *Tr. Vses. Inst. Gel'mintol. imeni K.I. Skryabina* **16**:249–252.

Tarakanov, V.I., and Krasnova, L.L., 1971, The *in vitro* cultivation of decapsulated *Trichinella spiralis* larvae in a system of constant flow nutrient medium, *Tr. Vses. Inst. Gel'mintol. K.I. Skryabina* **17**:229–231.

Teppema, J.S., Robinson, J.E., and Ruitenberg, E.J., 1973, Ultrastructural aspects of capsule formation in *Trichinella spiralis* infections in rats, *Parasitology* **66**:291–296.

Thomas, H., 1965, Beitrage zur Biologie und mikroskopischen Anatomie von *Trichinella spiralis* Owen, 1835, *Z. Tropenmed. Parasitol.* **16**:148–180.

Thornbury, F.J., 1897, The pathology of trichinosis: Original observations, *Univ. Med. Mag.* **10**:64–79.

Van Cott, J.M., and Lintz, W., 1914, Trichinosis, *J. Am. Med. Assoc.* **62**:680–684.

Van Someren, V.D., 1939, On the presence of a buccal stylet in adult *Trichinella*, and the mode of feeding of the adults, *J. Helminthol.* **17**:83–92.

Villella, J.B., 1958, Observations on the time and number of molts in the intestinal phase of *Trichinella spiralis*, *J. Parasitol.* **44**:41.

Villella, J.B., 1966, Morphologic criteria for distinguishing the sex of *Trichinella spiralis* larvae from muscle, *J. Parasitol.* **52**:908–910.

Villella, J.B., 1970, Life cycle and morphology, in: *Trichinosis in Man and Animals* (S.E. Gould, ed.), Charles C. Thomas, Springfield, Illinois, pp. 19–60.

Virchow, R., 1859, Recherches sur le development du *Trichina spiralis*, *C. R. Acad. Sci.* **49**:660–662.

Von Brand, T., Weinstein, P.P., Mellman, B., and Weinbach, E.C., 1952, Observations on the metabolism of bacteria-free larvae of *Trichinella spiralis*, *Exp. Parasitol.* **1**:245–255.

Wakelin, D., 1980, Genetic control of immunity to parasites. Infection with *Trichinella spiralis* in inbred and congenic mice showing rapid and slow responses to infection, *Parasite Immunol.* **3**:85–98.

Wassom, D.L., David, C.S., and Gleich, G.J., 1979, Genes within the major histocompatibility complex influence susceptibility to *Trichinella spiralis* in the mouse, *Immunogenetics* **9**:491–496.

Weller, T.H., 1943, The development of the larvae of *Trichinella spiralis* in roller tube tissue culture, *Am. J. Pathol.* **19**:502–515.

Wolfthugel, K., 1938, Wieviel eingekapselte Trichinen (*Trichinella spiralis*) erzeugt ein Muttertier?, *Z. Fleisch-Milchhyg.* **48**:301–302.

Wright, K., 1979, *Trichinella spiralis*: An intracellular parasite in the intestinal phase, *J. Parasitol.* **65**:441–445.

Wright, K.A., and Hope, W.D., 1968, Elaborations of the cuticle of *Acanthonchus duplicatus* Weiser, 1959 (Nematoda: Cyatholaimidae), as revealed by light and electron microscopy, *Can. J. Zool.* **46**:1005–1011.

Wu, L.Y., 1955a, Studies on *Trichinella spiralis*. I. Male and female reproductive system, *J. Parasitol.* **41**:40–47.

Wu, L.Y., 1955b, The development of the stichosome and associated structures in *Trichinella spiralis*, *Can. J. Zool.* **33**:440–466.

Wu, L.Y., and Kingscote, A.A., 1957, Studies on *Trichinella spiralis*. II. Times of final molts, spermatozoa formation, ovulation, and insemination, *Can. J. Zool.* **35**:207–211.

Zimmerman, E.A., Hsu, K.C., Robinson, A.G., Carmel, P.W., Franz, A.G., and Tannenbaum, M., 1973, Studies of neurophysin secreting neurons with immunoperoxidase techniques employing antibody to bovine neurophysin. I. Light microscopic findings in monkeys and bovine tissues, *Endocrinology* **92**:931–940.

Zimmermann, W.J., Hubbard, E.D., Schwarte, L.H., and Biester, H.E., 1962, *Trichinella spiralis* in Iowa wildlife during the years 1953 to 1961, *J. Parasitol.* **48**:429–432.

Zuckerman, B.M., (ed.), 1980, *Nematodes as Biological Models*, Vol. II, Academic Press, New York.

4

Biochemistry

GEORGE L. STEWART

1. INTRODUCTION

Most studies on the biochemistry of *Trichinella spiralis* have dealt with the muscle larva. This stage in the life cycle of the parasite has enjoyed the greatest amount of attention primarily for three reasons: First, it is relatively simple to isolate large numbers of muscle larvae for biochemical analyses. Second, the muscle larva establishes with the host striated myofiber one of the most intimate and complex relationships seen among intracellular helminth parasites (see Chapter 7). Finally, the muscle larva plays a major role in the development of the primary pathological lesions in trichinosis (myositis and myocarditis).

The few studies that have been conducted on adult worms clearly indicate that their biochemistry differs in some important ways from that of the muscle larvae. These findings emphasize the need for acquiring a more thorough understanding of the biochemistry of adult *T. spiralis*. No information is at present available on the biochemistry of newborn larvae. Since these forms are exposed during their migratory phase to a variety of environments (including those in which the adult worms and the muscle larvae are found), investigation of their biochemistry would be important.

GEORGE L. STEWART • Laboratory of Parasitology, Department of Biology, The University of Texas, Arlington, Texas 76019.

2. CARBOHYDRATES AND CARBOHYDRATE METABOLISM

2.1. Adult Worms

Total carbohydrates comprise 3.3% of the dry weight of adult *T. spiralis* (Ferguson and Castro, 1973). For some time, it has been known that adult worms contain little glycogen (Oliver-Gonzalez and Bueding, 1948; Kozar *et al.*, 1966). This was recently confirmed quantitatively by Ferguson and Castro (1973), who reported that glycogen accounts for only 1.3% and trehalose for only 1.7% of the dry weight of adult worms. These authors suggested that the paucity of stored carbohydrates in adult worms underlies their inability to survive in Krebs–Ringer bicarbonate buffer (KRB) for more than 12 hr in the absence of exogenous glucose. This explanation is supported by the finding that adult worms survive *in vitro* for at least 48 hr in KRB containing 5 mM glucose (Ferguson and Castro, 1973) and absorb substantial quantities of glucose during short-term incubations *in vitro* (Castro and Fairbairn, 1969c).

Excretion of volatile fatty acids by adult worms and their survival for 48 hr during incubation under anaerobic conditions in KRB (5 mM glucose present) indicate that adults are capable of obtaining energy through fermentations. Under anaerobic conditions, adult worms produce the same fermentation acids as do muscle larvae [formic, acetic, propionic, *n*-pentanoic (*n*-valeric), *n*-butyric, and *n*-hexanoic (*n*-caproic) acids]. However, the total amount of acid excreted by adult worms is approximately one third that produced by an equal number of larvae (Ferguson and Castro, 1973). These findings are in opposition to those of Oliver-Gonzalez and Bueding (1948), who were unable to demonstrate production of fatty acids by adult worms incubated in balanced salt solution containing glucose. It is of interest to note that volatile fatty acids are excreted by other adult nematodes during degradation of carbohydrates (see von Brand, 1979). Future studies on adult worms should include identification and characterization of enzymes of the glycolytic sequence as well as a search for the pathways by which fermentation acids are produced by this stage.

Evidence presented in Section 4.1 suggests that adult worms maintained under aerobic conditions are capable of utilizing fatty acids via the beta-oxidation pathway. Ferguson and Castro (1973) suggest that acetyl-CoA resulting from the latter pathway may be completely oxidized via the Krebs cycle, a situation similar to that seen in developing eggs of *Ascaris lumbricoides* (Ward and Fairbairn, 1970). However, before any firm conclusions can be drawn concerning the importance of the Krebs cycle in carbohydrate metabolism in adult worms, the enzymes involved in this pathway must be identified and characterized.

2.2. Muscle Larvae

Total carbohydrates make up 21.1% (according to Castro and Fairbairn, 1969b) or 19.8% (according to Kurylo-Borowska and Kozar, 1960) of the dry weight of muscle larvae. Several workers have reported that muscle larvae contain large amounts of glycogen (von Brand et al., 1952; Castro and Fairbairn, 1969b; De Nollin and Van den Bossche, 1973; Stewart, 1976). Castro and Fairbairn (1969b) found that 15.9% of larval dry weight is glycogen, while von Brand et al. (1952) reported that glycogen accounts for 12% of the dry weight of muscle larvae. Although the glycogen content of the larvae on their arrival in the host muscle fibers is unknown, Stewart (1976) showed an increase in the glycogen content of muscle larva between days 16 ($0.025/\mu g$ glycogen per larva) and 34 ($0.0595/\mu g$ glycogen per larva) postinfection. The greatest amount of glycogen is found in the muscle cells of the worm, while other organs that contain histochemically demonstrable glycogen include (in order of decreasing glycogen content) the stichosome, lateral lines, midgut, esophagus, hindgut, genital primordia, and dorsal and ventral lines (Beckett and Boothroyd, 1962). Fairbairn (1958) reported that free glucose accounts for 0.04% and trehalose for 1.76% of the dry weight of larvae, while Castro and Fairbairn (1969b) found that trehalose constitutes 4.8% of the dry weight of larvae, and glucose is present in "trace" amounts. The actual function and significance of trehalose are at present unknown and provide an interesting subject for future investigation.

Muscle larvae readily absorb glucose during incubation in KRB at 37°C (Castro and Fairbairn, 1969c; De Nollin and Van den Bossche, 1973). During 3-hr incubations in vitro in KRB containing labeled glucose, muscle larvae incorporate 98% of total radioactivity absorbed into acid-soluble glycogen, protein, and lipid fractions. A majority of label is found in the carbohydrate fraction (Castro et al., 1973b). There remains some question concerning the site of absorption of organic substances by muscle larvae. Castro and Fairbairn (1969a) suggest that the intestinal surface is the primary site for absorption of organic substances by parasitic nematodes, while the work of others (see von Brand, 1979) has emphasized the importance of the cuticular surface of nematodes in this regard. Larvae incubated in vitro in the absence of exogenous glucose rapidly break down endogenous stores of glycogen (von Brand et al., 1952; Castro and Fairbairn, 1969b) and trehalose (Castro and Fairbairn, 1969b). During aerobic or anaerobic incubation in vitro for 48 hr in KRB at 37°C, larvae utilize around 70% of their glycogen and about 60% of endogenous trehalose (Castro and Fairbairn, 1969b). Glycogen-consumption data in this study confirm those of von

Brand *et al.* (1952), who reported that larvae consume about 38% of their glycogen reserves during 24-hr aerobic or anaerobic incubation *in vitro*. Volatile fatty acids excreted during aerobic and anaerobic fermentations are quantitatively and qualitatively similar (von Brand *et al.*, 1952; Castro and Fairbairn, 1969b). These include *n*-valeric, *n*-caproic, acetic (von Brand *et al.*, 1952; Agosin and Aravena, 1959; Castro and Fairbairn, 1969b), formic, propionic, and *n*-butyric acids (von Brand *et al.*, 1952; Castro and Fairbairn, 1969b). In all studies, *n*-valeric acid was the predominant end product of aerobic and anaerobic fermentations. This fatty acid is readily demonstrable by gas–liquid chromatographic methods in the muscles of trichinous hogs (Hill *et al.*, 1970).

Traces of lactic acid are excreted during anaerobic (von Brand *et al.*, 1952; Agosin and Aravena, 1959) and aerobic (von Brand *et al.*, 1952) incubations. In larval homogenates, degradation of glucose to lactic acid appears to be an important pathway in carbohydrate catabolism (Goldberg, 1958b; Agosin and Aravena, 1959). A similar situation is seen with *A. lumbricoides* (von Brand, 1973; Fairbairn, 1970. Only traces of lactate are produced by intact *Ascaris* (von Brand, 1934), while homogenates of *Ascaris* muscle produce lactate as the major end product of fermentation (Bueding and Yale, 1951; Rathbone and Rees, 1954). In *Ascaris*, fatty acids are produced via "extended glycolysis" (see Fairbairn, 1970), which involves production of pyruvate from malate in the mitochondria of the worm. Pyruvate does not freely diffuse out of the mitochondrion and is not available to be reduced to lactate by lactate dehydrogenase (LDH) present only in the cytoplasm. However, on homogenization of *Ascaris*, this intracellular compartmentalization would be broken down, and increased amounts of lactic acid could be produced. A similar explanation may be offered for the differences seen in lactate production by intact *Trichinella* larvae as compared to larval homogenates.

As pointed out by Fairbairn (1970), it may be of considerable advantage to both the host and the parasite for the parasite to excrete weak acids such as succinic and the volatile fatty acids rather than lactic acid, a much stronger acid. This is an especially important point with regard to the larva of *T. spiralis*, which is restricted to the confines of a host myofiber for the entire life of the host (Fairbairn, 1970). On the other hand, von Brand (1970) points out that the final steps in the pathway leading to the formation of fermentation acids are more vulnerable to alteration during preparation of larval homogenates than is glycolysis itself.

The importance of the glycolytic sequence in the early phase of sugar catabolism is emphasized by the work of Goldberg (1958b), Agosin and Aravena (1959), and Ward *et al.* (1969). Goldberg (1958) demonstrated the presence of hexokinase, phosphofructokinase, aldolase, α-glycerophosphate dehydrogenase, glyceraldehyde-3-phosphate dehydrogenase, enolase, and LDH. Agosin and Aravena (1959) found that worm homogenates catalyze the phosphorylation of glucose, fructose, mannose, and glucosamine in the presence of ATP and Mg^{2+}. However, among these sugars, glucose is the preferred substrate for this reaction. These same authors confirmed the presence of the glycolytic enzymes identified by Goldberg (1958b). The ability of muscle larvae to carry out glycolytic phosphorylation is suggested by these studies with larval homogenates.

Ward *et al.* (1969) investigated the pathways involved in the production of fermentation acids in homogenates of muscle larvae. The activities of phosphoenolpyruvate (PEP) carboxylase and PEP carboxytransphosphorylase are very low. The activity of PEP carboxykinase in larval homogenates is very high, and the pyruvate kinase/PEP carboxykinase ratio is 0.31. In addition, homogenates exhibit very high malate dehydrogenase activity and a low malic enzyme and LDH activity. The quality and proportion of enzymes described above are reminiscent of those seen in several other parasitic helminths known to produce succinic and volatile fatty acids (see Ward *et al.*, 1969). From these findings, Ward *et al.* (1969) suggested that larvae possess a modification of the classic Embden–Meyerhoff pathway. The degradation of sugar proceeds via the glycolytic sequence to PEP. This substrate is converted to oxaloacetate by PEP carboxykinase. Oxaloacetate is in turn converted to malate by the highly active malate dehydrogenase with concomitant oxidation of the $NADH_2$ formed earlier during glycolysis. The formation of malate involves enzymes located in the cytoplasm. If this system is similar to the one described for *Ascaris* (Saz, 1971; Cheah, 1974), malate will cross over into the mitochondria, where some of this substrate is converted to pyruvate by malic enzyme and the remainder is converted to succinate (via fumarate) by the action of fumarate reductase. A link between fumarate reductase and the cytochrome system is present in muscle larvae in the form of a rhodoquinone (Allen, 1974). The pathway outlined above could play a role in the energy economy of muscle larvae, since in *Ascaris* the reduction of fumarate during succinate formation results in the generation of ATP. Pyruvate and succinate may serve as precursors in the formation of a variety of fatty acids (Saz, 1971).

Some evidence points to the presence of at least a partial pentose phosphate pathway in muscle larvae (Agosin and Aravena, 1959; Kozar *et al.*, 1965; Karpiak *et al.*, 1965; Boczon, 1974; Kozar and Seniuta, 1974). Of the numerous enzymes involved in the complete pathway, only 2-hexokinase (Agosin and Aravena, 1959), glucose-6-phosphate dehydrogenase (Agosin and Aravena, 1959; Boczon, 1974; Kozar and Seniuta, 1974), and phosphogluconate dehydrogenase (Boczon, 1974; Kozar and Seniuta, 1974) have been demonstrated. Kozar *et al.* (1965) reported greater stimulation of larval oxygen consumption by xylose and ribose-5-phosphate than by glucose. Kozar *et al.* (1965) have suggested that a partial pentose phosphate pathway may be operative in muscle larvae. However, the importance of the role played by this sequence in the metabolism of larvae remains undefined. The experimental approach that might provide conclusive proof for the existence of a pentose phosphate cycle in *T. spiralis* larvae was outlined earlier by von Brand (1979).

Goldberg (1957) demonstrated the presence of aconitase, isocitrate dehydrogenase, α-ketoglutarate dehydrogenase, succinate dehydrogenase, fumarase, and malate dehydrogenase in homogenates of *T. spiralis* larvae and reported the formation of citrate in larval homogenates exposed to oxaloacetate and acetate. In addition, oxygen uptake by homogenates is stimulated by succinate and α-ketoglutarate. On the other hand, Boczon (1967) found very low isocitrate dehydrogenase activity in larval homogenates (100 times lower than in mammalian tissues). Karpiak *et al.* (1965) suggest that the Krebs cycle is insignificant in larvae, while von Brand (1970) points out that the Krebs cycle may be involved in lipid or protein utilization by larvae rather than in the breakdown of carbohydrates. An alternative explanation for the apparent contradictions described above is offered by Fairbairn (1970). The presence of these components may reflect preparation by the muscle larva for rapid development to an adult worm that possesses a functional aerobic metabolism (Ferguson and Castro, 1973). Additional studies on the function of Krebs-cycle enzymes and cytochrome activity in larvae and adult worms are needed (Fairbairn, 1970).

More thorough analyses have been made of several enzymes found in larvae. The activity of ATPase in larval homogenates requires Mg^{2+}, while addition of Ca^{2+} and F^- in the presence of Mg^{2+} inhibits enzyme activity. The activities of hexokinase and phosphofructokinase in larval homogenates require Mg^{2+} and ATP. Phosphofructokinase exhibits the broad optimum pH range of 6–8.5. The effects of various metals on aldolase activity were investigated. Of the eight metals tested, none stimulates enzyme activity in larvae above the level seen in the absence of metals. In fact, complete suppression of aldolase activity occurs in the presence of Cu^{2+}, while Zn^{2+} and Fe^{2+} cause moderate suppression.

Metal-binding agents had no affect on aldolase activity. Larval glyceraldehyde-3-phosphate dehydrogenase is activated by cysteine, a situation similar to the one seen in yeast and in mammalian muscle. The activity of this enzyme is inhibited by 3.3×10^{-4} M iodoacetate (Agosin and Aravena, 1959). Phosphoglucose isomerase (PGI) was studied in some detail following a 48-fold concentration of the enzyme (Mancilla and Agosin, 1960). The PGI of muscle larvae differs substantially from that of host muscle. The optimum pH for this larval enzyme is 8.0 compared to 8.6 for the rabbit muscle enzyme. The parasite PGI shows greater heat stability than that from other sources. Finally, Mg^{2+} inhibits PGI from rabbit muscle, but has no effect on the larval enzyme. Dusanic (1966, 1967) found that saline extracts of larvae contain two electrophoretically separable isoenzymes of LDH. The larval enzyme has a lower optimum pH, is more heat-stable, and reacts differently with divalent cations compared to LDH recovered from rabbit muscle. Carboxykinase isolated from muscle larvae displays cation requirements and nucleotide specificity similar to those of the enzyme isolated from vertebrate tissue. Both enzymes require Mn^{2+} ions, and GDP and IDP are the most effective nucleotide cofactors (Ward et al., 1969).

It appears that muscle larvae rely heavily on a modification of the classic Embden–Meyerhoff pathway ["extended glycolysis" (Saz, 1971)] for energy production. A role for aerobic pathways in the energy economy of muscle larvae is questionable (see Section 3.2).

3. RESPIRATION

3.1. Adult Worms

Although cytochrome oxidase and cytochrome c reductase are present in homogenates of adult worms, they reportedly display lower activity than the enzymes present in larval homogenates (Goldberg, 1957). The presence of succinic dehydrogenase and cytochrome oxidase in adult worms was demonstrated in a histochemical study (Kozar et al., 1966). Oliver-Gonzalez and Bueding (1948) reported that the rate of oxygen uptake by adult worms is less than that for muscle larvae. Contrary to these findings, Ferguson and Castro (1973) observed no detectable oxygen uptake by muscle larvae, while adult worms took up about 14 μl O_2/mg protein per hr. Oxygen uptake by adults was completely inhibited by cyanide, and worms were more active in the presence than in the absence of oxygen. The fact that adult worms readily oxidize lipids indicates that oxygen is of physiological importance in their metabolism (Ferguson and Castro, 1973). In support of this hypothesis, Berntzen (1965) demonstrated that the development *in vitro* of adult worms proceeds best under aerobic conditions. Future work on adult worms should include a careful reexamination of the electron-transport system in adults as well as identification and analysis of the activities of enzymes involved in oxidative metabolic pathways.

3.2. Muscle Larvae

Stannard *et al.* (1938), von Brand *et al.* (1952), and Kozar *et al.* (1965) demonstrated oxygen uptake by intact muscle larvae. Stannard *et al.* (1938) found no difference in oxygen uptake of larvae at oxygen tensions ranging between 1 and 100% of an atmosphere. This same author reported that cyanide (even at 0.0001 M) strongly inhibits oxygen uptake by intact muscle larvae and reversibly blocks motility. Both CO and *p*-phenylenediamine stimulate rather than inhibit respiration in muscle larvae. Stimulation of respiration in homogenates of larvae by CO occurs in the dark and is reversed in the light (Goldberg, 1957). The latter phenomenon indicates that the normal inhibitory function of CO on respiration is not functional in larvae (von Brand, 1970). Inhibitors of glycolysis slowly depress oxygen uptake in larvae (Stannard *et al.*, 1938; Kozar *et al.*, 1965).

Absorption bands corresponding to cytochromes c, b, and a + a_3 have been demonstrated in intact larvae (Agosin, 1956) and in preparations of mitochondria from larvae (see Gerwel *et al.*, 1975). Larval homogenates are positive for cytochrome oxidase, cytochrome c reductase, and succinoxidase activities (Goldberg, 1957). Agosin (1956) reported that muscle larvae contain 2.73 μg cytochrome c/mg N and that the cytochrome system is particle-bound and is localized in the mitochondria of the worms. Allen (1974) demonstrated the presence of an ubiquinone and a rhodoquinone in larvae. The latter compound may be connected with the fumarate reductase involved in extended glycolysis (see Section 2.2).

Goldberg (1957) reported that oxygen uptake by homogenates of larvae is 7–10 times greater in the presence of succinate than in its absence. The increased respiration seen with succinate is abolished by addition of cyanide or malonate. Recent studies showed that a mitochondrial fraction isolated from *T. spiralis* larvae (Boczon, 1967, 1974) takes up oxygen. Maximal oxygen uptake occurs in the presence of succinate at a rate only one third that seen in rat muscle mitochondria.

More recently, Ferguson and Castro (1973) were unable to demonstrate oxygen uptake by muscle larvae. In addition, these same authors examined oxygen consumption by worms isolated from the host intestine at 24 and 48 hr postinfection ("juveniles") and at 96 hr postinfection (adults). The two intestinal stages took up similar amounts of oxygen. It may be hypothesized that at some point during the first 24 hr following their arrival in the host alimentary canal, infective larvae undergo profound changes in metabolism that result in activation of terminal oxidative pathways for energy production. Once these alterations in parasite metabolism have taken place, the worms must be considered juveniles rather than larvae, since they then exhibit a metabolism similar to that seen in mature adult worms.

To isolate muscle larvae for oxygen-uptake experiments, Ferguson and Castro (1973) incubated homogenates of trichinous mice at 37°C for 45 min (Castro and Fairbairn, 1969b). In experiments described above in which muscle larvae were reported to take up oxygen and possess a functional Krebs cycle or cytochrome system, larvae were isolated by incubating homogenates of trichinous mice for at least 3 hr (Stannard et al., 1938; von Brand et al., 1952; Agosin, 1956; Goldberg, 1957). Information on the duration of incubation of muscle homogenates was not obtained for studies by Kozar et al. (1965) and Boczon (1967, 1974). It is possible that muscle larvae exposed to digestive solution for some period of time exceeding 45 min may have changed over or begun to change over from larval metabolism to that typical of adults. This may explain why some workers have found evidence for a functional aerobic metabolism in "muscle larvae." They may have been measuring these parameters in juvenile worms possessing a metabolism characteristic of adults. It would be important to evaluate the effects of duration of exposure to digestive solution as well as the effects of length of time from initial contact with digestive solution on aerobic metabolism in muscle larvae. The latter point is especially important in experiments in which preparation of larvae may take several hours beyond the time during which they are exposed to digestive solution [e.g., von Brand et al. (1952) reported that isolation and preparation of larvae took 7 hr]. In addition, intestinal stages should be examined for evidence of aerobic metabolism at several time points before 24 hr postinfection. This would allow determination of the time following infection at which infective larvae undergo or begin to undergo a change in metabolism. It would be of great interest to compare the biochemistry and ultrastructure of worms isolated at points before and after they have undergone the hypothesized changes in metabolism.

4. LIPIDS AND LIPID METABOLISM

4.1. Adult Worms

The major components of the total lipids of adult worms are similar to those of muscle larvae and include phospholipids, monoglycerides, free fatty acids, sterols, diglycerides, triglycerides, and sterol esters. The major fatty acids recovered from total lipids of adults are qualitatively similar to those in rat intestinal mucosa. In support of these findings, similarities between the fatty acid composition of adult tapeworms and that of the host environment have been demonstrated (Ginger and Fairbairn, 1966; Buteau *et al.*, 1969). The major fatty acids isolated from muscle larvae and adult worms are qualitatively similar, but differ quantitatively. Around 50% of the total fatty acid content of adult worms consists of C_{18} acids, while this component accounts for only 40% of total fatty acids in muscle larvae. Larvae contain about equal amounts of unsaturated and saturated fatty acids, while in adult worms 63% of total fatty acids are unsaturated (Ferguson and Castro, 1973).

Exogenous palmitate is absorbed, incorporated, and oxidized to CO_2 by adult worms. The latter finding suggests that adults catabolize lipids via the beta-oxidation pathway (Ferguson and Castro, 1973). These authors suggest that this pathway may be tied into an active Krebs cycle in adult worms (see Section 2.1). These findings do establish that oxygen plays a physiological role in the metabolism of adult worms and that fat catabolism may be an important pathway for aerobic energy production in the adult parasite (Ferguson and Castro, 1973).

4.2. Muscle Larvae

Lipids constitute 5.5% (von Brand *et al.*, 1952), 18.3% (Kurylo-Borowska and Kozar, 1960), or 9.1% (Castro and Fairbairn, 1969b) of the dry weight of muscle larvae. As pointed out by von Brand (1970), differences in procedures for lipid extraction and determination may underlie these discrepancies. The distribution of lipids in muscle larvae is not known. However, Moore (1965) isolated lipids from the cuticle of muscle larvae.

Castro and Fairbairn (1969b) studied the lipid composition of muscle larvae. They found that phospholipids make up 72.2%, glycolipids 8.5%, and neutral lipids 19.3% of total lipids. The phospholipid fraction consists of 52% phosphatidylcholine, 20% phosphatidylethanolamine, 12% lysophosphatidyl ethanolamine, 10% phosphatidylserine, and 6% sphingomyelin. Neutral lipids consist of 48% cholesterol, 9% cholesterol esters, 20% triglycerides, 7% diglycerides, and 8% free fatty acids. About 50% of the total lipid fatty acids are saturated. Thirty-seven different fatty acids containing from 10 to 22 carbons were identified. The major fatty acids of mouse muscle lipids were qualitatively similar to, but differed quantitatively from, those in larvae. Neither total lipids nor any of the 10 fatty acids found in muscle larvae decreased during aerobic or anaerobic incubation *in vitro*. Von Brand *et al.* (1952) have reported the breakdown of endogenous lipids by muscle larvae incubated under aerobic conditions. These authors found that muscle larvae consume about 21% of their endogenous stores of lipids during 24-hr incubation *in vitro*. Since larvae are motile in the presence but not in the absence of oxygen, these authors postulated that larvae utilize lipid catabolism to provide energetic support for motility. However, as pointed out by Castro and Fairbairn (1969b), triglycerides are the usual source of substrates for fat catabolism, and this component comprises only 5% of the total lipids in muscle larvae. It is noteworthy that Castro and Fairbairn (1969b) reported that muscle larvae showed little motility when incubated under aerobic or anaerobic conditions. As reported above, von Brand *et al.* (1952) observed that under aerobic conditions, muscle larvae were highly active, while under anaerobic conditions, they showed little activity. Ferguson and Castro (1973) found that both juvenile and adult worms were very active under aerobic conditions and less active under anaerobic conditions. These observations on activity of worms would seem to support the suggestion made in Section 3.2 that "muscle larvae" used in some experiments may be juvenile worms.

Karpiak *et al.* (1965) found that oxygen uptake by muscle larvae increased by 20% in the presence of propionic and lauric acids (oxygen uptake was not affected by palmitate). In a more recent study (Ferguson and Castro, 1973), muscle larvae incubated aerobically in the presence of labeled palmitate failed to metabolize this compound (measured as $^{14}CO_2$ production). However, larvae do absorb and incorporate this fatty acid; 94% of total label in muscle larvae is recovered from free fatty acids, and 6% is found in the phospholipids of the worm.

In general, it has been found that production of energy via degradation of endogenous lipids occurs primarily in free-living stages in the life cycle of parasitic helminths (see Castro and Fairbairn, 1969b; von Brand, 1979). From results presented above, it appears that utilization of exogenous and endogenous lipids for energy production by *T. spiralis* muscle larvae remains an open question.

5. NUCLEIC ACIDS AND NUCLEIC ACID METABOLISM: MUSCLE LARVAE

Total nucleic acids make up 0.68% of the fresh substance of muscle larvae [0.45% RNA and 0.23% DNA (Kurylo-Borowska and Kozar, 1960)]. Goldberg (1958a) found that 35–40% of total phosphorus present in muscle larvae is attributable to RNA, while only 8% consists of DNA. Stewart and Read (1973) reported that between days 30 and 38 postinfection, the mean concentration of nucleic acid per unit protein in muscle larvae is 3.41 μg DNA/mg protein and 63.3 μg RNA/mg protein.

Despommier *et al.* (1975) reported that larvae undergo a period of rapid growth in the host muscle fiber between days 13 and 29 postinfection. Stewart and Read (1973) examined larvae for changes in the metabolism of some key macromolecules during a portion of this growth phase and beyond (days 23–38 postinfection). The protein content of muscle larvae more than doubles between days 23 (0.107 μg protein/larva) and 28 postinfection (0.265 μg protein/larva). The RNA content of larvae remains at high levels during the period of rapid growth (day 23: 0.027 μg RNA/larva; day 28: 0.027 μg RNA/larva), while the rate of incorporation *in vivo* of thymidine into DNA is highest on day 23 postinfection (15.72 pmoles thymidine incorporated into DNA/mg protein per hr). After the growth period (days 32–38), the protein content of larvae stabilizes (day 32: 0.270 μg protein/larva; day 38: 0.297 μg protein/larva), the RNA content of larvae decreases to 0.018 μg RNA/larva on day 38 postinfection, and the rate of incorporation of thymidine into larval DNA decreases substantially by day 38 postinfection (2.24 pmoles thymidine incorporated into DNA/mg protein per hr). These results confirm those of Zarzycki (1962), who found low levels of histochemically demonstrable RNA when larvae first arrive in host muscle. Later during the stay of larvae in muscle, the levels of RNA in larvae rise rapidly.

Feldman *et al.* (1975) reported that guanine plus cytosine (G+C) constitute 35% of total DNA of muscle larvae. These findings are in agreement with the findings of others for G+C content of several helminth parasites other than *Trichinella* (see von Brand, 1979).

No information is at present available on nucleic acids and nucleic acid metabolism in adult worms.

6. PROTEINS AND PROTEIN METABOLISM: MUSCLE LARVAE AND ADULT WORMS

Analyses of many of the proteins and glycoproteins of muscle larvae have been conducted in recent years in an effort to isolate, characterize, and purify protection-inducing antigens as well as antigens of immunodiagnostic importance. Results from these studies are presented in Chapter 9.

An increase in the protein content of muscle larvae (Stewart and Read, 1973) accompanies a period of rapid growth of the worms (see Section 5). Hemoglobin and oxyhemoglobin were identified in larvae. Unlike most other parasite hemoglobins (von Brand, 1979), the one found in larvae has a very low affinity for oxygen. Hemoglobin appears to accumulate gradually in larvae, and worms that have resided in muscle for more than 6 weeks have more hemoglobin than younger worms (Goldberg, 1957). Several cytochromes (see Section 3) occur in muscle larvae and in adult worms. Numerous enzymes involved in the pathways of carbohydrate metabolism have been identified, and several have been studied in detail (see Section 2). Young muscle larvae contain low levels of leucine aminopeptidase activity. As the larva grows, the amount of activity of this enzyme increases (Beckett, 1961). Bullock (1953), in a histochemical study of trichinous muscle, found no evidence of alkaline phosphatases in muscle larvae.

In animals maintained on diet containing ^{14}C-labeled amino acids, both encapsulating and encapsulated larvae incorporate label into several macromolecular fractions (predominantly the protein fraction). The actively growing larvae incorporate greater quantities of label than do encapsulated larvae. That larvae remain metabolically active well after encapsulation is suggested by their continued incorporation of labeled amino acids into protein at least to day 180 postinfection (Stoner and Hankes, 1955; Hankes and Stoner, 1958). The authors cited also studied incorporation of ^{14}C-labeled amino acids by worms maintained *in vitro* for 6, 24, or 48 hr in Krebs–Ringer solution (KR) or Krebs–Ringer solution supplemented with mouse serum (KR-S) (Hankes and Stoner, 1956; Stoner and Hankes, 1958). Larvae maintained in KR incorporated greater amounts of label into protein than did those incubated in KR-S. This may be due to uptake by larvae of some substitute in serum. Hankes and Stoner (1962) found that larvae isolated from mice injected intraperitoneally with either glycine-2-[^{14}C] or tryptophan-2-[^{14}C] incorporate the majority of total label absorbed (between 80 and 85%) into the protein fraction. Other fractions in which label is found include amino acids and peptides, lipid, and glycogen. Larvae with the aforedescribed distribution of label were placed *in vitro* in nonnutritive medium, and the redistribution of radioactivity was determined after 24 hr at 37°C. By the end of the period of incubation *in vitro*, larvae exposed *in vivo* to glycine-2-[^{14}C] show a decrease in the amount of label present in the lipid and glycogen fractions, while label in the amino acid–peptide fraction is unaltered. At the end of 24-hr incubation *in vitro* of larvae exposed *in vivo* to tryptophan-2-[^{14}C], the synthesis of proteins and perhaps lipids is evident. These changes are accompanied by recovery of lower levels of label from the glycogen and amino acid–peptide fractions. Isolation of larvae for incubation *in vitro* was accomplished by exposure of trichinous mouse homogenates to digestive solution for 3 hr. For reasons discussed in Section 3.2, the foregoing results from studies *in vitro* may be indicative of the metabolism of juvenile worms rather than of muscle larvae.

Haskins and Weinstein (1975a–c) conducted a quantitative evaluation of nitrogenous materials excreted by muscle larvae during 24-hr axenic, aerobic incubation in 0.7% NaCl. Several categories of nitrogenous excretions were identified: 33.3% ammonia, 7.4% volatile amines, 20.8% peptides, 28.5% amino acids, and 10% nitrogen not accounted for (Haskins and Weinstein, 1957a). In a later study, Haskins and Weinstein (1957b) identified amino acids excreted by larvae during incubation *in vitro* as glutamic acid, serine, glycine, alanine, tyrosine, valine, methionine, leucine, phenylalanine, and proline. In conducting a more detailed study of amines excreted by larvae (Haskins and Weinstein, 1956c), these same authors demonstrated the presence of methyl, ethyl, propyl, butyl, amyl, and heptyl amines, ethylenediamine, cadaverine, two hydroxyamines, ethanolamine, 1-amino-2-propanol, and allylamine. These latter findings were recently confirmed by Castro *et al.* (1973a).

As pointed out by von Brand (1970) and Haskins and Weinstein (1957a–c), the excretion of ammonia by muscle larvae may represent the terminal stage in catabolism of nitrogenous substances. Haskins and Weinstein (1956c) and von Brand (1970) suggest that at least some of the amines excreted *in vitro* by larvae may result from decarboxylation of α-amino acids. Castro *et al.* (1973a) suggest that such decarboxylations might help satisfy the CO_2 requirement imposed on larvae by their fermentative pathways (Ward *et al.*, 1969). However, the significance of excretion of amino acids and peptides by larvae is difficult to assess (von Brand, 1970). It is possible that these substances may leak from the intestine of the larva (Haskins and Weinstein, 1957a). Another possibility would be that amino acids and particularly peptides may come from secretory granules released from stichocytes of the muscle larvae (see Chapter 3).

The only information at present available on metabolism of nitrogenous substances in adult worms comes from the recent study of Castro *et al.* (1973a). These authors reported excretion of amines by adult worms including methyl-, ethyl-, *n*-propyl-, *n*-heptyl-, and *n*-hexylamine, as well as ethylenediamine and 1,5-pentanediamine. While previously reported from some adult nematodes parasitic in plants (Rogers, 1969), this is the first adult parasite of animals known to excrete amines. Larval *Taenia taeniaformis* and infective juveniles of *A. lumbricoides* and *Nippostrongylus muris* are also known to excrete amines (Haskins and Weinstein, 1957a; Haskins and Oliver, 1958). Castro *et al.* (1973b) showed that exposure to low pH (6.0–6.5) decreased the viability of juvenile and adult *Trichinella* by 50%. Intestinal inflammation accompanying trichinosis (Larsh, 1967) may induce numerous changes in the enteroenvironment including a reduction in pH and CO_2 tension. Castro *et al.* (1973a) suggest that the 3-fold increase in amine output by adult worms compared to larvae may be a developmental change in adult worms that allows them to respond to an environment rendered unsuitable by inflammation. Amine production resulting from decarboxylation of amino acids may also provide a source of CO_2 for fulfilling their metabolic needs for this gas during periods of anaerobiasis or when exogenous CO_2 tensions drop during inflammation (Menkin, 1956).

7. NUTRITION

7.1. Adult Worms

Little information is available on nutrition of adult worms. However, low levels of storage polysaccharides and the absence of evidence for ingestion of host blood suggest that, as is the case with many other adult intestinal helminth parasites (see von Brand, 1979), adult *T. spiralis* probably acquires nutrients from the contents of the host intestine or from the intestinal mucosal cells in which the worms reside. Malabsorption of host dietary components (Castro *et al.*, 1967; Olson and Richardson, 1968) by the host small intestine may confer on the parasite an advantage in its competition with the host for available nutrients.

Adult worms maintained *in vitro* absorb and catabolize glucose and fatty acids (see Sections 2.1 and 4.1). Rats given food and glucose solution *ad libitum* retain greater numbers of adult worms for a longer period of time and house greater numbers of muscle larvae than do rats given food and water *ad libitum* (Pawlowski, 1967). A similar response by the parasite was observed in mice rendered hyperglycemic by alloxan treatment (Spaldonova *et al.*, 1974). These results may be interpreted as evidence that increased nutrients in the form of glucose benefit the parasite. However, the effects of treatment on host response to infection and on the enteroenvironment were not assessed.

Castro *et al.* (1974) found a reduction in the number of adult worms when the rat host was placed on intravenous alimentation before infection. On the other hand, greater numbers of adult worms were recovered from the host intestine when rats were placed on intravenous alimentation after infection (Castro *et al.*, 1976). Reduced host response was thought to be responsible for the increased worm burden in the latter study. However, the authors demonstrated alterations in intestinal disaccharidase activity in infected, hyperalimented animals and pointed out that the absence of oral food intake would be expected to induce many changes in enterophysiology—some or all of which may influence the parasite. The reproductive potential of adult worms housed by hyperalimented hosts was not examined in these studies. Stewart *et al.* (1980) showed a reduction in fecundity of adult *T. spiralis* recovered from mice starved for 12 hr compared to that for worms isolated from mice fed *ad libitum*.

7.2. Muscle Larvae

Little is known concerning the nutritional requirements of muscle larvae. A number of workers (see below) have demonstrated that substances present in the host diet are incorporated into the tissues of larvae residing within host myofibers. In view of the tremendous growth undergone by the larva between the time it enters the host muscle fiber and the time it becomes encapsulated (Despommier *et al.*, 1975), it is reasonable to assume that the worm relies heavily on nutrients supplied by the host. The severe disruptions in the biochemistry and ultrastructure of the host myofiber in which the larva resides include alterations that might provide the parasite with needed nutrients (see Chapter 7). Around day 20 postinfection, the larva is surrounded by a double membrane thought to be of host origin (Despommier, 1975). Thus, substances that make contact with the mature muscle larva from host blood must first cross the collagenous capsule, the modified cytoplasm of the host myofiber [the "nurse cell" (Purkerson and Despommier, 1974)], and finally the double membrane surrounding the larva. Stewart and Giannini (1982) point out that this double membrane may possess permeability characteristics that enhance the influx of molecules required by the worm, while precluding the influx or promoting the efflux of substances harmful to the parasite.

Larvae encapsulated in the muscles of the host incorporate host dietary amino acids into protein, glycogen, and lipids (Stoner and Hankes, 1955; Hankes and Stoner, 1958) and take up large amounts of host dietary phosphorus (McCoy *et al.*, 1941). The incorporation of labeled host dietary cholesterol into lipids by encapsulated muscle larvae (Digenis *et al.*, 1970) is interesting in view of the fact that Meerovitch (1965) showed that larvae cultivated *in vitro* require cholesterol for prolonged survival. Finally, thymidine injected intraperitoneally into the host is incorporated into DNA by encapsulated and encapsulating muscle larvae (Stewart and Read, 1973). Uptake *in vitro* and utilization of sugars, fatty acids, and amino acids is suggested by work described above.

REFERENCES

Agosin, M., 1956, Studies on the cytochrome system of *Trichinella spiralis*, *Bol. Chil. Parasitol.* **11**:46–51.

Agosin, M., and Aravena, L.C., 1959, Anaerobic glycolysis in homogenates of *Trichinella spiralis* larvae, *Exp. Parasitol.* **8**:10–30.

Allen, P.C., 1974, Helminths: Comparison of their rodoquinone, *Exp. Parasitol.* **34**:211–220.

Beckett, E.B., 1961, Some histochemical changes in the protein of mouse skeletal muscle-fibres infected by *Trichinella spiralis*, *Ann. Trop. Med. Parasitol.* **55**:419–426.

Beckett, E.B., and Boothroyd, B., 1962, The histochemistry and electron microscopy of glycogen in the larva of *Trichinella spiralis* and its environment, *Ann. Trop. Med. Parasitol.* **56**:264–273.

Berntzen, A.K., 1965, Comparative growth and development of *Trichinella spiralis in vitro* and *in vivo*, with a redescription of the life cycle, *Exp. Parasitol.* **16**:74–106.

Boczon, K., 1967, Some data on bioenergetics of *Trichinella spiralis*, *Bull. Soc. Amis Sci. Lett. Poznan Ser. D* **50**:166–170.

Boczon, K., 1974, The tricarboxylic acid cycle and pentose pathway enzymes in *Trichinella spiralis* larvae, *Wiad. Parazytol.* **20**:29–39.

Bueding, E., and Yale, H.W., 1951, Production of α-methylbutyric acid by bacteria-free *Ascaris lumbricoides*, *J. Biol. Chem.* **193**:411–423.

Bullock, W., 1953, Phosphotases in experimental *Trichinella spiralis* infections in muscles, *Med. Parazitol.* **29**:183–186.

Buteau, G.H., Simmons, J.E., and Fairbairn, D., 1969, Lipid metabolism in helminth parasites. IX. Fatty acid composition of shark tapeworms and their hosts, *Exp. Parasitol.* **26**:269–273.

Castro, G.A., and Fairbairn, D., 1969a, Comparison of cuticular and intestinal absorption of glucose by adult *Ascaris lumbricoides*, *J. Parasitol.* **55**:13–16.

Castro, G.A., and Fairbairn, D., 1969b, Carbohydrates and lipids in *Trichinella spiralis* larvae and their utilization *in vitro*, *J. Parasitol.* **55**:51–58.

Castro, G.A., and Fairbairn, D., 1969c, Effect of immune serum on glucose absorption and infectivity of *Trichinella spiralis, J. Parasitol.* **55:**59–66.

Castro, G.A., Olsen, L.J., and Baker, R.D., 1967, Glucose malabsorption and intestinal histopathology in *Trichinella spiralis*-infected guinea pigs, *J. Parasitol.* **53:**595–612.

Castro, G.A., Ferguson, J.D., and Gorden, C.W., 1973a, Amine excretion in excysted larvae and adults of *Trichinella spiralis, Comp. Biochem. Physiol.* **45A:**819–828.

Castro, G.A., Cotter, M.V., Ferguson, J.D., and Gorden, C.W., 1973b, Physiologic factors possibly altering the course of infection, *J. Parasitol.* **59:**268–276.

Castro, G.A., Johnson, L.R., Copeland, E.M., and Dudrick, S.J., 1974, Development of enteric parasites in parenterally fed rats, *Proc. Soc. Exp. Biol. Med.* **146:**703–706.

Castro, G.A., Johnson, L.R., Copeland, E.M., and Dudrick, S.J., 1976, Course of infection with enteric parasites in host shifted from enteral to parenteral nutrition, *J. Parasitol.* **62:**353–359.

Cheah, K.S., 1974, Oxidative phosphorylation in *Ascaris* muscle mitochondria, *Comp. Biochem. Physiol.* **47B:**237–242.

De Nollin, S., and Van den Bossche, H., 1973, Biochemical effects of mebendazole on *Trichinella spiralis* larvae, *J. Parasitol.* **59:**970–976.

Despommier, D.D., 1975, Adaptive changes in muscle fibers infected with *Trichinella spiralis, Am. J. Pathol.* **78:**477–484.

Despommier, D.D., Aron, L., and Turgeon, L., 1975, *Trichinella spiralis*: Growth of the intracellular (muscle) larva, *Exp. Parasitol.* **37:**108–116.

Digenis, G.A., Konyalian, A., and Thorson, R., 1970, *In vivo* transfer of ^{14}C-4-cholesterol from mouse host to encapsulated *Trichinella spiralis* larvae, *Lipids* **5:**282–283.

Dusanic, D.G., 1966, Serologic and enzymatic investigations of *Trichinella spiralis*. I. Precipitin reactions and lactic dehydrogenase, *Exp. Parasitol.* **20:**288–294.

Dusanic, D.G., 1967, Serologic and enzymatic investigations of *Trichinella spiralis*. II. Characterization of larval lactate dehydrogenase, *Exp. Parasitol.* **20:**288–294.

Fairbairn, D., 1958, Trehalose and glucose in helminths and other invertebrates, *Can. J. Zool.* **36:**787–795.

Fairbairn, D., 1970, Biochemical adaptation and loss of genetic capacity in helminth parasites, *Biol. Rev.* **45:**29–72.

Feldman, A., Rosenkrantz, H.S., and Despommier, D., 1975, Guanine–cytosine content of DNA from the mature muscle larva of *Trichinella spiralis* as determined from buoyant density and thermal-helix coil transition measurements, *J. Parasitol.* **63:**570–571.

Ferguson, J.D., and Castro, G.A., 1973, Metabolism of intestinal stages of *Trichinella spiralis, Am. J. Physiol.* **225:**85–89.

Gerwel, C., Michejda, J., and Boczon, K., 1975, Biochemistry of *Trichinella spiralis, Wiad. Parazytol.* **21:**669–677.

Ginger, C.D., and Fairbairn, D., 1966, Lipid metabolism in helminth parasites. II. The major origins of the lipids of *Hymenolepis diminuta* (Cestoda), *J. Parasitol.* **52:**1097–1107.

Goldberg, E., 1957, Studies on the intermediary metabolism of *Trichinella spiralis, Exp. Parasitol.* **6:**367–382.

Goldberg, E., 1958a, The extraction and analyses of the nucleic acids of *T. spiralis* larvae, *J. Parasitol.* **44**(Sect. 2)(4):34.

Goldberg, E., 1958b, The glycolytic pathway in *Trichinella spiralis* larvae, *J. Parasitol.* **44:**363–370.

Hankes, L.V., and Stoner, R.D., 1956, *In vitro* metabolism of DL-alanine-2-C^{14} and glycine-2-C^{14} by *Trichinella spiralis* larvae, *Proc. Soc. Exp. Biol. Med.* **91:**443–446.

Hankes, L.V., and Stoner, R.D., 1958, Incorporation of DL-tyrosine-2-C^{14} and DL-tryptophan-2-C^{14} by encysted *Trichinella spiralis* larvae, *Exp. Parasitol.* **7**:92–98.

Hankes, L.V., and Stoner, R.D., 1962, *In vitro* metabolism of tryptophan-2-C^{14} and glycine-2-C^{14} by *Trichinella spiralis* larvae and chemical fractionation of C^{14}-labeled larvae, in: *Trichinellosis* (Z. Kozar, ed.), Polish Scientific Publications, Warsaw, pp. 313–318.

Haskins, W.T., and Oliver, L., 1958, Nitrogenous excretory products of *Taenia taeniaformis* larvae, *J. Parasitol.* **44**:569–573.

Haskins, W.T., and Weinstein, P.P., 1957a, Nitrogenous excretory products of *Trichinella spiralis* larvae, *J. Parasitol.* **43**:19–24.

Haskins, W.T., and Weinstein, P.P., 1957b, Amino acids excreted by *Trichinella spiralis* larvae, *J. Parasitol.* **43**:25–27.

Haskins, W.T., and Weinstein, P.P., 1957c, The amine constituents from the excretory products of *Ascaris lumbricoides* and *Trichinella spiralis*, *J. Parasitol.* **43**:28–32.

Hill, C.H., Baisden, L.A., and Smith, C., 1970, Relationship of *n*-valeric acid content and intensity of infection in trichinous hogs, *J. Parasitol.* **56**:265–270.

Karpiak, S., Kozar, Z., Krzyzanowski, M., and Kozar, M., 1965, Effect of some organic acids on the respiration of *Trichinella spiralis* larvae, *Acta Parasitol. Pol.* **13**:265–270.

Kozar, Z., and Seniuta, R., 1974, Histochemical examination in different developmental forms of *Trichinella spiralis*, *Wiad. Parazytol.* **20**:41–47.

Kozar, Z., Karpiak, S.E., Krzyzanowski, M., and Kozar, M., 1965, Observations on the carbohydrate metabolism of *Trichinella spiralis* muscular larvae, *Acta Parasitol. Pol.* **13**:259–264.

Kozar, Z., Karpiak, S.E., Krzyzanowski, M., and Kozar, M., 1966, Histochemische Untersuchen über die Darmphase der Trichinellos bei weissen Mäusen, *Z. Parasitenkol.* **27**:106–126.

Kurylo-Borowska, Z., and Kozar, Z., 1960, The general chemical composition of muscle *Trichinella spiralis* larvae (abstract), *Wiad. Parazytol.* **6**:357–359.

Larsh, J.E., Jr., 1967, The present understanding of the mechanisms of immunity to *Trichinella spiralis*, *Am. J. Trop. Med. Hyg.* **16**:123–132.

Mancilla, R., and Agosin, M., 1960, The phosphoglucose isomerase from *Trichinella spiralis* larvae, *Exp. Parasitol.* **10**:43–50.

McCoy, O.R., Downing, V.F., and Van Voorhis, S.N., 1941, The penetration of radioactive phosphorus into encysted *Trichinella* larvae, *J. Parasitol.* **27**:53–58.

Menkin, V., 1956, *Biochemical Mechanisms in Inflammation*, 1st ed., Charles C. Thomas, Springfield, Illinois.

Meerovitch, E., 1965, Studies on the *in vitro* axenic development of *Trichinella spiralis*. II. Preliminary experiments on the effects of farnesol, cholesterol and an insect extract, *Can. J. Zool.* **43**:81–85.

Moore, L.L.A., 1965, Studies in mice on the immunogenicity of cuticular antigens from larvae of *Trichinella spiralis*, *J. Elisha Mitchell Sci. Soc.* **81**:137–143.

Oliver-Gonzalez, J., and Bueding, E., 1948, Reduction in the number of adult *Trichinella spiralis* in rats after treatment with naphthoquinones, *Proc. Soc. Exp. Biol. Med.* **69**:569–571.

Olson, L.J., and Richardson, J.A., 1968, Intestinal malabsorption of D-glucose in mice infected with *Trichinella spiralis*, *J. Parasitol.* **54**:445–451.

Pawlowski, Z., 1967, Adrenal cortex hormones in intestinal trichinellosis. III. Effect of adrenalectomy and hydrocortisone, insulin, alloxan and glucose treatment on elimination of *Trichinella spiralis* adult in hooded rats, *Acta Parasitol. Pol.* **15**:179–189.

Purkerson, M., and Despommier, D.D., 1974, Fine structure of the muscle phase of *Trichinella spiralis* in the mouse, in: *Trichinellosis* (C. Kim, ed.), In text, New York, pp. 7–23.

Rathbone, L., and Rees, K.R., 1954, Glycolysis in *Ascaris lumbricoides* from the pig, *Biochim. Biophys. Acta* **15:**126–133.

Rogers, W.P., 1969, Nitrogenous components and their metabolism: Acanthocephala and Nematoda, in: *Chemical Zoology,* Vol. 3 (M. Florkin and B.T. Sheer, eds.), Academic Press, New York, pp. 379–428.

Saz, H., 1971, Anaerobic phosphorylation in *Ascaris* mitochondria and the effects of anthelmintics, *Comp. Biochem. Physiol.* **39B:**627–637.

Spaldonova, R., Komandarev, S., and Tomasovicova, O., 1974, The effect of alloxan diabetes on Intestinal and muscle trichinellosis, in: *Trichinellosis* (C.W. Kim, ed.), Intext, New York, pp. 149–154.

Stannard, J.N., McCoy, C.R., and Latchford, W.E., 1938, Studies on the metabolism of *Trichinella spiralis* larvae, *Am. J. Hyg.* **27:**666–682.

Stewart, G.L., 1976, Studies on biochemical pathology in trichinosis. II. Changes in liver and muscle glycogen and some blood chemical parameters in mice, *Rice Univ. Stud.* **62:**211–224.

Stewart, G.L., and Giannini, S.H., 1982, Intracellular parasites of striated muscle: A review, *Exp. Parasitol.* **53:**406–447.

Stewart, G.L., and Read, C.P., 1973, Deoxyribonucleic acid metabolism in mouse trichinosis, *J. Parasitol.* **59:**264–267.

Stewart, G.L., Kramar, G.W., Reddington, J.J., and Hamilton, A.M., 1980, Studies on *in vitro* larvaposition by adult *Trichinella spiralis, J. Parasitol.* **66:**94–99.

Stoner, R.D., and Hankes, L.V., 1955, Incorporation of ^{14}C-labeled amino acids by *Trichinella spiralis, Exp. Parasitol.* **4:**435–444.

Stoner, R.D., and Hankes, L.V., 1958, *In vitro* metabolism of DL-tyrosine-2-C^{14} and DL-tryptophan-2-C^{14} by *Trichinella spiralis* larvae, *Exp. Parasitol.* **7:**145–151.

Von Brand, T., 1934, Der Stoffwechsel von *Ascaris lumbricoides* bei Oxybiose und Anoxybiose, *Z. Vgl. Physiol.* **23:**220–235.

Von Brand, T., 1970, Physiology and biochemistry of *Trichinella spiralis,* in: *Trichinosis in Man and Animals* (S.E. Gould, ed.), Charles C. Thomas, Springfield, Illinois, pp. 81–90.

Von Brand, T., 1973, *Biochemistry of Parasites,* 2nd ed., Academic Press, New York.

Von Brand, T., 1979, *Biochemistry and Physiology of Parasites,* 1st ed., Elsevier/North-Holland, Amsterdam, 447 pp.

Von Brand, T., Weinstein, P.P., Mehlman, B., and Weinbach, E.C., 1952, Observations on the metabolism of bacteria-free larvae of *Trichinella spiralis, Exp. Parasitol.* **1:**245–255.

Ward, C.W., and Fairbairn, D., 1970, Enzymes of β-oxidation and their function during development of *Ascaris lumbricoides* eggs, *Dev. Biol.* **22:**366–387.

Ward, C.W., Castro, G.A., and Fairbairn, D., 1969, Carbon dioxide fixation and phosphoenolpyruvate metabolism in *Trichinella spiralis* larvae, *J. Parasitol.* **55:**67–71.

Zarzycki, J., 1962, Histochemical investigations on distribution of nucleic acids and inorganic salts in muscle tissue at the infection with *Trichinella spiralis,* in: *Trichinellosis* (Z. Kozar, ed.) Polish Scientific Publications, Warsaw, pp. 302–305.

5

Anatomical Pathology

NORMAN F. WEATHERLY

1. INTRODUCTION

The anatomical pathology, i.e., the gross and microscopic study of the effects of *Trichinella* infection on the organs and tissues of the host, is the subject of this chapter. The material presented is limited primarily to those studies that used small laboratory animals and conventional histological techniques. Ultrastructural changes, as detected by various electron-microscopic techniques, are described elsewhere.

The mouse and the rat have been by far the most popular animals for the study of experimental trichinosis. Guinea pigs, rabbits, and hamsters have also been used with some frequency. In addition, there are isolated reports in the literature on the use of young chickens, small pigs, and wild rodents. Because most recent investigators have used the mouse for both gross and microscopic study of infected organs and tissues, the histological changes in this animal species will be detailed, with studies in other experimental animals being compared to those in the mouse.

The anatomical changes produced by the preadults and adults in the gastrointestinal tract will be discussed first. Following this, the changes associated with invasion of striated muscle cells by larvae will be characterized. The last section of this chapter will deal with the pathological anatomy produced by invasive larvae in various organs, such as heart, liver, spleen, eyes, and central nervous system.

In reading this discussion of the histopathological changes in the

NORMAN F. WEATHERLY • Department of Parasitology and Laboratory Practice, School of Public Health, University of North Carolina, Chapel Hill, North Carolina 27514.

tissues and organs of experimental animals, the reader should keep in mind that although the basic mechanisms of pathogenesis and host defense response to infectious agents such as bacteria, protozoa, and helminths are similiar, *Trichinella* does have certain peculiarities that may make accurate interpretation of histopathological observations difficult. For example, compared to bacteria and protozoa, *T. spiralis* is a relatively large organism, has a relatively resistant outer cuticle, and has, at certain phases of its life, migrational abilities. Different antigenic compositions and different methods of feeding of preadult, adult, newborn larvae, and encysted larvae—in other words, factors that affect the nature of disease—are not well understood. Thus, the conventional understanding of the usual modes of immunoglobulin action, inflammation, complement activity, and cellular as well as cell-mediated immunity may not be appropriate when one attempts to unravel the specific mechanism of pathogenesis of an infection such as that caused by *T. spiralis*. For example, large amounts of immunoglobulins are produced by the host in response to infection with *T. spiralis*, yet the protective function of these immunoglobulins is in question. Rather than being beneficial to the host, they may contribute to the pathogenesis by causing immune-complex disorders. Also, the relatively recent discovery of certain immunosuppressive properties of *T. spiralis* has yet to be fully investigated.

Host factors are also important determinants of disease—numerous examples exist in which an infective agent causes little or no morbidity in one species of animal, yet leads to severe illness or death in another; individual variation exists within the same species, as well as among strains. In addition, it is imperative that this interaction between the two organisms not be viewed as a static relationship but, rather, as one that is constantly changing due to various parasite and host factors. Host factors known to influence the degree of morbidity caused by *T. spiralis* are age, sex, diet, general nutritional status, genetics, prior infection, and physiological stressful conditions such as pregnancy and lactation.

Finally, there are differences in virulence among various strains and isolates of *T. spiralis*. This, and the factors discussed above relating to both the host and the parasite, probably account for the various inconsistencies and discrepancies that have characterized the literature on the pathogenesis and host response to infection with *T. spiralis*.

2. GASTROINTESTINAL TRACT

This section deals with the morbidity associated with the development of the adult parasite within the tissues of the gastrointestinal tract.

The stomach, small intestine, and portions of the large intestine are involved, with the small intestine being the most affected. In all involved areas, there are histological changes as well as functional derangements.

2.1. Gross Changes

2.1.1. Stomach

Relatively little work has been reported that shows the degree of involvement of adult *T. spiralis* with the host stomach. This is unfortunate, because worms in this location may be missed when investigators attempt to recover adults. It is expected by those working with *Trichinella* that depending on numerous host factors such as species, age, and immune status, considerably less than 100% of the larvae in the infecting inoculum will be recovered as adult worms from the small bowels of animals. It is possible that a portion of these unaccounted for worms are present in the stomach and large intestine, organs that are not usually examined when adult worms are recovered for counting.

According to Gould (1970), Askanazy observed hemorrhages and hemorrhagic erosions of the gastric mucosa of infected rabbits that had died as a result of experimental infection. Gursch (1949) was surprised to find viable adults in the stomachs of rats that had been infected 15–16 days previously with 5000 larvae. Although not stated in the report, it is assumed that the worms were situated in the lumen of the stomach, since Gursch hypothesized that their presence in that organ possibly indicated a return from the intestine.

Most recent reviews of trichinosis in man fail to mention the involvement of the stomach. However, Cohnheim in 1865 and 1866, Ehrhardt in 1896, Flury in 1913, and Most and Abeles in 1937, according to Gould (1970), observed marked redness, small hemorrhagic ulcers, and pinpoint submucosal hemorrhages of various portions of the stomach.

In summary, the available literature fails to provide information as to whether or not the stomach and its tissues should be considered as a possible organ of habitation for adult worms in experimental animals. The indications are, however, that in man and in at least the rabbit and rat, the stomach is involved.

2.1.2. Small Intestine

There is little doubt that the small intestine is the primary site for the establishment, development, and maturation of adult *T. spiralis* in most animal species and strains tested so far; guinea pigs and young chickens are possible exceptions. There is considerable variation, however, regarding which portion of the small intestine is most severely affected (see Chapter 3). Regardless of the location, there seems to be general agreement regarding the gross changes that take place within the small intestine and its tissues.

Gastroenteritis and diarrhea are common symptoms of the intestinal phase of trichinosis. Constipation has also been noted, but this may be due to decreased food consumption rather than to altered bowel motility and organ dysfunction.

Penetration of small numbers of infective larvae into the mucosa causes little damage; minute ulcers and slight bleeding sometimes occur. With more severe infections, edema, marked cellular infiltration, and profuse hemorrhage may occur. Hyperemia, petechiae of the serosa, swollen and atrophied villi, excessive secretion of mucin, enlarged Peyer's patches, and dilatation of the loops of the bowel have all been reported. Catty (1969) reports that in guinea pigs, damage due to the invading larvae and the adult worms and their movements within the intestinal mucosa may even lead to tissue necrosis.

It is clear from the literature and from the author's own observations that the gross changes seen in the small bowel are directly related to the number of larvae that invade the intestinal tissues and the length of time the adults remain in the tissues. Immune animals manifest less intestinal damage due to the reduced longevity of the adults.

2.1.3. Large Intestine

Investigators have noted the presence of adult worms in the cecums and colons of infected mice in both primary and secondary infections (Kennedy, 1978; Beresantev, 1962). Gursch (1949) and Leonard and Beahm (1941), using only primary infections, noted the presence of worms in similar locations in rats. Golden hamsters (Boyd and Huston, 1954), guinea pigs (Roth, 1938), gophers of the species *Citellus richardsonii* (Offutt and McCoy, 1941), and young chickens (Marty, 1966) have also been shown to harbor adult *Trichinella* in various portions of the large intestine. From a study of the aforecited reports, one concludes that the cecal and colonic portions of the large intestine, along with the distal segment of the small intestine, are the preferred sites for tissue invasion in young chickens and guinea pigs. However, even though these sites may be inhabited, there are indications that the adults in these locations are abnormal. Kennedy (1978) suggests that in NIH mice, worms in the large intestine are effete due to host resistance or nutritional factors, and Roth (1938) provides evidence that adult female worms in the cecum are less fecund.

In none of the reports cited was there any mention of the gross pathological changes of the tissues of the large intestine. Perhaps changes somewhat similar to those that occur in the small intestine would be present. However, since there are indications that the adults that establish here are "abnormal," and considering the different physiological function and tissue organization of the large intestine as compared to the small bowel, the alterations could be quite distinct.

2.2. Microscopic Changes

2.2.1. Stomach and Large Intestine

As stated previously, no histopathological studies have been reported in the literature.

2.2.2. Small Intestine

Detailed studies on the microscopic changes that occur in the small bowel of mice during all enteral phases of a *T. spiralis* infection have been conducted by Larsh, Race, and their colleagues (Larsh, 1963; Larsh and Race, 1954; Larsh *et al.*, 1954; Race *et al.*, 1974, 1978). Although there has been some controversy as to the precise ecological niche of adult worms in the small intestine, Gardiner (1976) provided evidence that the preferred niche is within the epithelium at the base of the villi, in the glandular crypts, with an occasional worm embedded in the epithelium at the tip of a villus. This is important in relation to the degree of tissue damage produced by the worms. Gardiner (1976) also found that the worms were situated entirely within the epithelial layer, whereas Gursch (1949) considered the worms to be wound around the villi, Beresantev (1962) thought that only the anterior portions were embedded in the epithelium with the remainder free in the lumen, and Castro *et al.* (1974) reported that in their studies, the body of the worm was embedded within the mucosa with both ends free in the lumen.

Until recently, it was accepted that adult *T. spiralis* worms existed in extracellular sites within the intestinal tissues. Wright (1979), using electron-microscopic techniques, has shown that the adults may instead be intracellular. According to him, worms "lie directly in the cytoplasm, threaded through a serial row of enterocytes." In this location, they were observed to produce no distortion of the epithelium and little damage (Fig. 1 and Chapter 3, Fig. 3). This finding, if shown to be true for other experimental animals, will need to be considered when interpreting the results of future pathological and immunological studies.

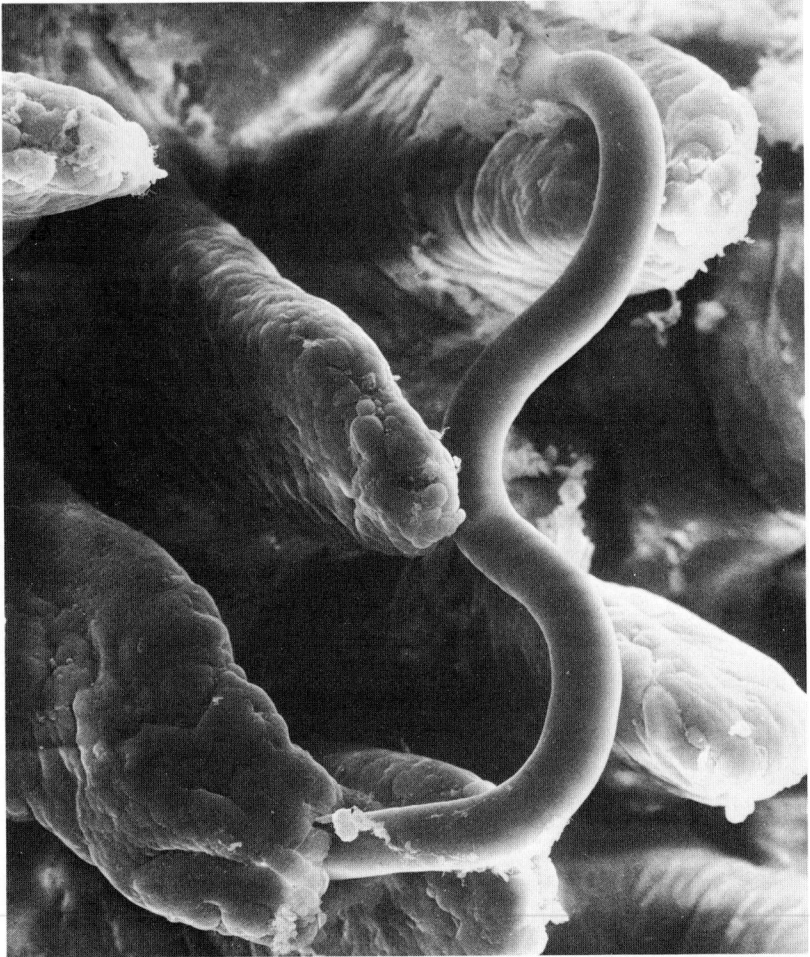

FIGURE 1. Scanning electron-microscopic view of an adult apparently emerging from the side of one villus and entering the tip of another. × 270. From Wright (1979), courtesy of the author and editor.

In mice heavily infected, the invading intestinal-phase worms may cause microscopic ulceration and bleeding. Mucosal hyperemia, punctate hemorrhages, and severe edema of the small bowel are evident. Depending on the number of larvae, death can occur as early as 1 day after infection. In the author's laboratory, using an outbred strain of Swiss mouse, the establishment of over 500–700 adult worms will cause death in 4–5 days.

Histopathological studies have also been conducted using immunosuppressed or immunodeficient mice. These studies will be discussed in the general description of the histopathology observed in nonimmune and immune mice (see below). Most evidence indicates that much of the pathological alteration of the small intestine is due to an allergic inflammation (Larsh and Race, 1975).

In a randomly outbred Swiss strain of laboratory mouse, with a moderate-level infection (150–300 adults establishing), histological examination of normal (nonimmunized) mice showed a minimal inflammatory response and little cellular infiltration during the first 4 days after infection. Some tissue sections, however, showed an increase in the numbers of plasma cells and lymphocytes (Race et al., 1974). In general, the damage produced by the invading worms during the first 4 days of infection was minimal, and was most likely of a mechanical nature.

At 6 days after infection, a mild inflammatory reaction with focal collections of moderate numbers of neutrophils and eosinophils was present. Large and small lymphocytes, plasma cells, and macrophages in increased numbers could be seen (Race et al., 1978). This mild inflammatory reaction indicates that the acute response is just beginning (Fig. 2).

The peak of the acute response occurred at around days 8–10, with the tissues showing considerable cellular infiltration. There seemed to be a panmucosal reaction, with focal areas containing large numbers of granulocytic cells (50% eosinophils), as well as plasma cells and lymphocytes. Race et al. (1978) have judged that there is present at this time a mixed acute and chronic inflammation (Fig. 3). The reaction remained at this level until about day 14, the point at which a majority of the adult worms had been expelled (Fig. 4).

At 22 days after infection, when nearly all the worms had been expelled, the tissue reaction had diminished greatly, with only a moderate degree of inflammation being present. Neutrophils and eosinophils were noted in moderate numbers in focal areas, but plasma cells and lymphocytes were the predominant types of cells in the infiltration, indicating a chronic type of inflammation. The mucosal inflammation continued to decrease, and by day 36, it consisted mostly of small numbers of plasma cells and large and small lymphocytes. Race et al. (1978) estimated that the inflammation had run its course by day 38, with the return of the normal architecture of the intestinal tissues.

The histopathological picture of the small intestine in immunized mice was similar to that of the nonimmunized mice, with the exception of timing. The acute inflammatory response was initiated within 24 hr

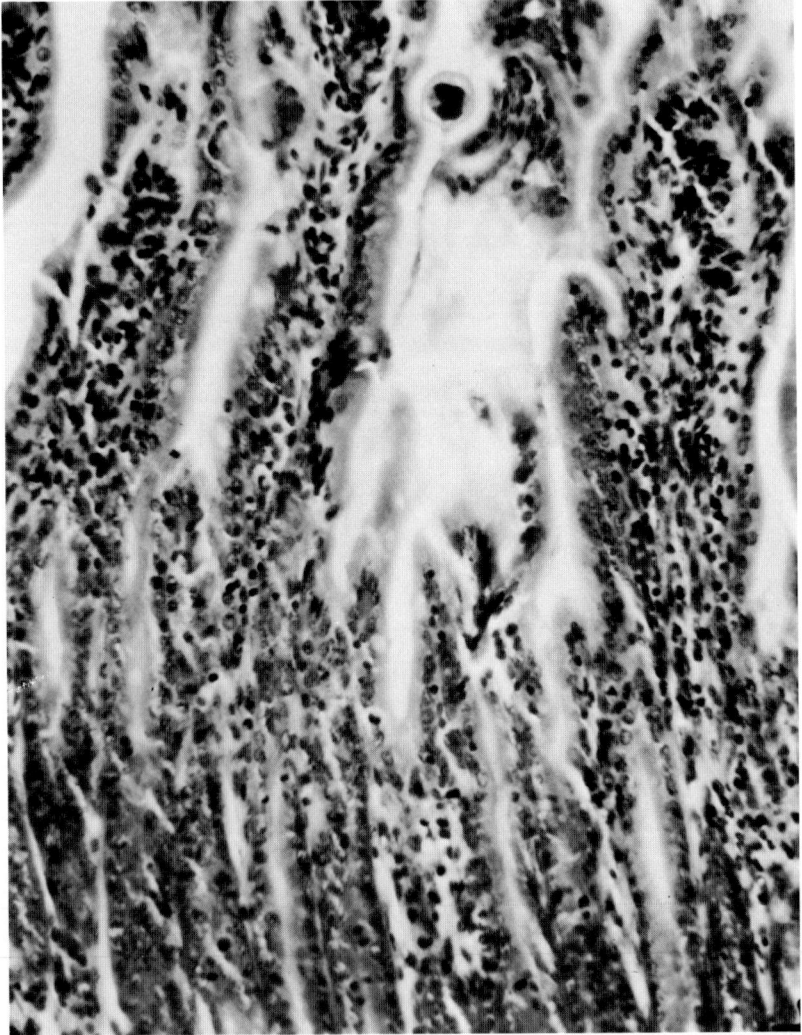

FIGURE 2. Section of intestine from nonimmunized mouse 6 days after infection. Note that the mucosa is mildly inflamed. × 171. From Larsh and Race (1954), courtesy of the University of Chicago Press.

of infection (Fig. 5). A mild panmucosal inflammation was noted, with neutrophils, eosinophils, plasma cells, and lymphocytes. The peak of the inflammatory response occurred during days 4–8. The cell types present in the infiltrate were the same as those listed as being present at day 1, but their numbers were greatly increased. Many large and small lymphocytes, and plasma cells, were present, indicating a mixed acute and chronic inflammation. Definite clusters of granulocytes could be seen (Fig. 6 and 7). It should be remembered that a significant number of adult worms is being expelled from immunized mice about day 8.

This moderately severe to severe inflammatory response subsided

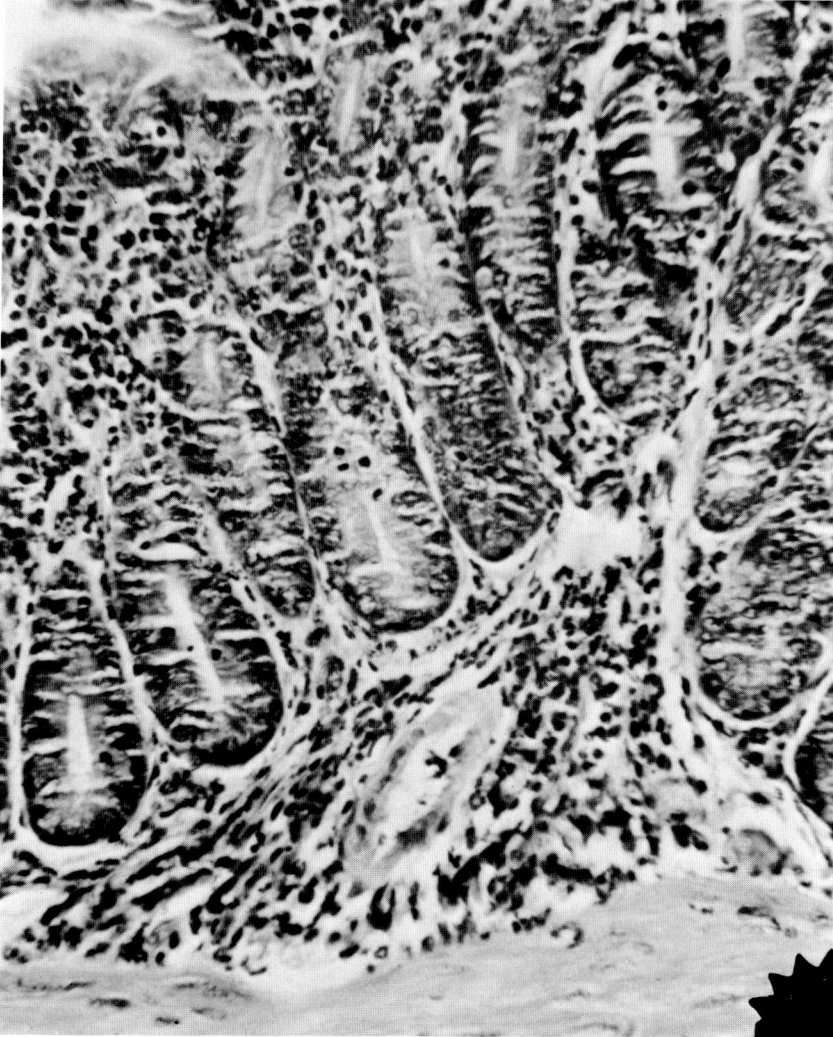

FIGURE 3. Section from intestine of nonimmunized mouse 8 days after infection. The mucosa and submucosa are intensely inflammed and infiltrated with neutrophils, eosinophils, lymphocytes, and plasma cells. ×280. From Larsh and Race (1954), courtesy of the University of Chicago Press.

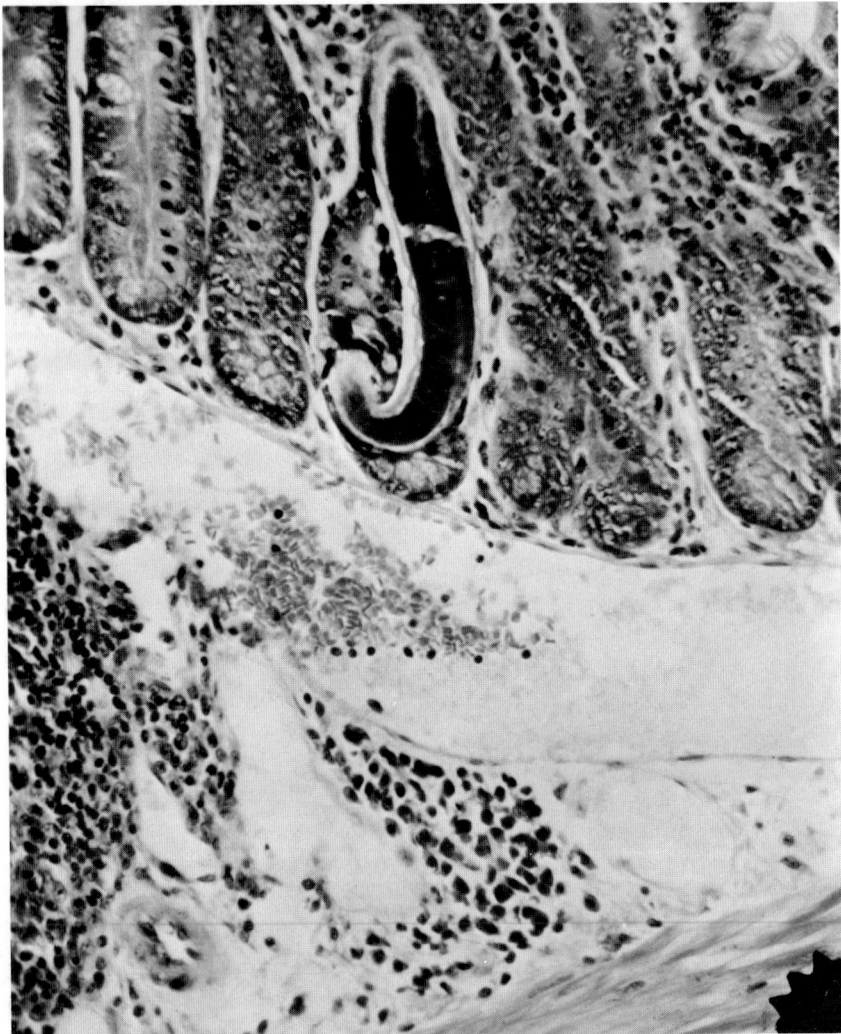

FIGURE 4. Section of intestine from nonimmunized mouse 14 days after infection. A mixed acute and chronic infiltrate is present at this time. × 171. From Larsh and Race (1954), courtesy of the University of Chicago Press.

by day 15. At this time, the mucosal infiltration was more diffuse. There was a continued resolution of the inflamed tissue so that by days 30–36, the intestine had reacquired its normal architecture.

Various investigators have described the tissue alterations produced in T-cell-deficient mice (Walls *et al.*, 1973; Ruitenberg and Elgersma,

1976; Ruitenberg *et al.*, 1977; Gustowski *et al.*, 1980), antithymocyte (ATS) serum-treated mice (Larsh *et al.*, 1974), and X-irradiated mice (Larsh *et al.*, 1962).

CBA/H male mice, 8 weeks old, were used by Walls *et al.* (1973). Experimental mice were thymectomized, irradiated with 850 rads whole-

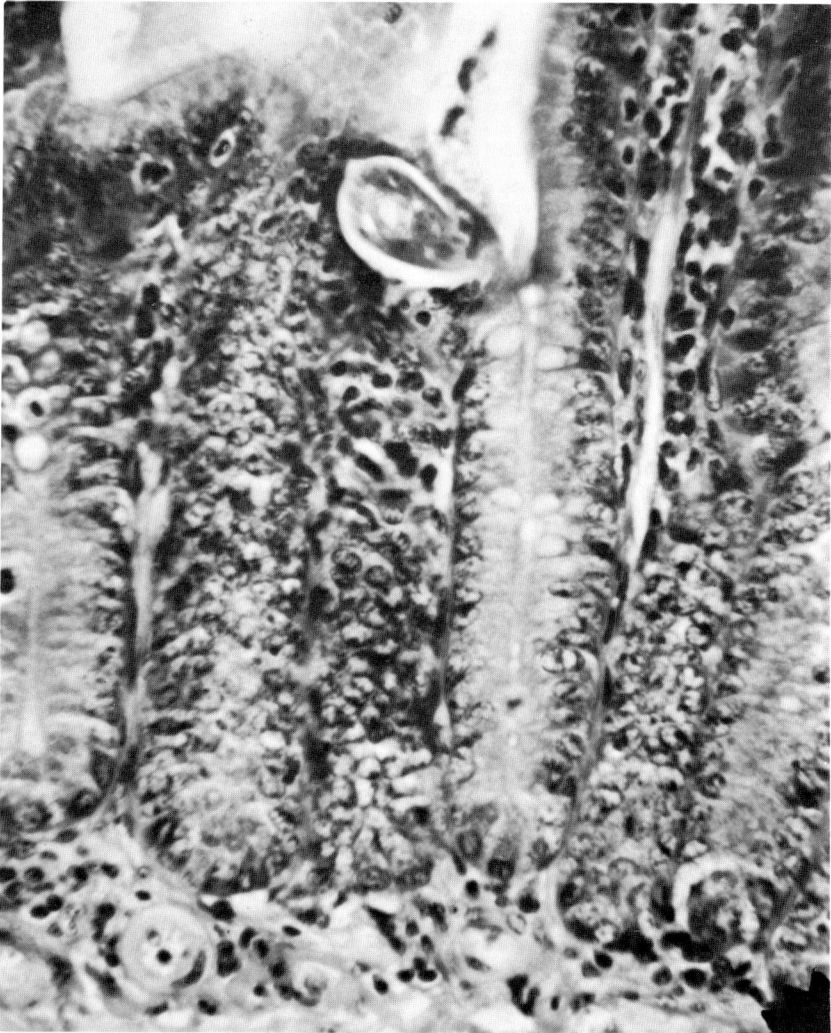

FIGURE 5. Section of intestine from immunized mouse 1 day after challenge. An acute inflammatory response has already been started. ×350. From Larsh and Race (1954), courtesy of the University of Chicago Press.

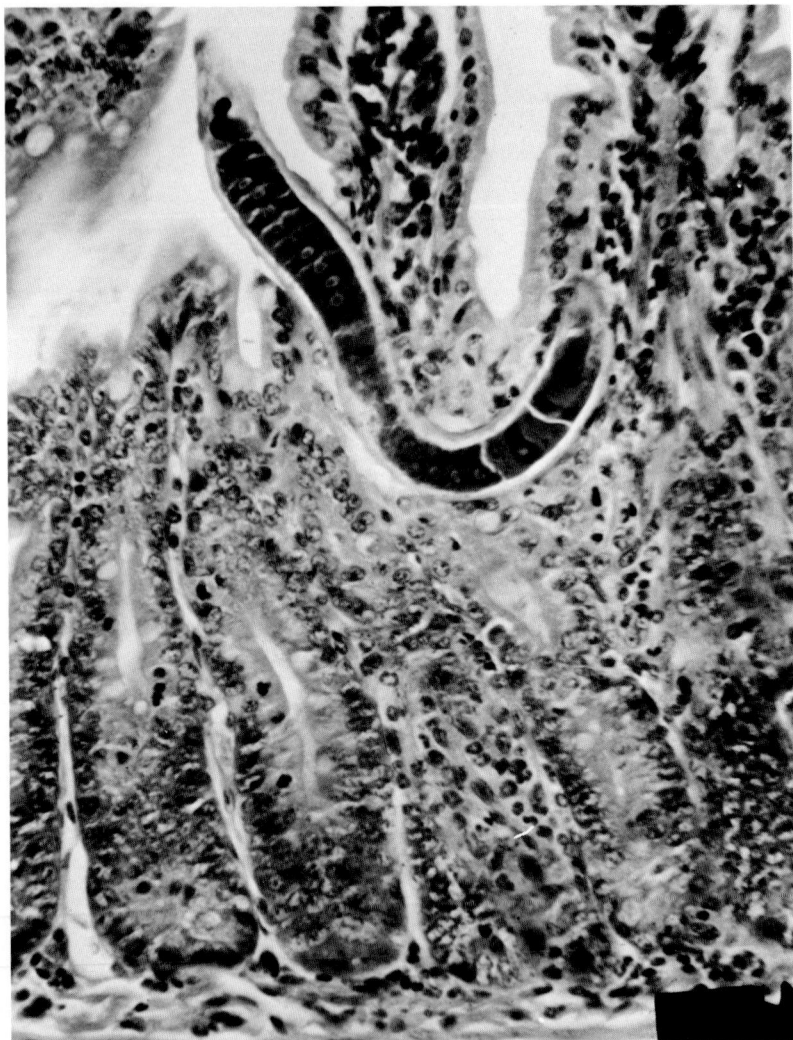

FIGURE 6. Section of intestine from immunized mouse 4 days after challenge. Note the worm and abundant cellular infiltrate (primarily polymorphonuclear leukocytes). ×350. From Larsh and Race (1954), courtesy of the University of Chicago Press.

body irradiation, and reconstituted with 5×10^6 syngeneic bone marrow cells. In control mice, a mild inflammatory infiltrate was present in the submucosa between days 3 and 10, consisting of neutrophils, eosinophils, lymphocytes, and macrophages. In the T-cell-deficient mice, inflammatory changes were negligible. Peyer's patches were smaller than those

of the controls, their edges were often hypocellular, and small collections
of eosinophils were seen at 10 and 15 days. In control mice, a few
worms were detected in tissue sections at day 7; none was seen later.
In immunodeficient mice, worms were noted at days 15 and 18 and
even at day 38.

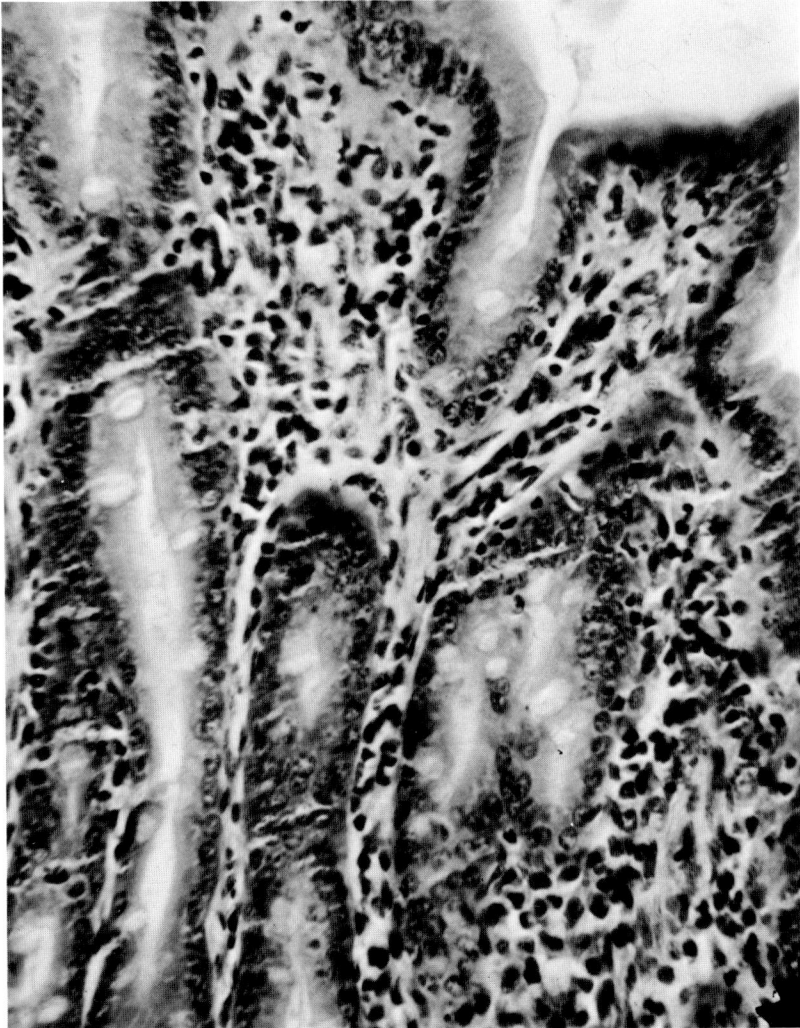

FIGURE 7. Section of intestine from immunized mouse 8 days after challenge. The
inflammatory reaction at this time is diminishing, and the predominant cells are mononuclear. ×270. From Larsh and Race (1954), courtesy of the University of Chicago
Press.

Ruitenberg *et al.* (1977) and Gustowski *et al.* (1980) used congenitally athymic (*nu/nu*) mice and their thymus-bearing heterozygous littermates (+/*nu*). Ruitenberg and colleagues monitored the effects of *T. spiralis* infection by determining the villus/crypt ratio and the mitotic index. The mucosa of noninfected mice was similar in both *nu/nu* and +/*nu* animals, with the villi being long and slender and showing distinct scalloping and crypts (ratio of villus length to depth of crypt being 3:1). After infection, both groups of mice manifested a shortening of the villi and a deepening of the crypts (ratio 2:1) due to hyperplasia. In general, no differences between the two groups were noted. On day 0 of the study, the mitotic index of the +/*nu* mice was significantly higher than that of the *nu/nu* animals. After infection, the mitotic index of the *nu/nu* mice was significantly higher on days 7–13 than that of their heterozygous littermates. Histological examination showed also that eosinophilia in the gut tissue of thymus-bearing mice occurred only during the early phase of infection, whereas in athymic mice, the mild increase that occurred was first noted on day 21 and continued until the end of the study at day 42.

The pattern of establishment, maintenance, and expulsion of *T. spiralis* in rats is very similar to that in mice. Gursch (1949) found that in an undesignated strain of rat, mucosal penetration by larvae had occurred by 4 hr after infection. During the next few days, as the worms matured, there was extensive damage of the intestinal villi. It was also observed that when adult worms reached the muscularis layer, they would turn about, thereby causing additional tissue destruction.

Leonard and Beahm (1941) have provided a clear description of the anatomical changes in the rat. Soon after penetration into the intestinal mucosa, there was a copious secretion of mucus and cells into the intestinal lumen. Most of the cells in this exudate were found to be polymorphonuclear leukocytes (PMNs). The inflammatory reaction in the mucosa varied, ranging from mild surface desquamation to intense interstitial inflammation. Mucosal glands were often collapsed, and epithelial cells showed degenerative changes. The submucosal tissues likewise showed varying degrees of inflammation, ranging from a low-grade vascular hyperemia with a mild infiltration of pus cells, including monocytes, to an intense PMN infiltration.

The deeper layers of the submucosa manifested less cellular infiltration, but edema with widening of the tissue layer and vascular hyperemia was marked; interstitial hemorrhages were also noted. Similiar changes were present in the muscularis mucosa. In their conclusion, Leonard and Beahm state:

> It was observed that the intensity of the reaction of the different layers of the gut was fairly uniform at any particular level. That is, if there was a

mild reaction in the mucosa the same held true for the other layers of the intestine. On the other hand if there was intense accumulation of pus at any particular level, there was usually an advanced infiltration of inflammatory cells in all the intestinal coats, but invariably the inflammatory reaction decreased in intensity from the lumen outward.

Ismail and Tanner (1972) found that in female Wistar rats weighing 200–250 g, an eosinophilic infiltration of the proximal small intestine occurred during infection. This infiltration occurred early, being quite prominent by day 6. Although clusters of eosinophils were commonly seen in the submucosa and in the lamina propria of the villi, infiltration was generally diffuse. Eosinophils were never found to aggregate around parasites. These researchers concluded that the eosinophil reaction was unrelated to the general inflammatory response. They based their conclusion on the observation that the latter reaction began after day 6 and was most prominent about days 10–12, a time when the eosinophil response was in its initial stage of decline.

As a result of intestinal infection of rodents with nematodes such as *T. spiralis* and *Nippostrongylus brasiliensis* (Ruitenberg and Elgersma, 1980), a proliferation of mast cells and globule leukocytes in the intestinal mucosa was noted. Both types of cells were located intraepithelially and are characterized by metachromatic granules; differentiation of these two types of cell requires special fixation and staining methods. The presence and proliferation of these cells are thought to be thymus-dependent, and although their origin and function are unclear, they are considered to be lymphoid blast-cell precursors of some sort. At one time, globule leukocytes were regarded as degranulated intestinal mast cells that migrate into the intestinal epithelial layer (Murray *et al.*, 1968). However, the recent work by Ruitenberg and Elgersma (1980) indicates that the two types of cells may represent independent populations. This conclusion was reached as a result of the active migration of globule leukocytes through the epithelial lining, differences in the timing of the appearance of both cell types, and their mitotic indexes.

The anatomical pathology of the intestinal phase of a *T. spiralis* infection in guinea pigs has been characterized by Castro *et al.* (1967), Catty (1969), and Lin and Olson (1970). Intestinal tissue from uninfected animals (Fig. 8), when compared to that of infected animals (Fig. 9), shows striking differences. In Fig. 8, it can be seen that the villi are well formed with deep intestinal crypts, whereas the tissue from the infected animals shows a very flattened mucosa with a much reduced villus-length to crypt-depth ratio. Microscopic examination showed that the shortened and blunted villi were apparently fused to form distinct transverse ridges across the gut surface. In addition, the diameter of

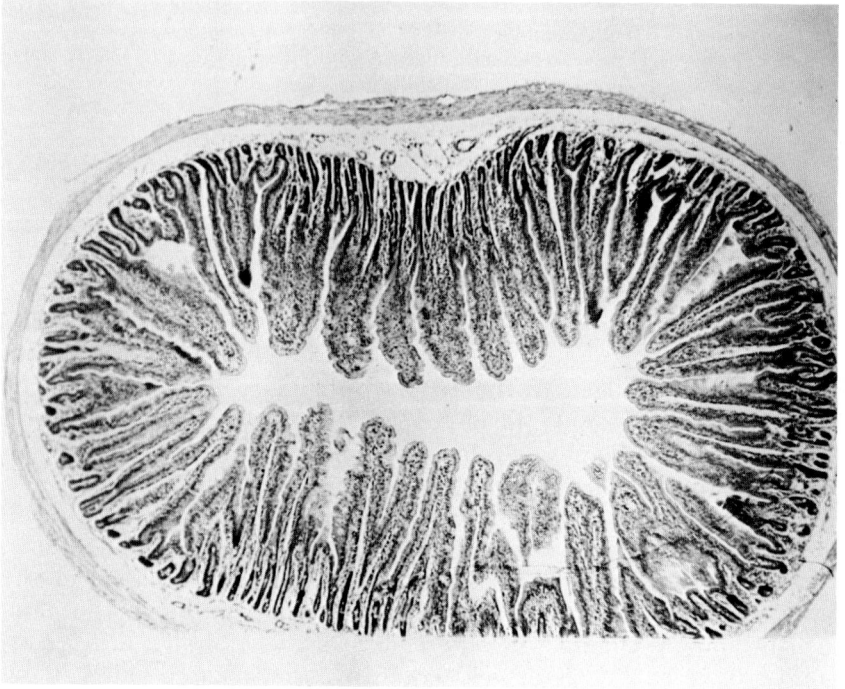

FIGURE 8. Section of intestine showing normal villus morphology of noninfected guinea pig. ×18. From Castro *et al.* (1967), courtesy of the author and editor.

the intestine of infected animals was much larger. The changes described above occurred in both the anterior and posterior portions of the small intestine. However, they occurred somewhat earlier in the anterior than in the posterior portion.

Changes were also noted in epithelial cells of the gut from infected animals when compared to control animals (Fig. 10 and 11). Cells from control animals can be seen to possess abundant cytoplasm above the nuclei, which are arranged in the typical palisade arrangement. Epithelial cells in tissues from infected animals have less cytoplasm, giving the cells a flattened or cuboidal appearance. Pyknotic nuclei are frequently seen. An extensive and intensive cellular infiltration was noted beneath the epithelial layer. According to Castro *et al.* (1967), this infiltrate consisted primarily of eosinophils, with substantial numbers of plasma cells and lymphocytes. It is surprising that no mention was made of increased numbers of neutrophils or macrophages, a characteristic of the cellular infiltrate in other *T. spiralis*-infected animals. Catty (1969)

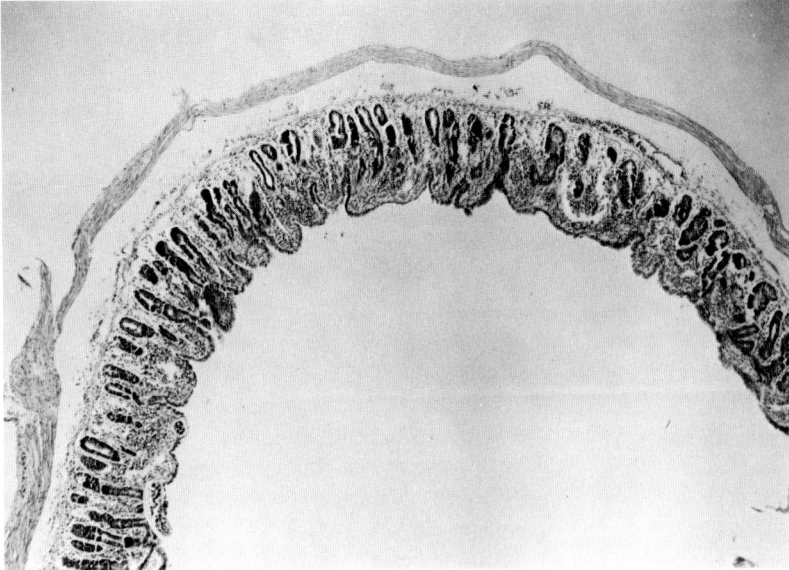

FIGURE 9. Section of intestine showing altered villus morphology of infected guinea pig × 18. From Castro *et al.* (1967), courtesy of the author and editor.

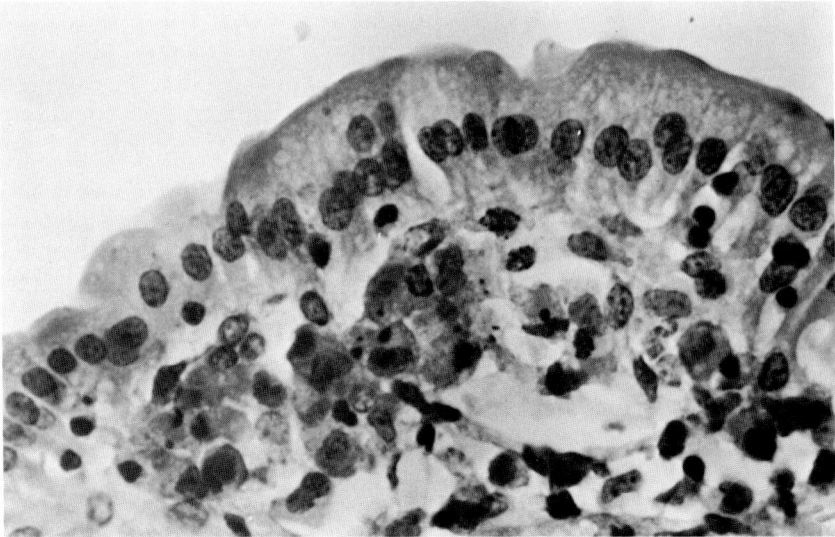

FIGURE 10. Section of villus tip showing columnar epithelial cells of noninfected guinea pig. × 325. From Castro *et al.* (1967), courtesy of the author and editor.

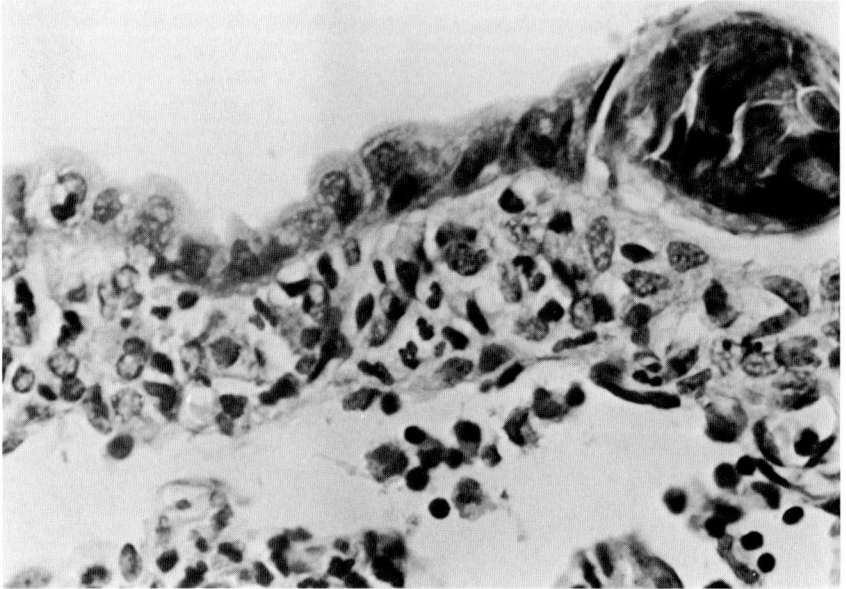

FIGURE 11. Section of villus showing altered epithelial cells of infected guinea pig. ×325. From Castro *et al.* (1967), courtesy of the author and editor.

found that eosinophils appeared first in the intestinal tissue, but by day 7 of infection, neutrophils were present in large numbers and formed a mixed infiltrate in all layers of the intestine. By day 8, extensive damage to the villi was noted, with acute hemorrhagic conditions present. Red cells were present in the interstitial tissues of the submucosa, and eosinophils, neutrophils, plasma cells, lymphocytes, and macrophages were "packed" into the villi. No specific migration or adherence of any cells within the infiltrate to the cuticle or orifices of the worms was noted. Normal villus architecture and tissue organization was restored by day 25. In the repair process, neutrophils and eosinophils disappeared first, leaving primarily macrophages and lymphocytes. These cells apparently remain in the tissues in elevated numbers until all worms have been expelled.

Hamsters have been used for pathological study of the muscle phase of trichinosis, but not the intestinal phase. This is unfortunate, since dramatic differences in response to infection between different species of hamsters are well known. For example, the Chinese hamster (*Cricetulus griseus*) will support the intestinal phase of *T. spiralis*, but is highly resistant to muscle invasion by larvae, whereas the golden hamster

(*Mesocricetus auratus*) supports both intestinal and muscular phases of the infection (Ritterson, 1957). Whether or not the resistance to muscle invasion in the Chinese hamster is due to some aspect of the intestinal phase is unknown. It is known, however, that the adult worms establish themselves in the anterior portion of the small intestine in the Chinese hamster as in rats and mice, whereas in the golden hamster, they are in the lower portion of the small intestine as in guinea pigs. The fact that rats, mice, and guinea pigs are susceptible to muscle invasion by larvae refutes the idea that a difference in the location of the adult worms in the intestine is the cause for the strong resistance to muscle invasion by the Chinese hamster.

Rabbits have not been widely used for the study of trichinosis. A search of the literature failed to reveal a single study that characterized the anatomical pathology of the intestinal phase. Both Catty (1969) and Tanner (1968) have successfully infected rabbits and studied various aspects of muscle invasion as well as adult longevity in the gut. It is interesting to note that both researchers found that despite the varying sizes of the infecting doses, no significant differences in the numbers of larvae in the musculature were detected. Again, as is the situation with hamsters, a detailed analysis of the intestinal pathology during the adult phase may shed light on this interesting finding. Tanner (1968) did note in his study that the marked blood eosinophilia that occurs in most animals is not a characteristic of trichinosis in rabbits. Whether or not an increase in the number of eosinophils is present in the intestinal tissue of infected rabbits is not known. It would be most surprising if it were not so, since most researchers have found a positive correlation between the presence of eosinophils and the expulsion of adult worms.

The microscopic changes associated with *T. pseudospiralis* have not yet been fully described. In monkeys, infection with *T. pseudospiralis* induced an inflammatory reaction similar to that induced by *T. spiralis*, and consisted of a slight decrease in villus crypt ratio, a slight increase in mitotic index, and an increase in the number of intestinal plasma cells and mast cells (Teppema *et al.*, 1981).

Larsh and Race (1975) have provided a unified hypothesis that links intestinal inflammation and pathology with the expulsion of adults from the intestinal tracts of animals. As a result of their own numerous studies and those of their colleagues, as well as those of others using laboratory animals, they have concluded that: (1) there is a close, direct association between the degree of sensitivity of the host at challenge and the timing and intensity of inflammation and loss of worms; (2) there is a similar association between the size of the challenging infection and the degree of resulting inflammation; and (3) there is a similar association between the persistence of worms and the absence of the characteristic acute inflammation. The inflammation resulting from the infection is due not only to the mechanical damage to cells and tissues caused by parasites, but also to a specific immune cellular response of the delayed-hypersensitivity type [allergic inflammation (see Chapter 8)]. As a consequence, the adults leave the intestinal tissues and move to the gut lumen in response to the unfavorable environment created by the inflammatory response.

3. STRIATED MUSCLE

According to Gould (1970), the muscle groups in man that are most frequently the sites of encystment of newborn larvae are the extraocular muscles, the masseters, the muscles of the tongue and larynx, the diaphragm, the muscles of the neck, the intercostal muscles, and the deltoids. In addition, the portions of the muscle fibers nearest to the sites of attachment to tendons and joints are most heavily involved. There is some indication that the more superficial muscles of the body are more heavily affected than those muscles that are deeply situated and that the encysted larvae are concentrated near the superficial surfaces rather than the deeper portions of the same muscle group.

In CD-1 mice, 8–10 weeks old, muscles involved in a descending order of predilection were found to be: masseters, diaphragm, biceps, pectoralis, gastrocnemius, triceps, vastus, tongue, and abdominal (Stewart and Charniga, 1980). There was a significantly greater mean number of larvae in the muscles situated cranial to the lower margin of the rib cage than was recovered from the muscles located below the rib cage.

Experimentally infected swine show a different pattern of larval encystment. Of 12 infected pigs, the diaphragm was the most heavily infected muscle in 7, and the tongue was the most heavily infected in 5. After the diaphragm and tongue, muscles invaded by larvae in order of preference were: masseters, the muscles of the neck, deltoids, pectoralis, abdominal, gluteus maximus, and muscles of the hindlimb (Olsen et al., 1964).

Roth (1939) found that in guinea pigs, the masseters and the diaphragm were most heavily infected. In rats, the diaphragm contained the most larvae (Roth, 1939), whereas in experimentally infected baboons and monkeys, the biceps were most involved, with the diaphragm containing the smallest mean larval density (Nelson and Mukundi, 1962).

The foregoing brief review of the muscles most heavily invaded by *T. spiralis* larvae illustrates the variation in muscle selection. In general, it appears that the muscles anterior to the posterior edge of the rib cage are most heavily involved. A review of the literature further suggests that the extraocular muscles may contain the greatest density of larvae, but these muscles were not examined by many of the researchers who have done such studies.

As pointed out by Gould (1970), it is generally believed that the most active muscles are those that have the most efficient blood supply and are most susceptible to invasion by larvae. Experimental evidence on this point is scarce. It does not appear that the invasion of muscle and the distribution of larvae reflect merely the mechanical factor of transportation by the vascular system.

3.1. Gross Changes

Human muscle has been studied most, and its gross appearance varies considerably. At autopsy, infected muscle has been characterized as tough and firm; others have described it as edematous and soft. The color of infected muscle at autopsy also varies; reports of color ranging from gray-red to red-brown with a tint of violet or blue have been published. Muscles during the 5th week of infection may manifest small gray streaks, and after 2–3 months, these change to small white specks. The speckled appearance intensifies 6–18 months later when the encysted larvae have been enclosed in calcified capsules (Gould, 1970).

3.2. Microscopic Changes

Surprisingly, very few studies have been done that characterize the inflammatory response in and around muscle fibers of laboratory animals. One gets the distinct impression from the literature that most comments relating to inflammation are attributable to the clinicians who studied human autopsy and biopsy specimens around the turn of the century. Whether or not these early observations can be applied to muscle tissue from laboratory animals is not known. Gould (1970) suggests that there are significant differences and that

> skeletal muscles of infected human beings, compared to those of animals, manifest more severe fatty metamorphosis, hyaline degeneration, hydropic degeneration, interstitial inflammation, and more frequent destruction of trichinae without encapsulation; in animals, there is said to be a relatively greater increase in the number of muscle nuclei. Human beings seem to withstand the effects of the intestinal stage of trichinosis better than experimental laboratory animals, and their defensive powers against muscular invasion by the parasites seem to be greater, as judged by the greater degree of inflammatory reaction and the relatively large number of trichinae destroyed.

No clear picture of inflammation in muscle tissue has been presented, and often there are conflicting reports in the literature. It is generally agreed, however, that as a result of ruptured capillaries and damage to the sarcolemma during the invasion process, small hemorrhages and accumulations of PMNs, lymphocytes, and tissue histiocytes are present in the interstitial connective tissue spaces. Such cells have also been reported to invade the muscle cells through the damaged sarcolemma (Gould, 1970).

Drachman and Tunchay (1965) noted in guinea pigs that damage to muscle fibers and the inflammatory infiltrate increased in severity up to day 20 after infection. Prominent perivasculitis, with interstitial collections of lymphocytes and PMNs, was evident. At day 25, perivascular inflammation was less prominent, and there were fewer accumulations of inflammatory cells. At 32 days after infection, some cysts were virtually free of surrounding inflammation, whereas others were surrounded by focal inflammatory infiltrates.

In CBA mice, the first changes in diaphragm muscle were seen on day 10, and in gastrocnemius muscle, on day 15. At these times, scattered inflammatory cells were noted. These soon formed discrete foci of inflammation, being composed of eosinophils, neutrophils, lymphocytes, and macrophages. Plasma cells and basophilic leukocytes were rarely seen. Eosinophil numbers declined after day 30, but eosinophils were still present in elevated numbers at 50 days. At this latter time, the sarcolemma and capsule had been breached, and inflammatory cells were noted next to degenerating larvae. Grove *et al.* (1977) report that in female Swiss albino mice, the marked muscular infiltrate observed at 4 weeks after infection had subsided at 8 weeks, and from 14 to 40 weeks, inflammation continued at a low, persistent level.

Increased vascularity in the immediate vicinity of muscle fibers infected with *T. spiralis* has been observed in human and mouse tissue derived postmortem and in living tissues of the cheek pouch of golden hamsters (Humes and Akers, 1952). According to these researchers, Pagenstecher in 1865 observed the extraordinary development of a mesh of blood vessels around infected muscle fibers. This increased vascularization was noted before the beginning of encapsulation. Ogielski (1949) noted in mice into the vascular system of which China ink had been injected a "netting of capillaries" at day 33 postinfection around infected muscle fibers.

Encysted larvae and the accompanying vascular changes can be observed in living hamsters. In this technique, the epithelial layers and connective tissue covering the thin, nonpigmented cheek pouch are carefully removed from anesthetized animals. When exposed, the muscle fibers that extend longitudinally from the open end of the pouch and the blood vessels that serve the muscle fibers can be seen. Humes and Akers (1952) report that in cheek-pouch preparations of golden hamsters made 3 days after infection, many white blood cells were observed rolling slowly along the internal surfaces of the veins in the cheek pouch. By day 6, veins and venules showed a distinct leukocytic pavement (mural thrombi). Such trombi were not seen in arterioles. On day 11, mural thrombi were still present in veins and venules; some were completely plugged, preventing the normal flow of blood. Mural thrombi continued to be present until day 36, after which vascular flow appeared to become normal.

A network of minute vessels around infected muscle fibers became apparent as early as day 19 following infection; this coincided with the beginning of the coiling of larvae that were in muscle fibers at this time. This increased vascularity persisted up to the 280th day, but at the 341st day, when opaque cyst walls (calcified?) were observed around the larvae, it had become inconspicuous, and vessels appeared smaller in size and number. According to Humes and Akers (1952), it is unknown whether or not the increased vascularity is due to enlargement of preexisting vessels, formation of new vessels, or a combination of both. They hypothesize that new vessels were indeed formed as response to stimulation of the capillary endothelium. These "new" vessels appeared sinusoidal in character and contained neither mural thrombi nor slowly moving leukocytes. Observations indicated that the network of vessels arose from arterioles by branching off at oblique angles and drained away from the infected fiber into one or more venules.

3.3. Encapsulation

Gould (1970) states that in man, encapsulation takes place after the 5th week of infection. In the rat, capsule formation is reported to begin on day 13 postinfection (Teppema et al., 1973), in the guinea pig on day 17 (Catty, 1969), and in the mouse on days 20–21 (Walls et al., 1973; Shanta and Meerovitch, 1967). Since Gould (1970) states that encapsulation at the 5th week is associated with a subsidence of the inflammatory process and formation of fibrous or scar tissue, it is evident that he was referring to the nearly complete process of encapsulation, whereas the other investigators were referring to its commencement. Thus, in man and in laboratory animals, encapsulation of a larva appears to be initiated around day 15 and is completed at 4–5 weeks postinfection. The microscopic appearance of encapsulated larvae in the muscle of pigs is shown in Figs. 12–15.

According to Gould (1970), the capsule enclosing a larva is com-

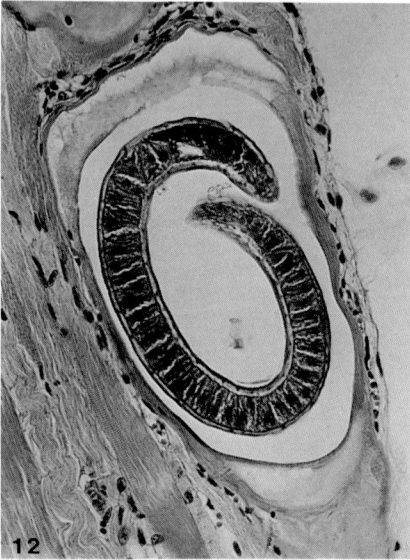

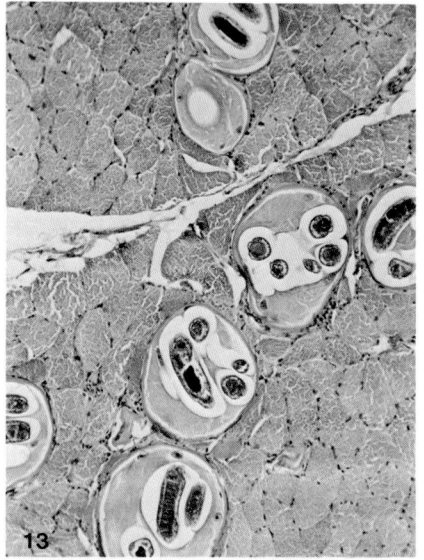

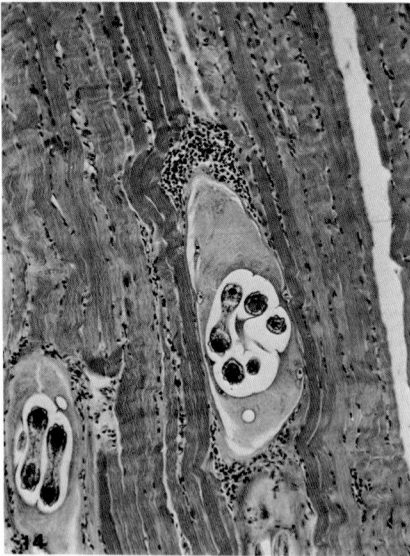

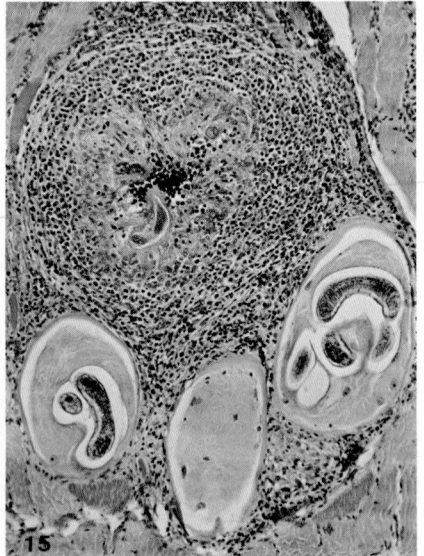

posed of an inner portion derived from the muscle fiber itself and an outer portion, homogeneous and hyaline in nature, derived from the sarcolemma.

Teppema *et al.* (1973), using SPF-raised Wistar rats, studied capsule formation with both light- and electron-microscopic techniques. They concluded that capsule formation began on day 13 postinfection, when a thin clear halo appeared around the larva. Coiling of the larva was completed at day 20, and at this time, a rapid extension of the capsule around the entire infected muscle fiber occurred. At 45–50 days after infection, the capsule had reached its maximum thickness. Within the capsule, the coiled larva was embedded in a clearly defined basophilic matrix that contained large nuclei. Lymphocytes, monocytes, and macrophages were also present in this matrix. As a result of electron-microscopic studies, these researchers state that the capsule is formed exclusively, or nearly so, from the infected muscle fiber; this conclusion is at variance with that of Bruce (1970), who suggested that the early capsule was formed of fibrils produced by connective tissue surrounding the infected muscle fiber. Collagen does appears to be a component of the capsule, but its origin is not known (Teppema *et al.*, 1973).

The fully formed capsule is somewhat lemon-shaped. Size varies with host animal (Table 1). According to Harley (1972), the variance in size of mature cysts suggests that cyst size is dependent more on the host's physiology than on the parasite's. Ordinarily, only one larva is present within a cyst; however, two larvae are frequently found and, occasionally, more than two. When more than one larva is present, they

←——————————————————————————————

FIGURE 12. Longitudinal section of encapsulated *Trichinella* larva in pig (42 days after inoculation). Section has cut mostly through stichosome region of larva. Most muscle shows minimal inflammatory reaction. Original magnification: ×300. Unpublished photograph, courtesy of Dr. W.C. Campbell.

FIGURE 13. Transverse section of several encapsulated *Trichinella* larvae in pig (77 days after inoculaton). A single capsule typically shows multiple sections of a single larva. Minimal cellular infiltration of host muscle. Original magnification: ×125. From Campbell and Cuckler (1966), by permission of the author and editor.

FIGURE 14. Encapsulated larva in muscle of pig (42 days after inoculation) showing moderate inflammation and characteristic infiltration of mononuclear cells at the poles of a capsule. Original magnification: ×125. From Campbell and Cuckler (1966), by permission of the author and editor.

FIGURE 15. Granuloma in muscle of pig, probably in response to spontaneous death of a larva (77 days after inoculation). Numerous fibroblasts and mononuclear leukocytes are present, as well as several giant cells and a central cluster of eosinophils. Adjacent to the granuloma are three typical *Trichinella* capsules. Original magnification: ×125. From Campbell and Cuckler (1966), by permission of the author and editor.

usually line up in tandem formation with little or no increase in cyst diameter.

Giant cells of the foreign-body type are sometimes observed on the outside of cyst walls. More frequently, giant cells are seen in association with necrotic muscle containing dead larvae that have not been encapsulated (Fig. 15). It is assumed that their function is the removal of the dead host tissue and parasites. Under some circumstances, fat cells concentrated at the poles of the lemon-shaped cyst may appear a few weeks after infection. According to Gould (1970), these cells are particularly well developed in the pig and cat, but are relatively inconspicuous in man. Little mention is made in the current literature of these fat-cell deposits in experimental animals.

In summary, the encapsulation process that results in the formation of a cyst suggests a specific alteration and adaptation of the infected muscle to the presence of the larva. Although most often referred to as a basophilic degenerative process, it is, in fact, a redifferentiation that probably serves a variety of necessary functions for the larva inasmuch as unencapsulated larvae quickly die and are resorbed (Teppema et al., 1973; Despommier, 1976).

While the pathogenesis of T. pseudospiralis infection has not yet been examined extensively, preliminary reports suggest that there is a striking lack of inflammatory response around the larvae in mice (Gabryel et al., 1978; Al Karmi and Faubert, 1981) and in monkeys (Teppema et al., 1981). Since evidence is emerging to show that T. pseudospiralis is primarily a parasite of birds, a comparison of pathogenesis in avian and mammalian hosts is needed.

TABLE 1
Size of Cyst

Animal	Length (mm)	Width (mm)	Author
Mouse	0.18–0.95	0.02 –0.06	Harley (1972)
	0.23	0.13	Gould (1970)
Rat	0.9 –1.28	0.035–0.04	Gould (1970)
	0.2 –1.3	0.02 –0.08	Harley (1972)
Guinea pig	0.15–0.80	0.01 –0.05	Harley (1972)
Pig	0.26–0.66	0.21 –0.31	Harley (1972)
	0.4	0.26	Harley (1972)
Polar bear	0.88	0.32	Gould (1970)
Man	0.4	0.26	Gould (1970)
	0.4 –0.6	0.2	Harley (1972)

TABLE 2
Time Required for Calcification of *Trichinella* Cysts[a]

Animal	Calcification first seen (months)	Complete calcification (months)
Man	5	18
Rat	2	2
Rabbit	3	7
Pig	5	9
Mouse	24	29

[a] Adapted from Gould (1970).

3.4. Calcification

According to Gould (1970), nothing is known of the mechanism of calcification of *Trichinella* cysts. A recent computer-based search of the literature indicates that the situation is still the same today. It has been reported that the administration of irradiated ergosterol or parathormone causes accelerated calcification of both host tissue and *Trichinella* cysts (Gould, 1970). Bullock (1953) suggests that the process of calcification of cysts and ossification of host tissues, and the presence of alkaline phosphatase, may be related. The report of Bullock (1953) does not, however, indicate a direct involvement of the enzyme in the deposition of calcium salts in the wall of the cyst.

It has long been known that larvae can remain viable for extended periods of time within calcified cysts. On death of the larva in a mature cyst, the larva, too, becomes calcified rather quickly. The process of calcification begins at one or both poles. This process is first noted as fine granules in the periphery or midportion of the cyst wall.

Information available in the literature regarding the time required for cyst calcification after infection is presented in Table 2. As can be seen, there is considerable variation in the time required for calcification among the various species of animals. It is not known why the time required for calcification of cysts in mice is over 10-fold longer than the time required in rats. These figures will most likely be adjusted after more careful study.

4. OTHER ORGANS INVOLVED

As previously stated, newborn larvae develop primarily in striated muscle of the skeletal system. However, they do occur with some frequency in other organs and tissues, where, most evidence indicates, they are transient in nature.

4.1. Heart

During autopsy, many investigators have noted characteristic macroscopic lesions and alterations of the hearts of *Trichinella*-infected human corpses. These lesions and alterations include a pericardial cavity containing blood-tinged or straw-colored fluid, a hyperemic pericardium and epicardium, fatty degeneration of the myocardium, flabby myocardium, altered colorations of myocardium (pale yellow to dark red-brown), and, occasionally, hemorrhagic extravasation of the endocardium with thrombosis (Gould, 1970). Microscopically, the pericardial fluid may contain a few newborn larvae. Mild edema, small focal hemorrhages, scattered focal necrosis of muscle fibers, and interstitial granulomas composed of neutrophils, eosinophils, lymphocytes, macrophages, and histiocytes may be seen in the myocardium. These lesions are usually most prominent beneath the endocardial or epicardial surfaces. Eosinophils are particularly abundant in some lesions. Although the myocardium is often involved in infections with *Trichinella* during the acute phase, cysts containing larvae never develop. It is thought that after newborn larvae invade the myocardium, they are either killed and resorbed, escape into the pericardial cavity, or enter into the cavity of the heart. Failure of the heart to support encystment has been attributed to: (1) paucity of connective tissue through which larvae were formerly thought to migrate; (2) the constant myocardial contractions, which interfere with localization in heart tissue; (3) the alleged absence of sarcolemma or the delicacy of the sarcolemmal sheaths, which are unable to retain the larvae inside the muscle fiber; and (4) a particularly strong inflammatory reaction in the myocardium.

Dunlap and Weller (1933) infected white rats with unknown numbers of infective larvae to determine whether the lesions of the myocardium and its surrounding tissues were similar to those reported for man. Their study showed that the alterative and exudative lesions in the rat were indeed comparable in all respects to those found in human hearts. Newborn larvae were found in heart tissues as early as 5 days after infection. In rats examined after active migration of larvae had stopped, the myocardium showed no reaction. In contrast, Leonard and Beahm (1941) found no larvae in tissue sections of heart muscle of rats, nor did they find any focal areas of inflammation indicative of larval invasion.

Pambuccian and Cironeanu (1961), although they did not find inflammatory infiltrates, did report the presence of dystrophic lesions of myocardial fibers in infected rats. These lesions were reported to be characterized by the presence of small vacuoles and changes in the size and shape of nuclei. The authors did not find any newborn larvae in the myocardium and, as a result, attributed the damage to a toxin produced by the infection.

Myocardial lesions similar to those in rats and man have been found in mice (Mauss and Otto, 1942), Chinese hamsters (Ritterson, 1957), and rabbits (Edwards and Hood, 1962). With regard to the last report, lesions were infiltrated with mononuclear cells and eosinophils, usually interstitial in location, and occasionally contained remains of dead larvae; necrosis of myocardial fibers in some lesions was noted. Edwards and Hood noted that the descriptions of the lesions they studied were identical to those reported for human heart muscle. Thus, it appears that newborn larvae do invade the tissues of the heart of experimental animals and do cause alterations in morphology, tissue organization, and physiology (Bernard and Sudak, 1960) similar to those seen in man. Also, the presence of the larvae in the heart is transient, with no encapsulation of larvae. Once the active migration of the newborn larvae has ended, no invasion of the myocardium occurs, and the heart muscle returns to normal.

4.2. Liver

Enlargement and marked fatty metamorphosis of the liver, similar to that caused by phosphorus poisoning, have been reported in humans who have died of acute trichinosis (Gould, 1970). Similar fatty changes in the liver of experimentally injected rats have also been reported.

Mikhail et al. (1978) observed lesions in the livers of rats infected with 100 or 500 larvae as early as 4 days after infection. On day 4, portal tracks representing migratory pathways of larvae showed dense lymphocytic infiltration proportionate to the level of infection. By day 10, liver parenchyma showed areas of focal fatty degeneration and necrosis. Necrosis was followed by regeneration nodules separated by fibrous trabeculae. Sometimes diffuse and severe fatty metamorphosis was evident in some liver 2.5 months after infection, but by the 4th month, the livers of infected animals had regained their normal architecture. Similar findings were reported by Pambuccian and Ciro-neanu (1961). In addition to the aforedescribed observations, these latter authors noted enlargement of the liver with yellow spots. Hyper-emia was evident at all times; sometimes it was severe.

Other studies have indicated that larvae may be present in the livers of mice (Mauss and Otto, 1942), pigs (Hill, 1957), cats, guinea pigs, and young dogs (Matoff and Komandarev, 1964). No mention was made in any of these reports as to whether or not pathological changes were present; it is likely that there would be changes similar to those reported for rats and man.

4.3. Spleen

The tissues of the spleen of experimental animals do not appear to be invaded by newborn larvae; Gould (1970) reports the same finding for man. However, there is an indirect involvement of the spleen, since enlargement, hyperplasia, and hyperemia are common observations. These conditions are considered to be a consequence of the general inflammatory process and the development of immunity to antigens of *Trichinella*.

4.4. Kidneys

Studies have revealed the presence of newborn larvae in the kidneys of mice (Mauss and Otto, 1942) and rats (Mikhail *et al.*, 1978). Other studies have failed to show the presence of larvae in the kidneys of rabbits (Edwards and Hood, 1962) and rats (Leonard and Beahm, 1941). However, the kidneys, like the spleen, are involved. Pambuccian and Cironeanu (1961) report inflammatory infiltrations, sometimes of a nodular nature, and dystrophic alterations of the tubular epithelium with swelling and granulovascular degenerescence. In severe infections, rats may manifest tubuloglomerulonephritis with a prevailing epithelial component; these authors have referred to this condition as trichinosic nephritis.

In man, according to Gould (1970), the usual change in the kidney consists of cloudy swelling and distinct opacity of the cortex. The renal parenchyma is normal in consistency, and fatty metamorphosis may or may not be observed. Swelling may be intracapsular, intratubular, and interstitial in location. Focal hemorrhages and infarction may also be seen.

The etiology of the changes and lesions in the kidney is not known. It is possible that they reflect damage due to the invasion of kidney tissue by a few newborn larvae or to inflammation and immunity of the hypersensitive type (immune complex).

4.5. Eyes

Edema of the eyelids, most notable in humans, is an early finding in trichinosis. This may be followed by conjunctival edema or hemorrhage. Hyperemia, linear hemorrhages of the retina with focal inflammatory cellular infiltrates, and myositis of the extraocular muscles are other manifestations (Gould, 1970).

Gould (1954) infected white rats and rabbits with heavy and lethal doses of *Trichinella* larvae. Subsequent to inoculation and up to 33 days postinfection, he studied the eye and its tissues histologically. In the rats, extreme dehydration was seen in the ocular apparatus as a result of the drying of the secretions in the conjunctival sacs and precipitation of the secretions of the lacrimal glands. Chronic edema of the eyelids and conjunctivae of rabbits was seen. Microscopically, the edema was frequently accompanied by cellular infiltrates.

Schoop and colleagues observed unencapsulated newborn larvae in the retina or choroid of one third of all experimentally infected rats, mice, and rabbits. They concluded from their study that most ocular manifestations resulted from invasion of the inner tissues of the eye, and not from toxic products of larvae being carried there by the vascular system (Gould, 1970).

4.6. Lungs

Opie (1904) observed hemorrhagic foci in the lungs of infected guinea pigs 4 weeks after infection. At times, the interalveolar capillaries were very dilated, and red blood corpuscles had escaped into the alveoli. In one instance, fibrin was also present, and leukocytes, with eosinophil granulations, had accumulated in the periphery of the focus. In two experiments, the lungs contained small nodules of consolidated tissue in which eosinophil cells were massed in immense numbers. The alveolar walls were thickened, and the alveoli were either filled by large desquamated epithelial cells or replaced by fibrous tissue. In the center of the nodule, eosinophils were so closely packed that in sections stained with eosin, the tissue had an almost homogeneously red color. In the walls of the adjacent alveoli, eosinophil cells were scattered in countless numbers. Opie did not find larvae in any of these lesions.

Askanazy found in recently infected rabbits disseminated subpleural and pulmonary hemorrhages and hemorrhagic foci in small bronchioles and groups of alveoli. He was consistently able to demonstrate *Trichinella* larvae within these hemorrhagic foci and attributed their presence to capillary obstruction and rupture (Gould, 1970). Edwards and Hood (1962), on the other hand, were unable to find any indication of the presence of larvae in squash preparations of rabbit lung. Although Mauss and Otto (1942) made no mention of lesions, they did find newborn larvae in the lungs of recently infected mice.

4.7. Central Nervous System

Encephalitis or encephalomeningitis is usually a consequence of severe infection in man, and larvae have frequently been found in cerebrospinal fluid. Microscopically, the brain tissues may be edematous and hyperemic. Punctate hemorrhages in both the cortical and medullary portions of the cerebrum are common findings. There may be perivascular infiltrations composed of lymphocytes, neutrophils, eosinophils, fibroblasts, and plasma cells. Although larvae are rarely found within the area of cellular infiltration, the neurological changes have been attributed to the presence of larvae and not to a toxin (Most and Abeles, 1937).

Edwards and Hood (1962) induced cerebral lesions in rabbits by infecting them with 40,000 or 2600 larvae. The resulting lesions were located usually in the white matter, but also in the cortex and basal ganglia. They varied from perivascular cuffing with small cells, resembling lymphocytes, to cuffing with large mononuclear cells and formation of diffusely distributed collections of cells in the parenchyma and compact granulomas, sometimes with central necrosis. Astrocytes, microglia, and mononuclear cells in varying proportions comprised these granulomas. The authors believed that the lesions bear a temporal relationship to the appearance of circulating larvae and circulating antilarval antibodies. They concluded that these lesions, as well as those in the heart, are most likely related either to the toxic effects of larvae and their metabolites or to toxic products produced in the course of the host reaction, rather than to the formation of antilarval antibodies and a subsequent antigen–antibody reaction in the tissues.

4.8. Bone Marrow

The report by Foldes (1953) is the only one known that indicates the finding of newborn larvae in bone marrow. In this instance, a larva was found in the marrow of a 13-year-old girl who died from myocarditis and pneumonia 32 days after infection.

4.9. Other Locations

It seems that the presence of larvae in any tissue other than skeletal muscle is of a transient nature. Larvae have been observed in virtually every tissue, body fluid, and organ of the body, including lymph nodes, pancreas, urine, placenta, mammary gland tissue, milk, bile, pleural and peritoneal cavities, and skin, and in arterial and venous blood, in addition to the tissues discussed previously.

Numerous authors have mentioned the possibility that infection with *T. spiralis* may somehow induce cancer (Gould, 1970). Cancer of the diaphragm in a heavily infected rat and carcinoma of the larynx in a patient who suffered from acute trichinosis have been reported (Kean, 1966). At this time, however, there is no evidence that these malignancies were caused by the infection.

REFERENCES

Al Karmi, T.O., and Faubert, G.M., 1981, Comparative analysis of mobility and ultra-structure of intramuscular larvae of *Trichinella spiralis* and *Trichinella pseudospiralis, J. Parasitol.* **67:**685–691.

Beresantev, Y.-A., 1962, On the relationship of trichinellae to the wall of the intestine, *Wiad. Parazytol.* **8:**57–61.

Bernard, G.R., and Sudak, F.N., 1960, Experimental trichinosis in the golden hamster. II. Electrocardiographic changes, *Am. Heart J.* **60:**88–93.

Boyd, E.M., and Huston, E.J., 1954, The distribution, longevity, and sex ratio of *Trichinella spiralis* in hamsters following an initial infection, *J. Parasitol.* **40:**686–690.

Bruce, R.G., 1970, The structure and development of the capsule of *Trichinella spiralis, J. Parasitol.* **56:**38–39.

Bullock, W.L., 1953, Phosphatases in experimental *Trichinella spiralis* infections in the rat, *Exp. Parasitol.* **2:**150–162.

Campbell, W.C., and Cuckler, A.C., 1966, Further studies on the effect of thiabendazole on trichinosis in swine, with notes on the biology of the infection, *J. Parasitol.* **52:**260–279.

Castro, G.A., Olson, L.J., and Baker, R.D., 1967, Glucose malabsorption and intestinal histopathology in *Trichinella spiralis*-infected guinea pigs, *J. Parasitol.* **53:**595–612.

Castro, G.A., Johnson, L.R., Copeland, E.M., and Dudrick, S.J., 1974, Development of enteric parasites in parenterally fed rats, *Proc. Soc. Exp. Biol. Med.* **146:**703–706.

Catty, D., 1969, The immunology of nematode infections: Trichinosis in guinea pigs as a model, in: *Monographs in Allergy*, Vol. 5 (P. Kallos, M. Hasek, T.M. Inderbitzin, P.A. Miescher, and B.K. Waksman, eds.), S. Karger, Basel, pp. 1–134.

Despommier, D., 1976, Musculature, in: *Ecological Aspects of Parasitology* (C.R. Kennedy, ed.), North-Holland, Amsterdam, pp. 269–285.

Drachman, D.A., and Tunchay, T.O., 1965, The remote pathology of trichinosis, *Neurology* **15:**1127–1135.

Dunlap, G.L., and Weller, C.V., 1933, Pathogenesis of trichinous myocarditis, *Proc. Soc. Exp. Biol. Med.* **30:**1261–1262.

Edwards, J.L., and Hood, C.I., 1962, Studies on the pathogenesis of cardiac and cerebral lesions of experimental trichinosis in rabbits, *Am. J. Pathol.* **40:**711–717.

Foldes, J., 1953, Acute trichinosis with finding of larva in bone marrow, *Am. J. Clin. Pathol.* **23:**918–920.

Gabryel, P., Gustowski, L., Blotna-Filipiak, M., and Rauhut, W., 1978, Pathomorphology of mouse muscle tissue during *Trichinella pseudospiralis* (light- and electronmicroscopic observations), in: *Trichinellosis*, Proceedings of the Fourth International Conference on Trichinellosis (C.W. Kim and Z.S. Pawlowski, eds.), University Press of New England, Hanover, New Hampshire, pp. 281–294.

Gardiner, C.H., 1976, Habitat and reproductive behavior of *Trichinella spiralis, J. Parasitol.* **62:**865–870.

Gould, S.E., 1954, The eye and orbit in trichinosis, *Bull. N. Y. Acad. Med.* **30:**726–729.

Gould, S.E. (ed.), 1970, *Trichinosis in Man and Animals*, Charles C. Thomas, Springfield, Illinois.

Grove, D.I., Hamburger, J., and Warren, K.S., 1977, Kinetics of immunological responses, resistance to reinfection, and pathological reactions to infection with *Trichinella spiralis*, *J. Infect. Dis.* **136:**562–570.

Gursch, O.F., 1949, Intestinal phase of *Trichinella spiralis* (Owen, 1835) Railliet, 1895, *J. Parasitol.* **35:**19–26.

Gustowski, L., Ruitenberg, E.J., and Elgersma, A., 1980, Cellular reactions in tongue and gut in murine trichinellosis and their thymus-dependence, *Parasite Immunol.* **2:**133–154.

Harley, J.P., 1972, Size of *Trichinella spiralis* (Nematoda) muscle cysts in the rat, mouse, and guinea-pig, *Experientia* **28:**486–487.

Hill, C.H., 1957, Distribution of larvae of *Trichinella spiralis* in the organs of experimentally infected swine, *J. Parasitol.* **43:**574–577.

Humes, A.G., and Akers, R.P., 1952, Vascular changes in the cheek pouch of the golden hamster during infection with *Trichinella spiralis* larvae, *Anat. Rec.* **114:**103–111.

Ismail, M.M., and Tanner, C.E., 1972, *Trichinella spiralis*: Peripheral blood, intestinal, and bone-marrow eosinophilia in rats and its relationship to the inoculating dose of larvae, antibody response and parasitism, *Exp. Parasitol.* **31:**262–272.

Kean, H., 1966, Cancer and trichinosis of the larynx, *Laryngoscope* **76:**1766–1768.

Kennedy, M.W., 1978, Kinetics of establishment, distribution, and expulsion of the enteral phase of *Trichinella spiralis* in the NIH strain of mouse, in: *Trichinellosis*, Proceedings of the Fourth International Conference on Trichinellosis (C.W. Kim and Z.S. Pawlowski, eds.), University Press of New England, Hanover, New Hampshire, pp. 193–205.

Larsh, J.E., 1963, Experimental trichiniasis, in: *Advances in Parasitology*, Vol. 1 (B. Dawes, ed.), Academic Press, New York, pp. 213–286.

Larsh, J.E., and Race, G.J., 1954, A histopathologic study of the anterior small intestine of immunized and nonimmunized mice infected with *Trichinella spiralis*, *J. Infect. Dis.* **94:**262–272.

Larsh, J.E., and Race, G.J., 1975, Allergic inflammation as a hypothesis for the expulsion of worms from tissues: A review, *Exp. Parasitol.* **37:**251–266.

Larsh, J.E., Race, G.J., and Jeffries, W.B., 1954, The association in young mice of intestinal inflammation and the loss of adult worms following an initial infection with *Trichinella spiralis*, *J. Infect. Dis.* **99:**63–71.

Larsh, J.E., Race G.J., and Yarinsky, A., 1962, A histopathologic study in mice immunized against *Trichinella spiralis* and exposed to total-body X-irradiation, *Am. J. Trop. Med. Hyg.* **11:**633–640.

Larsh, J.E., Race, G.J., Martin, J.H., and Weatherly, N.F., 1974, Studies on delayed (cellular) hypersensitivity in mice infected with *Trichinella spiralis*. VIII. Serologic and histopathologic responses of recipients injected with spleen cells from donors suppressed with ATS, *J. Parasitol.* **60:**99–109.

Leonard, A.B., and Beahm, E.H., 1941, Studies on the distribution of *Trichinella* larvae in the albino rat, *Trans. Kansas Acad. Sci* **44:**429–433.

Lin, T.-M., and Olson, L.J., 1970, Pathophysiology of reinfection with *Trichinella spiralis* in guinea pigs during the intestinal phase, *J. Parasitol.* **56:**529–539.

Marty, W.G., 1966, The intestinal phase of experimental infection of chicks with *Trichinella spiralis*, *J. Parasitol.* **52:**903–907.

Matoff, K., and Komandarev, S., 1964, Further investigations into the problem of muscle trichinae occurrence in organs devoid of striated muscles, *Wiad. Parazytol.* **10:**639–650.

Mauss, E.A., and Otto, G.F., 1942, The occurrence of *Trichinella spiralis* larvae in tissues other than skeletal muscles, *J. Lab. Clin. Med.* **27**:1384–1387.

Mikhail, E.G., Milad, M., Sabet, S., and Abdallah, A., 1978, Experimental trichinosis. I. A pathological study of hepatic, renal, and gonadal involvement, *J. Egypt. Public Health Assoc.* **53**:327–340.

Most, H., and Abeles, M.M., 1937, Trichiniasis involving the nervous system: A clinical and neuropathologic review, with report of two cases, *Arch. Neurol. Psychiatry* **37**:589–616.

Murray, M., Miller, H.R.P., and Jarrett, W.F.H., 1968, The globule leucocyte and its derivation from the subepithelial mast cell, *Lab. Invest.* **19**:222–234.

Nelson, G.S., and Mukundi, J., 1962, The distribution of *Trichinella spiralis* larvae in the muscles of primates, *Wiad. Parazytol.* **8**:629–632.

Offutt, E.P., and McCoy, O.R., 1941, The "gopher," *Citellus richardsonii* (Sabine) as an experimental host for *Trichinella spiralis*, *J. Parasitol.* **27**:535–538.

Ogielski, L., 1949, Reaction of the vascular vessels against an invasion of the larvae of *Trichinella spiralis*, *Zool. Pol.* **5**:34–42.

Olsen, B.S., Villella, J.B., and Gould, S.E., 1964, Distribution of *Trichinella spiralis* in muscles of experimentally infected swine, *J. Parasitol.* **50**:489–495.

Opie, E.L., 1904, An experimental study of the relation of cells with eosinophil granulation to infection with an animal parasite (*Trichinella spiralis*), *Am. J. Med. Sci.* **127**:477–493.

Pambuccian, G., and Cironeanu, I., 1961, Observations on experimental trichinellosis in white rats: A pathological and clinical study, *Rum. Med. Rev.* **6**:8–13.

Race, G.J., Larsh, J.E., Martin, J.H., and Weatherly, N.F., 1974, Light and electron microscopy of the intestinal tissue of mice parasitized by *Trichinella spiralis*, in: *Trichinellosis*, Proceedings of the Third International Conference on Trichinellosis (C.W. Kim, ed.), Intext, New York, pp. 75–100.

Race, G.J., Larsh, J.E., Martin, J.H., Weatherly, N.F., and Goulson, H.T., 1978, Histopathologic observations of mice after expulsion of *Trichinella spiralis*, in: *Trichinellosis*, Proceedings of the Fourth International Conference on Trichinellosis (C.W. Kim and Z.S. Pawlowski, eds.), University Press of New England, Hanover, New Hampshire, pp. 239–261.

Ritterson, A.L., 1957, The Chinese hamster (*Cricetulus griseus*) as an experimental host for *Trichinella spiralis*, *J. Parasitol.* **43**:542–547.

Roth, H., 1938, On the localization of adult trichinae in the intestine, *J. Parasitol.* **24**:225–331.

Roth, H., 1939, Experimental studies on the course of trichina infection in guinea pigs. II. Natural susceptibility of the guinea pig to experimental trichina infection, *Am. J. Hyg.* **29**:89–104.

Ruitenberg, E.J., and Elgersma, A., 1976, Absence of intestinal mast cell response in congenitally athymic mice during *Trichinella spiralis* infection, *Nature (London)* **264**:258–260.

Ruitenberg, E.J., and Elgersma, A., 1980, Study of the kinetics of globule leucocytes in the intestinal epithelium of rats after single or double infection with *Trichinella spiralis*, *Br. J. Exp. Pathol.* **61**:285–290.

Ruitenberg, E.J., Leenstra, F., and Elgersma, A., 1977, Thymus dependence and independence of intestinal pathology in a *Trichinella spiralis* infection: A study in congenitally athymic (nude) mice, *Br. J. Exp. Pathol.* **58**:311–314.

Shanta, C.S., and Meerovitch, E., 1967, The life cycle of *Trichinella spiralis*. II. The muscle phase of development and its possible evolution, *Can. J. Zool.* **45**:1261–1267.

Stewart, G.L., and Charniga, L.M., 1980, Distribution of *Trichinella spiralis* in muscles of the mouse, *J. Parasitol.* **66**:688–689.

Tanner, C.E., 1968, Relationship between infecting dose, muscle parasitism, and antibody response in experimental trichinosis in rabbits, *J. Parasitol.* **54:**98–107.

Teppema, J.S., Robinson, J.E., and Ruitenberg, E.J., 1973, Ultrastructural aspects of capsule formation in *Trichinella spiralis* infection in the rat, *Parasitology* **66:**291–296.

Teppema, J.S., Blomjous, F.J.E.M., Elgersma, A., and Ruitenberg, E.J., 1981, *Trichinella pseudospiralis* and *T. spiralis* infections in monkeys. III. Pathological aspects, in: *Trichinellosis*, Proceedings of the Fifth International Conference on Trichinellosis (C.W. Kim, E.J. Ruitenberg, and J.S. Teppema, eds.), Reedbooks, Chertsey, Surrey, England, pp. 209–214.

Walls, R.S., Carter, R.L., Leuchars, E., and Davies, A.J.S., 1973, The immunopathology of trichiniasis in T-cell deficient mice, *Clin. Exp. Immunol.* **13:**231–242.

Wright, K.A., 1979, *Trichinella spiralis:* An intracellular parasite in the intestinal phase, *J. Parasitol.* **65:**441–445.

6

Pathophysiology of the Gastrointestinal Phase

GILBERT A. CASTRO and GRAHAM R. BULLICK

1. FORMAT OF THIS REVIEW

Physiological alterations associated with the gastrointestinal (GI) phase of trichinosis are considered using a format based on several physiological and pathological principles. Since physiology involves a study of structure–function relationships, and abnormal biochemistry and physiology generally accompany abnormal morphology, both structural and functional tissue changes are considered. Qualitative and quantitative aspects of pathogenesis of infection with *Trichinella spiralis* are conditioned by prior contact with the parasite. Because of this, some attention is given to the onset and expression of structural–functional changes as they occur in primary as compared with secondary infection. Although it is quite evident that the degree of pathological damage in trichinosis is influenced in part by the intensity of infection, pathophysiological changes are considered primarily with regard to their presence in the host, not with regard to the size of the infective inoculum.

Pathogenesis of trichinosis may be expressed differently among the many individual species that can serve as host to *T. spiralis*. Nevertheless, the authors have opted not to present a species-by-species account, but to review categorically parasite-induced changes that influence the primary function of the GI tract—food assimilation. This

GILBERT A. CASTRO and GRAHAM R. BULLICK • Department of Physiology and Cell Biology, University of Texas Medical School at Houston, Houston, Texas 77025.

involves changes in smooth muscle motor function, secretory activity, and terminal digestive and absorptive processes at the level of the brush border. Different levels of activity for specific functions exist along the length of the GI tract and within the depth of the tract wall. Therefore, for the sake of convenience, pathophysiology is presented with reference to spatial distribution along the length and among successive layers, i.e., epithelium, lamina propria, and smooth muscle, of various organs that comprise the GI tract.

2. GASTROINTESTINAL SYMPTOMS

Gould (1970a) tabulated 18 symptoms and physical signs associated with the intestinal phase of trichinosis in humans. Of these, loss of appetite, constipation, abdominal cramps and pain, nausea, and weight loss are generally considered to be caused by parasite-induced physiological changes referable to the GI tract. On the basis of available experimental evidence, however, diarrhea is the only symptom to which a physiological basis can be ascribed with some degree of certainty. The primary reason is that diarrhea is the only symptom listed above for which a general understanding of the physiological etiology exists.

Diarrhea may be caused by several malfunctions. Osmotic retention of water in the gut lumen is one. To understand how this might induce diarrhea, a general understanding of the volume and origin of fluid entering the GI tract on a daily basis is necessary, as is a working knowledge of the dynamics of bidirectional fluid movement in the intestine and colon. Such an understanding can be gained from any number of reviews in this area (e.g., Binder, 1979; Field *et al.*, 1980). An important underlying principle is that diarrhea is caused ultimately by the retention of abnormal amounts of water in the lumen of the GI tract, which overwhelms the maximum absorptive capacity of the colon. Water, in response to osmotic pressure caused by ions or other solutes, fluxes into and out of the lumen. It becomes clear, then, that impaired digestive activity can lead to failure in removing osmotically active molecules from the intestinal lumen. The classic example of diarrhea caused by this mechanism is lactase deficiency, i.e., a deficiency in a brush-border enzyme.

The prototype of diarrhea due to active secretion of ions and fluid is that caused by the bacterium *Cholera vibrio*. This organism, through action of a toxin, stimulates NaCl and water flux from the epithelium to the lumen by activating an adenylate-cyclase-modulated secretory mechanism (Field, 1980). The possibility that *T. spiralis* could induce diarrhea through moderate degrees of stimulation of this same mechanism is supported by the observations that other stimulants such as vasoactive intestinal polypeptide and prostaglandins induce intestinal electrolyte and water secretion via a pathway similar to that activated by *C. vibrio* toxin.

Another factor that can contribute to diarrhea is a change in intestinal motor activity (intestinal motility) that increases intestinal transit, thus decreasing the time of contact between luminal solutions and the absorbing surface. This would lead to a decrease in the amount of fluid taken up by the mucosa. As will be seen from the following considerations, *T. spiralis* causes changes in GI physiology that may contribute to diarrhea through each or all of these mechanisms.

Loss of weight or failure to maintain normal weight patterns is an obvious symptom of infection with *T. spiralis* (Castro and Olson, 1967) and is common to intestinal parasitism in general. This may originate from metabolic changes within the host or from a decreased capacity to assimilate nutrients. Weight loss, however, can be more easily accounted for by another symptom of infection—decreased food intake, or anorexia. Despite the importance of anorexia in parasitism, no relationship between loss of appetite and GI physiology has been established.

3. MORPHOLOGICAL CHANGES

3.1. Macroscopic

Lesions of the GI tract of man due to trichinosis, even when accompanied by death, appear insignificant. Small ulcerations and, rarely, small hemorrhagic erosions are present (Gould, 1970b). The ileum is most severely affected, with the stomach, duodenum, jejunum, and colon less often involved. In experimental animals, the duodenum and jejunum are most severely affected.

Small-bowel pathology in infected rats, as described by Pambuccian and Cironeanu (1961), was insignificant even in cases of severe outward signs of disease. Some microscopic ulcerations accompanied by slight bleeding were present in animals that died within the first week of infection.

More general changes of the infected intestine included an increased mass, due in part to edema, as judged by an increase in the tissue weight/dry weight ratio, and to an increase in tissue cellularity, as measured by an increase in total mucosal DNA and dry weight. In rats in which these measurements were made, the changes were most marked in the proximal half of the intestine (Smith and Castro, 1978).

3.2. Histological

3.2.1. Mucosa—General

Lin and Olson (1970) reported graded changes in villous patterns in the intestine of previously infected guinea pigs that were challenged. These changes ranged from normal, fingerlike villi to villi that were shortened and arranged in convoluted ridges. Similar changes were noted in primarily infected hosts; however, the changes in sensitized, challenged animals had an earlier onset.

Mice infected with *T. spiralis* show what has been described as "hobnail" and convoluted-mosaic villous atrophy (Olson and Richardson, 1968). Disappearance of the normal villous pattern was most pronounced in the proximal fourth of the small intestine, less obvious in the second quarter, and absent in the distal half of the gut.

Examination of histological sections of small intestine from *T. spiralis*-infected guinea pigs revealed a dilated intestine with a flattened mucosa lacking a normal villous pattern in some areas (Castro *et al.*, 1967). Similar changes have been reported for infected mice (Olson and Richardson, 1968). The histological picture described here is similar to that reported for other intestinal nematode infections (Symons and Fairbairn, 1962; Sheehy *et al.*, 1962; Barker, 1973) and in other diseases in which inflammatory changes in the lamina propria are prominent (Takeuchi *et al.*, 1965). These tissue changes, therefore are not pathognomonic of trichinosis.

Reduced villus/crypt ratios were observed in rats and guinea pigs infected with *T. spiralis* (Pambuccian and Cironeanu, 1961; Castro *et al.*, 1967; Lin and Olson, 1970). Ruitenberg *et al.* (1977a,b) examined the nonspecific histological changes of the proximal jejunum in congenitally athymic mice (nude, *nu/nu*) and their thymus-bearing littermates (+/*nu*) infected with *T. spiralis*. In noninfected +/*nu* and *nu/nu* mice, the villus/crypt ratio was approximately the same (3:1), but the villus/crypt ratio after infection was reduced (2:1) in both groups. The reduction of the ratio was due primarily to a shortening of the villi and a concurrent hyperplasia of the crypts. The villi in both groups of mice before infection were long and slender with distinct scalloping (folding or indentations). After infection, the villi appeared shorter, and scalloping had disappeared. These effects lasted for approximately 10 days in the thymus-bearing mice and for 13 days in athymic mice. By 16 days postinfection (PI), the villus/crypt ratio had returned to essentially normal values even though adult worms were still present in athymic mice. Ruitenberg *et al.* (1977b) thus concluded that these nonspecific changes were thymus-independent, i.e., were not dependent on the immunological status of the host. This conclusion is in opposition to that of Manson-Smith (1979) (1975), whose experiments indicated that villi/crypt ratios and other nonspecific histopathological changes were thymus-dependent in mice infected with *T. spiralis.*

3.2.2. Epithelium

According to Pambuccian and Cironeanu (1961), the penetration of *T. spiralis* into the intestinal mucosa of rats causes desquamation of epithelium. This appears to be the only report of such a drastic epithelial response to infection. In guinea pigs, which show marked histological responses to infection, epithelial desquamation was not present. However, several changes were noted. Control gut exhibited an orderly arrangement of columnar epithelial cells lining the surface of the villi. There was an abundance of cytoplasm above the nuclei, which were located in the palisades near the base of the cells. In contrast, infected gut revealed cuboidal epithelial cells with an apparent reduction in the volume of cytoplasm (Castro and Olson, 1967). The cells stained darker than normal and had pyknotic nuclei that varied in size. Epithelial morphology remained altered even when villous patterns had returned to normal 21 days PI. Lin and Olson (1970) showed that heavy challenge doses in sensitized guinea pigs led to disruption of the brush-border membrane, reflected in the loss of microvilli. Since these latter changes occurred only when animals were challenged with extremely high doses of larvae, the importance of this structural change in the pathogenesis of infection must be considered cautiously. Caution is warranted, since impaired glucose absorption occurred in infected guinea pigs even when the brush border appeared structurally "normal."

An increase in goblet-cell numbers and mucus secretion in the *T. spiralis*-infected host is part of the intestinal response to the parasite. The work of Lin and Olson (1970) with guinea pigs shows an increase in the number of goblet cells elicited by primary infection and an anamnestic elevation in the number of these cells following secondary infection. Whereas there is little doubt that inflammatory reactions elicited are catarrhal in nature, as reflected in increased goblet-cell numbers, mucus secretion *per se* elicited by *T. spiralis* has not been measured quantitatively, nor has the quality of mucus secreted been examined.

3.2.3. Lamina Propria

Reasons for epithelial changes in trichinosis are not clear, but both morphological and functional alterations generally occur in response to some degree of inflammation in the lamina propria. Factors responsible for homing of cells into the lamina propria are poorly understood. The accumulation of various cells in the intestinal tissues of infected animals, however, has been demonstrated conclusively (Larsh, 1963). Quantitation of cell types using chemical markers has been performed in a few studies. Lymphoid cells and plasma cells containing specific immunoglobulins to *T. spiralis* have been detected by immunofluorescence techniques (Kozek and Crandall, 1974). Elevated mucosal myeloperoxidase activity has been correlated with myeloid-cell influx (Castro *et al.*, 1974; Smith and Castro, 1978). Lysophospholipase activity has been directly related to the presence of eosinophils in intestinal tissue (Larsh *et al.*, 1974).

Larsh and Race (1954), Larsh (1963), and Race *et al.* (1974) described the inflammatory reaction to *T. spiralis* in some detail. They documented inflammatory changes of both primary and secondary infections in mice. Major differences are that the severity and intensity of the inflammatory reaction are greater and the reaction reaches its zenith more rapidly following challenge of previously infected hosts as compared with mice infected for the first time.

In nonimmunized mice, an early reaction developed consisting of an increase in the numbers of polymorphonuclear leukocytes (PMNs) in the mucosa, especially centered around the worms. The migration by PMNs continued until a peak was reached at day 8 PI. At this time, a severe panmucosal and submucosal inflammatory reaction existed accompanied by extensive edema. Subsequent to this peak, the inflammatory reaction diminished and a mixed cell population consisting of plasmacytes, lymphocytes, and macrophages began to replace the earlier infiltrating myeloid cells, which were primarily neutrophils. Larsh and Race (1954) rarely observed eosinophils, a cell so characteristic of tissue reaction to nematodes (Leid and Williams, 1979). In guinea pigs, an extensive infiltration of eosinophils into the lamina propria and submucosa of the anterior gut was observed by Castro *et al.* (1967) and Catty (1969). This eosinophilia peaked at day 3 PI and was moderate on days 7 and 14 and absent on days 21 and 28. In the posterior small intestine of guinea pigs, a similar eosinophilia occurred, but was slightly delayed and did not reach a maximum until day 7. Leonard and Beahm

(1941) observed infiltrates of monocytes and PMNs, including eosinophils, in the intestinal mucosa of rats 2–8 days PI.

Tissue eosinophilia in athymic (*nu/nu*) mice infected with *T. spiralis* has been studied by Ruitenberg and co-workers. Ruitenberg *et al.* (1977a) found that intestinal eosinophilia and intestinal plasma-cell production were not observed in *nu/nu* infected mice, but these responses were observed in the thymus-bearing (+/*nu*) mice. Consequently, it was concluded that the eosinophil and plasma cell response were T-cell-dependent. Gustowska *et al.* (1980) reported the return of a minor cellular inflammatory reaction (involving eosinophils, mononuclear cells, and mast cells) beginning 3 weeks PI in *nu/nu* mice. This indicates partial thymus independence of the inflammatory reaction as the infection progresses.

Another cell that appears in increased numbers in the intestinal wall is the macrophage. Ruitenberg and Elgersma (1976) and Ruitenberg *et al.* (1979) have also examined intestinal mastocytosis and globular leukocytosis in *T. spiralis* infections. These workers established primarily through work with thymus-bearing rats and in athymic mice that the intestinal mast-cell population is distinct from those in other tissues. The intestinal mast-cell response to *T. spiralis* in the rat is thymus-independent; the origin of the mast cells is thymus-dependent. In contrast, the globular leukocyte response to *T. spiralis* is thymus-dependent, and its origin is thymus-independent. In mice, the globule leukocyte and mast-cell response (Fig. 1) are influenced by the thymus (Ruitenberg and Elgersma, 1976; Ruitenberg *et al.*, 1980) and are probably independent cell populations (Ruitenberg *et al.*, 1979; Ruitenberg and Elgersma, 1979).

Responses that attract or draw cells into the intestine are a matter of controversy. Warren *et al.* (1976) reported that components of *T. spiralis* larvae promote migration of eosinophils. However, Wine *et al.* (1977) and Jensen and Castro (1981) found that worms alone were not chemotactic for these cells. Warren *et al.* (1976) drew conclusions using a technique that did not differentiate random from directed migration, whereas Jensen and Castro (1981) used a technique that would specifically detect true chemotaxis. This may account for the different conclusions in the two studies. Crandall (1965) and Jensen and Castro (1981) reported that rabbit neutrophils and rat eosinophils, respectively, were attracted by metabolic products of *T. spiralis* in the presence of immune serum. The chemotaxis of eosinophils was dependent on the worm stage, which serves as the source of metabolites, infective larvae being more effective than juvenile and adult stages.

Several authors have attempted to quantify the number of cells in the mucosa of *T. spiralis*-infected animals by taking advantage of their

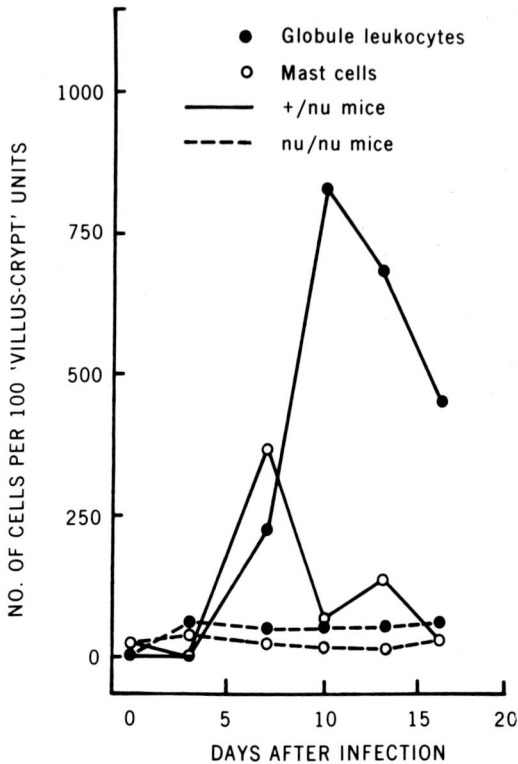

FIGURE 1. Mean number of intestinal mast cells and globule leukocytes in a 10-cm portion of proximal jejunum in groups of 4–5 +/nu (thymus-bearing) or nu/nu (athymic) mice infected with 100 T. spiralis larvae/mouse. From Ruitenberg and Elgersma (1976).

association with certain chemical markers. The major techniques are those of Larsh et al. (1974), who used lysophospholipase B as a marker for eosinophils, and Castro et al. (1974), who used mucosal peroxidase activity as a marker for myeloid cells. Larsh et al. (1974) reported changes in lysophospholipase B in challenged mice and rats. They indicated that coupled with increased bone marrow and intestinal eosinophilia, lysophospholipase B levels increased 5 days PI and remained high until 29 days PI in mice. In rats, lysophospholipase B levels increased between 4 and 18 days PI from resting levels. The discrepancy in timing between the two species was related to a difference in expulsion time of adult worms (rats 9–12 days PI and mice 11–14 days PI).

Castro et al. (1974) found that in rats, the flux of cells into the lamina propria is paralleled by an increase in peroxidase activity (Castro *et al.*, 1974; Smith and Castro, 1978). This increased enzyme activity was most prominent in the proximal jejunum, where the majority of adult worms resided. Increased peroxidase activity during infection results from increased numbers of PMNs, monocytes, and young monocyte-derived macrophages present in the mucosa and submucosa. Leukocyte peroxidase is present within each of these cells (Furth *et al.*, 1970). Histological observations confirm these results, with inflammatory cells increasing drastically in the lamina propria an submucosa (Fig. 2). The activity of peroxidase increased 4 to 10-fold in *Trichinella*-infected rats 7–10 days after exposure to infective larvae of *T. spiralis*. This method of indirectly measuring myeloid-cell influx in the lamina propria has also been employed to estimate intestinal inflammation in the mouse (Kramar *et al.*, 1981; Charniga *et al.*, 1981).

3.2.4. Muscularis Externa

A striking change in the small intestine of infected hosts involves the smooth muscle layers. Although a wealth of information concerning the changes in skeletal muscle is available, the intestinal smooth muscle has largely escaped attention. This layer clearly increases in thickness (Castro *et al.*, 1976a; Lin and Olson, 1970) during infection and, as will be shown below, is associated with functional alterations. It is not known whether this increase in muscle mass is due to edema, hypertrophy, or hyperplasia. Whatever the cause of this change, it exerts its effect within a few days after primary infection. Examination of histological sections of intestine published by Castro (1976) and Smith and Castro (1978) reveals obvious changes within 3–7 days PI (Fig. 3). Lin and Olson (1970) noted that in guinea pigs, an increase in muscle thickness was due to changes in the inner longitudinal rather than the circular layer and that secondary infections induced an increase in mass much earlier than did primary infections of equal size.

4. PHYSIOLOGICAL CHANGES

4.1. Epithelium-Related

4.1.1. Gastric Secretion

The gastric mucosa and exocrine pancreas secrete enzymes that are involved in cavital digestion. A cholinergic reflex activated by HCl

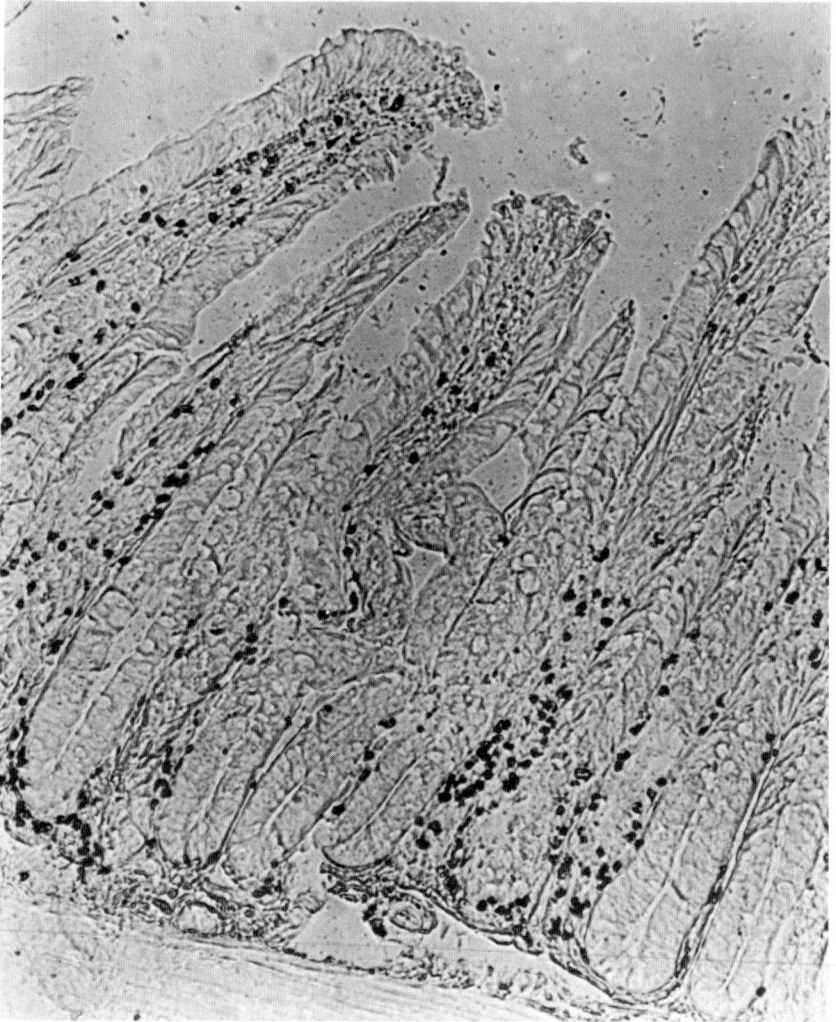

FIGURE 2. Jejunal section of *T. spiralis*-infected rat demonstrating localization of dark-staining, peroxidase-positive cells [diaminobenzadine reaction (Graham and Karnovsky, 1966)] in the lamina propria 7 days after infection with 7.5×10^3 *T. spiralis* larvae. From Smith and Castro (1978).

partially regulates secretion of pepsinogen by chief cells. Conversion of this precursor to active pepsin depends on a low pH, also provided by HCl. Thus, the physiological role of acid in the stomach is evident. Gastric acid secretion in dogs is caused, in part, by the hormone gastrin.

This gastrin-stimulated component of secretion is suppressed by another hormone, secretin. Secretin is released under physiological conditions by H^+ entering the small intestine from the stomach and contacting the duodenal mucosal surface (Johnson and Grossman, 1968, 1969). In dogs infected with *T. spiralis*, secretin regulation of gastrin-stimulated acid secretion is altered because of impaired release of secretin (Dembinski *et al.*, 1979a). The conclusion that altered regulation was due to impaired secretin release rather than an impairment in target-organ response rests on the finding that secretin, given by intravenous injection, carried out its expected regulatory role (Fig. 4).

4.1.2. Pancreatic Secretion

Control of water and bicarbonate secretion by duct cells of the exocrine pancreas as well as stimulation of enzyme secretion by acinar cells is a major function of secretin. Pancreatic enzyme secretion, however, is stimulated to a greater degree by another GI hormone, cholecystokinin (CCK), which is released from the duodenal mucosa. Major stimuli for CCK release are peptic hydrolysates of dietary protein and fat (Vagne and Grossman, 1968).

Dogs infected with *T. spiralis* displayed normal pancreatic secretion of fluid, bicarbonate, and enzymes when stimulated by exogenous secretin or CCK administered intravenously. However, when the duodenum of these hosts was perfused with H^+ or fat, the physiological stimulants for release of the two hormones, pancreatic secretion was not stimulated as it was in uninfected hosts. Pancreatic secretion was decreased during the first week of a primary infection, but was at the preinfection level when studied 3 weeks PI. Contrary to observations after primary infection, dogs given a secondary infection and examined within 1 week PI secreted normal levels of fluid, HCO_3^-, and enzymes (Dembinski *et al.*, 1979b). From these findings (Fig. 5), it was concluded that pancreatic secretion was impaired during the intestinal phase of primary infection with *T. spiralis*. Since the reaction induced by primary infection was not elicited by a secondary infection, it was proposed that this reflected the immunizing effect of prior contact with the parasite.

4.1.3. Intestinal Secretion

Infection with *T. spiralis* caused a decrease in net fluid absorption or caused net secretion in the small intestine. This was determined in rats through use of a perfusion and marker dilution technique to measure net intestinal fluid flux (Castro *et al.*, 1979a). Worm-induced

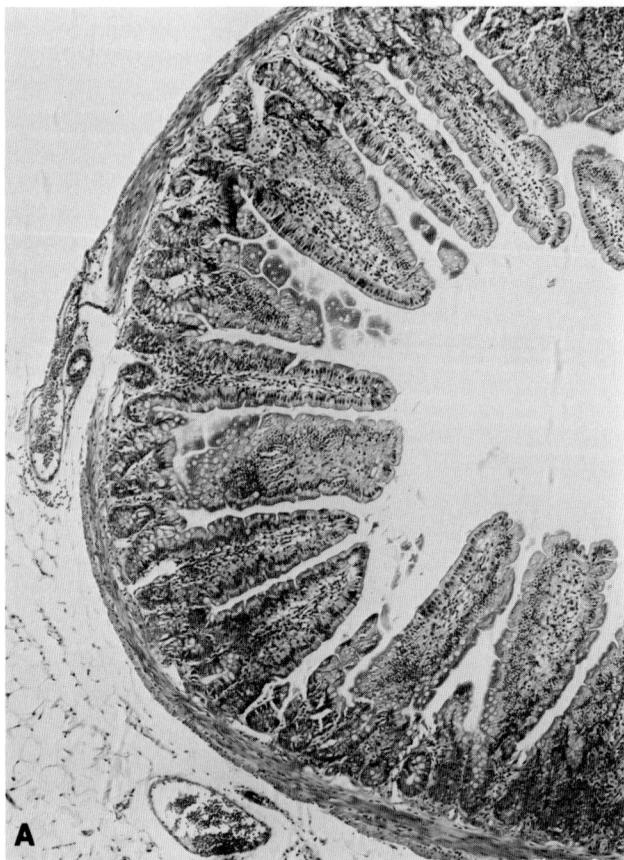

FIGURE 3. Histological section of small intestine from an uninfected rat (A) and an infected rat (8 × 10³ larvae) (B) killed 4 days PI. From Castro (1976).

changes in net fluid flux were evident within 3 days after primary infection, but within minutes after secondary infection (Fig. 6). The mechanism underlying the accumulation of fluid in the gut lumen was not determined, but it was suggested that a variation of the cyclic-nucleotide-mediated secretory process that occurs in *C. vibrio* infection (Field, 1980) should be considered.

4.1.4. Membrane Digestion

Examination of tissue from the small intestines of hosts infected with *T. spiralis* has revealed a general depression in the activity of

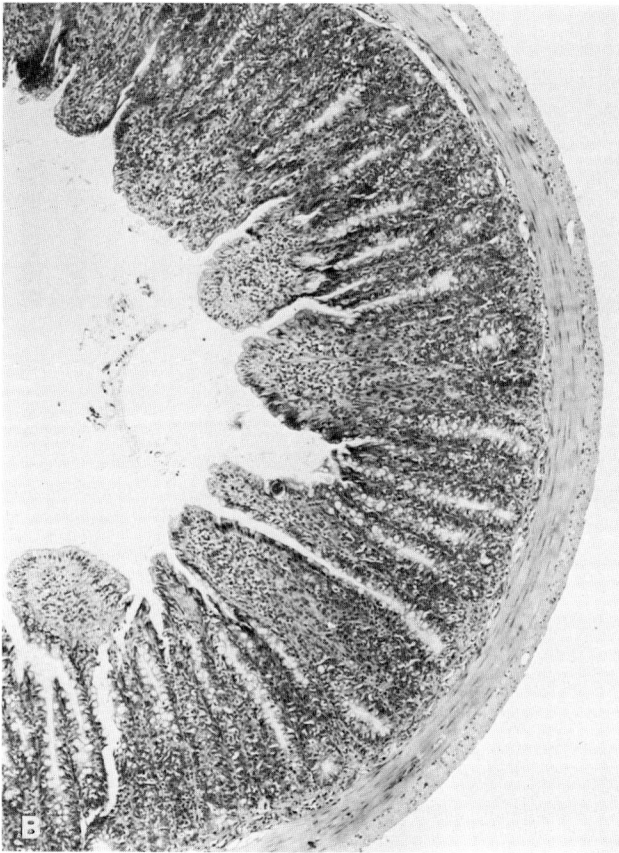

FIGURE 3. (*Continued*)

enzymes associated with the epithelial brush border, i.e., a decrease in membrane digestive capacity. Measurements made in the proximal half of the guinea pig small intestine showed a 50–90% decrease in the specific activities of maltase, sucrase, trehalase, and isomaltase (Castro and Gentner, 1972). Similar enzyme changes in terms of both specific and total activities paralleled the course of intestinal inflammation in *T. spiralis*-infected rats (Smith and Castro, 1978; Castro *et al.*, 1979b).

Mucosal peroxidase activity, used as a marker for inflammation in rats, showed that decreased activities of brush-border enzymes were closely associated with the spatial and temporal distribution of the parasite—the inflammatory stimulus. In short, the relationship between peroxidase and disaccharidase activities was an inverse one; when

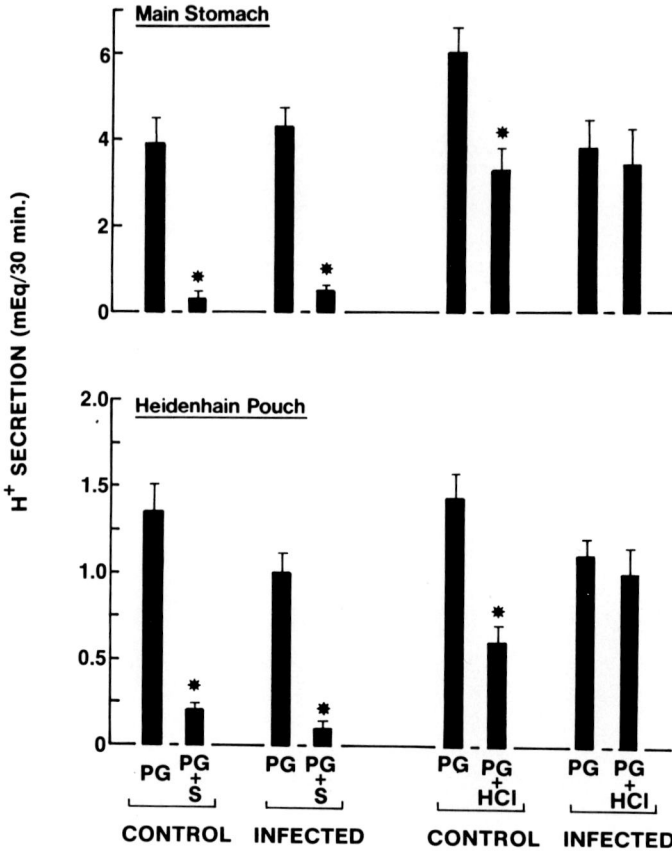

FIGURE 4. Maximum inhibitory effects of secretin (S) and HCl on pentagastrin (PG) induced acid (H^+) secretion from the main stomach and from surgically isolated pouches (Heidenhain) before and during the first week of infection with *T. spiralis* in dogs. The infective dose of 10^4 larvae/kg body weight was administered orally. PG (1.0 μg/kg-hr) was administered intravenously throughout the period of S (4 unit/kg-hr) infusion, given intravenously, and HCl (16 meq/hr) infusion, administered intraduodenally. Results show that infection does not inhibit the regulatory role of S when the exogenous hormone is given by vein, but the S inhibitory effect on H^+ secretion is prevented due to a depressed release of endogenous S by its physiological secretagogue. (*) Significantly different ($P <$ 0.5) from PG stimulation alone for respective group. From Dembinski *et al.* (1979a).

peroxidase levels (inflammation) were high, disaccharidase activities were low, and vice versa (Fig. 7).

In rats administered secondary infections, intestinal inflammation was induced at a faster rate and peaked earlier, although the maximal intensity was unchanged as compared with a primary infection (Russell and Castro, 1979). During primary infection, inflammation was detectable at day 2 PI, was maximal between days 7 and 14 PI, and declined to control levels by day 21 PI. The peroxidase peak occurred earlier (day 4 PI) following challenge infection and brush-border disaccharidases were depressed earlier as compared with the primary infection.

4.1.5. Intestinal Absorption

Several studies involving a variety of methods have demonstrated impaired absorption during the intestinal phase of trichinosis. Rogers (1942) reported a decrease in intestinal calcium uptake in rats 4–8 days PI. Guinea pigs, studied by means of the *in vitro* everted sac and *in vivo*

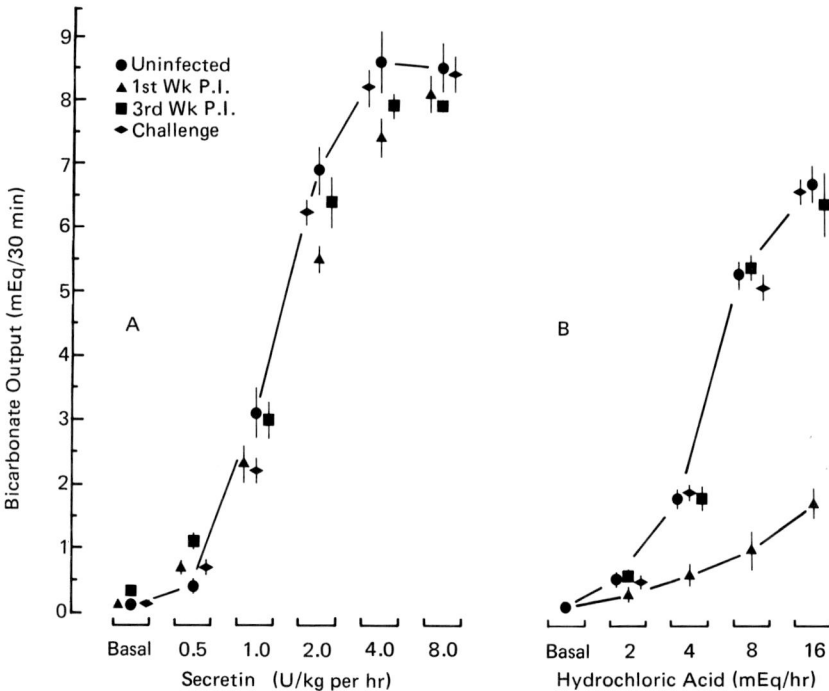

FIGURE 5. Pancreatic bicarbonate output in response to intravenous administration of secretin (A) and to intraduodenal instillation of HCl (B) to release endogenous secretin in dogs with primary and secondary *T. spiralis* infections. Infective dose was 10^4 larvae/kg body weight administered orally. Note the distinct effect of early infection on HCl-stimulated secretion. From Dembinski *et al.* (1979b).

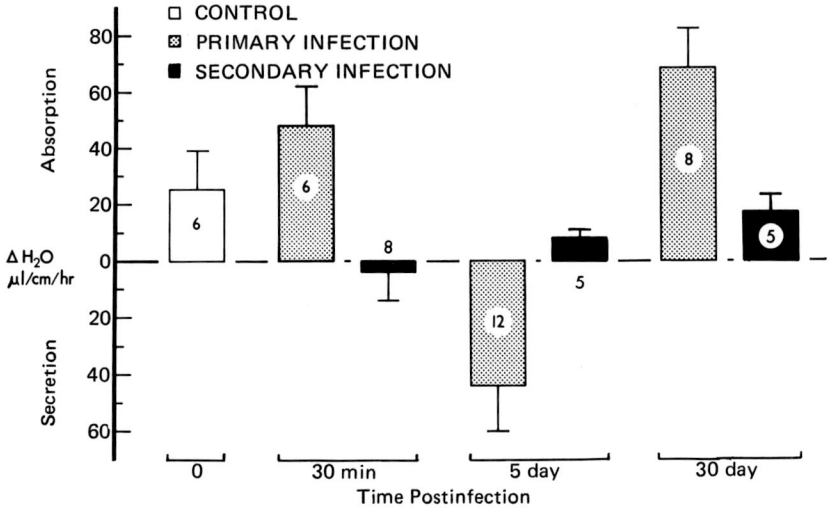

FIGURE 6. Net intestinal fluid movement as a function of time in control (uninfected) rats and in rats following infection with 7×10^3 T. *spiralis* larvae. From Castro *et al.* (1979a).

perfusion methods, were unable to absorb glucose normally when infected with *T. spiralis* (Castro *et al.*, 1967). The anterior region of the small intestine, where worms were present in large numbers, was the area in which uptake was most drastically depressed by infection. However, all areas of the intestine were affected at one time or another in the course of infection. Impaired glucose uptake occurred earlier following a secondary as compared with a primary infection (Lin and Olson, 1970). Olson and Richardson (1968) used an *in vivo* perfusion method to show glucose malabsorption associated with intestinal trichinosis in mice.

Related studies have been performed in rats. With the use of an *in vitro* tissue accumulation technique measuring sugar uptake under conditions of substrate saturation, it was found that the proximal intestine of infected hosts was unable to absorb β-methyl-D-glucoside (a nonmetabolizable analogue of glucose absorbed by the same mechanism as glucose) at normal rates (Castro *et al.*, 1979b). Hessel *et al.*, (1981), also using a tissue accumulation technique, demonstrated that β-methyl-D-glucoside uptake by intestinal epithelium was impaired within 30 min after a secondary infection, but not after a primary infection studied during the same time frame. This suggested immune-mediated influences with regard to control or regulation of epithelial transport.

Bullick *et al.* (1981), using an "Ussing" chamber technique (Ussing and Zerahn, 1951) to determine transepithelial electrical potential difference (PD), resistance, and short-circuit current [(Isc) a measurement for ion transport] in rats, corroborated the finding of absorptive changes immediately following challenge. The addition of β-methyl-D-glucoside to the mucosal half-chamber caused a rise in Isc in uninfected rats and in rats examined 30 min after primary infection. This was due to an increase in net hexose/Na$^+$ transport. Sugar and Na$^+$ are coupled (Schultz and Zelusky, 1964), and their transfer from the mucosal to the serosal side of the gut is electrogenic, i.e., generates a change in PD and its correlate, the Isc. The rise in Isc, indicative of active sugar transport, failed to appear in rats given a primary infection, challenged 30 days later, and examined within 30 min postchallenge. In short, the response was indicative of reduced Na$^+$/hexose transport triggered by an immunological reaction.

This reduction in absorption rate following challenge may be significant in explaining rapid changes in net intestinal fluid transport noted above in immunized rats after secondary infection (Castro *et al.*, 1979a). Fluid movement in the intestine is bidirectional and follows osmotic forces set up by nutrient and ion movement. Reduced β-methyl-D-glucoside uptake immediately following challenge infection suggests decreased lumen-to-tissue movement of solutes. The osmotic effect of these solutes may contribute to the accumulation of luminal fluid, i.e., a decrease in net absorption, or even net secretion.

4.2. Smooth-Muscle-Related

Changes that *T. spiralis* induces in smooth muscle tissue of the GI tract may be important in explaining some symptoms of trichinosis,

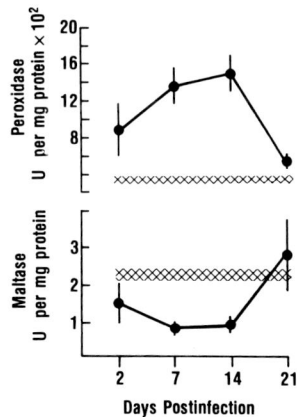

FIGURE 7. Mucosal peroxidase and maltase activities seen in the proximal quarter of the small intestine of rats infected with *T. spiralis.* Cross-hatched horizontal bars indicate mean ± S.E. for uninfected rats.

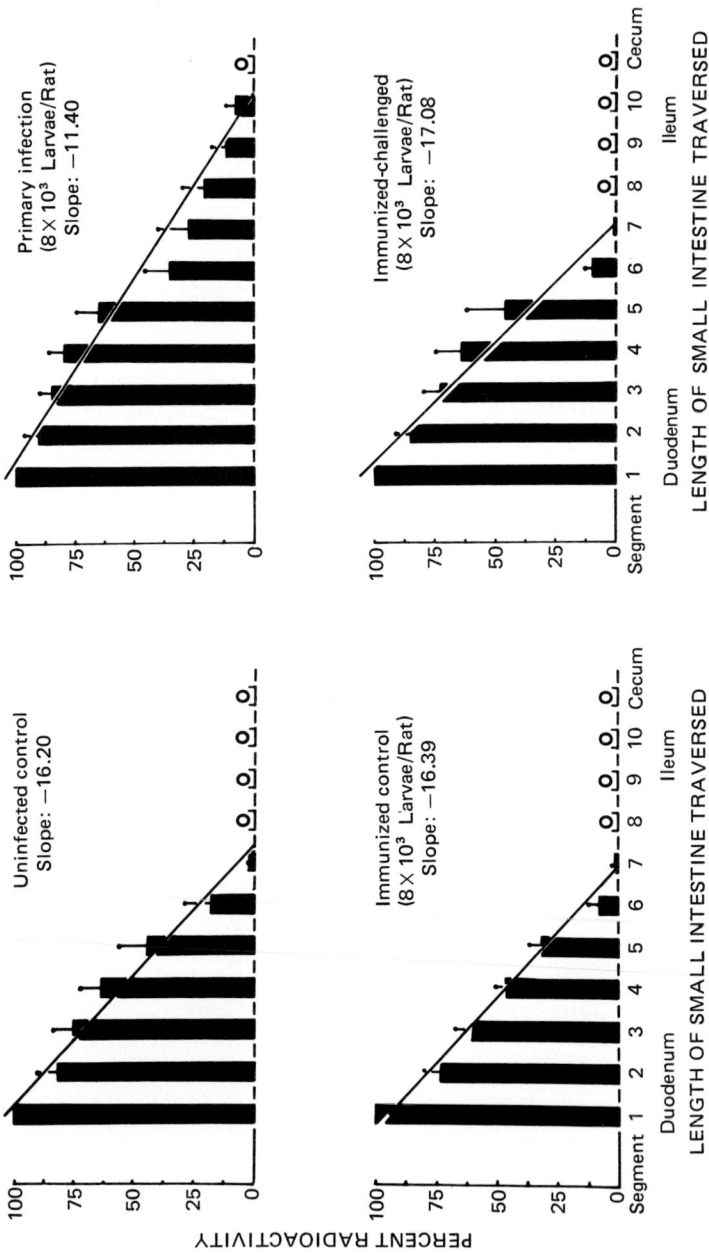

FIGURE 8. Intestinal transit in rats as measured by the distribution of a radioactive marker (^{51}Cr) passing through or present in a given segment of the small intestine during a 15-min test period. The marker was added by intraduodenal injection. Rats were studied prior to a primary infection (Uninfected control), 3–5 days post primary infection (Primary infection), 30 days post primary infection (Immunized control), and 3–5 days after a secondary infection (Immunized-challenged). Results show that only the animals examined during the 1st week of a primary infection showed alterations in transit as compared to uninfected rats. From Castro *et al.* (1977).

such as abdominal pain and diarrhea. Of interest in the overall host–parasite interaction is that enhanced intestinal transit has been suggested to be responsible for expulsion of a secondary inoculum of *T. spiralis* larvae in immunized hosts (McCoy, 1940) and for differences in the intestinal distribution patterns of worms between young and old mice (Larsh and Henricks, 1949). In support of the latter contention, a marked concentration of worms was noted in the anterior small intestines of "young" mice treated with morphine to suppress transit. This was compared with the distribution pattern seen in untreated mice. The influence of morphine on transit was measured by observing the passage of carbon ink through the small intestine following stomach intubation of the marker (Larsh, 1947). The influence of morphine on gastric emptying was not controlled in this study, whereas the inhibiting effect of morphine on transit is well known (Weisbrodt *et al.*, 1977).

During the first week of infection, rats show a significantly shorter intestinal transit time as compared with uninfected animals, as evident from faster orad-to-caudad propulsion of a radioactive marker injected into the duodenum (Castro *et al.*, 1976a). The moving front and total amount of the marker traversing the midpoint of the intestine were endpoints for measurement (Fig. 8). The shortened transit time in primary infection is accompanied by inflammation, reduced brush-border disaccharidase activity, and net intestinal secretion (Castro *et al.*, 1976a, 1979a). Previously immunized rats did not show altered intestinal transit when challenged and examined within a similar time frame (Castro *et al.*, 1977; Russell and Castro, 1979).

Intestinal motility changes caused by *T. spiralis* in dogs following secondary and primary infections have been reported (Schanbacher *et al.*, 1978). Motility was monitored by measuring intestinal myoelectric activity in fasted and fed hosts. Alterations in characteristic relationships between electrical slow waves and spiking occurred as early as 18 hr after primary infection. These deviations were marked 3–4 days PI, a period during which dogs were diarrheic. The major alteration involved a shift from the regular periodic spiking pattern to one of continuous spiking during the fasted state. This parasite-induced pattern resembled that seen in fed dogs. Patterns were normal 11–15 days PI. A secondary infection, given 6 weeks after the first, failed to elicit outward signs of disease (e.g., diarrhea) and did not produce changes in the normal myoelectric patterns (Fig. 9). These latter findings were attributed to immunity elicited by the first infection.

Measurements of intestinal myoelectric activity were made recently in rats. Findings included a decreased contractile state, impairment of contractile behavior, and the appearance of unusual myoelectric events.

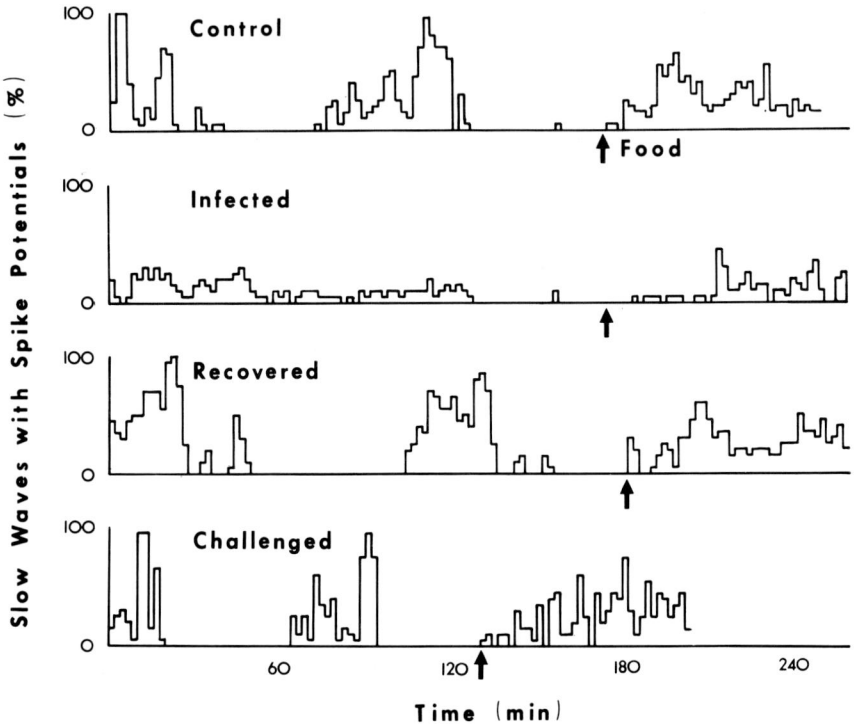

FIGURE 9. Intestinal myoelectric activity in dogs. Histogram patterns of motility in the proximal small intestine prior to infection (Control), 3 days after administration of 2×10^4 *T. spiralis* larvae/kg body weight (Infected), 11 days post primary infection (Recovered), and 3 days after secondary infection (Challenged) with 2×10^4 larvae/kg body weight. Dogs were challenged 6 weeks after the primary infection. Data from motility tracings, measured directly from serosally implanted electrodes, are plotted as the percentage of slow waves with superimposed spike potentials per 2-min intervals during fasted and fed states. (↑) Time when dog was fed one can of food. From Schanbacher *et al.* (1978).

Parasite-induced changes were indicated by decreases in electrical slow-wave frequency and mean spiking activity that were maximal 8–12 days PI. The appearance and frequency of normal migrating myoelectric complexes decreased during infection. This decrease in coordinated activity coincided with the onset of unusual electrical events, designated as migrating action potential complexes, that swept down the bowel rapidly and occurred with greatest frequency 2–6 days PI (Palmer *et al.*, 1981).

Results from *T. spiralis*-infected dogs and rats using two different methods of assay indicate that motility changes occur and are influenced by host immunity. Despite observations of distinct myoelectric patterns in dogs that were diarrheic (Schanbacher *et al.*, 1978), the relationship between specific electrical patterns and the etiology of this symptom remains obscure.

5. BASES FOR FUNCTIONAL CHANGES

5.1. Direct Action of Parasite

Once *T. spiralis* gains access to the host GI tract, the degree of pathological damage produced depends in part on the agressive action of the parasite, involving direct traumatic or lytic damage to the host tissues. However, since the parasite is microscopic in size and the area of the mucosal surface inhabited is quite small in relation to the total area, it is reasonable to assume that tissue changes result primarily from an amplified host response to noxious somatic components or metabolic products of the parasite. Well-known metabolic excretory–secretory (ES) products of intestinal stages of *T. spiralis* include fermentation acids (von Brand *et al.*, 1952; Castro and Fairbairn, 1969), aliphatic amines (Haskins and Weinstein, 1957a; Castro *et al.*, 1973), and antigenic molecules (Ewert and Olson, 1961; Campbell, 1955; Mills and Kent, 1965; Tanner and Gregory, 1961). The production and release of these compounds are considered in other chapters. Except for host reactions to antigenic components, little is known regarding the possible role of ES products in influencing host tissue responses. Consequently, this area remains speculative.

5.2. Influence of Lamina Propria

Gross changes in mucosa and smooth-muscle layers of the intestine may have their basis in inflammation in the lamina propria. Details of the inflammatory response were considered in an earlier section of this chapter. The stimulus for this reaction may be nonspecific on initial contact with the parasite. However, specific immune mediation may come into play during late primary and subsequent infections. The general observations that the GI tract responds to diverse stimuli in a similar manner (Sprinz, 1962) and that this response includes inflammation in the lamina propria indicate that lesions observed in intestinal trichinosis are predictable but are not unique.

Potential influence of lamina propria cells on GI pathophysiology is based more on inferential than on real observations. The way in which the various cells involved in the lamina propria response to *T. spiralis* influence the physiology of epithelial and smooth-muscle layers of the intestine are not clear. Some insight might be gained from an examination of results obtained from studies of another host–parasite system, i.e., *Nippostrongylus brasiliensis* infection in the rat. Here, it has been shown that infection causes an increase in epithelial goblet-cell number and that the capacity for goblet-cell hyperplasia can be transferred to uninfected hosts by passage of lymphocytes (Miller and Nawa, 1979). Ferguson and MacDonald (1979) have suggested, on the basis of studies in thymectomized rats, that crypt hyperplasia, increased epithelial-cell turnover, and villous atrophy associated with nippostrongylosis result from cell-mediated immune reactions. Although inconclusive, some evidence indicates that villous atrophy and crypt hyperplasia in the small intestines of *T. spiralis*-infected rats are T-cell-mediated. This was concluded from the finding that in thymectomized mice, villous atrophy and crypt hyperplasia are delayed or absent. Adoptive immunization of these hosts with mesenteric lymph-node cells enhances onset of crypt hyperplasia (Manson-Smith, 1979; Ferguson and Jarrett, 1975).

The Schultz–Dale phenomenon, or *in vitro* anaphylaxis (Coulson, 1953), results from effects of antigen-stimulated mast-cell degranulation and resultant effects of mediator substances on intestinal smooth muscle. Analogous reactions have not been demonstrated *in vivo*, but the likelihood is high that immediate hypersensitivity reactions could play a role in pathophysiological changes (Olson and Schultz, 1963; Ivey, 1965) in the intestine. Whereas the Schultz–Dale reaction provides insight into potential effects of anaphylactic reactions on smooth muscle, the question must be asked: what are the effects of immediate hypersensitivity on epithelium? The answer is not known. An intriguing prospect for consideration in this regard arises from the report that mast-cell granules contain, in addition to several well-recognized pharmacological agents, the candidate hormone, vasoactive intestinal polypeptide (VIP). This "hormone," which has been localized in endocrine cells and nerves of the GI tract and from pancreatic islets (Polak *et al.*, 1974), is liberated by mast cells following their degranulation (Cutz *et al.*, 1978). VIP stimulates intestinal secretion (Schwartz *et al.*, 1974) by a cyclic-nucleotide-mediated mechanism in a similar manner to *C. vibrio* toxin (Kimberg *et al.*, 1971). These observations may provide some insight into how pathophysiological changes are triggered in hosts whose tissues have been sensitized by contact with the parasite.

5.3. Endocrine Disturbances

Trichinella spiralis may cause pathophysiological changes in its various hosts by influencing functions regulated by GI hormones. Although information in this area is tentative at this time and hormone-related changes in host physiology may be due directly or indirectly to inflammation-induced lesions, this topic will be considered briefly because of its relative novelty at this stage of our knowledge. The first observation of GI hormone alterations in trichinosis came from studies in rats fed chronically by parenteral means. Infection in such hosts caused a rise in serum concentrations of gastrin (Castro *et al.*, 1976b). Unfortunately, the source of this increase was not directly determined; however, possible explanations can be offered. Despite the antral mucosa being the primary source of gastrin, this hormone in the rat is secreted by crypt cells (G cells) in the small intestine (Lichtenberger *et al.*, 1975). Lichtenberger and Graziani (1981) showed that ammonia, a by-product of protein hydrolysis, influences gastrin release. Such a release mechanism is interesting because major nitrogenous excretions of *T. spiralis* are ammonia and aliphatic amines (Haskins and Weinstein, 1957b). It is possible, therefore, that these excretions stimulate gastrin release. An alternate explanation is that during intestinal trichinosis, a gastrin-release regulatory mechanism reportedly associated with the small bowel (Bowen *et al.*, 1978) is functionally repressed by some component in mucosal inflammation.

Whereas the serum gastrin in rats was elevated by infection, in parasitized dogs, the levels of the hormones secretin and CCK were reduced. The etiology of these alterations remains obscure, as does the physiological effect of these changes on host homeostasis.

6. HOST–PARASITE INTERRELATIONSHIPS

Structural alterations in the GI tract caused by *T. spiralis* are more easily recognized than are functional changes. Thus, to attain an accurate picture of host–parasite interactions, attention must be paid to the basic axiom in pathology that biochemical and functional lesions underlie anatomical ones. From this, one is compelled to acknowledge that during the incubation period of trichinosis as well as during periods of marked histopathology, physiological changes are taking place in intestinal tissues that are beyond or have evaded present means of detection. The onset of pathogenesis and the decrease or increase in severity of symptoms are influenced by previous contact with *T. spiralis*. This points to the role of specific anamnestic responses in regulating or influencing pathology. An overview of the various factors in primarily and secondarily infected hosts that bear on the onset and severity of disease produced can be gained from Fig. 10.

7. RELATIONSHIPS BETWEEN PATHOPHYSIOLOGY AND SYMPTOMS

Except in situations involving loss of genetic capacity to perform a given physiological task, as in genetically based enzyme deficiencies, GI functions vary over a wide range, even on a daily basis. Differences in the magnitude of physiological activities within the GI tract may be enormous depending on whether an animal is in a fasted or fed state. The capacity of the GI tract to perform physiological work is determined genetically. However, expression of maximal capacity for work may occur only when an animal is stressed. This is evident in hypertrophic tissue changes and elevated digestive and absorptive activities seen in the remaining small intestine when a portion of it is removed surgically (Dowling and Riecker, 1973). In addition to these adaptive changes, it should be understood that under physiological circumstances, the GI tract does not have to function at maximal levels to maintain homeostasis. This statement is supported by the fact that the small intestine has the capacity to absorb several thousand times the glucose load placed on it in one day (Crane, 1975) and the amount of enzymes released by the

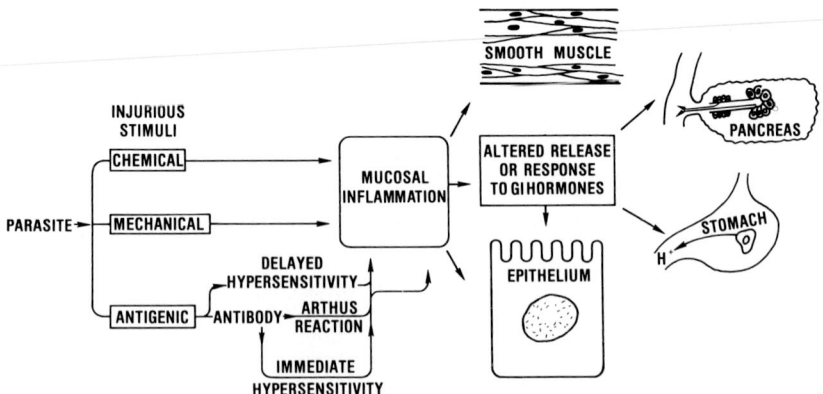

FIGURE 10. Summary of interrelationships among parasite-induced morphological and physiological changes during intestinal trichinosis. Adapted from Castro (1976).

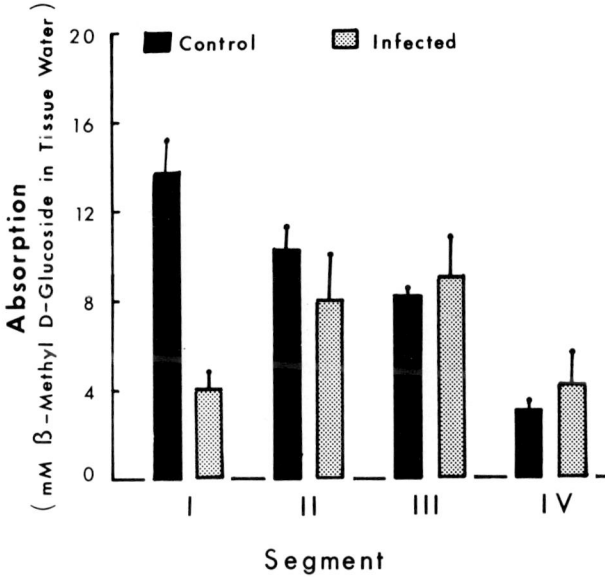

FIGURE 11. Uptake of β-methyl-D-glucoside by segments from each quarter of small intestine from control (uninfected) and *T. spiralis*-infected rats. Values are means ± S.E. From Castro *et al.* (1979b).

exocrine pancreas in response to stimulation by a meal is several fold greater than that necessary to carry out luminal digestion (Snook, 1973). The former example is clearly demonstrated in experiments in which a standardized liquid diet, in which glucose was the major caloric source, was infused intraduodenally into *T. spiralis*-infected rats for 1 week. Despite a drastically decreased capacity for glucose absorption in the proximal intestine of the parasitized host (Fig. 11), these animals maintained the same weight pattern as uninfected animals fed similarly and infected animals fed intravenously (Castro *et al.*, 1979b). A noteworthy observation in this study was that a group of rats allowed to drink the liquid diet *ad libitum* lost significant weight as compared with the intraduodenally and intravenously fed groups and with a noninfected group fed *ad libitum* (Table 1). Weight loss was due to a decrease in food consumption. Collectively, these findings point to a decrease in food intake, rather than metabolic or intestinal pathophysiological changes, in parasitized hosts as the major factor in causing weight loss.

The foregoing accounts indicate that the mere observation of altered GI function cannot be equated with a pathological state. These

TABLE 1
Body Weight of Rats on Stock or Liquid Diet[a]

Feeding regimen	Mean ($\pm$ S.E.) body weight (g)		Change (%)
	Initial	Final	
Stock diet			
Control ($N = 5$)	224 ± 5	279 ± 8^b	$+14.0 \pm 0.8$
Infected ($N = 5$)	240 ± 1	$188 \pm 5^{b,c}$	-21.8 ± 1.7^b
Liquid diet			
Orally			
Control ($N = 6$	224 ± 4	237 ± 4^b	$+6.8 \pm 2.0$
Infected ($N = 6$) 2.0	230 ± 4	$181 \pm 7^{b,c}$	-21.3 ± 2.8^c
Intraduodenally			
Control ($N = 6$)	210 ± 3	214 ± 3	$+2.7 \pm 2.4$
Infected ($N = 6$)	210 ± 6	208 ± 4	-0.7 ± 3.6
Intravenously			
Control ($N = 5$)	208 ± 2	219 ± 6	$+5.4 \pm 10.5$
Infected ($N = 5$)	201 ± 4	215 ± 7	$+6.8 \pm 5.9$

[a] From Castro *et al.* (1979b). Initial body weight was taken when the specific feeding regimen was started. Final weight was taken 7 or 8 days later.
[b] Indicates significant difference ($p < 0.05$) compared with initial weight.
[c] Indicates significant difference as compared with weights of controls.

alterations must be evaluated along with the adaptive potential and functional reserve capacity of the GI tract. Thus, the association of changes in GI motility, digestion, absorption, and secretion with symptoms of disease is at present only suggestive of possible cause–effect relationships.

8. SUMMARY

A clear association between infection with *T. spiralis* and physiological changes in the GI tract exists. The extent to which these changes contribute to pathology and symptoms of disease cannot be categorically stated. To firmly establish that a particular alteration contributes to the pathogenesis of disease, studies are needed to demonstrate that the magnitude of change caused by the parasite is beyond the range to which the host can adapt to maintain homeostasis.

A virgin area for future consideration in dealing with the intestinal phase of infection concerns inflammatory changes in the lamina propria. These changes, once initiated, clearly influence the structure and function of deeper smooth-muscle layers and the overlying epithelial tissue. How is this influence mediated? Another fertile area concerns the physiology of appetite control. A hallmark of parasitism is weight loss in the host. Considerable direct and indirect evidence suggests that the major contributing factor is loss of appetite. What regulates satiety? The broad host range of *T. spiralis* and its highly predictable life cycle can be used to advantage in pursuing answers to these questions. Acquisition of answers will not only clarify components in the pathogenesis of trichinosis, but also provide evidence or clues to the mechanisms by which GI-related functions are controlled.

REFERENCES

Barker, I.K., 1973, Scanning electron microscopy of the duodenal mucosa of lambs infected with *Trichostrongylus colubriformis, Parasitology* **67**:307–314.

Binder, H.J. (ed.), 1979, *Mechanisms of Intestinal Secretion,* Kroc Foundation Series, Vol. 12, Alan R. Liss, New York.

Bowen, J.C., Paddack, G.L., Bush, J.C., Wilson, R.J., and Johnson, L.R., 1978, Comparison of gastric responses to small intestinal resection and bypass in rats, *Surgery* **83**:402–405.

Bullick, G., Frizzell, R., and Castro, G.A., 1981, Change in epithelial transport with rapid immune rejection of *Trichinella spiralis,* Program and abstracts, 56th Annual Meeting of the American Society of Parasitologists, Abstract No. 13.

Campbell, C.H., 1955, The antigenic role of the excretions and secretions of *Trichinella spiralis* in the production of immunity in mice, *J. Parasitol.* **41**:483–491.

Castro, G.A., 1976, Spatial and temporal integration of host responses to intestinal stages of *Trichinella spiralis*: Retro- and prospective views, in: *Biochemistry of Parasites and Host–Parasite Relationships* (H. Van den Bossche, ed.), North-Holland, New York, pp. 343–358.

Castro, G.A., and Fairbairn, D., 1969, Carbohydrates and lipids of *T. spiralis* larvae and their utilization *in vitro, J. Parasitol.* **55**:51–58.

Castro, G.A., and Gentner, H., 1972, Disaccharidase deficiency associated with the intestinal phase of trichinosis in guinea pigs, *Proc. Soc. Exp. Biol. Med.* **140**:342–345.

Castro, G.A., and Olson, L.J., 1967, Relationship between body weight and food and water intake in *Trichinella spiralis*-infected guinea pigs, *J. Parasitol.* **53**:589–594.

Castro, G.A., Olson, L.J., and Baker, R.D., 1967, Glucose malabsorption and intestinal histopathology in *Trichinella spiralis*-infected guinea pigs, *J. Parasitol.* **53**:595–612.

Castro, G.A., Ferguson, J.D., and Gorden, C.W., 1973, Amine excretion in excysted larvae and adults of *Trichinella spiralis, Comp. Biochem. Physiol.* **45A**:819–828.

Castro, G.A., Roy, S.A., and Stockstill, R., 1974, *Trichinella spiralis*: Peroxidase activity in isolated cells from the rat small intestine, *Exp. Parasitol.* **36**:307–315.

Castro, G.A., Badial-Aceves, F., Smith, J.W., Dudrick, S.J., and Weisbrodt, N.W., 1976a, Altered small bowel propulsion associated with enteric parasitism, *Gastroenterology* **71**:620–625.

Castro, G.A., Copeland, E.M., Dudrick, S.J., and Johnson, L.R., 1976b, Serum and antral gastrin levels in rats infected with intestinal parasites, *Am. J. Trop. Med. Hyg.* **25**:848–853.

Castro, G.A., Post, C.A., and Roy, S.A., 1977, Intestinal motility during the enteric phase of trichinellosis in immunized rats, *J. Parasitol.* **63**:713–719.

Castro, G.A., Hessel, J.J., and Whalen, G., 1979a, Altered intestinal fluid movement in response to *Trichinella spiralis* in immunized rats, *Parasite Immunol.* **1**:259–266.

Castro G.A., Copeland, E.M., Dudrick, S.J., and Ramaswamy, K., 1979b, Enteral and parenteral feeding to evaluate malabsorption in intestinal parasitism, *Am. J. Trop. Med. Hyg.* **28**:500–507.

Catty, D., 1969, The immunology of nematode infections: Trichinosis in guinea pigs as a model, in: *Monograph in Allergy*, Vol. 5 (P. Kalles, M. Hasek, T.M. Inderbitzen, P.A. Miescher, and B.H. Waksman, eds.), S. Karger, New York, p. 134.

Charniga, L., Stewart, G.L., Kramar, G.W., and Stanfield, J.S., 1981, The effects of host sex on enteric response to infection with *Trichinella spiralis*, *J. Parasitol.* **67**:917–922.

Coulson, E.J., 1953, The Schultz–Dale technique, *J. Allergy* **24**:458–473.

Crandall, R.B., 1965, Chemotactic response of polymorphonuclear leukocytes to *Trichinella spiralis* and *Ascaris suum* extracts, *J. Parasitol.* **51**:397–404.

Crane, R.K., 1975, The physiology of the intestinal absorption of sugars, in: *Physiological Effects of Food Carbohydrates*, American Chemical Symposium Series No. 15 (A. Jeanes and J. Hodge, eds.), American Chemical Society, Washington, D.C., pp. 1–37.

Cutz, E., Chan, W., Track, N.S., Goth, A., and Said, S.I., 1978, Release of vasoactive intestinal polypeptide in mast cells by histamine liberators, *Nature (London)* **275**:661–662.

Dembinski, A.B., Johnson, L.R., and Castro, G.A., 1979a, Influence of parasitism on secretin-inhibited gastric secretion, *Am. J. Trop. Med. Hyg.* **28**:854–859.

Dembinski, A.B., Johnson, L.R., and Castro, G.A., 1979b, Influence of enteric parasitism on hormone-regulated pancreatic secretion in dogs, *Am. J. Physiol.* **237**:R232–R238.

Dowling, R.H., and Riecker, E.O., 1973, *Intestinal Adaptation*, Proceedings of the International Conference on the Anatomy, Physiology and Biochemistry of Intestinal Adaptation, Titisee, Germany (May 1973), Schattauer, New York, p. 271.

Ewert, A., and Olson, L.J., 1961, The use of a mouse LD_{50} to evaluate the immunogenicity of *Trichinella spiralis* metabolic antigens, *Tex. Rep. Biol. Med.* **19**:580–584.

Ferguson, A., and Jarrett, E.E., 1975, Hypersensitivity reactions in the small intestine. I. Thymus dependence of experimental partial villous atrophy, *Gut* **16**:114–117.

Ferguson, A., and MacDonald, T.T., 1979, Effects of local delayed hypersensitivity on the small intestine, in: *Symposium on Immunology of the Gut*, Ciba Foundation Symposium, 46, New Series, Elsevier/North-Holland, New York, pp. 305–327.

Field, M., 1980, Regulation of small intestinal ion transport by cyclic nucleotides and calcium, in: *Secretory Diarrhea* (M. Field, J.S. Fordtran, and S. Schultz, eds.), American Physiological Society, Bethesda, Maryland, pp. 21–30.

Field, M., Fordtran, J.S., and Schultz, S. (eds.), 1980, *Secretory Diarrhea*, American Physiological Society, Bethesda, Maryland.

Furth, R.J. van, Hirsh, J.G., and Fedorko, M.E., 1970, Morphology and peroxidase cytochemistry of mouse promonocytes, monocytes, and macrophages, *J. Exp. Med.* **132**:794–812.

Gould, S.E., 1970a, Clinical manifestations, A. Symptomatology, in: *Trichinosis in Man and Animals* (S.E. Gould, ed.), Charles C. Thomas, Springfield, Illinois, pp. 269–306.

Gould, S.E., 1970b, Anatomic pathology, in: *Trichinosis in Man and Animals* (S.E. Gould, ed.), Charles C. Thomas, Springfield, Illinois, pp. 147–189.

Graham, R.C., Jr., and Karnovsky, M.J., 1966, The early stages of absorption of injected horseradish peroxidase in the proximal tubules of mouse kidney: Ultrastructural cytochemistry by a new technique, *J. Histochem. Cytochem.* **14:**291–302.

Gustowska, L., Ruitenberg, E.J., and Elgersma, A., 1980, Cellular reactions in tongue and gut in murine trichinellosis and their thymus dependence, *Parasite Immunol.* **2:**133–154.

Haskins, W.T., and Weinstein, P.P., 1957a, The amine excretory products of *Ascaris lumbricoides* and *Trichinella spiralis* larvae, *J. Parasitol.* **43:**28–32.

Haskins, W.T., and Weinstein, P.P., 1957b, Nitrogenous excretory products of *Trichinella spiralis* larvae, *J. Parasitol.* **43:**19–24.

Hessel, J.J., Ramaswamy, K., and Castro, G.A., 1982, Rapid change in enterocyte absorptive capacity in immune hosts after challenge with *Trichinella spiralis, J. Parasitol.* **68:**202–207.

Ivey, M.H., 1965, Immediate hypersensitivity and serological responses in guinea pigs infected with *Toxocara canis* or *Trichinella spiralis, Am. J. Trop. Med. Hyg.* **14:**1044–1051.

Jensen, L.J., and Castro, G.A., 1981, *Trichinella spiralis:* Generation *in vitro* of factors chemotactic for rat cells in the presence of rat serum, *Exp. Parasitol.* **52:**53–61.

Johnson, L.R., and Grossman, M.I., 1968, Secretin, the enterogasterone released by acid in the duodenum, *Am. J. Physiol.* **215:**885–888.

Johnson, L.R., and Grossman, M.I., 1969, Characteristics of inhibition of gastric secretion by secretin, *Am. J. Physiol.* **217:**1401–1404.

Kimberg, D.V., Field, M., Johnson, J., Henderson, A., and Gershow, E., 1971, Stimulation of intestinal adenylate cyclase by cholera enterotoxin and prostaglandins, *J. Clin. Invest.* **50:**1218–1230.

Kozek, W.J., and Crandall, R.B., 1974, Intestinal and serum immunoglobulins and antibodies in mice infected with *Trichinella,* in: *Trichinellosis,* Proceedings of the 3rd International Conference on Trichinellosis (C.W. Kim, ed.), Intext, New York, pp. 157–164.

Kramar, M., Stewart, G.L., and Charniga, L., 1981. Comparative study of *Trichinella spiralis* (Owen, 1835) and *Trichinella pseudospiralis* (Garkavi, 1972), *J. Parasitol.* **67:**911–916.

Larsh, J.E., Jr., 1947, The relationship in mice of intestinal emptying time and natural resistance to *Hymenolepis, J. Parasitol.* **33:**79–84.

Larsh, J.E., Jr., 1963, Experimental trichinosis, *Adv. Parasitol.* **1:**213–286.

Larsh, J.E., Jr., and Hendricks, J.R., 1949, The probable explanation for the difference in the localization of adult *Trichinella spiralis* from rats, *J. Parasitol.* **35:**101–106.

Larsh, J.E., Jr., and Race, G.J., 1954, A histopathological study of the anterior small intestine of immunized and non-immunized mice infected with *Trichinella spiralis, J. Infect. Dis.* **38:**262–272.

Larsh, J.E., Jr., Ottolenghi, A., and Weatherly, N.F., 1974, *Trichinella spiralis:* Phospholipase in challenged mice and rats, *Exp. Parasitol.* **36:**299–306.

Lee, G.B., and Ogilvie, B.M., 1980, The mucus layer in nematode infections, in: *The Mucosal Immune System in Health and Disease,* Proc. 81st Ross Conf. on Pediatric Res. Ross Laboratories, Columbus, Ohio, pp. 175–182.

Leid, R.W., and Williams, J.F., 1979, Helminth parasites and the host inflammatory system, *Chem. Zool.* **11:**229–266.

Leonard, A.B., and Beahm, E.H., 1941, Studies on the distribution of *Trichinella* larvae in the albino rat, *Trans. Kans. Acad. Sci.* **44:**419–433.

Lichtenberger, L.M., and Graziani, L.A., 1981, Possible importance of dietary ammonia (NH3) in the postprandial release of gastrin (G), *Gastroenterology* **30**(Pt. 2):1212.

Lichtenberger, L.M., Lechago, J., and Johnson, L.R., 1975, Depression of antral and serum gastrin concentration by food deprivation in the rat, *Gastroenterology* **68**:1473–1479.

Lin, T.-M., and Olson, L.J., 1970, Pathophysiology of reinfection with *Trichinella spiralis* in guinea pigs during the intestinal phase, *J. Parasitol.* **56**:529–539.

Manson-Smith, D.F., 1979, Villous atrophy and expulsion of intestinal *Trichinella spiralis* are mediated by T cells, *Cell. Immunol.* **47**:285–292.

McCoy, O.R., 1940, Rapid loss of trichinella larvae fed to immune rats and its bearing of the mechanism of immunity, *Am. J. Hyg.* **32**:105–116.

Miller, H.R.P., and Nawa, T., 1979, *Nippostrongylus brasiliensis*: Intestinal goblet cell response in adoptively immunized rats, *Exp. Parasitol.* **47**:81–90.

Mills, C.K., and Kent, N.H., 1965, Excretions and secretions of *Trichinella spiralis* and their role in immunity, *Exp. Parasitol.* **16**:300–310.

Olson, L.J., and Richardson, J.A., 1968, Intestinal malabsorption of D-glucose in mice infected with *Trichinella spiralis*, *J. Parasitol.* **54**:441–451.

Olson, L.J., and Schultz, C.W., 1963, Nematode induced hypersensitivity reactions in guinea pigs: Onset of eosinophilia and positive Schultz–Dale reactions following graded infections with *Toxocara canis*, *Ann. N.Y. Acad. Sci.* **113**:440–445.

Palmer, J.M., Weisbrodt, N.W., and Castro, G.A., 1981, Small intestinal myoelectric activity during intestinal trichinellosis in the rat, Program and abstracts, 56th Annual Meeting of the American Society of Parasitologists, Abstract No. 154.

Pambuccian, G., and Cironeanu, F.I., 1961, Observations on experimental trichinellosis in white rats, *Rum. Med. Rev.* **6**(2):8–13.

Polak, J.M., Pearse, A.G.E., Garaud, J.C., and Bloom, S.R., 1974, Cellular localization of a vasoactive intestinal peptide in the mammalian and avian gastrointestinal tract, *Gut* **15**:720–724.

Race, G.J., Larsh, J.E., Jr., Martin, J.H., and Weatherly, N.F., 1974, Light and electron microscopy of the intestinal tissue of mice parasitized by *Trichinella spiralis*, in: *Trichinellosis*, Proceedings the 3rd International Conference on Trichinellosis (C.W. Kim, ed.), Intext, New York, pp. 75–100.

Rogers, W.P., 1942, The metabolism of trichinosed rats during the intermediate phase of the disease, *J. Helminthol.* **20**:139–158.

Ruitenberg, E.J., and Elgersma, A., 1976, Absence of intestinal mast cell response in congenitally athymic mice during *Trichinella spiralis* infection, *Nature (London)* **264**:258–260.

Ruitenberg, E.J., and Elgersma, A., 1979, A response of intestinal globule leucocytes in the mouse during a *Trichinella spiralis* infection and its dependence on intestinal mast cells, *Br. J. Exp. Pathol.* **60**:246–251.

Ruitenberg, E.J., Elgersma, A., Kruizinga, W., and Leenstra, F., 1977a, *Trichinella spiralis* infection in congenitally athymic (nude) mice; Parasitological, serological and haematological studies with observations on intestinal pathology, *Immunology* **33**:581–587.

Ruitenberg, E.J., Elgersma, A., Kruizinga, W., and Leenstra, F., 1977b, Thymus dependence and independence of intestinal pathology in a *Trichinella spiralis* infection: A study in congenitally athymic (nude) mice, *Br. J. Exp. Pathol.* **58**:311–314.

Ruitenberg, E.J., Elgersma, A., and Kruizinga, W., 1979, Intestinal mast cells and globule leukocytes: Role of the thymus on their presence and proliferation during a *Trichinella spiralis* infection in the rat, *Int. Arch. Allergy Appl. Immunol.* **60**:302–309.

Ruitenberg, E.J., Perrudet-Badoux, A., Boussac-Aron, Y., and Elgersma, A., 1980, *Trichinella spiralis* infection in animals genetically selected for high and low antibody production: Studies on intestinal pathology, *Int. Arch. Allergy Appl. Immunol.* **62**:104–110.

Russell, D.A., and Castro, G.A., 1979, Physiological characterization of a biphasic immune response to *Trichinella spiralis* in the rat, *J. Infect. Dis.* **139**:304–312.

Schanbacher, L.M., Nations, J.K., Weisbrodt, N.W., and Castro, G.A., 1978, Intestinal myoelectric activity in parasitized dogs, *Am. J. Physiol.* **234**:R188–R195.

Schultz, S.G., and Zelusky, R., 1964, Ion transport in isolated rabbit ileum. I. Short-circuit current and Na fluxes, *J. Gen. Physiol.* **47**:567–584.

Schwartz, C.J., Kimberg, D.V., Sheerin, H.E., Field, M., and Said, S.I., 1974, Vasoactive intestinal peptide stimulation of adenylate cyclase and active electrolyte secretion in intestinal mucosa, *J. Clin. Invest.* **54**:536–544.

Sheehy, T.W., Meroney, W.H., Cox. R.S., Jr., and Sola, J.E., 1962, Hookworm disease and malabsorption, *Gastroenterology* **42**:148–156.

Smith, J.W., and Castro, G.A., 1978, Relation of peroxidase activity in gut mucosa to inflammation, *Am. J. Physiol.* **234**:R72–R79.

Snook, J.T., 1973, Protein digestion in nutritional metabolic considerations, in: *World Review of Nutrition and Dietetics,* Vol. 18 (G.H. Bourne, ed.), S. Karger, New York, pp. 121–176.

Sprinz, H., 1962, Morphological response of intestinal mucosa to enteric bacteria and its implication in sprue and Asiatic cholera, *Fed. Proc. Fed. Am. Soc. Exp. Biol.* **21**:57–64.

Symons, L.E.A., and Fairbairn, D., 1962, Pathology, absorption, transport and activity of digestive enzymes in rat jejunum parasitized by the nematode *Nippostrongylus brasiliensis, Fed. Proc.* **21**:913–918.

Takeuchi, A., Sprinz, H., Labrec, E.H., and Formal, S.B., 1965, Experimental bacillary dysentery, *Am. J. Pathol.* **47**:1011–1044.

Tanner, C.E., and Gregory, J., 1961, Immunochemical study of the antigens of *Trichinella spiralis.* I. Identification and enumeration of antigens, *Can. J. Microbiol.* **7**:473–481.

Ussing, H.H., and Zerahn, K., 1951, Active transport of sodium as the source of electric current in the short circuited isolated frog skin, *Acta Physiol. Scand.* **23**:110–127.

Vagne, M., and Grossman, M.I., 1968, Cholecystokinetic potency of gastrointestinal hormones and related peptides, *Am. J. Physiol.* **215**:881–884.

Von Brand, T., Weinstein, P.P., Mehlman, B., and Weinbach, E.C., 1952, Observations on the metabolism of bacteria-free larvae of *Trichinella spiralis, Exp. Parasitol.* **1**:245–255.

Warren, K.S., Karp, R., and Pelly, R.P., 1976, The eosinophil stimulation promoter in murine and human *Trichinella spiralis* infection, *J. Infect. Dis.* **134**:277–280.

Weisbrodt, N.W., Badial-Aceves, F., Dudrick, S.J., Burks, T., and Castro, G.A., 1977, Tolerance to the effect of morphine on intestinal transit, *Proc. Soc. Exp. Biol. Med.* **154**:587–590.

Wine, A.C., Stone, M.K., and Mahmond, A.A.F., 1977, Eosinophil chemotaxis by products of antigen-stimulated spleen cells, *Clin. Res.* **25**:351A.

7

Pathophysiology of the Muscle Phase

GEORGE L. STEWART

1. INTRODUCTION

Since Paget (1866) discovered *Trichinella spiralis* muscle larvae during a human autopsy, numerous studies have focused on myopathophysiology in trichinosis. From these studies, it soon became apparent that some of the more outstanding clinical manifestations and the primary causes of mortality in this disease were related to parasitism of striated skeletal muscle and invasion of the myocardium (see Chapter 11). Evidence was also provided establishing the intracellular existence of the muscle larva and revealing that the parasite induced many dramatic alterations in the chemical and physical nature of the host cell. Many of the myopathophysiological changes in trichinosis result from the process by which the parasite establishes with the host striated myofiber one of the most intimate and complex host–helminth relationships in nature. This chapter addresses pathophysiology of the muscle phase with emphasis on the roles played by these lesions in the evolution of the aforementioned relationship.

GEORGE L. STEWART • Laboratory of Parasitology, Department of Biology, The University of Texas, Arlington, Texas 76019.

2. PARASITE-INDUCED MODIFICATIONS IN HOST STRIATED SKELETAL MUSCLE

2.1. Alterations Induced in the Host Myofiber during Contact and Entry by the Newborn First-Stage Larva

Although the newborn first-stage (L_1) larva of *Trichinella* will pass through or remain for short periods of time in a variety of cell types in the mammalian host (see Chapter 3), it is well established that the parasite will complete its development only in striated skeletal myofibers (see Ribas-Mujal, 1971). Carried by the general circulation throughout the body of the host, the greatest number of newborn L_1 larvae enter the muscles of the anterior half of the host (Stewart and Charniga, 1980). The most active muscles appear to receive the greatest burden of larvae (Staubli, 1905a,b; Lewis, 1928a,b; Ogielski, 1949). This apparent preference for more active muscles may be determined in part by the larva's positive taxis to a 120-mV stimulus (the action potential for striated muscle), or by the increased negativity of the sarcolemma seen in more active muscles, or by both (Hughes and Harley, 1977). *Trichinella* does not appear to exhibit any predilection for a particular type of muscle fiber; both oxidative and glycolytic human muscle fibers are invaded randomly (Ochoa and Pallis, 1980).

Prior to penetration, the newborn L_1 larva becomes closely associated with the sarcolemma of a striated myofiber, attaching to and causing an indentation in this structure (Despommier, 1976). Complete penetration of a host muscle cell is accomplished within 10 min, presumably by mechanical means. Invaded host myofibers can be identified by the presence of a gaping tear in the sarcolemma (Fig. 1).

Immediately following its entrance into a host muscle cell, the newborn larva, moving just beneath the sarcolemma, begins to migrate away from the point of entrance. During migration, the newborn larva creates an open tunnel behind it that eventually closes, isolating the larva from the extracellular environment (Despommier, 1976). Larval migration away from the point of entrance may be in response to the worm's need for an isolated intracellular niche in which to exert its influence over the metabolic machinery of the host muscle cell and in which it may avoid contact with elements of the host's response.

2.2. Alterations in Host Muscle during Growth and Development of the Muscle Larva

During its growth and development in the intracellular niche, the muscle larva induces a variety of profound changes in the chemical and

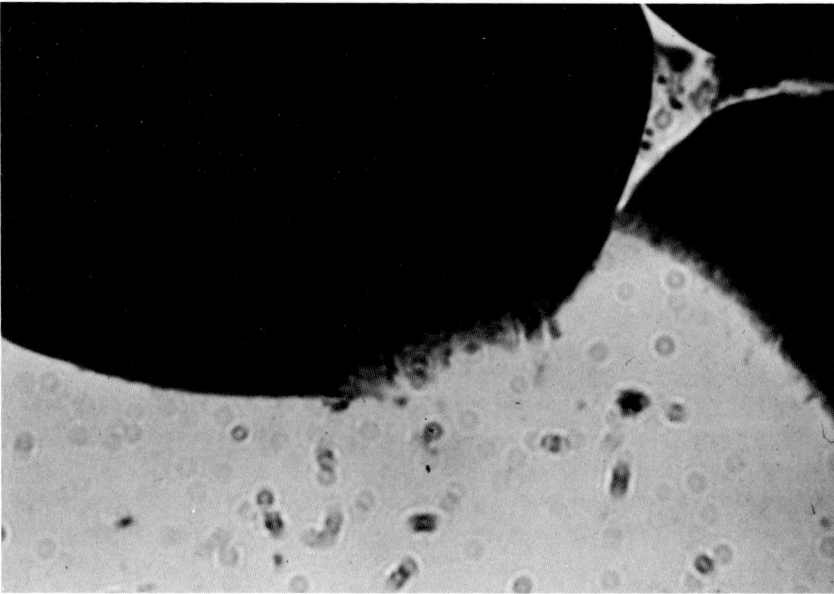

FIGURE 1. Gaping tear in the sarcolemma of a host myofiber following penetration by a newborn L_1 larva of *T. spiralis.* ×1700. After Despommier (1976).

structural makeup of the host striated myofiber. Collectively, these changes result in the formation of a dramatically different type of host cell that houses, protects, and nurtures the larva. This new cell type has been termed the "Nurse cell" (Purkerson and Despommier, 1974).

Despommier *et al.* (1975) described the growth pattern of *Trichinella* from newborn L_1 larva to mature muscle larva (see Chapter 3). From the standpoint of chronological accuracy of microarchitectural modifications in the host myofiber, the studies of Purkerson and Despommier (1974) and Despommier (1975) are most reliable. These workers studied the system in question during development of muscle larvae injected as newborn L_1 larvae into host muscle. This technique ensured that all invaded myofibers were at approximately the same point in their development to a Nurse cell.

Disruption of contractile filaments within the immediate vicinity of the larva are the only changes induced in the host myofiber during the first 2 days postpenetration (PP) of the muscle cell (Despommier, 1975, 1976). Between days 2 and 4 PP, host myofibers housing a larva undergo several structural perturbations. The striations seen in normal host myofibers disappear (Drachman and Tunchay, 1965; Gabryel and

Gustowska, 1967; Gould, 1970; Teppema *et al.*, 1973) at the same time that disorganization of contractile filaments begins (Fasske and Themann, 1961; Ribas-Mujal and Rivera-Pomar, 1968; Backwinkle and Themann, 1972; Teppema *et al.*, 1973; Despommier, 1975, 1976).

Dramatic changes are initiated in the nuclei of infected myofibers during this stage of larval development. An increase in the size (Fig. 2) and number of these nuclei and a change in their position have been observed (Fielder, 1864; Ehrhardt, 1896; Graham, 1897; Langerhans, 1892; Hemmert-Halswick and Bugge, 1934; Beckett and Boothroyd, 1961; Fasske and Themann, 1961; Gabryel and Gustowska, 1967; Ribas-Mujal and Rivera-Pomar, 1968; Backwinkle and Themann, 1972; Teppema *et al.*, 1973; Despommier, 1975). Eventually, there occurs a 4- to 9-fold increase in the number of nuclei per infected myofiber (Graham, 1897; Hemmert-Halswick and Bugge, 1934; Despommier, 1975, 1976). In infected muscle fibers, one or more enlarged nucleoli are seen in the hypertrophied nuclei (Fig. 2) (Fasske and Themann, 1961; Beckett and Boothroyd, 1961; Ribas-Mujal and Rivera-Pomar, 1968; Teppema *et al.*, 1973; Despommier, 1975), which migrate from their normal subsarcolemmal position to assume a more central location within the myofiber (Fielder, 1864; Ehrhardt, 1896; Graham, 1897; Langerhans, 1892; Hemmert-Halswick and Bugge, 1934; Fasske and Themann, 1961; Gabryel and Gustowska, 1967; Ribas-Mujal and Rivera-Pomar, 1968; Backwinkle and Themann, 1972; Teppema *et al.*, 1973; Despommier, 1975). Stewart and Read (1973a) reported that between days 1 and 20 PP, trichinous muscle incorporates 200% more [^{3}H]thymidine into DNA than does uninfected muscle. By day 12 PP, the DNA content of trichinous muscle is 3-fold above that for muscle from uninfected mice. A significant proportion of autoradiographically demonstrable incorporation of [^{3}H]thymidine is confined to the hypertrophied nuclei of infected myofibers (Gabryel and Gustowska, 1967).

Several workers have reported an increase in the amount of sarcoplasmic matrix and in the size of the infected portion of the muscle cell (Fasske and Themann, 1961; Ribas-Mujal and Rivera-Pomar, 1968; Ribas-Mujal, 1971; Backwinkle and Themann, 1972; Teppema *et al.*, 1973; Purkerson and Despommier, 1974; Despommier, 1975).

Between days 4 and 19 PP, the larva grows at an exponential rate, increasing its volume by about 40% per day (Despommier *et al.*, 1975). Larval growth and development are completed by day 20 PP. It is during this exponential growth phase of the larva that the majority of changes in the macromolecular and microanatomical constitution of the host myofiber take place (Stewart and Read, 1973b; Despommier, 1975, 1976).

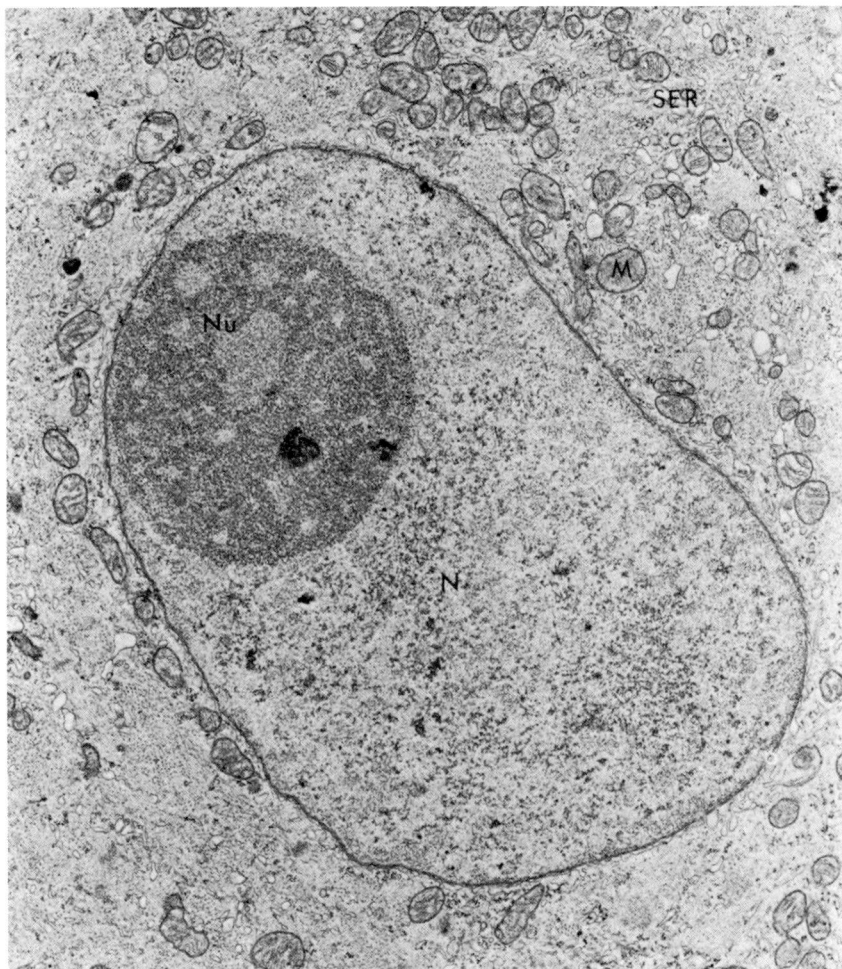

FIGURE 2. Nucleus of host myofiber 5 days PP. The nucleus (N) has enlarged and developed a prominent nucleolus (Nu) by this point during infection. The chromatin is sparse and patchy. In addition, dense inclusions are seen in both the nucleoplasm and the nucleolus. (M) Mitochondria; (SER) sarcoplasmic reticulum. × 15,100. After Despommier (1975), courtesy of Harper and Row, New York.

Disappearance of myofilaments in infected myofibers (Fasske and Themann, 1961; Ribas-Mujal and Rivera-Pomar, 1968; Backwinkle and Themann, 1972; Teppema, *et al.*, 1973; Despommier, 1975, 1976) is chronologically coincident with a chemically demonstrable decrease in myofibrillar proteins (Stewart and Read, 1974) and with a histochemically evident decrease in the protein content of trichinous muscle (Beckett, 1961). Disappearance of myofilaments is heralded by disruption of the structural integrity of the Z bands. Loss of myofilaments occurs in a random fashion (Fig. 3). Areas of the sarcoplasm devoid of myofilaments appear next to others in which dissolution is in the early stages, while in still other sarcoplasmic zones of an infected myofiber, the myofilaments remain intact (Fasske and Themann, 1961; Ribas-Mujal and Rivera-Pomar, 1968; Backwinkle and Themann, 1972; Teppema *et al.*, 1973; Despommier, 1975). Disruption of the structural components of contraction is accompanied by dramatic reductions in several key chemical elements that play an integral role in the contractile function of muscle (Garbulinski *et al.*, 1965; Stewart and Read, 1974). Significant decreases occur in the ATP (Garbulinski *et al.*, 1965),

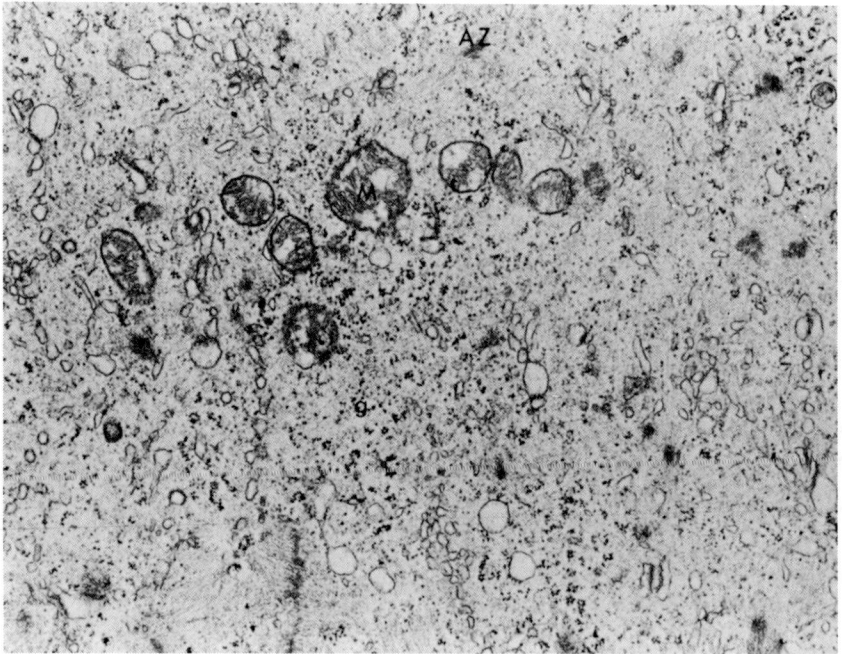

FIGURE 3. By day 6 PP, the triads have become indistinguishable from the rest of the sarcoplasm. Remnants of actin filaments attached to Z bands (AZ) are still present. Mitochondria (M) continue to exhibit vacuolation. Glycogen (g) is still present in quantity throughout the sarcoplasm. The sarcoplasmic reticulum has not yet filled in the areas vacated by myofilaments. ×41,800. After Despommier (1975), courtesy of Harper and Row, New York.

phosphocreatine (Garbulinski *et al.*, 1965; Stewart and Read, 1974), and creatine and myoglobin (Stewart and Read, 1974) content of infected muscle. The latter authors observed close to a 50% decrease in the myoglobin, creatine, and phosphocreatine content of trichinous muscle by day 6 PP. Although Garbulinski *et al.* (1965) reported an elevation in the rates of incorporation of ^{32}P into ATP, ADP, AMP, and phosphocreatine in trichinous campared to uninfected muscle, the work of Rogers (1942) demonstrates that these changes may be due in large part to enhanced phosphate turnover in infected muscle. In addition, Stewart *et al.* (1978) noted an approximate 2.5-fold increase in serum creatine phosphokinase activity during the same period of time in which the aforedescribed perturbations in the chemical and structural elements supporting contraction were occurring. Alterations in structural and chemical components playing a role in the mechanical, energetic, and aerobic economy of muscular contraction underlie significant changes in the kinetics of contraction of trichinous muscle (Farris and Harley, 1977; Casey and Harley, 1978). Trichinous muscle shows a reduction in the efficiency and strength of contraction and an increase in excitability compared to uninfected muscle (Farris and Harley, 1977). These changes are thought not to be due to chemical blockage of the neuromuscular junction of infected host myofibers (Farris and Harley, 1977). In addition, infected muscle is characterized by a significantly lower membrane potential than that seen in uninfected muscle (Casey and Harley, 1978). Nicoleso *et al.* (1962) reported increased innervations of infected host myofibers. This event is difficult to interpret given that studies on the kinetics of trichinous muscle have failed to demonstrate alterations in the integrity of neuromuscular junctions in infected myofibers (Farris and Harley, 1977).

Flury (1913) and Nevinny (1927) described a "basophilic halo" surrounding the *Trichinella* muscle larva. Using histochemical techniques, Maier and Zaiman (1966), Drachman and Tunchay (1965), Gabryel and Gustowska (1967), and Zarzycki (1962) showed that this sarcoplasmic basophilia is due to an increase in the amount of RNA present in infected muscle fibers. The latter workers reported the uptake of ^{35}S by this basophilic material. Electron-microscopic studies have revealed a dramatic increase in smooth sarcoplasmic reticulum at the outer edge of the infected fiber and within the vicinity of the triads around day 5 PP. By day 10 PP, intense proliferation of rough endoplasmic reticulum, smooth sarcoplasmic reticulum, and free ribosomes is evident throughout the cytoplasm of the infected muscle cell (Despommier, 1975). Similar findings have been reported by others (Fasske and Themann, 1961; Ribas-Mujal and Rivera-Pomar, 1968;

Backwinkle and Themann, 1972; Teppema *et al.*, 1973; Purkerson and Despommier, 1974; Despommier, 1976). These changes parallel in time a dramatic elevation in the RNA content of trichinous mouse diaphragm and pectoralis muscle and an increase in the rate of incorporation of [^{14}C]uridine into RNA of infected diaphragm muscle. By day 18 PP, the RNA content of trichinous muscle decreases somewhat, but remains greater than that of uninfected muscle for at least the first 40 days of infection.

A change in the number and the size of mitochondria in trichinous myofibers (Fasske and Themann, 1961; Ribas-Mujal and Rivera-Pomar, 1968; Backwinkle and Themann, 1972; Teppema *et al.*, 1973; Despommier, 1975) is paralleled by a rise in histochemically demonstrable succinic acid dehydrogenase activity (Zarzycki, 1963; Bruce, 1970b) around the forming *Trichinella* capsule wall in infected fibers. The hyperplastic mitochondria of the infected myofiber appear smaller to some workers (Teppema *et al.*, 1973; Purkerson and Despommier, 1974; Despommier, 1975), while others report them as being hypertrophied compared to those from uninfected myofibers (Fasske and Themann, 1961; Ribas-Mujal and Rivera-Pomar, 1968). Although the cristae of the hyperplastic mitochondria of trichinous myofibers appear normal, the inner regions of the mitochondria are highly vacuolated (Fig. 4) (Teppema *et al.*, 1973; Purkerson and Despommier, 1974; Despommier, 1975). Structural alterations in host-cell mitochondria are accompanied by profound changes in bioenergetics in these organelles. Oxidative phosphorylation is uncoupled (Boczon *et al.*, 1967; Michejda and Boczon, 1972), and there occurs an inhibition of glutamate, malate, and pyruvate oxidation and stimulation of succinate oxidation. No differences in enzymatic activities involved in the oxidation and reduction of cytochrome c occur between mitochondria isolated from infected and those isolated from uninfected rat muscle (Boczon, 1967; Boczon *et al.*, 1967; Hryniewiecka *et al.*, 1970; Michejda and Boczon, 1972). Karpiak *et al.* (1963) showed that trichinous guinea pig muscle takes up less oxygen and produces less carbon dioxide than does uninfected muscle. In addition, these authors reported that an increase in fat synthesis parallels a decrease in glycogen content (see below) in infected muscle. Oxygen uptake by infected muscle is stimulated to the greatest degree by succinate and propionate, while other Krebs-cycle intermediates inhibit oxygen uptake in trichinous guinea pig muscle (Kozar *et al.*, 1965).

Enhanced thiamine pyrophosphatase activity (Maier *et al.*, 1962; Maier and Zaiman, 1966) accompanies an increase in the size and

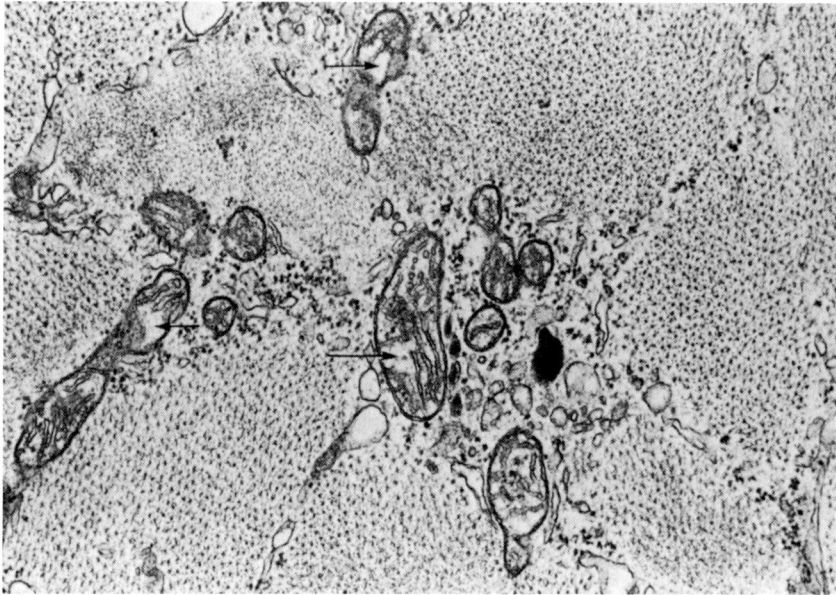

FIGURE 4. The triad regions of the infected muscle cell at 3 days after infection have begun to fill in with sarcoplasm. The inner matrix of most mitochondria has become vacuolated (arrows). ×42,100. After Despommier (1975), courtesy of Harper and Row, New York.

number of Golgi bodies in trichinous myofibers (Fasske and Themann, 1961; Ribas-Mujal and Rivera-Pomar, 1968; Backwinkle and Themann, 1972; Teppema *et al.*, 1973). Maier *et al.* (1962) and Maier and Zaiman (1966) demonstrated the presence of acid phosphatase, esterase, and aminopeptidase activities in infected but not in uninfected muscle fibers. Beckett (1961) and Bruce (1970b) reported the presence of leucine aminopeptidase activity in infected host myofibers. The observation of "lysosomelike" bodies in ultrastructural studies (Teppema *et al.*, 1973) offers one explanation for the presence of these enzymes.

Extensive growth of tubules of the T-system as well as elaborate infoldings of the sarcolemma of infected myofibers have been observed by several workers (Fig. 5) (Fasske and Themann, 1961; Ribas-Mujal and Rivera-Pomar, 1968; Backwinkle and Themann, 1972; Teppema *et al.*, 1973; Despommier, 1975). Ribas-Mujal and Rivera-Pomar (1968) provide a most detailed description of changes in these organelles in the trichinous myofiber. A dramatic enhancement of histochemically demonstrable alkaline phosphatase activity (Bullock and Gangi, 1950; Bullock, 1953; Stoyanov and Nenov, 1965; Schanzel and Holman, 1966; Kozar *et al.*, 1967; Bruce, 1970b; Seniuta, 1971; Ribas-Mujal, 1971) is associated with proliferating elements of the T-tubular system (Borgers *et al.*, 1975).

Formation of a host-derived double unit membrane immediately around the larva occurs about 10 days PP (see Chapter 3). Development of the capsule that will eventually enclose the mature Nurse cell first becomes evident around day 9 PP (Fig. 6) (Teppema *et al.*, 1973; Despommier, 1975). The capsule continues to increase in thickness well past the point when larval growth ceases on day 20 PP (Teppema *et al.*, 1973; Despommier, 1975). Several studies have established that the capsule is composed primarily of collagen (Frothingham, 1906; Beckett and Boothroyd, 1962; Ritterson, 1966; Bruce, 1970b; Teppema *et al.*, 1973). Considerable controversy surrounds the origin of the capsule. Some authors have suggested that the capsule consists of an inner portion derived from the sarcoplasm of the invaded muscle fiber and an outer portion consisting of the hypertrophied sarcolemma of the infected fiber (Virchow, 1860a,b; Nevinny, 1927; Gould, 1945). Nevinny (1927) and Loeschke (1927) hypothesized that the aforementioned thickening of the sarcolemma is due to an antigen–antibody reaction. Bischoff (1840), Leuckart (1860), and other authors supported the view that the parasite secretes the capsular material. Frothingham (1906) and others presented the view that the capsule is composed of collagen produced by fibroblasts surrounding the invaded muscle cell. Bruce (1970a,b) concluded that the capsule consists of an outer region composed of tightly compacted fibrils and an inner region of fibrils more loosely arranged within the peripheral cytoplasm of the infected myofiber. The same author suggested that capsule fibers were produced not only by the infected host muscle cell but also by fibroblasts lying outside the invaded myofiber. Fielder (1864), Durante (1902), Beckett and Boothroyd (1962), and Teppema *et al.* (1973) have concluded that the capsule is formed by the infected host muscle fiber. Beckett and Boothroyd (1961) described the capsule as "a tangled network of collagen fibrils which vary in thickness." They found "collagen precursor" closest to the sarcoplasm of infected myofibers, whereas the thickest, and presumably the oldest, collagen was located within the outer layers of the capsule. Most recently, Teppema *et al.* (1973) conducted a detailed light- and electron-microscopic study of capsule formation. These authors also concluded that the capsule was laid down almost exclusively by the infected myofiber. They found no evidence for involvement of fibroblasts in the process of capsule formation. Their study suggested

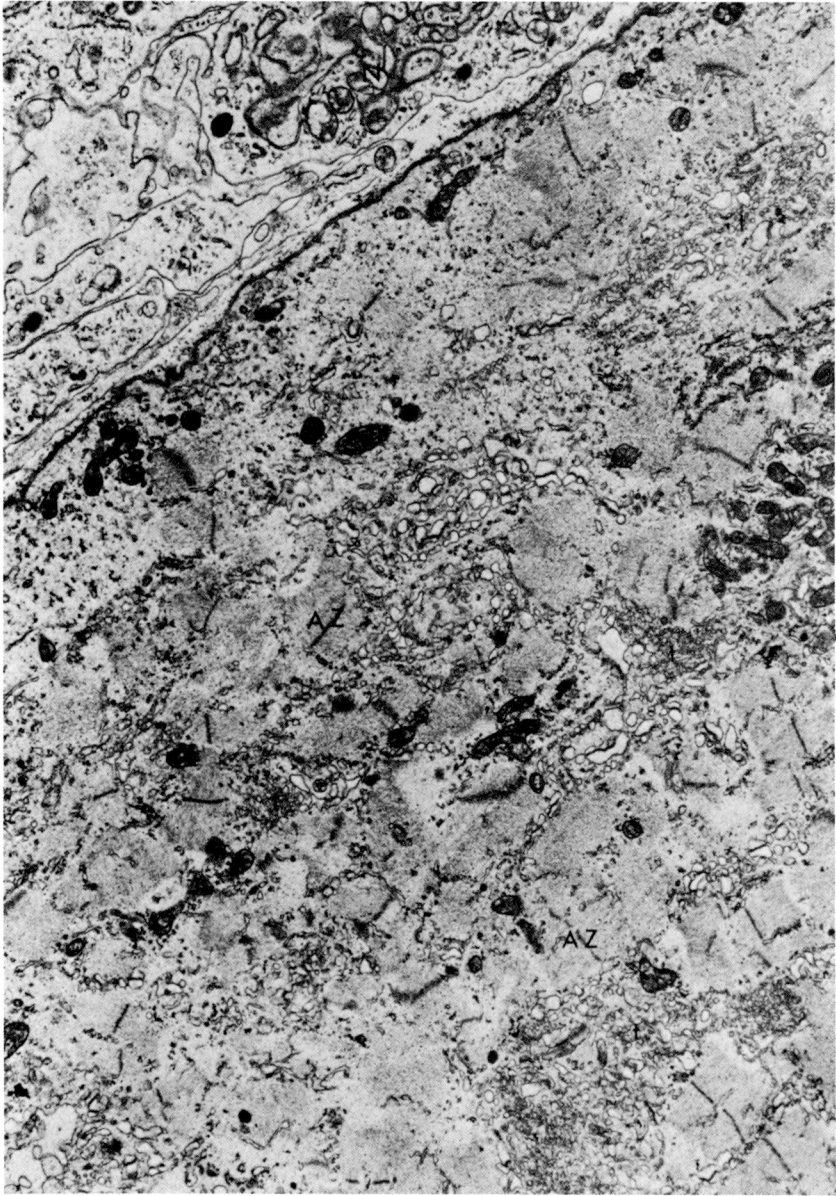

FIGURE 5. The few actin filaments attached to Z bands (AZ) that remain intact at 8 days after infection are sequestered to either end of the Nurse cell. Proliferation of the T-tubule system (t) is evident. The sarcolemma is unchanged. (N) Nerve. ×43,400. After Despommier (1975), courtesy of Harper and Row, New York.

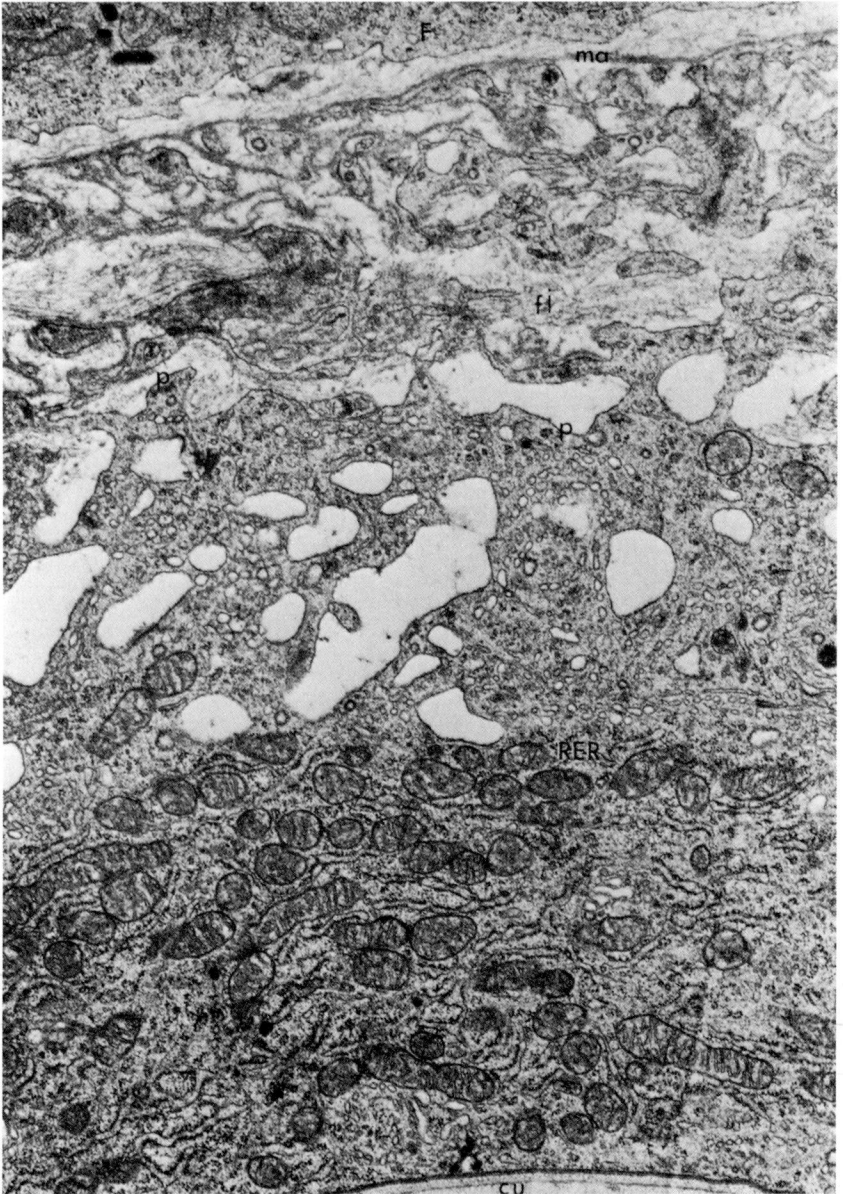

FIGURE 6. By day 10 PP, the plasma membrane (p) has undergone extensive involution. Increases in the amount of fibrous (fi) and matrix (ma) portions of the glycocalyx are associated with the plasma membrane. Rough endoplasmic reticulum (RER) is present near the larval–cuticular interface. The mitochondria are vacuolated. Note the close position of sarcoplasm next to the larval cuticle (cu). A portion of a fibroblast (F) is seen outside the glycocalyx. ×27,200.

that material packaged in vesicles within the sarcoplasm of the infected host cell was later deposited between the sarcolemma and the basal lamina of the invaded host myofiber, resulting in formation of the *Trichinella* capsule.

Alterations in the chemistry and structure of infected host myofibers described above indicate dramatic changes in the quality and quantity of structural proteins and enzymes required by *Trichinella*-infected muscle fibers. Fulfillment of these requirements is reflected by significant adjustments in protein metabolism in infected muscle. The period of infection during which the larva is growing most rapidly and the infected myofiber is undergoing its most dramatic changes in chemistry and structure (days 4–20 PP) witnesses an outstanding increase in the rates of incorporation of a variety of amino acids (methionine, alanine, glycine, proline, and tryptophan) into protein of infected as compared to uninfected muscle (Stewart and Read, 1972b; Stewart, 1973).

Using histochemical techniques, several workers have reported an increase in the glycogen content of infected myofibers before day 10 PP. This event is followed by a rapid decrease in the level of this polysaccharide to that seen in uninfected muscle cells (Zarzycki, 1956; Beckett and Boothroyd, 1962; Karpiak et al., 1963). These findings have been confirmed on the ultrastructural (Beckett and Boothroyd, 1962) and biochemical levels (Stewart, 1976). In the latter study, glycogen content of muscle larvae and of trichinous muscle was determined. Total glycogen in infected muscle rose between days 6 and 14 PP to a peak at approximately 40% above that seen in uninfected muscle. Between days 14 and 18 PP, a period of time during which larval glycogen stores increase rapidly, the glycogen content of trichinous muscle drops to levels similar to that seen in uninfected muscle. Serum glucose, pyruvate, and lactate, and liver glycogen stores, are within normal limits during this period of breakdown in muscle glycogen (Stewart, 1976; Stewart et al., 1978).

2.3. Mature Nurse Cell

Larval growth and evolution of the Nurse cell is complete by 20 days PP (see Chapter 3). The Nurse cell resulting from the complex series of chemical and microanatomical changes described above provides the larva with an optimal environment for extended survival. Ultrastructural and chemical findings (McCoy et al., 1941; Stoner and Hankes, 1955; Hankes and Stoner, 1958; Fasske and Themann, 1961; Karpiak et al., 1963; Stewart and Read, 1972a; Stewart, 1973; Purkerson and Despommier, 1974) demonstrate that the Nurse cell continues to maintain for long periods of time (presumably for the life of the larva) a level of metabolism quite unlike that of the uninfected myofiber. That the larva–Nurse cell complex can be isolated as a unit from the surrounding host tissues (Despommier, 1976) supports its hypothesized role as a chemically and physically independent entity.

2.4. Hypothesis: A Possible Mechanism by Which the Parasite Initiates Redifferentiation in the Host Myofiber

A number of workers have viewed the trichinous myofiber as a degenerative cell (Gould, 1945; Bullock and Gangi, 1950; Bullock, 1953; Beckett, 1961; Fasske and Themann, 1961). Others have suggested that the sarcoplasm of the infected myofiber enclosed within the capsule is a large phagocytic cell that either originated through reorganization of the enclosed sarcoplasm or arose from surrounding connective tissue (Staubli, 1909; Graham, 1897; Flury, 1913; Nevinny, 1927; Hemmert-Halswick and Bugge, 1934). More recently, several workers have postulated that the ultrastructural, histochemical, and biochemical changes that occur in the infected myofiber are indicative of a process of active reorganization, rather than a process of degeneration (Zarzycki, 1963; Maier and Zaiman, 1966; Ribas-Mujal and Rivera-Pomar, 1968; Ribas-Mujal, 1971; Stewart, 1973; Stewart and Read 1973b; Despommier, 1975, 1976; Stewart and Giannini, 1982).

Maier and Zaiman (1966) commented on similarities between some of the changes undergone by trichinous myofibers during evolution of the Nurse cell and those that occur in striated muscle fibers undergoing regeneration. Stewart and Read (1973b) presented a detailed comparison of ultrastructural and biochemical changes that occur during the two aforementioned processes (Table 1) and found them to be remarkably similar. These authors noted that in most forms of chemical and physical damage and disease that affect vertebrate striated muscle, altered myofibers either undergo complete degeneration and death or reestablish some degree of normal function through the process of regeneration. In this regard, trichinous myofibers are quite unique. Rather than degenerating or undergoing complete regeneration, host myofibers invaded by *Trichinella* undergo a process of reorganization resulting in the formation of a chemically and structurally new type of host cell (the Nurse cell). In view of the dramatic similarities between the early changes in the chemistry and structure of trichinous myofibers and those that occur in regenerating muscle cells, Stewart and Read (1973b) hypothesized that regeneration plays a significant role in the initial development of the Nurse cell. Damage done to the host myofiber by the invading newborn L_1 larva induces the cell to enter into a state

TABLE 1

Comparison of Ultrastructural and Biochemical Alterations Known to Occur in Host Striated Skeletal Myofibers Infected with *Trichinella spiralis* and Those That Occur in Striated Skeletal Myofibers Undergoing Regeneration

Biochemical or ultrastructural change	Trichinous myofiber	Regenerating myofiber
1. Increase in amount of sarcoplasmic matrix	+	+
2. Increase in size and number of nuclei; migration of nuclei from periphery to center of muscle fiber	+	+
3. Increase in free ribosomes and intense proliferation of rough endoplasmic reticulum and smooth sarcoplasmic reticulum	+	+
4. Intense proliferation of T-tubules	+	+
5. Increase in the size of affected myofiber	+	+
6. Increase in the number of mitochondria	+	+
7. Increase in the number of Golgi bodies	+	+
8. Increases in DNA and RNA content	+	+
9. Elevation in the rates of incorporation of thymidine into DNA and of uridine into RNA	+	+
10. Increase in the rates of incorporation of amino acids into protein	+	+
11. Onset of first ultrastructural changes from time of cell trauma	2 days	2 days
12. Duration of abnormal metabolic activity	For the life of the larvae	1 month
13. Disposition of myofibrils	Indiscriminately destroyed in all or part of fiber; no reconstitution of same	Only myofibrils damaged by trauma are destroyed; eventual reconstitution of same

of regeneration (Fig. 7). At some point following initiation of this process, the larva redirects regeneration from repair of damage to construction of a chemically and anatomically optimal niche for the long-term existence of the parasite. It may be speculated that this reorganization probably results from a complex series of chemical messages exchanged between the parasite and the host myofiber at key points during development of the Nurse cell (Read, 1970; Despommier, 1976; Stewart and Giannini, 1982).

Induction of such profound alterations in the trichinous myofiber suggests that the intracellular niche initially offered to the larva is unsuitable for its growth and development. The nature and magnitude of many of the changes in the chemistry and structure of the muscle fiber imply that the larva is somehow able to affect the quality and quantity of genetic information actively involved in determining the structure and function of the host cell.

An important area for future research is that dealing with the nature of the information exchanged between the muscle larva and the host myofiber during growth of the larva and modification of the host muscle fiber. It has been speculated that messages from the larva to the host cell may be in the form of low-molecular-weight compounds such as n-valeric acid (Stewart and Read, 1973b) or of macromolecules such as DNA (Despommier, 1975, 1976).

2.5. Benefits Derived by the Muscle Larva from Pathophysiological Alterations in Host Muscle

2.5.1. Nutrition

In terms of nutrition of the muscle larva, one of the most interesting alterations induced in the microarchitecture of the host muscle fiber is intense proliferation of the T-tubular system and widespread involution of the sarcolemma (Fasske and Themann, 1961; Ribas-Mujal and Rivera-Pomar, 1968; Teppema et al., 1973; Despommier, 1975). Such changes

---

FIGURE 7. Hypothesized events leading to reorganization of a vertebrate striated myofiber infected with *T. spiralis* into a Nurse cell. The host myofiber reacts to damage resulting from invasion by a newborn L_1 larva by entering into a state of regeneration. Chemical messages from the larva to the host myofiber redirect regeneration from repair of parasite-induced damage to the modification of the myoenvironment. The major benefits derived by the larva from such alterations in the host cell include: (1) enhancement of parasite nutrition; (2) stabilization of the myoenvironment; and (3) protection of the larva. All these events play a role in evolution of the Nurse cell.

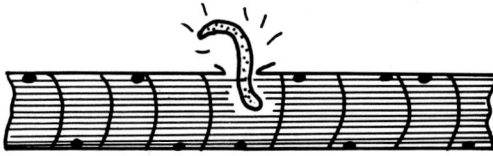

INVASION OF HOST MYOFIBER

HOST MYOFIBER REACTS TO INJURY
(INITIATION OF REGENERATION)

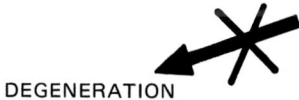

DEGENERATION

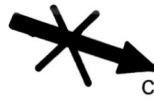

COMPLETE
REGENERATION

CHEMICAL INFORMATION FROM THE LARVA
REDIRECTS REGENERATION

SYNTHESIS OF STRUCTURAL PROTEINS AND ENZYMES
BY HOST MYOFIBER FOR MODIFICATION OF MYOENVIRONMENT

NUTRITION

STABILIZATION OF
THE MYOENVIRONMENT

PROTECTION OF
THE LARVA

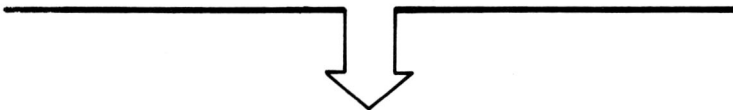

EVOLUTION OF THE NURSE CELL

translate into a significant increase in the surface area of infected fibers. Early in infection, there occurs a profound increase in the level of nonspecific alkaline phosphatase activity on the surfaces of the hyperplastic T-tubule membranes of trichinous host myofibers (Bruce, 1970a; Seniuta, 1971; Borgers *et al.*, 1975). Alkaline phosphatase is in general thought to be involved in active transport of molecules across biological membranes. The aforementioned changes in the T-tubule system of the infected myofiber may represent a highly significant increase in the absorptive capacity of the trichinous muscle cell. Such changes may be required to support the markedly enhanced rates of macromolecular synthesis that occur in parasitized muscle fibers and to satisfy the nutritional requirements of the rapidly growing muscle larva. Proliferation of T-tubules and enhancement of pinocytosis at the sarcolemmal and T-tubular membrane surfaces (Teppema *et al.*, 1973) and the increased alkaline phosphatase activity associated with T-tubular membranes should dramatically alter the quality as well as the quantity of nutrients available to the rapidly growing parasite. In addition, the double membrane formed around the larva may possess permeability characteristics that enhance the influx of essential molecules into the enclosed worm, while depressing the influx, or promoting the efflux, of substances harmful to the parasite (Stewart and Giannini, 1982).

Total glycogen of trichinous muscle, minus larval glycogen, rose well above that of uninfected tissue during the first 14 days PP. Between days 14 and 18 PP, total glycogen in infected muscle returned to the level seen in uninfected muscle. During this period of rapid diminishment in glycogen stores of infected tissue, the glycogen content of muscle larvae increased dramatically (days 10–18 PP) (Stewart, 1976). During the period of infection when muscle glycogen decreased, no changes were seen in serum glucose, lactate, or pyruvate, or in the glycogen content of liver in the trichinous host (Stewart, 1976; Stewart *et al.*, 1978). It may be that larvae make use of the glucose released during degradation of host muscle glycogen to increase their own polysaccharide reserves.

2.5.2. Stabilization of the Myoenvironment

Despommier (1976) described the physical and chemical environment offered by a vertebrate striated myofiber to an invading parasite. He pointed out that the muscle cell has a highly ordered physical composition, a rather narrow chemical composition with regard to the variety of biochemical components, and a metabolism that can vary enormously over short periods of time. The muscle fiber would appear to be a considerably less hospitable intracellular niche for parasites than most other mammalian cells. This view is supported by the fact that although muscle comprises a large percentage of the wet weight of vertebrates, few parasites assume an intracellular existence in this tissue. Study of intracellular parasites of vertebrate striated skeletal muscle has revealed that successful occupation of this niche requires that the parasite induce significant alterations in the biochemistry or structure, or both, of the host cell (Stewart and Giannini, 1982).

Included among the changes that occur in the trichinous myofiber is the appearance of lysosomes, which is preceded by dissolution of myofilaments (Teppema *et al.*, 1973). This event would remove space-occupying structures from the larval niche, making room for larval growth and for the intense hyperplasia of key organelles in the host myofiber. In addition, destruction of myofilaments (Fasske and Themann, 1961; Ribas-Mujal and Rivera-Pomar, 1968; Teppema *et al.*, 1973; Despommier, 1975) and loss of several chemicals (Stewart and Read, 1974) that support contraction (e.g., myoglobin, creatine phosphate, creatine) would avoid the severe mechanical stresses and changes in pH, ionic composition, and energy economy that occur within the host myofiber during muscular activity.

2.5.3. Protection of the Larva

The altered metabolic state of the trichinous myofiber is probably directed in part toward synthesis of collagen for capsule formation and toward construction of the double membrane of host origin that surrounds the larva. Both these structures may afford the enclosed larva some degree of protection from cellular and immune elements of the host response (see Gould, 1970; Ribas-Mujal, 1971).

3. CARDIOPATHOPHYSIOLOGY IN TRICHINOSIS

Numerous workers have observed *Trichinella* larvae in the myocardium of both experimental animals and man (Graham, 1897; Frothingham, 1906; Zoller, 1927; Horlick and Bicknell, 1929; Dunlap and Weller, 1933; Hemmert-Halswick and Bugge, 1934; Terry and Work, 1940; Edwards and Hood, 1962; and others). Despite the apparent ability of the newborn L_1 larvae to invade the myocardium, the worm never becomes encapsulated in this tissue (Gould, 1970; Ribas-Mujal, 1971). According to the former author, the larvae, after invading the heart muscle, are either destroyed by the intense myocarditis precipitated by their presence, migrate into the pericardial cavity, or reenter the circulation. The apparent inability of the larva to complete its development in the myocardial fiber has been postulated to be due to: (1) the continuous and vigorous myocardial contractions; (2) the fact that invasion by the larva destroys the integrity of the relatively weak sarcolemma of the myocardial fiber (Staubli, 1909); (3) the fact that myocardial fibers possess insufficient amounts of connective tissue to support migration of larvae; and (4) the fact that the heart is refractory to infection (Weller and Shaw, 1932) by virtue of some "special evolutionary endowment of heart muscle with antiparasitic powers" (Gould, 1970).

The nuclei of invaded myocardial fibers show an increase in both size and number (Gould, 1945, 1970), a situation similar to that seen in striated skeletal muscle (see Section 2.2). However, none of the other alterations in structure or chemistry that occur in trichinous striated myofibers has been observed in myocardial fibers from the trichinous host. Stewart (1973) found no significant difference between the RNA content of whole heart muscle from infected and that of heart muscle from uninfected hosts. On the other hand, a process of fatty degeneration of invaded myocardial fibers has been reported (Cohnheim, 1865; Howard, 1899; Knorr, 1912; Wehrmann, 1927). It is of interest to note that in numerous myopathies that affect both heart and skeletal muscle fibers, the former sometimes fail to display the capacity for regeneration seen in the latter tissue (Bourne, 1973). It may be hypothesized that the quality or quantity of damage done to a myocardial fiber by the invading larva may be inappropriate for induction of regeneration (see above). In the absence of regeneration, the larva is unable to modify the myocardial fiber in the way in which it does the skeletal muscle fiber and is therefore precluded from completing its development.

REFERENCES

Backwinkle, K.D., and Themann, H., 1972, Elektronmikroscopische Untersuchungen über die Pathomorphologie der Trichinellose, *Beitr. Pathol.* **146:**259–271.

Beckett, E.B., 1961, Some histochemical changes in the protein of mouse skeletal muscle fibers infected by *Trichinella spiralis, Ann. Trop. Med. Parasitol.* **55:**419–426.

Beckett, E.B., and Boothroyd, B., 1961, Some observations on the mature larva of the nematode *Trichinella spiralis, Ann. Trop. Med. Parasitol.* **55:**116–124.

Beckett, E.B., and Boothroyd, B., 1962, The histochemistry and electron microscopy of glycogen in the larva of *Trichinella spiralis* and its environment, *Ann. Trop. Med. Parasitol.* **56:**264–273.

Bischoff, T.L.W., 1840, Ein Fall von *Trichina spiralis*, *Heidelh. Med. Ann.* **6**:232–238.

Boczon, K., 1967, Some data on bioenergetics of the larvae of *Trichinella spiralis*, *Bull. Soc. Amis Sci. Lett. Poznan Ser. D* **8**:165–170.

Boczon, K., Michejda, J.W., and Hryniewiecka, L., 1967, Changes in bioenergetics of mitochondria and on lactate-NAD-oxidoreductase activity in rat skeletal muscle during experimental trichinosis, Proceedings of the 4th Meeting of the Federation of European Biochemical Societies, Oslo, Sweden, pp. 128.

Borgers, M., DeNollen, S., and Thone, F., 1975, The development of alkaline phosphatase in trichinous muscle, *Histochemistry* **43**:257–267.

Bourne, G.H., 1973, *The Structure and Function of Muscle*, Vols. I–IV, Academic Press, New York.

Bruce, R.G., 1970a, The structure and development of the capsule of *Trichinella spiralis*, *J. Parasitol.* **56**:38–39.

Bruce, R.G., 1970b, The structure and composition of the capsule of *Trichinella spiralis* in host muscle, *Parasitology* **60**:223–227.

Bullock, W. L., 1953, Phosphatases in experimental *Trichinella spiralis* infections in the rat, *Exp. Parasitol.* **12**:150–162.

Bullock, W.L., and Gangi, D.P., 1950, The distribution of alkaline glycerophosphatase in the muscle of rats infected with *Trichinella spiralis*, *J. Parasitol.* **36**:Suppl. 30.

Casey, M.A., and Harley, J.P., 1978, *Trichinella spiralis*: Skeletal muscle membrane potentials in infected and uninfected mice, *Exp. Parasitol.* **44**:66–71.

Cohnheim, J., 1865, Todtliche Trichinose mit parenchymatoser Degeneration von Leber, Herz und Nieren, *Virchows Arch. Pathol. Anat.* **33**:447–451.

Despommier, D.D., 1975, Adaptive changes in muscle fibers infected with *Trichinella spiralis*, *Am. J. Pathol.* **78**:477–496.

Despommier, D.D., 1976, Musculature, in: *Ecological Aspects of Parasitology* (C.R. Kennedy, ed.), North-Holland, Amsterdam, pp. 269–285.

Despommier, D.D., Aron, L., and Turgeon, L., 1975, *Trichinella spiralis*: Growth of the intracellular (muscle) larva, *Exp. Parasitol.* **37**:108–116.

Drachman, D.A., and Tunchay, T.O., 1965, The remote myopathy of trichinosis, *Neurology* **15**:1127–1135.

Dunlap, G.L., and Weller, C.V., 1933, Pathogenesis of trichinous myocarditis, *Proc. Soc. Exp. Biol. Med.* **30**:1261–1262.

Durante, G., 1902, Anatomie pathologique des muscles, in: *Manuel d'Histologie Pathologique* (F. Cornil and G. Ranvier, eds.), Masson, Paris, pp. 18–44.

Edwards, J.L., and Hood, C.I., 1962, Studies on the pathogenesis of cardiac and cerebral lesions of experimental trichinosis in rabbits, *Am. J. Pathol.* **40**:711–717.

Ehrhardt, P., 1896, Zur Kenntniss der Muskelveränderungen bei der Trichinose des Menschen, *Beitr. Pathol. Anat.* **20**:1–42.

Farris, K., and Harley, J.P., 1977, *Trichinella spiralis*: Alteration of gastrocnemius muscle kinetics in the mouse, *Exp. Parasitol.* **41**:17–30.

Fasske, E., and Themann, H., 1961, Elektronmicroskopische Befunde an der Muskelfaser nach Trichinbefall, *Virchows Arch. Pathol. Anat.* **334**:459–474.

Fielder, A., 1864, Uber die Kernwucherung in der Muskeln bei der Trichinenkrankheit, *Virchows Arch. Pathol. Anat.* **30**:461–468.

Flury, F., 1913, Beitrage zur Chemie und Toxokologie der Trichinin, *Arch. Exp. Pathol. Pharmakol.* **53**:164–213.

Frothingham, C., Jr., 1906, A contribution to the knowledge of the lesions caused by *Trichina spiralis*, *J. Med. Res.* **15**:483–490.

Gabryel, P., and Gustowska, L., 1967, Veränderungen der quergestreiften Muskelfasern im frühen Stadium einer *Trichinal spiralis* Infektion, Gegenbauers Morph. Jahrb. **111:**174–180.

Garbulinski, T., Kozar, Z., Bubien, Z., Debowy, J., and Biblinski, E., 1965, ^{32}P-Incorporation into energetic phosphates of the heart and skeletal muscles in rats infected with *Trichinella spiralis, Acta Parasitol. Pol.* **13:**275–281.

Gould, S.E., 1945, Pathology, in: *Trichinosis* (S.E. Gould, ed.). Charles C. Thomas, Springfield, Illinois, pp. 73–132.

Gould, S.E., 1970, Anatomic pathology, in: *Trichinosis in Man and Animals* (S.E. Gould, ed.), Charles C. Thomas, Springfield, Illinois, pp. 147–189.

Graham, J.Y., 1897, Beiträge zur Naturgeschichte der *Trichina spiralis, Arch. Mikrosk. Anat.* **50:**219–275.

Hankes, L.V., and Stoner, R.D., 1958, Incorporation of DL-tyrosine-2-C-14 and DL-tryptophan-2-C-14 by encysted *Trichinella spiralis* larvae, *Exp. Parasitol.* **7:**82–89.

Hemmert-Halswick, A., and Bugge, G., 1934, Trichinen und Trichinose, *Ergebn. Allg. Pathol.* **28:**313–319.

Horlick, S.S., and Bicknell, R.E., 1929, Trichiniasis with wide-spread infestation of many tissues, *N. Engl. J. Med.* **201:**816–819.

Howard, W.T., Jr., 1899, Report of a fatal case of trichinosis without eosinophilia but with large numbers of eosinophilic cells in the muscle lesions; with remarks on the origin of eosinophilic cells in trichinosis, *Philadelphia Med. J.* **4:**1085–1087.

Hryniewiecka, L., Boczon, K., and Michejda, J.W., 1970, *Trichinella spiralis*: Enzymes reducing and oxidizing cytochrome c in rat muscle, *Exp. Parasitol.* **28:**544–550.

Hughes, W.L., and Harley, J.P., 1977, *Trichinella spiralis*: Taxes of first stage migratory larvae. *Exp. Parasitol.* **42:**363–373.

Karpiak, S.E., Kozar, Z., and Krzyanowski, M., 1963, Changes in the metabolism of the skeletal muscles of guinea pigs caused by the invasion of *Trichinella spiralis*. I. Influence of the invasion on the carbohydrate metabolism of muscles, *Wiad. Parazytol.* **9:**435–446.

Knorr, H., 1912, Bietrag zur Kenntnis der Trichinellen Krankheit des Menschen, Dtsch. Arch. Klin. Med. **108:**137–159.

Kozar, Z., Karpiak, S.E., and Krzyzanowski, M., 1965, Changes in the metabolism of the skeletal muscles of guinea pigs caused by the invasion of *Trichinella spiralis*. II. Effect of invasion on the metabolism of organic acids, *Acta Parasitol. Pol.* **13:**271–274.

Kozar, Z., Zarzycki, J., Seniuta, R., and Martynowicz, T., 1967, Histochemical study of drug effects on mice infected with *Trichinella spiralis*, *Exp. Parasitol.* **21:**177–185.

Langerhans, R., 1892, Ueber regressive Veränderungen der Trichinen und ihre Kapseln, *Virchows Arch. Pathol. Anat.* **130:**205–216.

Leuckart, R., 1860, Untersuchungen über *Trichina spiralis*, Leipzig, Winter. pp. 57.

Lewis, J.H., 1928a, Studien über den Mechanismus der Trichinelleninfektion. II. Der Einfluss des Glykogens auf die Muskelinvasion, *Zentralbl. Bakteriol.* **107:**114–126.

Lewis, J.H., 1928b, Influence of glycogen on the infection of muscle with trichinae, *Trans. Chicago Pathol. Soc.* **13:**12–15.

Loeschke, H., 1927, Vorstellungen über das Wesen von Hyalin und Amyloid auf Grund von serologischen Versuchen, *Beitr. Pathol. Anat.* **77:**231–239.

Maier, D.M., and Zaiman, H., 1966, The development of lysosomes in rat skeletal muscle in trichinous myositis, *J. Histochem. Cytochem.* **14:**396–400.

Maier, D.M., Zaiman, H., and Howard, R., 1962, Histochemical changes in muscle degeneration, *Lab. Invest.* **11:**667 (abstract).

McCoy, O.R., Downing, V.F., and van Voorhis, S.N., 1941, The penetration of radioactive phosphorus into encysted *Trichinella* larvae, *J. Parasitol.* **27**:53–58.

Michejda, J.W., and Boczon, K., 1972, Changes in bioenergetics of skeletal muscle mitochondria during experimental trichinosis in rats, *Exp. Parasitol.* **3**:161–171.

Nevinny, H., 1927, Uber die Veränderungen der Skelettmuskulatur bei Trichinose, *Virchows Arch. Pathol. Anat.* **266**:185–238.

Nicolesco, S., Onicesco, D., Gavat, V., and Simionesco, V., 1962, A propos de la signification de certaines lesions nerveuses déterminées par les parasites animaux a localisation musculaire, *Acta Morphol. Acad. Sci. Hung.* **11**:257–266.

Ochoa, J., and Pallis, C., 1980, *Trichinella* thrives in both oxidative and glycolytic human muscle fibers, *J. Neurol. Neurosurg. Psychiatry* **43**:281–282.

Ogielski, L., 1949, Reaction of the vascular vessels against invasion of the larvae of *Trichinella spiralis*, *Zool. Pol.* **5**:35–42.

Paget, J., 1866, On the discovery of trichina, *Lancet* **1**:269–270.

Purkerson, J., and Despommier, D., 1974, Fine structure of the muscle phase of *Trichinella spiralis* in the mouse, in: *Trichinellosis* (C. Kim, ed.), Intext, New York, pp. 7–23.

Read, C.P., 1970, Chemical pathology, in: *Trichinosis in Man and Animals* (S.E. Gould, ed.), Charles C. Thomas, Springfield, Illinois, pp. 91–101.

Ribas-Mujal, D., 1971, Trichinosis, in: *Pathology of Protozoal and Helminthic Diseases*, Williams and Wilkins, Baltimore, pp. 677–710.

Ribas-Mujal, D., and Rivera-Pomar, J.M., 1968, Biological significance of the early structural alterations in skeletal muscle fibers infected by *Trichinella spiralis*, *Virchows Arch. Pathol. Anat.* **345**:154–168.

Ritterson, A.L., 1966, Nature of the cyst of *Trichinella spiralis*, *J. Parasitol.* **52**:157–161.

Rogers, W.P., 1942, The metabolism of trichinosed rats during the early phase of the disease, *J. Helminthol.* **20**:139–158.

Schanzel, H., and Holman, J., 1966, Lokalisation der alkalischen Phosphatase in der *Trichinella* befallenden Muskulatur, *Angew. Parasitol.* **7**:252–259.

Seniuta, R., 1971, Histochemical investigations of the activity of some phosphates in skeletal muscles of mice under the influence of infection with *Trichinella spiralis*, *Fol. Histochem. Cytochem.* **9**:95–116.

Staubli, C., 1905a, Klinische und experimentelle Untersuchengen über Trichinosis, *Verhandl. Kongr. Inn. Med.* **22**:353–362.

Staubli, C., 1905b, Klinische und experimetelle Untersuchungen über Trichinose und über die Eosinophilie in Allgemeinen, *Virchows Arch. Pathol. Anat. Physiol.* **85**:286–341.

Staubli, C., 1909, *Trichinosis*, J.F. Bergmann, Wiesbaden, 295 pp.

Stewart, G.L., 1973, Studies on chemical pathology in trichinosis, Doctoral thesis, Rice University, Houston, Texas, 85 pp.

Stewart, G.L., 1976, Studies on biochemical pathology in trichinosis. II. Changes in liver and muscle glycogen and some blood chemical parameters in mice, *Rice Univ. Stud.* **62**:211–223.

Stewart, G.L., and Charniga, L.M., 1980, Distribution of *Trichinella spiralis* in muscles of the mouse, *J. Parasitol.* **66**:688–689.

Stewart, G.L., and Giannini, S., 1982, Intracellular parasites of striated muscle: A review, *Exp. Parasitol.* **53**:406–447.

Stewart, G.L., and Read, C.P., 1972a, Ribonucleic acid metabolism in mouse trichinosis, *J. Parasitol.* **58**:252–256.

Stewart, G.L., and Read, C.P., 1972b, Some aspects of cyst synthesis in mouse trichinosis, *J. Parasitol.* **58**:1061–1064.

Stewart, G.L., and Read, C.P., 1973a, Deoxyribonucleic acid metabolism in mouse trichinosis, *J. Parasitol.* **59**:264–267.

Stewart, G.L., and Read, C.P., 1973b, Changes in RNA in mouse trichinosis, *J. Parasitol.* **59**:997–1005.

Stewart, G.L., and Read, C.P., 1974. Studies on biochemical pathology in trichinosis. I. Changes in myoglobin, free creatine, phosphocreatine and two protein fractions of mouse diaphragm muscle, *J. Parasitol.* **60**:996–1000.

Stewart, G.L., Fisher, F.M., Jr., Ribelles, E., Chiapetta, V., and LaBrum, R., 1978, *Trichinella spiralis*: Alterations of blood chemistry in the mouse, *Exp. Parasitol.* **45**:287–297.

Stoner, R.D., and Hankes, L.V., 1955, Incorporation of C^{14} labeled amino acids by *Trichinella spiralis, Exp. Parasitol.* **4**:435–444.

Stoyanov, D.P., and Nenov, St. D. 1965, Some histochemical changes in tissues of guinea pigs infected with *Trichinella spiralis, Med. Parazytol.* **34**:392–396.

Teppema, J.S., Robinson, J.E., and Ruitenberg, E.J., 1973, Ultrastructural aspects of capsule formation in *Trichinella spiralis* infection in the rat, *Parasitology* **66**:291–296.

Terry, L.L., and Work, J.L., 1940, Trichinosis of the myocardium: Report of a case with autopsy findings, *Am. Heart J.* **19**:478–485.

Virchow, R., 1860a, Uber *Trichina spiralis, Virchows Arch. Pathol. Anat.* **18**:330–346.

Virchow, R., 1860b, Vorläufige Nachricht über neue trichinen Fütterungen, *Virchows Arch. Pathol. Anat.* **18**:535–536.

Wehrmann, O., 1927, Beitrag zur pathologischen Anatomie der Trichinose des Menschen, *Virchows Arch. Pathol. Anat.* **263**:584–589.

Weller, C.V., and Shaw, M., 1932, Myocardial failure due to trichinosis, *Trans. Assoc. Am. Physicians* **47**:31–46.

Zarzycki, J., 1956, Histologic investigations on the glycogen content in striated muscle infected with trichinellae, *Med. Weter.* **12**:328–332.

Zarzycki, J., 1962, Histochemical investigations on distribution of nucleic acids and inorganic salts in muscle tissue at the infection with *Trichinella spiralis* in: *Trichinellosis, Proceedings of the 1st International Conference on Trichinellosis* (Z. Kozar, ed.), Polish Scientific Publications, Warsaw, pp. 302–305.

Zarzycki, J., 1963, Studies on distribution and activity of succinic dehydrogenase in muscle tissue during infection with *Trichinellae, Wiad. Parazytol.* **9**:459–464.

Zoller, H., 1927, Uber Herzmuskelentzündung im Verlauf der Trichinose, *Virchows Arch. Pathol. Anat.* **265**:430–443.

8

The Immune Response

DEREK WAKELIN and DAVID A. DENHAM

1. INTRODUCTION

Trichinella spiralis is a highly successful parasite in that it can establish, develop, and reproduce in a wide range of vertebrate hosts. This low host specificity implies that the organism has the ability to adapt to a variety of environmental conditions and hence is relatively unaffected by many of those aspects of natural immunity that impose a more rigid specificity on other species. However, in common with all metazoan parasites, *T. spiralis* presents the host with a complex antigenic stimulus and thus evokes a powerful immune response. The complexity of the stimulus arises not only from the diversity of antigens present at any one time, but also from the fact that antigens may show stage specificity, changing qualitatively and quantitatively throughout development, and may be released in different tissues of the body. Many components of the immunological response probably have little or no effect on either host or parasite, though they may prove useful in diagnosis; some are deleterious to the parasite and provide protective resistance against infection, yet others are actually or potentially harmful to the host, either from their involvement in immunopathological reactions or through their modulation of unrelated immune responses. This chapter will concentrate on those responses that confer resistance on the host; immune responses in the contexts of diagnosis and pathology are dealt

DEREK WAKELIN • Department of Zoology, University of Nottingham, Nottingham, England. DAVID A. DENHAM • London School of Hygiene and Tropical Medicine, London WC1E 7HT, England.

with elsewhere in this volume. Discussion will be limited to experimental data obtained from work with mice, rats, and rabbits.

2. IMMUNITY AND THE INTESTINAL PHASE

The intestine is the initial site of parasitization and is the initial site of the immune response. In naïve hosts, the time taken to generate responses is such that the preadult stages of the worm cannot be affected by host resistance, and it is the adult worms that first show the effects of the immune response. In previously infected hosts, this may also be the case, but in some hosts, and under certain circumstances, the preadult worms are very strongly affected.

2.1. Immunity against Adult Worms in Primary Infections

The duration of the intestinal phase in an initial infection is variable among species of hosts and among strains of host species. For example, it has been estimated that adult worms persist in man for 6 weeks or more, in guinea pigs for 30–40 days, and in mice and rats (depending on the strain concerned) for 10–20 days. The intestinal phase is terminated by a sudden or gradual loss of worms, and it has been shown clearly, e.g., by treatment with immunosuppressive drugs (Coker, 1955; Markell, 1958), that worm loss is the result of immunologically mediated responses. Loss of worms from the intestine is, however, only the culmination of a sequence of host responses, and other effects of immunity are apparent in the worm well before expulsion takes place. These effects include a reduction in fecundity of adult females (Denham and Martinez, 1970; Despommier et al., 1977a), the appearance of cytopathological changes in both somatic and reproductive cells (Love et al., 1976; Kennedy and Bruce, 1981), and displacement of the worm population within the intestine (Larsh et al., 1952; Kennedy, 1980) (Fig. 1), although this is also strain-dependent, at least in mice (Denham, 1968).

It is unlikely that the ability of the host to respond protectively is wholly dependent on a single mechanism; in all probability, resistance is the outcome of a complex interplay involving several responses, each of which may independently be capable of producing resistance. However, under particular circumstances, specific manifestations of resistance may reflect the activity of specific responses. Such an assumption underlies much of the experimental analysis of immunity that has been undertaken in the mouse and in the rat. In both species, protective

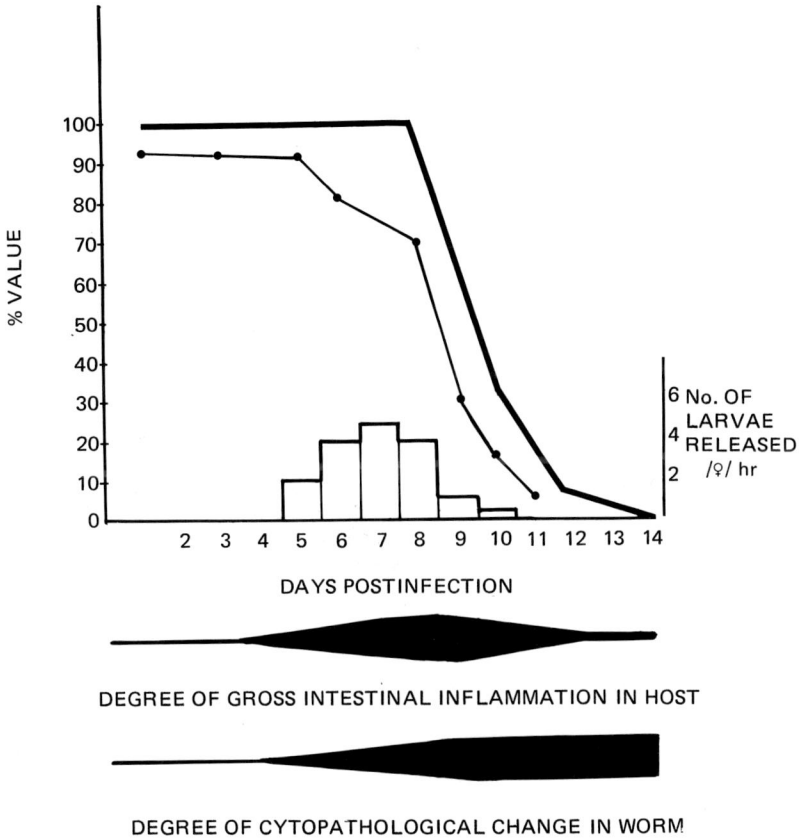

FIGURE 1. Diagrammatic representation of events that occur during primary infection of NIH mice by *T. spiralis*. (———) Number of worms as percentage of maximum recovered; (●—●) percentage of worms in anterior half of intestine.

immunity is dependent on the activity of thymus-derived (T) lympho-cytes, and infections are prolonged in thymus-deficient (Ruitenberg and Steerenberg, 1974; Perrudet-Badoux *et al.*, 1980), thymus-deprived (Walls *et al.*, 1973; Gore *et al.*, 1974; Manson-Smith *et al.*, 1979a), or T-cell-depleted hosts (Kozar *et al.*, 1971; Dinetta *et al.*, 1972; Machnicka, 1972), although antiparasite responses may still persist (Ljungström and Ruitenberg, 1976). The precise roles of T cells in immunity to *T. spiralis* have yet to be defined, but there is substantial evidence, particularly in the mouse, to implicate such cells in the initiation of intestinal inflammatory reactions (Ruitenberg *et al.*, 1977a; Wakelin and

Wilson, 1979a, 1980), and it may be assumed that they have in addition a helper function in the formation of antiparasite antibody responses.

2.1.1. Mouse

Immunity to *T. spiralis* in the mouse was described by Culbertson (1942) and has been extensively investigated by Larsh and co-workers in a long series of papers (reviewed by Larsh, 1963, 1970; Larsh and Race, 1975). This work defined many of the parameters of infection, showed that immunity was transferable with lymphoid cells, and described the close association of worm expulsion with inflammatory changes in the intestine. Failure to achieve passive transfer of immunity with serum led Larsh (1967) to the initial conclusion that expulsion resulted from delayed-hypersensitivity-induced changes in the intestine, a conclusion that was later modified into the concept of a T-cell-mediated "allergic inflammation" in the intestine (Larsh and Race, 1975; Larsh and Weatherly, 1975). Now that much more detail is known of the response of the mouse to *T. spiralis,* there is no doubt that this view of the way that intestinal immunity acts to expel the worm is substantially correct.

All of Larsh's work was carried out in a strain of mouse (inbred Swiss albino) that is a relatively poor responder to infection, responding slowly to initial infections and requiring several immunizing infections to stimulate strong challenge immunity. Much of what is now known of the mechanisms involved in immunity in the mouse has come from studies made in NIH mice, a strain that responds much more rapidly to infection. An early consequence of infection (2–4 days) is a marked lymphoblast response to infection (Rose *et al.*, 1976; Grencis and Wakelin, 1982; Wakelin *et al.*, 1982), and large numbers of dividing T cells appear in the mesenteric lymph node. Clearly, this response will be to all the antigens presented by the worm, but among the total dividing cell population are cells that are concerned specifically with the development of protective immunity. This can be shown in a direct fashion by transfer of immune mesenteric lymph node cells (IMLNC) from infected to naïve mice (Wakelin and Lloyd, 1976a; Wakelin and Wilson, 1977a). The cell recipients acquire a "ready-made" immunity that is expressed against infection in terms of reduced worm growth and fecundity and in an accelerated expulsion from the intestine (Table 1). Coincident with the lymphoblast response is a change in homing patterns of T lymphoblasts originating in the gut-associated lymphoid tissues. This change, which is not antigen-specific, and which is independent of altered vascular supply to the infected intestine, results in

TABLE 1
Adoptive Transfer of Immunity to _T. spiralis_ in NIH Mice: Effects of Immune Mesenteric Lymph Node Cells Taken from Donors Infected 8 Days Previously[a]

| Group | Cells | Worms recovered 8 days after infection with 350 larvae | | Fecundity (larvae/♀/hr) | Female length (mm) |
| | | Number | | | |
		Mean	S.D.		
1	None	174	28	2.5	2.6
2	IMLNC (4×10^7)	36[b]	19	0.3[b]	2.0[b]

[a] Data based on Wakelin and Wilson (1977a).
[b] Significantly lower than corresponding controls.

an increased accumulation of lymphoblasts in the intestinal mucosa (Rose _et al._, 1976; Ottaway _et al._, 1980).

Cells capable of transferring immunity appear in the mesenteric lymph nodes early in primary infection, but disappear once the worm population is expelled (Wakelin and Wilson, 1977a; Grencis and Wakelin, 1982). Adoptive transfer is not possible with cells taken 2 days after infection, but can be achieved with cells taken at day 4. The decline in availability of cells begins between days 8 and 12 of infection, during which time most of the worms are expelled, and transfers are generally unsuccessful with cells taken later than days 18–21 (Fig. 2). The capacity to transfer immunity is associated specifically with dividing lymphocytes (Wakelin _et al._, 1982). Cells from donors that have been treated with vinblastine (a mitotic inhibitor) do not transfer immunity, and when cell suspensions are fractionated on density gradients, the most effective fractions are those that contain the highest proportions of dividing cells. Cell-separation procedures have shown that the capacity to transfer accelerated worm expulsion is limited to T cells (Wakelin and Wilson, 1979a). Whereas a minimum of 1×10^7 unseparated cells is required to transfer immunity, as few as 3×10^6 T-enriched cells are effective. Fractions enriched in B cells, if adequately purified, appear to exert no effect on worm numbers in the intestines of recipients, but may transfer an immunity that is reflected in a lowered worm fecundity.

T cells _per se_ are not the direct cause of worm expulsion, since prior irradiation of the recipients of immune T cells abolishes their ability to express this form of resistance. Restoration of worm expulsion in such circumstances can be achieved only by providing irradiated recipients

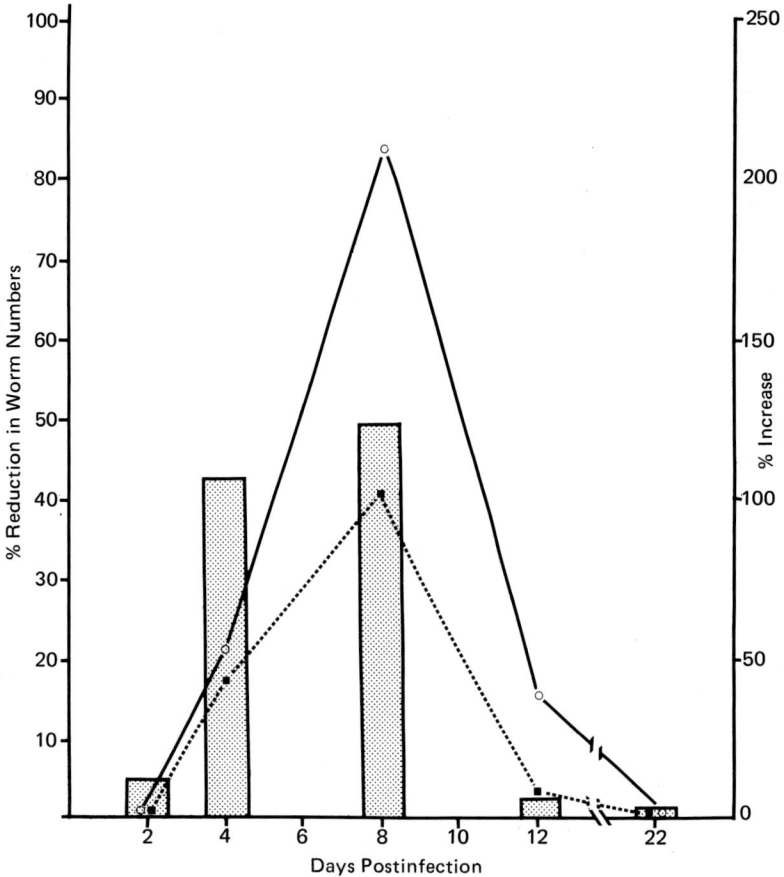

FIGURE 2. Cellular kinetics throughout a primary infection with *T. spiralis* in NIH mice. (O—O) Total number of nucleated cells in mesenteric lymph node (MLN) as percentage increase over uninfected control; (■┄┄┄■) level of incorporation of [^{125}I]iododeoxyuridine by MLN blast cells as percentage increase over control; ▨ ability of MLN cells to transfer immunity adoptively, measured by degree of worm expulsion at day 8 in recipient mice. Data from Grencis and Wakelin (1982).

with both immune lymphocytes and bone-marrow stem cells (Wakelin and Wilson, 1977b, 1980) (Table 2). There is strong presumptive evidence for concluding that the latter restore some nonlymphoid (myeloid) cell population that is required for the development of intestinal inflammatory changes in response to signals from the lymphocytes. The evidence for causal relationship between inflammation

TABLE 2

Adoptive Transfer of Immunity to *T. spiralis* in Irradiated NIH Mice: Requirement for Bone Marrow-Derived (BM) Cells in Worm Expulsion after Transfer of 2×10^7 Immune Mesenteric Lymph Node Cells[a]

		Worms recovered after infection with 200 larvae					
		Day 8			Day 12		
Group	Cells	Mean	S.D.	Fecundity (larvae/♀/hr)	Mean	S.D.	Fecundity (larvae/♀/hr)
Unirradiated mice							
1	None	81	17	3.7	—	—	—
2	IMLNC	47[b]	24	0.9[b]	—	—	—
Irradiated mice[c]							
3	BM cells	127	8	6.3	104	20	6.3
4	BM cells + IMLNC	123	15	4.8[b]	46[b]	30	2.7[b]
5	IMLNC	—	—	—	112	19	2.5[b]

[a] Data from Wakelin and Wilson (1982). [b] Significantly lower than corresponding controls.
[c] Irradiated at 600 rad.

and expulsion is based on many circumstantial correlations between the two events (Larsh and Race, 1975) and on direct observations of the inability of worms to establish and survive in the intestine once that organ is inflamed (Kennedy *et al.*, 1979; Wakelin and Wilson, 1979b). It is possible to transplant adult worms from one host directly into the intestines of another. When the recipient is uninfected, the transplanted worms establish perfectly well and survive for a period that is equivalent to the duration of an infection established by the oral route. However, if the recipient is given a prior oral infection and worms are transplanted at the time that gross inflammatory changes appear in the intestine, i.e., shortly before worm expulsion would occur, the transplanted worms establish but are expelled together with those from the initial infection. This suggests that extensive prior damage to the worms is not a necessary precondition for expulsion to occur.

This evidence of a functional association between inflammation and expulsion of worms from the intestine raises the question of what precise aspects of inflammation are involved. A considerable body of data is available concerning the changes that occur in the intestine, although there is no clear understanding of the relationship of these changes to protective resistance. The most pronounced of these changes are the infiltration of the mucosa by a variety of cells, alterations in mucosal architecture and cell kinetics, increases in the levels of a number of enzymes of leukocyte origin, and changes in net fluid flux across the mucosa.

Cellular infiltration is apparent within a few days of infection, the earliest changes involving neutrophils, i.e., cells associated with acute inflammatory changes. However, the most marked cellular infiltration involves mast cells and, to a lesser degree, eosinophils (Karmanska *et al.*, 1973; Ruitenberg *et al.*, 1977a; Tronchin *et al.*, 1979; Alizadeh and Wakelin, 1982a). In rapidly responding mice, mast cells become apparent from the 4th day of infection; their numbers rise considerably, peak at about the time of worm expulsion, and then decline (Fig. 3). Although it has been suggested that there is a correlation between the mast-cell response and worm expulsion (Karmanska *et al.*, 1973), there is little evidence to link intestinal mastocytosis directly with worm loss, and indeed the temporal association between the two events varies widely among different strains of mice. It seems reasonable to assume only that there must be some significant correlation between the presence of large numbers of mast cells and the inflammatory changes that are involved in expulsion. The increase in mast-cell numbers, intestinal inflammation, and worm expulsion are thymus-dependent phenomena (Ruitenberg and Elgersma, 1976; Ruitenberg *et al.*, 1977b;

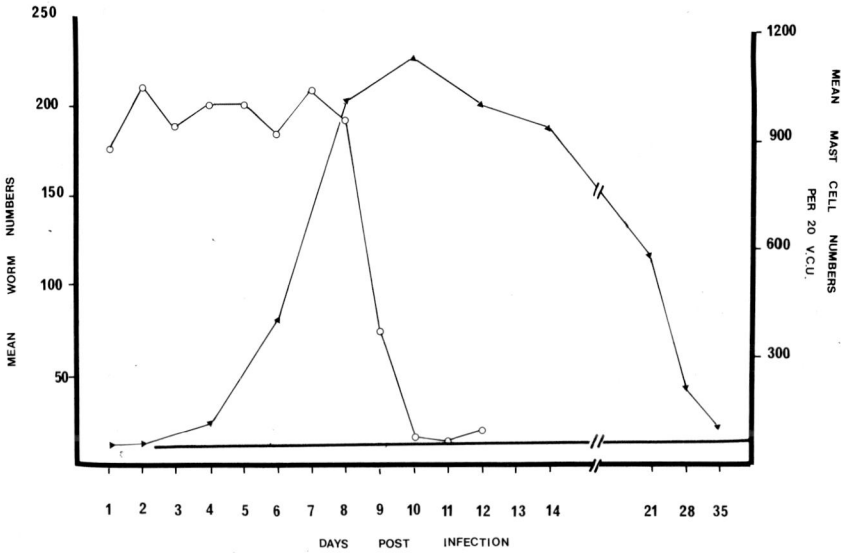

FIGURE 3. Numbers of mucosal mast cells during primary infection of *T. spiralis* in NIH mice. (O—O) Number of intestinal worms; (▶—▶) number of mucosal mast cells per 20 villus crypt units (V.C.U.); (———) number of mast cells in uninfected control mice. Data from Alizadeh and Wakelin (1982a).

Manson-Smith *et al.*, 1979a; Brown *et al.*, 1981), and the rise in mast cells can be accelerated by the adoptive transfer of mesenteric-node lymphocytes (Alizadeh and Wakelin, 1981). An important limiting factor in present understanding is an inability to assess the dynamics of mast-cell changes and to distinguish among degranulating, regranulating, newly formed, and effete cells. The static picture obtained by conventional histology does not allow mast-cell numbers to be related to their function. Nevertheless, a number of speculations concerning the consequences of the presence of this cell type can be put forward. Degranulation of mast cells, either directly by products of the worms themselves or through antigen linking to membrane-bound immunoglobulin E (IgE) or IgG$_1$, would result in the release of a variety of mast-cell factors, including the vasoactive amines histamine and 5-hydroxy-tryptamine (5-HT). These would exert profound effects on vascular and mucosal permeability (Murray, 1972), causing mucosal edema and plasma leakage into the lumen and facilitating the infiltration of leukocytes responding to T-cell lymphokines (Askenase, 1979). The presence of relatively large amounts of histamine, a known modulator of many cellular functions, could also exert a variety of effects on the intestine and on associated tissues. One specific effect of significance could be to increase the production and release of mucus from goblet cells (Lake *et al.*, 1980) and thus change substantially one of the important physicochemical parameters of the intestinal environment. There is no direct evidence to support the involvement of any of these mechanisms in worm expulsion, but it is relevant that antigen-induced anaphylaxis in infected animals results in intestinal changes and that injection of histamine and 5-HT into the body has been shown to have some effect on worm loss (Briggs and Degiusti, 1966); conversely, prolonged feeding of antihistamine and anti-5-HT compounds delays worm expulsion (Campbell *et al.*, 1963a) as, to some extent, does treatment with sodium dichromoglycate, an inhibitor of mast-cell degranulation (Michalska and Karmanska, 1976).

Trichinella spiralis is a potent inducer of IgE antibodies, and these are often detectable serologically as early as the 2nd week after infection (Mota *et al.*, 1969; Rivera-Ortiz and Nussenzweig, 1976; Gabriel and Justus, 1979; Ruitenberg *et al.*, 1980). Connective-tissue mast cells rapidly become sensitized to worm antigens (Briggs, 1963; Briggs and Degiusti, 1966), and it may be assumed that mucosal mast cells are similarly primed. Although this has not been formally demonstrated in the mouse, IgE has been identified on mucosal mast cells in *T. spiralis*-infected rats (Ruitenberg *et al.*, 1978).

Infiltration of the mucosa by granulocytes, though not as extensive as that by mast cells, is also characteristic of the intestinal response to *T. spiralis*. One consequence of this infiltration is an elevation, both in the mucosa and in the lumen, of lysosomal enzymes associated with such cells. Two in particular have been studied, myeloperoxidase and lysophospholipase B (Larsh *et al.*, 1974; Stewart, personal communication). Levels of both enzymes rise during the course of primary infections, and it is suggested that one result may be further damage to the mucosa itself or directly to the worms present. Phospholipases are known to be associated with the formation of prostaglandins (by breakdown of arachidonic acid), which have been implicated in expulsion of other nematodes (Kelly and Dineen, 1976). However, injection of prostaglandins (PgE$_1$ and PgE$_2$) directly into the intestine failed to accelerate expulsion of *T. spiralis* from mice; rather, it had the opposite effect (Karmanska and Michalska, 1977; Dutoit *et al.*, 1979). Although the probable source of intestinal lysophospholipase B is eosinophils, depletion of these cells has no major effect on worm expulsion (Grove *et al.*, 1977a).

Inflammatory changes during infection are not restricted to alterations in physicochemical parameters. Infection exerts, either directly or via the immune responses that it provokes, a profound influence on epithelial-cell kinetics, increasing the rate of cell division and shortening cell transit time from crypt to villus. As a consequence, crypt hyperplasia and villus atrophy are prominent during the height of the inflammatory response, and the structural organization of the mucosa alters radically (Richardson and Olson, 1974; Ruitenberg et al., 1977a; Grove and Civil, 1978; Manson-Smith et al., 1979a).

Although the transplantation studies described above show that expulsion is not dependent on prolonged prior exposure of the worm to the developing immunity of the host, in the normal course of infection worms are affected structurally and functionally by this immunity. It is likely that these changes in the worm, though not themselves the immediate cause of expulsion, are symptomatic of a reduced ability to withstand the changes in the intestinal environment. There is evidence that these changes can arise from the operation of direct antiworm immune responses, although it is probable that profound physicochemical changes in the intestine also bring them about. When immune cells are adoptively transferred into irradiated recipients, immunity is not expressed in the form of worm expulsion, but the worms fail to grow or reproduce normally (Table 3). Similarly, there is evidence that when a B-cell-enriched fraction of immune lymphocytes

TABLE 3
Adoptive Transfer of Immunity to *T. spiralis* in NIH Mice: Effects of Immune Mesenteric Lymph Node Cells on Worm Survival, Reproduction, and Growth[a]

| Group | Cells | Worms recovered 8 days after infection with 315 larvae | | | |
| | | Number | | Fecundity (larvae/♀/hr) | Female length (mm) |
		Mean	S.D.		
Unirradiated mice					
1	None	192	24	4.8	2.1
2	1×10^8 IMLNC	50[b]	40	1.2[b]	1.5[b]
Irradiated mice					
3	None	209	32	5.4	2.6
4	1×10^8 IMLNC	196	35	1.7[b]	1.5[b]

[a] Data from Wakelin and Wilson (1980).
[b] Significantly lower than corresponding controls.
[c] Irradiated at 400 rad.

is transferred, the major expression of immunity is a reduction of worm fecundity.

Structural changes in the worms are apparent by (and probably before) the 8th day of infection and take the form of disruption of the normal organization of the intestinal cells and the appearance of lipid droplets. Similar changes occur in somatic cells, and there is depletion of glycogen reserves (Kennedy and Bruce, 1981). Preceding these structural alterations is a reduction in fecundity, as measured by *in vitro* output of newborn larvae, and it seems probable that this in turn reflects an earlier reduction in oocyte production by the ovary (Fatunmbi, 1978).

Worms remaining in the intestine 8–10 days after oral infection are severely damaged, both structurally and functionally, by host responses (Kennedy and Bruce, 1981), yet can survive and repair this damage if transplanted into naïve recipients (Kennedy *et al.*, 1979).

The simplest explanation for these effects is the operation of antiworm antibodies, directed either at stichosomal antigens, and therefore perhaps interfering with nutrition, or directed against surface antigens.

Although many attempts to do so have failed, it is possible to transfer immunity passively with serum, and maternal transfer of immunity has also been described (Denham, 1969; Duckett *et al.*, 1972; Perry, 1974). In contrast to transfer with immune cells, transfer with serum is less reliable or less complete or both (Wakelin and Lloyd, 1976b), and interpretation of the results of such transfers is difficult for many reasons. It is *a priori* more probable that antiworm antibodies are produced locally in the intestine than systemically (though this may not apply to IgE), and thus the identity and specificity of antibodies present in serum from immune animals and their activity within the intestine are open to question. Certainly serum antibodies do react with surface antigens, internal antigens, and secretory material, and form plugs at body openings, but the direct effects on the viability of worms are relatively minor (Castro *et al.*, 1973). It is possible that the effects of serum antibodies on worms may be indirect, for example, through their involvement in intestinal Arthus reactions (Briggs and Degiusti, 1966; Perry, 1974), through mediation of intestinal hypersensitivity (see above), or through an effect on intestinal mastocytosis, as has been demonstrated in the rat–*Nippostrongylus brasiliensis* model by Befus and Bienenstock (1979) and Miller (1979). Recent work with *T. spiralis* has shown that is is possible to transfer immunity with serum containing both IgG_1 and IgE antibodies; and this result, if confirmed, must imply an indirect action (Gabriel and Justus, 1979).

Infection is associated with an increase in number of plasma cells present in the lamina propria, in particular those that produce IgM and IgG$_1$ (Crandall and Crandall, 1972). Crandall and Crandall found that the numbers of IgA plasma cells did not change significantly even though the anti-*T. spiralis* antibodies present in intestinal contents were predominantly of this isotype. It is interesting, in this respect, that IgA is the only immunoglobulin so far shown to have a direct effect on worm function. Material extracted from the intestinal secretions of infected animals, and enriched in this isotype, significantly depressed the fecundity of worms maintained *in vitro* (Jacqueline *et al.*, 1978).

It is unlikely that antiworm antibodies contribute nothing to immunity against the adult worm, but it may well be that their role is essentially secondary, at least in terms of worm expulsion, and that events mediated more directly by T cells are primarily responsible for inflammation and expulsion. While there are several lines of evidence to support this suggestion, it has to be admitted that some experimental data argue against it. For example, treatment of mice with the compound niridazole, a proven suppressant of cell-mediated responses, had no obvious effects on the expulsion of adult worms (Grove and Warren, 1976). However, such is the complexity of the responses that lead to expulsion that individual components can be ablated without substantially interfering with the overall end result.

2.1.2. Rat

The kinetics of primary infections in rats resemble those in rapidly responding mice, and there are many features in common; e.g., expulsion is preceded by structural and functional changes in the worms (Love *et al.*, 1976) and is associated with rapid cellular responsiveness (Ottesen *et al.*, 1975; Levin *et al.*, 1976) and with gross inflammation in the intestine (Castro, 1976). The inflammatory changes that occur include extensive infiltration of the mucosa, especially by mast cells (Ruitenberg *et al.*, 1979; Alizadeh and Wakelin, 1981a), alteration of mucosal architecture (Smith and Castro, 1978), alteration of lymphoblast homing (Love and Ogilvie, 1977), elevation of levels of lysosomal enzymes (Smith and Castro, 1978), and altered fluid flux (Castro *et al.*, 1979). Despite these similarities, however, it cannot necessarily be assumed that the underlying mechanisms of resistance are similar in mice and rats. Indeed, there is some evidence that distinct mechanisms may be operative.

Transfer of immunity has been achieved using both serum and lymphoid cells from immune donors (Table 4). Each component works

TABLE 4
Transfer of Immunity to *T. spiralis* in PVG/c Rats with Immune Serum or Immune Mesenteric Lymph Node Cells or Both[a]

Group	Treatment	Number of worms recovered on day 6 after infection with 500 larvae	
		Mean	S.E.
1	None	475	31
2	Immune serum[b]	286[d]	45
3	Immune cells[c]	346[d]	76
4	Immune serum[b] + immune cells[c]	85[d]	45

[a] Data from Love *et al.* (1976).
[b] 5 ml/100 g body weight on day 0.   [c] 2.5 × 10[8] cells on day 0.
[d] Significantly lower than untreated controls.

separately, but a greater transfer of immunity is achieved if both are given. Analysis of the cells involved in adoptive transfer has been carried out using thoracic-duct lymphocytes from rats exposed to multiple-drug-abbreviated infection (Crum *et al.*, 1977; Despommier *et al.*, 1977b). Under these conditions, immunity, as measured by worm expulsion, was transferred rather more effectively by B cells than by T cells. An inference that can be drawn from this is that since the majority of thoracic-duct B cells are known to be committed to the production of IgA in the intestinal lamina propria, resistance may involve antiworm IgA. However, if this is so, no mechanism can as yet be proposed. As in the mouse, it has been shown that IgA from the intestinal secretions of infected rats can reduce the ability of female worms to liberate larvae in culture (Jacqueline *et al.*, 1978), but it is unlikely that this is relevant to worm expulsion.

The physicochemical changes induced in the rat intestine by *T. spiralis*, and those coincident with worm expulsion, have been extensively studied by Castro (see Chapter 6). Infection is associated with an increase in peroxidase activity in the intestine, and this appears to be directly related to the numbers of leukocytes present in the lamina propria (Smith and Castro, 1978). Peak peroxidase levels coincide with depressed epithelial-cell brush-border disaccharidase activity and with changes in mucosal architecture, although there may be no causal correlation, each reflecting aspects of intestinal response to infection. The inflamed gut shows increased peristaltic activity, resulting in faster transit of material along its length (Castro *et al.*, 1976), and there is a marked change in fluid flux across the mucosa, changing from net absorption in the uninfected state to net secretion at the height of the inflammatory response (Castro *et al.*, 1979).

There is no doubt that these pathophysiological changes are in large part due to the immune response to the worm, the potent immunological stimulus provided by *T. spiralis* leading to a cascade of inflammatory events. As in mice, it is difficult to prove that the changes are a direct cause of worm expulsion, but the intestinal environment alters so profoundly that it is difficult to resist this conclusion. An important observation that has been made recently is that infection stimulates pronounced blood eosinophilia and basophilia (Ogilvie *et al.*, 1980). The latter cell type has previously been considered unimportant in inflammatory reactions in the rat, although it is known to play a significant role in other hosts (Askenase, 1979), and has been implicated in immunity to *Trichostrongylus colubriformis* in guinea pigs (Rothwell *et al.*, 1974). Basophils are an important element in the development of delayed-type inflammatory responses and therefore may well have a role in mediating the intestinal responses associated with loss of *T. spiralis*.

2.2. Immunity against Adult Worms in Reinfections

Exposure to a primary infection confers strong immunity to reinfection. In rats and, under certain conditions, in mice, this immunity is expressed primarily against the preadult stages of the challenge infection, the majority of worms being expelled very rapidly (see Section 2.3). However, immunity against challenge infections may also be expressed against the adult stages. This appears to be the normal pattern of reinfection immunity in mice, in which it takes the form of an accelerated version of the events that occur during the course of a primary infection. Worms show structural changes at an early stage, they fail to grow normally, and their reproduction is reduced in comparison with primary-infection worms (Denham and Martinez, 1970; Kennedy, 1980; Kennedy and Bruce, 1981). The inflammatory responses that accompany expulsion occur earlier in a challenge infection than in a primary infection (Larsh and Race, 1954), as do the cellular events that underlie them. In NIH mice, for example, the mesenteric-node T-lymphoblast response is well developed at 2 days after challenge, and unlike the situation in primary infections, it is possible to transfer immunity adoptively with T lymphocytes taken at this time. The availability of cells capable of transferring immunity then falls off rapidly (Fig. 4). Although mice retain the ability to mount an

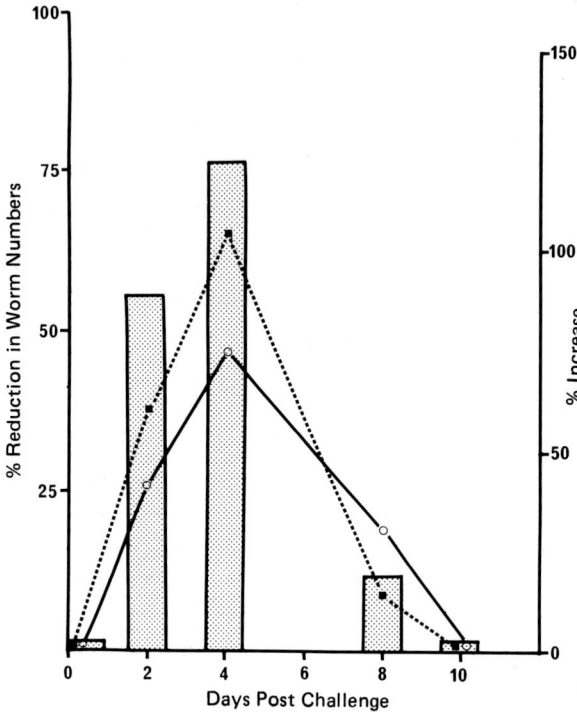

FIGURE 4. Cellular kinetics throughout a secondary infection with *T. spiralis* in NIH mice. (O—O) Total number of nucleated cells in mesenteric lymph node (MLN) as percentage increase over uninfected control; (■·······■) level of incorporation of [^{125}I]iododeoxyuridine by MLN blast cells as percentage increase over control; (▨) ability of MLN cells to transfer immunity adoptively, measured by degree of worm expulsion at day 8 in recipient mice. Data from Grencis and Wakelin (1982).

accelerated response to challenge for a considerable time after primary infection (several months), adoptive transfer is successful only when blast-cell activity is evoked by infection (Grencis and Wakelin, 1982); on the whole, cells taken from unchallenged immune animals fail to transfer immunity (Wakelin and Lloyd, 1976b). Thus, it can be inferred that the anamnestic response to *T. spiralis* is the property of memory cells that can be very rapidly mobilized.

Expression of challenge immunity may be modified by the immunomodulatory influences exerted by muscle larvae. At certain times after an initial infection, expulsion of a challenge infection is not markedly more rapid than expulsion of the primary infection, but even under these circumstances, the reproductive ability of the worms is still impaired (Faubert, 1977; Grove *et al.*, 1977b). This may reflect the continued operation of distinct, antibody-mediated, antiworm responses.

Although in rats the rapid expulsion response removes the majority of challenge worms, a small number survive to maturity (Russell and Castro, 1979), and these are subjected to an accelerated-primary-type immunity. It has been demonstrated that this immunity is the product of separate responses induced in a stage-specific manner (Bell *et al.*, 1979). Thus, exposure in a primary infection to the preadult stages only (i.e., those that develop during the first 24–48 hr of infection) stimulates responses that strongly depress adult-worm fecundity in an adult infection and contribute to worm expulsion. Exposure to the adult stages *per se* (by means of direct introduction into the intestine) stimulates responses that contribute primarily to adult-worm expulsion, but that also affect fecundity. Whereas these latter responses will operate directly against a challenge with implanted adult worms, those evoked by exposure to preadult worms operate only against the preadult stages of a challenge infection, although the expression of this immunity is not seen until the adults have matured.

2.3. Immunity against Preadult Stages—Rapid Expulsion

Early studies on reinfections in rats showed that a majority of the challenge worms were expelled very rapidly at the early preadult stage, only 7–24% persisting for more than 24 hr (McCoy, 1940). The worms when expelled were still alive and capable of infecting another host. This phenomenon, now termed rapid expulsion, has recently received a great deal of attention, directed both at complete description and analysis and at identification of the causal mechanisms.

Rapid expulsion can be induced most effectively by exposure to complete infections, but it can also be induced by exposure to specific stages. Thus, preadult and adult worms are each capable of stimulating the response, as are the parenteral stages, though less effectively (Bell and McGregor, 1979a,b). The response is present soon after appropriate stimulation, e.g., by day 6 of an enteral infection, and persists for a considerable time (Bell and McGregor, 1979b; Alizadeh and Wakelin, 1982a). Rapid expulsion appears to act specifically against the preadult stages, and adult worms transplanted directly into primed hosts survive unaffected, as they do when a larval infection is superimposed onto an adult infection (Bell and McGregor, 1979a,b).

A series of elegant experiments utilizing parabiotic rats has demonstrated that priming for rapid expulsion requires two separate stimuli to the host. One is immunological and specific to *T. spiralis*, while the other, which is a locally acting priming of the intestine, can be induced nonspecifically and is probably not immunological (Bell and McGregor, 1980a). If one animal of a parabiotic pair is infected with *T. spiralis* and the other with *Heligmosomoides polygyrus*, the immunological stimulus provided by *Trichinella* primes both partners, but the intestinal stimulus comes from *Trichinella* in one animal and from *H. polygyrus* in the other. On challenge, both show rapid expulsion of larvae (Fig. 5). In a complete infection with *T. spiralis*, the specific stimulus is probably supplied by antigens of the preadult stages and the nonspecific intestinal stimulus by the adults. Under experimental conditions, the specific stimulus can be provided by immunization with an antigen extract of muscle larvae and the intestinal stimulus by infection with an unrelated intestinal nematode (Bell and McGregor, 1980b).

The very speed of rapid expulsion is suggestive of an immediate hypersensitivity response, the larvae of the challenge infection triggering rapid changes in the intestine and being removed by these changes within a short period of time. Although the components necessary for such a response are present, i.e., intestinal mast cells (Alizadeh and Wakelin, 1982a; Ruitenberg *et al.*, 1979) and IgE antibodies (Williams *et al.*, 1972; Perrudet-Badoux *et al.*, 1976), there is no direct evidence that immediate hypersensitivity is involved in rapid expulsion, and there is some evidence against this concept, in that rapid expulsion cannot be prevented by drugs known to affect mast cells or to inhibit release of amines or block their activity, nor can it be induced by an unrelated anaphylactic response in the intestine (Lee and Ogilvie, 1981a). Many of the pathophysiological changes associated with loss of primary infections are not observed during rapid expulsion (Russell and Castro, 1979), but it has been reported that challenge provokes a rapid alteration in fluid flux across the mucosa leading to net fluid secretion (Castro *et al.*, 1979), and this may interfere with establishment and survival.

A likely explanation of rapid expulsion, and one supported by experimental data (Table 5), is that early in infection, the challenge larvae become trapped in intestinal mucus, fail to penetrate the mucosa, and are removed from the gut by peristalsis (Lee and Ogilvie, 1981a,b). The data shown in Table 5 were obtained using a series of recovery techniques that enabled the position of larvae to be detected in the various regions of the gut (lumen, mucus layers, and mucosal epithelium) and gave results rather different from those obtained by the

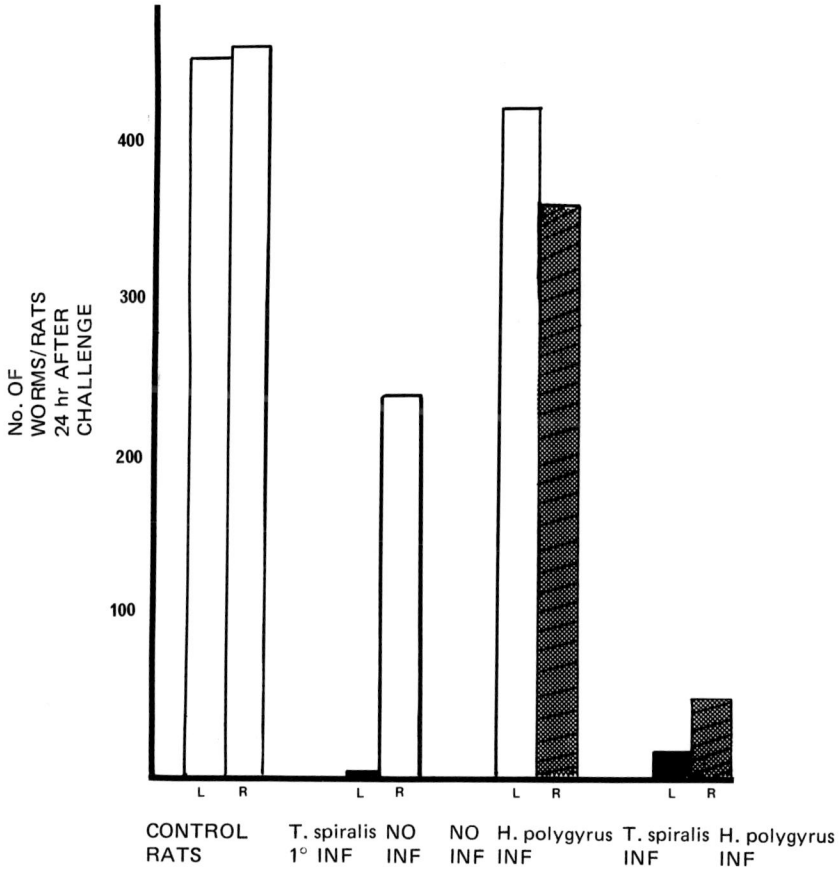

FIGURE 5. Rapid expulsion of *T. spiralis* from parabiotic rats. Rats were primed by exposure to 2000 larvae of *T. spiralis* or to 1000 larvae of *H. polygyrus*. The *T. spiralis* infection was limited to the intestinal stages by feeding thiabendazole in the diet and was terminated by treatment with methyridine after 10 days. All rats were challenged with 700 larvae of *T. spiralis* 17 days after initial infection (5 parabiotic pairs/group). Data from Bell and McGregor (1980b).

conventional Baermann technique of worm recovery. As can be seen, only about 30–40% of larvae in previously infected rats succeed in reaching the mucosa (regions 4 and 5) compared with 70–80% in controls. The longer-term fate of these worms (most of which are not recovered by conventional techniques) is uncertain, but they may be removed by an accelerated primary-type response. *In vitro* studies show

TABLE 5
Recovery and Distribution of *T. spiralis* Larvae from the Small Intestines of Control and Previously Infected (Immune) Rats after Direct (Intraduodenal) Injection of 3000 Larvae[a]

Time after injection	Group[b]	Total larvae recovered	Larvae recovered (% of total)				
			Free in lumen	Superficial mucus globules	Intermediate mucus	Deep mucus and epithelium	
90 min	Control	1875	11	2	4	83	
	Immune	1942	3	56	2	39	
3 hr	Control	2033	21	2	5	72	
	Immune	1628	27	41	2	31	

[a] Data from Lee and Ogilvie (1981b). [b] There were 5 rats in each group.

that trapping in mucus is enhanced equally by preincubation of larvae in fresh control serum and in fresh or inactivated immune serum, suggesting that activation of complement by, or adherence of antibodies to, the worm's cuticle may be an integral part of the phenomenon. The relationship of these studies to the *in vivo* situation, however, has still to be clarified, in particular the relationship of trapping to the type and volume of mucus present in immune hosts. While there is an increase in goblet-cell numbers during primary infection, and this increase persists for some time (Alizadeh and Wakelin, 1982a), it may be that the important change involved in trapping is qualitative rather than quantitative and that the qualitative change may involve both alterations in the mucus itself and potentiated release of antiworm antibodies with specificity for antigens present on the worm's cuticle.

In the mouse, rapid expulsion is a less significant component of immunity to reinfection. In NIH mice, rapid expulsion *per se* can be elicited only when challenge is made within a few days of the end of the primary infection. After this period, immunity to challenge takes the form of an accelerated version of the events that occur during initial infection (Alizadeh and Wakelin, 1982a). In other strains, rapid expulsion is more persistent (Bell and McGregor, 1980c). As in rats, rapid expulsion (as assessed by the Baermann recovery technique) is very efficient, removing some 90% of the challenge between 6 and 24 hr after infection. At present, there is no satisfactory explanation of the underlying mechanisms, but although there is no reason for the mechanisms necessarily to resemble those in the rat, it may well be that some form of mucus trapping is involved. Rapid expulsion can be demonstrated for only a short period, and this period coincides with the time at which the numbers of mucosal mast cells and goblet cells are elevated. Although equivalent numbers of larvae can be recovered from control and challenged mice at 1.5 hr after infection, it is not known whether this represents a fully normal establishment within the mucosa. Certainly there is little evidence that the challenge given under these circumstances elicits a "normal" lymphoblast response (Grencis, unpublished) or produces any significant change in lymphoblast homing (Alizadeh, 1981), implying that mucosal and immune changes, if they do occur, are qualitatively different from those in challenge infections given later after a primary infection.

3. IMMUNITY AND NEWBORN LARVAE

The preceding sections indicated the enormous interest that has been taken in the immune response associated with the intestinal phase of *Trichinella*. It is really only in the last ten years that work has been performed with the parenteral stages, although the techniques for such studies have been available for many years. For example, Doerr and Schmidt (1930) and Matoff (1943) showed that encysted larvae developed in the muscles of animals when newborn larvae were injected into the blood. Thus, it was possible to isolate any immune response involving the parenteral phase from the response stimulated by the enteral phase. However, it was not until the development of *in vitro* systems for maintaining fecund adult females that any progress was made in the investigation of the immune response to, or generated by, the parenteral stages. Methods for collecting adult females from rats, sterilizing them, culturing them for a few hours *in vitro*, and collecting the larvae produced were described by Denham (1967) and Dennis *et al.* (1970). There is no essential difference between these methods, and the paper by Dennis *et al.* (1970) is much more readily available. To produce newborn larvae, rats are infected with 7000–10,000 infective larvae; adult worms are collected 7 days later and then maintained in culture overnight. Large numbers of newborn larvae are produced and can be collected and injected intravenously (they will not migrate from the peritoneal cavity). Some 50–70% of newborn larvae injected into the bloodstream develop into muscle larvae.

3.1. Active Immunity in Mice and Rats

Despommier (1971) inoculated rats intravenously with newborn larvae produced *in vitro* and challenged half of these and normal controls with infective muscle larvae. The recovery of challenge larvae from the rats that had been previously infected was only 5% of that obtained from the normal controls. Ruitenberg and Steerenberg (1976) immunized rats with newborn larvae and found a high degree of resistance to challenge with this stage, immune rats harboring only 12% of the number of larvae that developed in controls. Similar experiments were performed by James and Denham (1974) in mice, and they likewise found complete resistance to infection after three previous injections of newborn larvae.

James and Denham (1974) immunized mice with three infections each of about 500 normal infective larvae, which were terminated 5 days later with methyridine (Denham, 1965) so that the mice were exposed only to the intestinal phase, and found no resistance to intravenous challenge with newborn larvae. Mice immunized in the same way and challenged with infective larvae were 87% resistant, presumably because of the effect of the immunization procedure on the longevity and fecundity of the enteral phase (see Section 2.1.1).

James *et al.* (1977) carried out three experiments in which mice were immunized with four injections of newborn larvae and challenged either with newborn larvae intravenously or with infective larvae *per os*. In each experiment, strong resistance to challenge with newborn larvae was demonstrated, but much less resistance was seen when a *per os* challenge was used. In one experiment, it was clearly shown that although the survival of adult worms was not affected by the "immunization" procedure, the mean resistance as judged by the number of muscle larvae was 51%. However, this was very much lower than the level of resistance to intravenous challenge (on average 85%). One reason for this difference in resistance to the establishment of muscle larvae might be the large quantitative difference in the size of the challenge. The challenge with newborn larvae resulted in means of 1605, 5150, and 4360 larvae in the controls in the three experiments, whereas challenge with infective larvae resulted in means of 67,500, 21,300, and 12,000 larvae in controls. Perhaps these much higher challenges were able to overcome the resistance generated by relatively light immunizing infections (which gave mean infections of 571, 3320, and 3320, respectively). Support for this suggestion comes from the fact that in the first experiment with the highest challenge level, the apparent immunity was 28%, whereas in the other two experiments it was 62%. Another explanation might be that the adult worms, which are antigenically dissimilar to the newborn larvae (see Section 5 and Chapter 9) and are also known to be immunosuppressive, may suppress the host's response to the antigens associated with the newborn larvae. If true, this would represent an exquisite example of the evolution of a mechanism for ensuring survival of reproductive stages in the fact of the host's immune response.

Despommier (1971) attempted to immunize rats against challenge with newborn larvae by placing 200–300 infective larvae in diffusion chambers in the peritoneal cavity, but found no difference between the "immunized" and control animals. This held true even though when such animals were challenged *per os*, they exhibited a 72% reduction in the number of muscle larvae that developed, again presumably because the immune response was affecting the survival or fecundity of the intestinal phase.

Despommier (1971) suggested that this lack of an effect on the newborn larvae may show that "newborn larvae of *T. spiralis* do not possess antigens to which the host produces antibodies during the natural course of infection." Now Despommier would probably not make this suggestion. James and Denham (1975) showed that if newborn larvae were incubated in immune rabbit serum, precipitates were produced around them and these precipitates reacted in the indirect fluorescent-antibody test with antirabbit antibodies. The precipitates were particularly prominent around the oral apertures of the newborn larvae, perhaps associated with an enzyme that these larvae secrete to pierce the muscle-cell wall. The work of Philipp *et al.* (1981) and Jungery and Ogilvie (1981) also shows antibody recognition of surface antigens of newborn larvae.

Some of the experiments reported in the following sections unequivocally prove that antibodies to newborn larvae not only exist in infected animals but also are of great importance in preventing the successful invasion of the muscle cells by intravenously injected newborn larvae.

3.2. Passive Immunity in Mice

Moloney and Denham (1979) showed that mice could be protected against challenge with newborn larvae if serum from immunized mice was injected before challenge. If the serum was taken from mice injected with newborn larvae, there was a mean 70% reduction in the number of newborn larvae in treated mice. If, however, the serum came from mice given four normal (i.e., *per os*) infections, there was a reduction of over 99% in the number of muscle larvae. Spleen cells from mice immunized with newborn larvae also conferred roughly the same degree of protection as serum, but there was no additive effect if the mice were given both cells and serum.

The passive protection conferred by immune serum was shown only if serum was given before challenge with newborn larvae. In one experiment, Moloney and Denham (1979) obtained 50% protection when the serum was given 2 hr before challenge and no protection when it was given 2 hr after challenge.

If newborn larvae were incubated in serum from immunized mice before being injected into mice, their infectivity was very considerably reduced. If, however, the immune serum was preabsorbed with large numbers of newborn larvae, this effect was not seen. Similarly, absorption of serum with newborn larvae partially removed its ability to protect mice passively against challenge with newborn larvae.

These experiments strongly suggest that immunity to newborn larvae is antibody-mediated and that the antibody attaches to the surface of the worms. As larvae incubated in immune serum become less infective, it is likely that they become coated or opsonized and when injected into normal mice are attacked by a nonspecific killer cell. However, evidence suggests that this attack is possible only while the larvae are in the bloodstream. Presumably, the reason that immune serum has no effect if given after the injection of newborn larvae is that the worms have penetrated into the striated muscle cells and therefore occupy a privileged site.

3.3. Effects of Cells and Serum Components *in Vitro*

Kazura and Grove (1978) showed that peritoneal-exudate cells adhered to and killed newborn larvae in the presence of serum from infected mice. The antibody that was responsible for this adherence and killing was first detected in the 4th week of infection; (detection was not attempted in the 3rd week). Incubation with newborn larvae absorbed out the ability of sera to mediate this reaction.

If a population of peritoneal-exudate cells with only 2% eosinophils was used, there was no significant destruction of larvae, but when the level of eosinophils reached 20%, nearly all the larvae were killed. Similarly, if the cell mixture was preincubated with antieosinophil serum and complement, the ability of the cell mixture to kill worms was lost, but if the proportion of eosinophils was raised by density-gradient centrifugation, killing was enhanced. It was noteworthy that eosinophils from the peritoneal cavities of mice infected with *Schistosoma mansoni* were not as effective as those from mice infected with *Trichinella*.

Mackenzie *et al.* (1978) confirmed that serum from infected rats would mediate cell killing of newborn larvae, but also demonstrated that the degree of killing was enhanced by complement. In the presence of immune rat serum, cells killed 94% of newborn larvae, whereas when the same serum was heated, only 67% of the larvae were killed. However, complement alone did not mediate cell adherence, showing that the surface of newborn larvae did not activate complement, whereas infective larvae did. Biologically, this is a completely logical finding, for if newborn larvae did activate complement, then they would presumably do so *in vivo* and be attacked by cells while migrating through the lymphatics and blood vessels. Mackenzie *et al.* (1978) found that the antibody that mediated cell adherence appeared in the blood of rats before 20 days.

Mackenzie *et al.* (1980) added further evidence that the killer cell *in vitro* was the eosinophil. For example, a cell population containing 90% eosinophils killed 98% of newborn larvae and one with 65% eosinophils killed 86% of larvae, while one with only 2% eosinophils killed only 5%. It is likely that the major basic protein found in eosinophil granules is a key component in this killing. Wassom and Gleich (1979) found that when newborn larvae were cultured in the presence of this protein, they were damaged within 2 hr and then killed rapidly.

4. GENETIC INFLUENCES ON IMMUNITY TO *TRICHINELLA*

Responses to infection with *T. spiralis* vary considerably, both among inbred strains of a given host species and among individuals of outbred strains (Wakelin and Lloyd, 1976a; Wakelin, 1978, 1980a), and thus are under genetic control. This is particularly true of the mouse, in which extensive variation has been recorded, but less so of the rat, in which greater uniformity seems to prevail.

In the mouse, variation is apparent both in protective resistance and in the immunological and pathological phenomena that accompany resistance. In primary infections, the duration of the intestinal phase, the period of female worm fecundity, and the number of resultant muscle larvae all show strain variability (Stefanski and Kozar, 1969; Wakelin and Lloyd, 1976a; Wassom *et al.*, 1979; Wakelin, 1980a), although this has not always been found to be the case (Tanner, 1978). Rapid responsiveness to primary infection is correlated with a rapid response to reinfection, in terms of both the accelerated primary-type response and rapid expulsion (Bell and McGregor, 1980c; Wakelin, 1980a), and greater responsiveness is inherited in F_1 progeny as a dominant characteristic.

Wassom *et al.* (1979, 1980) have shown that overall responsiveness to primary infection (measured by total muscle larval recovery) is controlled both by genes linked to the mouse major histocompatibility complex (*H-2*) and by genes outside this complex. Certain haplotypes (e.g., H-2^q and H-2^s) are associated with relative resistance, others (e.g., H-2^k) with relative susceptibility. Mapping studies have shown that some of the *H-2*-linked genes involved lie in the *I-A* and *I-B* subregions of the *H-2* complex. However, expression of resistance genes can be modified by other loci, especially at the *D* region of the *H-2*. For example, while the *s* and *q* alleles are associated with resistance, the presence of a *d* allelle in the *D* region results in increased susceptibility to infection (Table 6).

As far as immunity acting against the intestinal phase of infection is concerned, genetic control seems to operate primarily through non-*H-2*-linked genes. Thus, whereas NIH, SWR, and DBA₁ mice (all H-2^q) are rapid responders, expelling worms within about 12 days of infection, all mice carrying the C57BL/10 genetic background are slow responders, expelling worms after 14 days, even when, as in the B10.G congenic strain, the H-2^q haplotype is present (Wakelin, 1980a). It is apparent that this genetic control could be expressed through the immune components of the intestinal response, through the inflammatory components, or through both. A series of adoptive-transfer

TABLE 6
H-2-Linked Genetic Control of Resistance to *T. spiralis* in Mice: Evidence That *D*-End Genes Can Modify Expression of Resistant Alleles[a]

Strain of mouse	*H-2* haplotype								Muscle larval count 30 days after infection with 150 larvae (mean ± S.D.)	Status
	K	A	B	J	E	C	S	D		
B10.BR	k	k	k	k	k	k	k	k	30,286 ± 1291	Susceptible
B10.S	s	s	s	s	s	s	s	s	15,050 ± 1024	Resistant
B10.S(7R)	s	s	s	s	s	s	s	d	23,489 ± 1549	Intermediate
B10.DA	q	q	q	q	q	q	q	s	19,860 ± 2221	Resistant
B10.T(6R)	q	q	q	q	q	q	q	d	33,100 ± 2382	Susceptible

[a] Data from Wassom *et al.* (1980). There were 8–10 mice in each group.

experiments, using the histocompatible rapid-responder NIH and slow-responder B10.G mice, have shown that control is expressed through nonlymphoid cells and therefore influences the induction or development of inflammation. Thus, in reciprocal cell transfers, rapid responders showed accelerated expulsion whether given homologous or heterologous cells. Conversely, although accelerated expulsion was observed after adoptive transfer into slow-responder mice, the time at which this expulsion occurred was later than in rapid responders and was the same whether slow- or rapid-responder cells were transferred (Wakelin and Donachie, 1980). Confirmation of this interpretation of genetic control has come from experiments involving radiation chimaeras, i.e., mice restored with histocompatible bone-marrow cells from another strain after lethal irradiation. Chimaeras made from rapid-responder NIH (or NIH × B10.G F₁) mice behaved on infection as rapid responders if given NIH bone marrow, but as slow responders if given B10.G bone marrow, and this difference was maintained even when the mice were given IMLNC from rapid-responder (NIH) donors (Table 7).

The precise point of expression is as yet unclear, but it is known that many aspects of the immune and inflammatory responses to *T. spiralis* are under direct genetic control. Distinct strain differences occur in the pattern of lymphoblast response to infection and in mucosal changes that influence lymphoblast homing (Manson-Smith *et al.*, 1979b; Wakelin, 1980b). The mast-cell response to infection also occurs more quickly and intensely in rapid responders than in slow responders (Alizadeh and Wakelin, 1982b; Brown *et al.*, 1981), although there are

TABLE 7

Adoptive Transfer of Immunity in B10.G × NIH F₁ Mice Reconstituted after Irradiation with Slow-Responder B10.G or Rapid-Responder NIH Bone Marrow[a]

			Number of worms recovered after infection with 300 larvae			
			Day 7		Day 11	
Group	Bone marrow	IMLNC	Mean	S.D.	Mean	S.D.
Unirradiated mice						
1	—	—	137	26	—	—
Irradiated mice						
2	B10.G	–	143	40	121	48
3	B10.G	+	134	22	11[b]	11
4	NIH	–	146	18	32[b]	22
5	NIH	+	29[b]	23	—	—

[a] Data from Wakelin and Donachie (1981). Radiation dosage was 850 rads. Mice were given 3×10^7 IMLNC from NIH donors and infected 15 weeks after irradiation.
[b] Significantly lower than corresponding controls.

also distinct differences among slow responders. The extent of the response is characteristic of the strain even when adoptive transfer of IMLNC (known to transfer increased mastocytosis) is carried out. Thus, rapid-responder NIH mice continue to show higher mast-cell levels than B10.G mice even when both are given NIH or B10.G immune cells (Alizadeh and Wakelin, 1982b). A difference in mast-cell response has also been reported to occur between Biozzi high- and low-level antibody responder strains of mice (Ruitenberg *et al.*, 1979) when these are infected with *T. spiralis*, and this likewise appears to be independent of lymphocyte status. Both sets of observations may suggest that the genetic control of mast-cell responsiveness to *T. spiralis* operates at the level of nonlymphoid (?bone-marrow) cell populations, as other data also imply (Kitamura *et al.*, 1979).

Genetically determined variation has also been shown to exist in the IgG₁ and IgE antibody responses to infection. Mouse strains in general differ widely in the timing and level of the responses (Rivera-Ortiz and Nussenzweig, 1976), and there is some evidence of *H-2* linkage; marked differences have also been recorded between the lines of Biozzi mice (Ruitenberg *et al.*, 1979). Rivera-Ortiz and Nussenzweig failed to show a correlation between level of antibody response and kinetics of adult worm expulsion, but did find that good responders harbored fewer muscle larvae. A similar situation occurs in the Biozzi strains. Low-responder mice, which produce a lower IgE response, have twice as many muscle larvae after a primary infection as do high responders, although the former appear better able to resist a challenge infection (Perrudet-Badoux *et al.*, 1975, 1978). These differences in reagin response may simply reflect overall antibody responsiveness (Biozzi *et al.*, 1971) or differences in the level of cellular regulation of this isotype (Chiorazzi *et al.*, 1977). However, there are also examples where variation in antibody responsiveness appears to involve specific recognition of *T. spiralis* antigens. Mice are known to make antibody responses to the stage-specific antigens present on the cuticles of larval, preadult, and adult stages (Philipp *et al.*, 1980), and these responses can be measured both by immunoprecipitation of the antigens and by the ability of the antibody to mediate attachment of eosinophils (Jungery and Ogilvie, 1981). NIH mice, which respond rapidly to infection, recognized the antigens of infective larvae and day 2 adults earlier and more completely than did slow-responder C$_3$H mice, and NIH antibody to the adults mediated eosinophil attachment well before antibody from C$_3$H.

Knowledge of the existence of genetic variation makes it possible to reconcile some of the discrepancies evident in the extensive literature on immunity to *T. spiralis* and also suggests that it is unwise to extrapolate too freely from studies made with any particular strain of host. A further corollary is that in order to investigate particular aspects of the host–parasite relationship successfully, it may well be necessary to choose hosts that possess appropriate response characteristics. This should not be seen as a restriction on research; indeed, the usefulness of *T. spiralis* for studying purely immunological problems (e.g., aspects of intestinal responsiveness) makes it likely that infections with this nematode in genetically defined host strains may play a valuable role in unravelling some of the complexities of genetic control of immunity to infectious organisms.

5. STAGE SPECIFICITY OF THE IMMUNE RESPONSE

Nearly all nematodes have five life-cycle stages, but usually only three stages occur in the mammalian host. In *Trichinella*, all five life-cycle stages occur in one host and are completed within a few days. Consequently, there has been much confusion over the details of the life cycle, although it is now accepted that the infective form is an L$_1$ larva and that four molts occur within 2 days after the infective larva enters the intestine (see Chapter 3). Theoretically, the second generation of worms developing in the host should be subject to an immunological attack stimulated by the presence of the first generation, either still present or recently expelled, unless some form of protection against this response were evolved by the parasite. One way of achieving this would be for the parenteral stages to be antigenically distinct from the intestinal forms. Jośe Oliver-Gonzalez proposed that this was so in what, especially considering the state of immunological knowledge in 1940, is one of the landmarks in the study of the immune response to *Trichinella*.

The purpose of this section of our chapter is to review the accumulated evidence for the hypothesis that immunological stage specificity exists in the relationship between *Trichinella* and its hosts.

5.1. "Dual-Antibody" Hypothesis of Oliver-Gonzalez

In 1941, Oliver-Gonzalez published his paper (Oliver-Gonzalez, 1941) outlining the "dual-antibody" hypothesis. He obtained antisera from rabbits infected once or six times with *Trichinella*. When infective larvae and adult worms were exposed to this antiserum *in vitro*, precipitates formed on and around the worms. Figure 6 shows some of these precipitates as illustrated by Oliver-Gonzalez (1940). Precipitates formed around the mouths of both infective larvae and adult worms and also around the vulvas and anuses of the adults. Infective larvae were killed in immune serum, whereas adults were not affected. Most precipitates were obtained with the serum of rabbits that had been multiply infected.

If sera were absorbed with either whole living adults or infective larvae, they no longer reacted with that stage but still produced precipitates with the other stage. This showed, therefore, that in immune sera there were two types of reacting material (?antibodies), one that precipitated around adults but not around larvae and one that precipitated around larvae but not around adults.

As will be seen, Oliver-Gonzalez was accurately prophetic when he said that not only were there antigens that were individual to the two stages but also

> it is probable, on the one hand, that the two stages of the parasite have common antigens and, on the other hand, that each type [i.e. of precipitating serum] may represent a group of antibodies.

> And:

> In contrasting the anti-adult with the anti-larval antibody, it is not intended to imply that there are only two qualitatively distinguishable antibodies arising as the result of two single dissimilar antigens . . . each stage of the worm must contain many antigens only a few of which are probably involved in the present study.

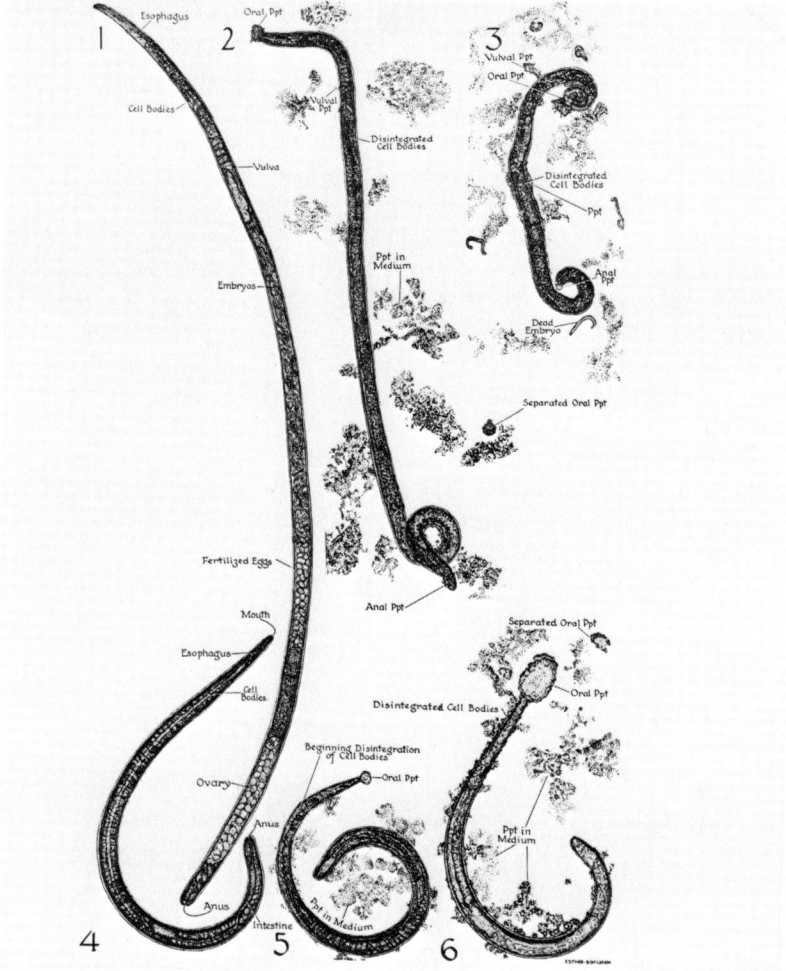

FIGURE 6. Immunoprecipitates around larvae of *T. spiralis*. Reproduced from Oliver-Gonzalez (1940) with the permission of the University of Chicago Press.

5.2. Immunological Evidence

The dual-antibody hypothesis was investigated further by Oliver-Gonzalez and Levine (1962), who used the Ouchterlony technique to analyze antigen–antibody reactions. They found different numbers of lines on their plates depending on whether they used adult or larval extracts as antigen and showed that the absorption of the serum with

one extract still left antibodies that reacted with the other extract.
Jackson (1959) used the fluorescent-antibody technique to study precipitates of antibody on various stages, but his results did not provide
a basis for assessing the antibody hypothesis. Rather oddly, in view of
later findings, a reaction between antibody and the cuticle of the
infective larva could not be demonstrated in his study.

In 1980, Philipp *et al.* (1980) reported their experiments using ^{125}I
labeling of the surface of different stages of *Trichinella*. They found
that the antigens present on the cuticular surface were extraordinarily
simple. If one considers the stages used by Oliver-Gonzalez (1941), i.e.,
infective larvae and 6-day-old adults, then Philipp and colleagues were
able to show that no surface antigens were shared between these two
stages. Newborn larvae shared no surface antigens with adults. These
results are shown in Fig. 7.

The infective larvae are characterized by a pair of antigens with
molecular weights of 90,000 and 105,000, which are not shared with
any other life-cycle stage, and another pair with molecular weights of

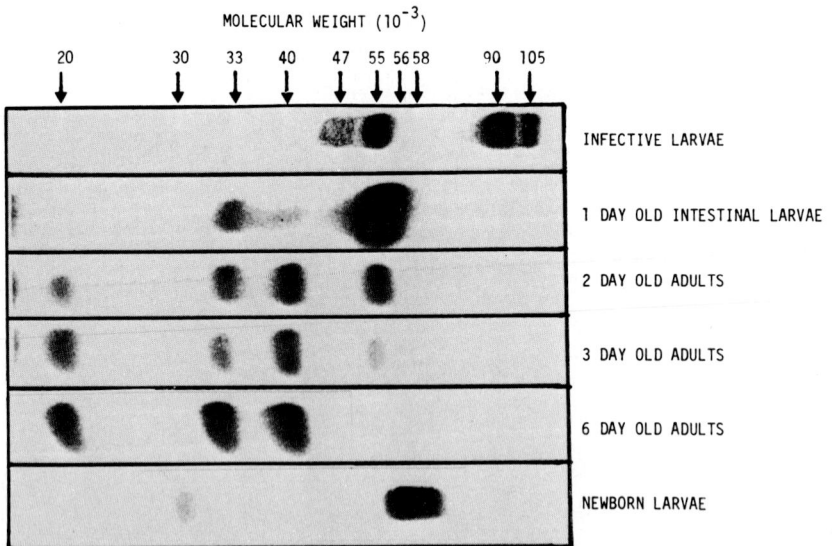

FIGURE 7. Sodium dodecyl sulfate–polyacrilamide gel electrophoresis of [^{125}I]chloro-
amine T–labeled *T. spiralis* life-cycle stages. From data supplied by M. Philipp, R.M.E. Parkhouse, and B.M. Ogilvie. Reproduced with the kind permission of the authors.

47,000 and 55,000, which again are unique. The couplet with the higher molecular weights was lost within 24 hr after the worms were fed to mice, but a new antigen had appeared with a molecular weight of 33,000. On the 2nd day, four antigens were seen with molecular weights of 56,000, 40,000, 33,000, and 20,000. Since these 2-day-old worms can be assumed to be fifth-stage (Ali Khan, 1966; Kozek, 1971), it is surprising that their surface antigens continued to change. The antigen with a molecular weight of 56,000 was less evident at 3 days and disappeared by day 6.

Parkhouse *et al.* (1981) have further characterized the surface antigens of infective larvae. Each couplet of antigens consists of a lentil-lectin-adherent glycoprotein and a slightly larger lentil-lectin-nonadherent protein. The bands at molecular weights of 90,000 and 105,000 were shown to be dimers of the two smaller units. The glycoprotein of molecular weight 90,000 also polymerized into a form of much higher molecular weight by disulfide bonding.

It is worth noting that the antigen of molecular weight 56,000 for the young intestinal worms and the antigen of molecular weight 55,000 are biochemically and immunologically distinct. The former binds to lentil lectin, i.e., has a carbohydrate moiety, whereas the latter does not. In addition, absorption of immune rat serum (which has antibodies to both antigens) with 2-day-old worms removes activity only against the homologous antigen.

This modern immunochemical approach supports nearly everything that Oliver-Gonzalez suggested 40 years ago. However, it must be recognized that the surface antigens discussed so far have been defined immunochemically, and we have not yet considered antibody recognition of them. Philipp *et al.* (1981) studied this aspect. Sera were collected sequentially from infected rats and studied by immunocoprecipitation and the eosinophil-adherence test (Mackenzie *et al.*, 1980) using newborn larvae, infective larvae, and adult worms as antigen. If one again considers the stages used by Oliver-Gonzalez, antibodies reacting with adult worms appeared at about the same time as those reacting with infective larvae. The titer of coprecipitating antibody against labeled infective-larval surface antigens continued to rise until the end of the observations at 40 days of infection, whereas that of antibodies reacting with adult antigens fell after 20 days. When immune serum was absorbed with living adult worms, the immunoprecipitation antibody reaction with infective larval antigen was not removed, whereas that reacting with the adult surface antigens decreased by three quarters. Antibody reacting with newborn larvae appeared several days after those reacting with the other two stages. Gel analysis showed that when the rat recognized any surface antigen on a particular life-cycle stage, it recognized all antigens although the strength of the reaction with different surface antigens did change.

All the evidence accumulated with this surface-labeling technique confirms that the antigens on the surface of not only the adults and infective larvae but also the newborn larvae are unique to that stage, i.e., are stage-specific.

5.3. Parasitological Evidence

Although the dual-antibody hypothesis concerns antibodies and their recognition of antigens associated with specific life-cycle stages, it can have no relevance whatsoever to the host–parasite relationship unless there are also resistance responses that affect individual stages of the life cycle. From this point of view, it is of little importance to consider the responses of the host to the adult worm and the encysted infective stage because once the larva is in the striated muscle (and especially after the muscle cell has become the nurse cell), it cannot be affected to any extent by the host's immune response, even if it can be damaged *in vitro*. It is of much greater significance to see whether there is an immune reaction that adversely affects either the adult worm or the newborn larva but does not affect the other stage.

To study this point, it is necessary to be able to immunize some animals with infections entirely composed of the parenteral phase and other animals with the intestinal phase but no parenteral phase. Then it is necessary to challenge with the heterologous and homologous stages. The technique for producing pure parenteral infections was described in Section 3.1.

There are several ways in which animals can be immunized against the intestinal phase of the infection without the development of any parenteral worms. Ionizing irradiation, whether by X-rays or ^{60}Co, can be used to sexually sterilize larvae that will nevertheless grow into the adult form. Many workers have shown that such sexually sterilized adults stimulate a strong immune response (Culbertson, 1942; Gould *et al.*, 1955). Another approach has been to use infections that have been terminated with an anthelmintic. This method has also demonstrated that preadult and adult stages are immunogenic (Campbell *et al.*, 1963b; Campbell, 1965; Denham, 1966a,b; Despommier *et al.*, 1977b).

James *et al.* (1977) immunized mice with newborn larvae and challenged some with newborn larvae and others with infective larvae. These mice were 85% resistant to newborn larvae, but there was no difference in the rate of expulsion of intestinal worms. It must be recognized, however, that the number of larvae used to immunize in this experiment was comparatively small (only 6000 newborn larvae were inoculated), and it is possible that a much larger inoculum would induce more rapid expulsion of adult worms of the challenge infection.

James and Denham (1975) performed the reverse of this experiment. They immunized mice with either methyridine-terminated infections or irradiated larvae, thus restricting the stimulus to that generated by the intestinal phase, and then challenged with newborn larvae intravenously. Although the mice were resistant to challenge with infective larvae, demonstrating the effectiveness of the immunizing procedure, they were completely susceptible to challenge with newborn larvae.

There seems to be good evidence from these parasitological experiments that the enteral and parenteral stages are treated as different animals by the host and that immunity produced against one stage has no adverse effect on the other.

5.4. A Revision of the Dual-Antibody Hypothesis

While the general ideas put forward by Oliver-Gonzalez have stood up to the rigorous test of immunochemists, immunologists, and parasitologists, it it perhaps now time to reevaluate and restate the hypothesis.

Oliver-Gonzalez recognized (see the quotation in Section 5.1) that there were multiple antibody responses to the adult and larval stages; we must now recognize that there are responses to more stages than the adult and infective larvae originally studied. Since *Trichinella* has all five of its life-cycle stages in the same host, it is possible that each elicits stage-specific responses. Indeed, since the L_1 larva has two antigenically distinct phases (see the surface proteins of the newborn and infective larvae in Fig. 7), it is possible that these quintuple stage-specific responses are more finely subdivided, possibly sextuple responses.

It is difficult to see what evolutionary advantage there is for the worm in maintaining antigenic dissimilarities among the second, third, and fourth stages, since the process of maturation is so rapid. There is, however, some advantage in having different antigens in the preadult and adult stages, since a response to the former will influence the survival of the latter, the reproductive stage. The most obvious advantages come from the differences between the infective larvae and the newborn larvae and between the adult worms and the newborn larvae. These differences ensure that the immune response stimulated by the intestinal phase of the infection, which is already stimulated by the time reproduction commences, does not interfere with the migration and establishment of the newborn larvae in the muscles.

Our revision of the hypothesis is therefore that there are antibodies that recognize not two but three sets of crucial stage-specific antigens, those of the infective larvae, adult worms, and newborn larvae. These antigens may well be primarily surface antigens, though a role for secreted antigens cannot be excluded. The biological advantage to the worm in maintaining different antigens at each stage is to allow the migration of newborn larvae to the muscles, without intereference from host immune responses generated by earlier stages, and thus allow the primary generation to reproduce successfully.

REFERENCES

Ali Khan, Z., 1966, The post embryonic development of *Trichinella spiralis* with special reference to ecdysis, *J. Parasitol.* **52:**248–259.

Alizadeh, H., 1981, Intestinal immune and inflammatory responses of mice to infection with the nematode *Trichinella spiralis*, Ph.D. thesis, University of Glasgow.

Alizadeh, H., and Wakelin, D., 1981, Mechanism of rapid expulsion of *Trichinella spiralis* from mice, in: *Trichinellosis* (C.W. Kim, E.J. Ruitenberg and J.S. Teppema, eds.), Proceedings of Fifth International Conference on Trichinellosis, Reedbooks, England, pp. 81–84.

Alizadeh, H., and Wakelin, D., 1982a, Comparison of rapid expulsion of *Trichinella spiralis* in mice and rats, *Int. J. Parasitol.* **12:**65–73.

Alizadeh, H., and Wakelin, D., 1982b, Genetic factors controlling the intestinal mast cell response in mice infected with *Trichinella spiralis*. *Clin. Exp. Immunol.* **49:**331–337.

Askenase, P.W., 1979, Immunopathology of parasitic diseases: Involvement of basophils and mast cells, *Springer Semin. Immunopathol.* **2:**2–59.

Befus, A.D., and Bienenstock, J., 1979, Immunologically mediated intestinal mastocytosis in *Nippostrongylus brasiliensis*-infected rats, *Immunology* **38:**95–101.

Bell, R.G., and McGregor, D.D., 1979a, *Trichinella spiralis*: Expression of rapid expulsion in rats exposed to an abbreviated enteral infection, *Exp. Parasitol.* **48:**42–50.

Bell, R.G., and McGregor, D.D., 1979b, *Trichinella spiralis*: Role of different life cycle phases in induction, maintenance and expression of rapid expulsion in rats, *Exp. Parasitol.* **48:**51–60.

Bell, R.G., and McGregor, D.D., 1980a, Requirement for two discrete stimuli for induction of the intestinal rapid expulsion response against *Trichinella spiralis* in rats, *Infect. Immun.* **29:**186–193.

Bell, R.G., and McGregor, D.D., 1980b, Rapid expulsion of *Trichinella spiralis*: Coinduction by using antigenic extracts of larvae and intestinal stimulation with an unrelated parasite, *Infect. Immun.* **29:**186–193.

Bell, R.G., and McGregor, D.D., 1980c, Variation in anti-*Trichinella* responsiveness in inbred strains, in: *Genetic Control of Natural Resistance to Infection and Malignancy* (E. Skamene, P.A.L. Kongshavn, and M. Landy, eds.), Academic Press, New York, pp. 67–73.

Bell, R.G., McGregor, D.D., and Despommier, D.D., 1979, *Trichinella spiralis*: Mediation of the intestinal component of protective immunity in the rat by multiple, phase-specific antiparasite responses, *Exp. Parasitol.* **47**:140–157.

Biozzi, G., Stiffel, C., Mouton, D., Bouthillier, Y., and Decreusefond, C., 1971, Genetic regulation of the function of antibody producing cells, in: *Progress in Immunology* (B. Amos, ed.), Academic Press, London and New York, pp. 529–545.

Briggs, N.T., 1963, Hypersensitivity in murine trichinosis: Some responses of *Trichinella*-infected mice to antigen and 5-hydroxytryptophan, *Ann. N. Y. Acad. Sci.* **113**:456–466.

Briggs, N.T., and Degiusti, D.L., 1966, Generalized allergic reactions in *Trichinella* infected mice: The temporal association of host immunity and sensitivity to exogenous antigens, *Am. J. Trop. Med. Hyg.* **15**:919–929.

Brown, P.J., Bruce, R.G., Manson-Smith, D.F., and Parrott, D.M.V., 1981, Intestinal mast cell response in thymectomized and normal mice infected with *Trichinella spiralis*, *Vet. Immunol. Immunopathol.* **2**:189–198.

Campbell, W.C., 1965, Immunizing effect of enteral and enteral–parenteral infections of *Trichinella spiralis* in mice, *J. Parasitol.* **51**:185–194.

Campbell, W.C., Hartman, R.K., and Cuckler, A.C., 1963a, Effect of certain antihistamine and antiserotonin agents upon experimental trichinosis in mice, *Exp. Parasitol.* **14**:23–28.

Campbell, W.C., Hartman, R.K., and Cuckler, A.C., 1963b, Induction of immunity to trichinosis in mice by means of chemically abbreviated infections, *Exp. Parasitol.* **14**:29–36.

Castro, G.A., 1976, Spatial and temporal integration of host responses to intestinal stages of *Trichinella spiralis*: Retro and prospective views, in: *Biochemistry of Parasites and Host–Parasite Relationships* (H. van den Bossche, ed.), Elsevier/North-Holland, Amsterdam, pp. 343–358.

Castro, G.A., Cotter, M.V., Ferguson, J.D., and Gordon, G.W., 1973, Trichinosis: Physiologic factors possibly altering the course of infection, *J. Parasitol.* **59**:268–276.

Castro, G.A., Badial-Aceves, F., Smith, J.W., Dudrick, S.J., and Weisbrodt, N.W., 1976, Altered small bowel propulsion associated with parasitism, *Gastroenterology* **71**:620–625.

Castro, G.A., Hessel, J.J., and Whalen, G., 1979, Altered intestinal fluid movement in response to *Trichinella spiralis* in immunized rats, *Parasite Immunol.* **1**:259–266.

Chiorazzi, N., Fox, D.A., and Katz, D.H., 1977, Hapten-specific IgE antibody responses in mice. VII. Conversion of IgE "non-responder" strains to IgE "responders" by elimination of suppressor T cell activity, *J. Immunol.* **118**:48–54.

Coker, C.M., 1955, Effects of cortisone on *Trichinella spiralis* infections in non-immunized mice, *J. Parasitol.* **41**:498–504.

Crandall, R.B., and Crandall, C.A., 1972, *Trichinella spiralis*: Immunologic response to infection in mice, *Exp. Parasitol.* **31**:378–398.

Crum, E.D., Despommier, D.D., and McGregor, D.D., 1977, Immunity to *Trichinella spiralis*. I. Transfer of resistance by two classes of lymphocytes, *Immunology* **33**:787–795.

Culbertson, J.T., 1942, Active immunity in mice against *Trichinella spiralis*, *J Parasitol.* **28**:197–202.

Denham, D.A., 1965, Studies with methyridine and *Trichinella spiralis*. 1. Effect upon the intestinal phase in mice, *Exp. Parasitol.* **17**:10–14.

Denham, D.A., 1966a, Immunity to *Trichinella spiralis*. I. The immunity produced by mice to the first four days of the intestinal phase of the infection, *Parasitology* **56**:323–327.

Denham, D.A., 1966b, Immunity to *Trichinella spiralis*. II. Immunity produced by the adult worm in mice, *Parasitology* **56**:745–751.

Denham, D.A., 1967, Application of the *in vitro* culture of nematodes especially *Trichinella spiralis*, in: *Problems of in Vitro Culture* (A.E.R. Taylor, ed.), Blackwell, London, pp. 49–60.

Denham, D.A., 1968, Immunity to *Trichinella spiralis*. III. The longevity of the infection in mice. *J. Helminth.* **42**:257–268.

Denham, D.A., 1969, Immunity of *Trichinella spiralis*. IV. Passive immunity in mice, *Folia Parasitol.* **16**:183–187.

Denham, D.A., and Martinez, A.R., 1970, Studies with methyridine and *Trichinella spiralis*. II. The use of the drug to study the rate of larval production in mice, *J. Helminthol.* **44**:357–363.

Dennis, D.T., Despommier, D.D., and Davis, N., 1970, Infectivity of the newborn larva of *Trichinella spiralis* in the rat, *J. Parasitol.* **56**974–977.

Despommier, D.D., 1971, Immunogenicity of the newborn larva of *Trichinella spiralis*, *J. Parasitol.* **57**:531–535.

Despommier, D.D., Campbell, W.C., and Blair, L.S., 1977a, The *in vivo* and *in vitro* analysis of immunity to *Trichinella spiralis* in mice and rats, *Parasitology* **74**:109–119.

Despommier, D.D., McGregor, D.D., Crum, E.D., and Carter, P.B., 1977b, Immunity to *Trichinella spiralis*. II. Expression of immunity against adult worms, *Immunology* **33**:797–805.

Dinetta, J., Katz, F., and Campbell, W.C., 1972, Effect of heterologous antilymphocyte serum on the spontaneous cure of *Trichinella spiralis* infections in mice, *J. Parasitol.* **58**:636–637.

Doerr, R., and Schmidt, G.W., 1930, Studien über den Mechanismus der trichinellen Infektion. VII. Experimentelle Beeinflussung der Trichinewanderung der natürlichen Immunität des Hundes, *Zentralbl. Bakteriol.* **115**:427–437.

Duckett, M.G., Denham, D.A., and Nelson, G., 1972, Immunity to *Trichinella spiralis*. V. Transfer of immunity against the intestinal phase from mother to baby mice, *J. Parasitol.* **58**:550–555.

Dutoit, E., Tronchin, G., Vernes, A., and Biguet, J., 1979, The influence of prostaglandins and vasoactive amines on the intestinal phase of experimental trichinellosis in CBA mice and Wistar rats, *Ann. Parasitol. Hum. Comp.* **54**:465–474.

Fatunmbi, O.O., 1978, Studies on some aspects of the development of *Trichinella spiralis* in mice, M. Sc. thesis, University of Glasgow.

Faubert, G.M., 1977, *Trichinella spiralis*: Immunosuppression in challenge infections of Swiss mice, *Exp. Parasitol.* **43**:336–341.

Gabriel, B.W., and Justus, D.E., 1979, Quantitation of immediate and delayed hypersensitivity responses in *Trichinella*-infected mice, *Int. Arch. Allergy* **60**:275–285.

Gore, R.W., Bürger, H.-J., and Sadun, E.H., 1974, Humoral and cellular factors in the resistance of rats to *Trichinella spiralis*, in: *Trichinellosis* (C.W. Kim, ed.), Intext, New York, pp. 367–382.

Gould, S.E., Gomberg, H.J., Bethell, F.H., Villella, J.B., and Heity, C.S., 1955, Studies on *Trichinella spiralis*. I. Concerning the time and site of insemination of females of *Trichinella spiralis*: II. Time of initial recovery of larvae of *Trichinella spiralis* from blood of experimental animals; III. Effect on the intestinal phase of trichinosis of feeding massive numbers of irradiated *Trichinella* larvae; IV. Effect of feeding irradiated *Trichinella* larvae on production of immunity to re-infection; V. Tests for a strain of trichina larvae resistant to radiation, *Am. J. Pathol.* **31**:933–963.

Grencis, R.K., and Wakelin, D., 1982, Short lived, dividing cells mediate adoptive transfer of immunity to *Trichinella spiralis* in mice. I. Availability of cells in primary and secondary infections in relation to cellular changes in the mesenteric lymph node, *Immunology* **46**:443–450.

Grove, D.I., and Civil, R.H., 1978, *Trichinella spiralis*: Effects on the host–parasite relationship in mice of BCG (attenuated *Mycobacterium bovis*), *Exp. Parasitol.* **44**:181–189.

Grove, D.I., and Warren, K.S., 1976, Effects on murine trichinosis of niridazole, a suppressant of cellular but not humoral immunological responses, *Ann. Trop. Med. Parasitol.* **70**:449–453.

Grove, D.I., Mahmoud, A.A.F., and Warren, K.S., 1977a, Eosinophils and resistance to *Trichinella spiralis*, *J. Exp. Med.* **145**:755–759.

Grove, D.I., Hamburger, J., and Warren, K.S., 1977b, Kinetics of immunological responses, resistance to reinfection and pathological reactions to infection with *Trichinella spiralis*, *J. Infect. Dis.* **136**:562–570.

Jackson, G.J., 1959, Fluorescent antibody studies of *Trichinella spiralis* infections, *J. Infect. Dis.* **105**:97–117.

Jacqueline, E., Vernes, A., Bout, D., and Biguet, J., 1978, *Trichinella spiralis*: Facteurs immunitaires inhibiteurs de la production de larves. II. Premier analyse *in vitro* des facteurs humoraux et secretoires actifs chez les souris, le rat, et la miniporc infestes ou immunises, *Exp. Parasitol.* **45**:42–54.

James, E.R., and Denham, D.A., 1974, The stage specificity of the immune response to *Trichinella spiralis*, in: *Trichinellosis* (C.W. Kim, ed.), Intext, New York, pp. 367–382.

James, E.R., and Denham, D.A., 1975, Immunity to *Trichinella spiralis*. VI. The specificity of the immune response stimulated by the intestinal stage, *J. Helminthol.* **49**:43–47.

James, E.R., Moloney, A., and Denham, D.A., 1977, Immunity to *Trichinella spiralis*. VII. Resistance stimulated by the parenteral stages of the infection, *J. Parasitol.* **63**:720–723.

Jungery, M., and Ogilvie, B.M., 1982, Antibody response to stage-specific *Trichinella spiralis* surface antigens in strong and weak responder mouse strains. *J. Immunol.* **129**:839–843.

Karmanska, K., and Michalska, Z., 1977, Influence of prostaglandin E$_2$ (PGE$_2$) on mast cells, histopathological changes and parasites in the course of trichinellosis in mice, *Wiad. Parazytol.* **23**:725–735.

Karmanska, K., Kozar, Z., Seniuta, R., and Dlugiewicz-Bolla, M., 1973, The influence of antilymphocyte and anti-macrophage serum on mast cells in experimental trichinellosis in mice, *Acta Parasitol. Pol.* **21**:173–182.

Kazura, J.W., and Grove, D.I., 1978, Stage-specific antibody-dependent eosinophil-mediated destruction of *Trichinella spiralis*, *Nature* (*London*) **274**:588.

Kelly, J.D., and Dineen, J.K., 1976, Prostaglandins in the gastrointestinal tract—evidence for a role in worm expulsion, *Aust. Vet. J.* **52**:391–397.

Kennedy, M.W., 1980, Effects of the host immune response on the longevity, fecundity and position in the intestine of *Trichinella spiralis* in mice, *Parasitology* **80**:49–60.

Kennedy, M.W., and Bruce, R.G., 1981, Reversibility of the effects of the host-immune response on the intestinal phase of *Trichinella spiralis* in the mouse, following transplantation to a new host, *Parasitology* **82**:39–48.

Kennedy, M.W., Wakelin, D., and Wilson, M.M., 1979, Transplantation of adult *Trichinella spiralis* between hosts: Worm survival and immunological characteristics of the host–parasite relationship, *Parasitology* **78**:121–130.

Kitamura, Y., Shimada, M., Go, S., Matsuda, H., Hatanaka, K., and Seki, M., 1979, Distribution of mast cell precursors in haematopoietic and lymphopoietic tissues of mice, *J. Exp. Med.* **150**:482–490.

Kozar, Z., Karmanska, K., Kotz, J., and Seniuta, R., 1971, The influence of antilymphocytic serum (ALS) on the course of trichinellosis in mice, *Wiad. Parazytol.* **17**:541–548.

Kozek, W.J., 1971, The moulting pattern in *Trichinella spiralis*. 1. A light microscope study, *J. Parasitol.* **57**:1015–1028.

Lake, A.M., Bloch, K.J., Sinclair, K.J., and Walker, W.A., 1980, Anaphylactic release of intestinal mucus, *Immunology* **39**:173–178.

Larsh, J.R., 1963, Experimental trichiniasis, *Adv. Parasitol.* **1**:213–286.

Larsh, J.E., 1967, Delayed (cellular) hypersensitivity in parasitic infections, *Am. J. Trop. Med. Hyg.* **16**:735–745.

Larsh, J.E., 1970, Immunity, in: *Trichinosis in Man and Animals* (S.E. Gould, ed.), Charles C. Thomas, Springfield, Illinois, pp. 129–146.

Larsh, J.E., and Race, G.J., 1954, A histopathologic study of the anterior small intestine of immunized and non-immunized mice infected with *Trichinella spiralis*, *J. Infect. Dis.* **94**:262–272.

Larsh, J.E., and Race, G.J., 1975, Allergic inflammation as a hypothesis for the expulsion of worms from tissues: A review, *Exp. Parasitol.* **37**:251–266.

Larsh, J.E., and Weatherly, N.F., 1975, Cell-mediated immunity against certain parasitic worms, *Adv. Parasitol.* **13**:183–222.

Larsh, J.E., Jr., and Gilchrist, H.B., and Greenberg, B.G., 1952, A study of the distribution and longevity of adult *Trichinella spiralis* in immunized and non-immunized mice, *J. Elisha Mitchell Sci. Soc.* **68**:1–11.

Larsh, J.E., Ottolenghi, A., and Weatherly, N.F., 1974, *Trichinella spiralis*: Phospholipase in challenged mice and rats, *Exp. Parasitol.* **36**:299–306.

Lee, G.B., and Ogilvie, B.M., 1981a, The mucus layer in intestinal nematode infections, in: *The Mucosal Immune System in Health and Disease* (P.L. Ogra and J. Bienenstock, eds.), Ross Laboratories, Columbus, Ohio, pp. 175–187.

Lee, G.B., and Ogilvie, B.M., 1981b, The mucus layer of the small intestine—its protective effect in rats immune to *Trichinella spiralis*, in: *Trichinellosis* (C.W. Kim, E.J. Ruitenberg, and J.S. Teppema, eds.), Proceedings of the Fifth International Conference on Trichinellosis, pp. 91–95.

Levin, D.M., Ottesen, E.A., Reynolds, H.Y., and Kirkpatrick, C.H., 1976, Cellular immunity in Peyer's patches of rats infected with *Trichinella spiralis*, *Infect. Immun.* **13**:27–30.

Ljungström, I., and Ruitenberg, E.J., 1976, A comparative study of the immunohistological and serological response of intact and T cell-deprived mice to *Trichinella spiralis*, *Clin. Exp. Immunol.* **24**:146–156.

Love, R.J., and Ogilvie, B.M., 1977, *Nippostrongylus brasiliensis* and *Trichinella spiralis*: Localization of lymphoblasts in the small intestine of parasitized rats, *Exp. Parasitol.* **41**:124–132.

Love, R.J., Ogilvie, B.M., and McLaren, D.J., 1976, The immune mechanism which expels the intestinal stage of *Trichinella spiralis* from rats, *Immunology* **30**:7–15.

Machnicka, B., 1972, *Trichinella spiralis*: Influence of antilymphocytic serum on mouse infections, *Exp. Parasitol.* **31**:172–177.

Mackenzie, C.D., Preston, P.M., and Ogilvie, B.M., 1978, Immunological properties of the surface of nematodes, *Nature (London)* **276**:826.

Mackenzie, C.D., Jungery, M., Taylor, P.M., and Ogilvie, B.M., 1980, Activation of complement, the induction of antibodies to the surface of nematodes and the effect of these factors and cells on worm survival *in vitro*, *Eur. J. Immunol.* **10**:594–601.

Manson-Smith, D.F., Bruce, R.G., and Parrott, D.M.V., 1979a, Villous atrophy and expulsion of intestinal *Trichinella spiralis* are mediated by T-cells, *Cell. Immunol.* **47:**285–292.

Manson-Smith, D.F., Bruce, R.G., Rose, M.L., and Parrott, D.M.V., 1979b, Migration of lymphoblasts to the small intestine. III. Strain differences and relationship to distribution and duration of *Trichinella spiralis* infection, *Clin. Exp. Immunol.* **38:**475–482.

Markell, E.K., 1958, The effect of cortisone treatment upon the longevity and productivity of *Trichinella spiralis* in the rat, *J. Infect. Dis.* **102:**158–161.

Matoff, K., 1943, Altersimmunität und parenterale erzeugte Muskeltrichinellose beim Hunde, *Zentralbl. Bakteriol. Parasitenkd.* **150:**328–336.

McCoy, O.R., 1940, Rapid loss of *Trichinella* larvae fed to immune rats and its bearing on the mechanisms of immunity, *Am. J. Hyg.* **32:**105–116.

Michalska, Z., and Karmanska, K., 1976, Influence of inhibition of degranulation of mast cells by Intal (disodium cromoglycate) on the course of trichinellosis in mice, *Acta Parasitol. Pol.* **24:**69–80.

Miller, H.R.P., 1979, Passive transfer of the mucosal mast-cell response, its relationship to goblet cell differentiation, in: *The Mast Cell* (J. Pepys and A.M. Edwards, eds.), Pitman Medical, pp. 738–742.

Moloney, A., and Denham, D.A., 1979, Effects of immune serum and cells on newborn larvae of *Trichinella spiralis, Parasite Immunol.* **1:**3–12.

Mota, I., Sadun, E., Bradshaw, R.M., and Gore, R.W., 1969, The immunological response of mice infected with *Trichinella spiralis, Immunology* **16:**71–81.

Murray, M., 1972, Immediate hypersensitivity effector mechanisms. II. *In vivo* reactions, in: *Immunity to Animal Parasites* (E.J.L. Soulsby, ed.), Academic Press, New York, pp. 155–190.

Ogilvie, B.M., Askenase, P.W., and Rose, M.E., 1980, Basophils and eosinophils in three strains of rats and in athymic (nude) rats following infection with the nematodes *Nippostrongylus brasiliensis* or *Trichinella spiralis, Immunology* **39:**385–389.

Oliver-Gonzalez, J., 1940, The *in vitro* action of immune serum on the larvae and adults of *Trichinella spiralis, J. Infect. Dis.* **67:**292–300.

Oliver-Gonzalez, J., 1941, The dual antibody basis of acquired immunity in trichinosis, *J. Infect. Dis.* **69:**254–270.

Oliver-Gonzalez, J., and Levine, D.M., 1962, Stage specific antibodies in experimental trichinosis, *Am. J. Trop. Med. Hyg.* **11:**241–244.

Ottaway, C.A., Manson-Smith, D.F., Bruce, R.G., and Parrott, D.M.V., 1980, Regional blood flow and the localization of lymphoblasts in the small intestine of the mouse. II. The effect of a primary enteric infection with *Trichinella spiralis, Immunology* **41:**963–971.

Ottesen, E.A., Smith, T.K., and Kirkpatrick, C.H., 1975, Immune response to *Trichinella spiralis* in the rat. I. Development of cellular and humoral responses, *Int. Arch. Allergy Appl. Immunol.* **49:**396–410.

Parkhouse, R.M.E., Philipp, M., and Ogilvie, B.M., 1981, Characterization of surface antigens of *Trichinella spiralis* infective larvae, *Parasite Immunol.* **3:**339–352.

Perrudet-Badoux, A., Binaghi, R.A., and Biozzi, G., 1975, *Trichinella* infestation in mice genetically selected for high and low antibody production, *Immunology* **29:**387–390.

Perrudet-Badoux, A., Binaghi, R.A., and Boussac-Aron, Y., 1976, Production of different classes of immunoglobulins in rats infected with *Trichinella spiralis, Immunochemistry* **13:**443–445.

Perrudet-Badoux, A., Binaghi, R.A., and Boussac-Aron, Y., 1978, *Trichinella spiralis* infection in mice: Mechanism of the resistance in animals genetically selected for high and low antibody production, *Immunology* **35**:519–522.

Perrudet-Badoux, A., Boussac-Aron, Y., Ruitenberg, E.J., and Elgersma, A., 1980, Preliminary studies on the course of a *Trichinella spiralis* infection in athymic, nude rats, *J. Parasitol.* **66**:671–673.

Perry, R.H., 1974, Transfer of immunity to *Trichinella spiralis* from mother to offspring, *J. Parasitol.* **60**:460–465.

Philipp, M., Parkhouse, R.M.E., and Ogilvie, B.M., 1980, Changing proteins on the surface of a parasitic nematode, *Nature (London)* **257**:538–540.

Philipp, M., Taylor, P.M., Parkhouse, R.M.E., and Ogilvie, B.M., 1981, Immune response to stage-specific surface-antigens of the parasitic nematode *Trichinella spiralis*, *J. Exp. Med.* **154**:210–215.

Richardson, J.A., and Olson, L.J., 1974, Murine trichinellosis: Changes in glucose absorption and intestinal morphology, in: *Trichinellosis* (C.W. Kim, ed.), Intext, New York, pp. 61–73.

Rivera-Ortiz, C.-I., and Nussenzweig, R., 1976, *Trichinella spiralis*: Anaphylactic antibody formation and susceptibility in strains of inbred mice, *Exp. Parasitol.* **39**:7–17.

Rose, M.L., Parrott, D.V.M., and Bruce, R.G., 1976, Migration of lymphoblasts to the small intestine. I. Effect of *Trichinella spiralis* infection on the migration of mesenteric lymphoblasts and mesenteric T lymphoblasts in syngeneic mice, *Immunology* **51**:723–730.

Rothwell, T.L.W., Prichard, R.K., and Love, R.J., 1974, Studies on the role of histamine and 5-hydroxytryptamine in immunity against the nematode *Trichostrongylus colubriformis*. I. *In vivo* and *in vitro* effects of the amines, *Int. Arch. Allergy Appl. Immunol.* **46**:1–13.

Ruitenberg, E.J., and Elgersma, A., 1976, Absence of intestinal mast cell response in congenitally athymic mice during *Trichinella spiralis* infection, *Nature (London)* **264**:258–260.

Ruitenberg, E.J., and Steerenberg, P.A., 1974, Intestinal phase of *Trichinella spiralis* in congenitally athymic (nude) mice, *J. Parasitol.* **60**:1056–1057.

Ruitenberg, E.J., and Steerenberg, P.A., 1976, Immunogenicity of the parenteral stages of *Trichinella spiralis*, *J. Parasitol.* **62**:164–166.

Ruitenberg, E.J., Elgersma, A., Kruizinga, W., and Leenstra, F., 1977a, *Trichinella spiralis* infection in congenitally athymic (nude) mice, *Immunology* **33**:581–587.

Ruitenberg, E.J., Leenstra, F., and Elgersma, A., 1977b, Thymus dependence and independence of intestinal pathology in a *Trichinella spiralis* infection: A study in congenitally athymic (nude) mice, *Br. J. Exp. Pathol.* **58**:311–314.

Ruitenberg, E.J., Elgersma, A., and Lamer, C.H.J., 1978, Thymus dependence and kinetics of intestinal mast cells and globule leucocytes, *Z. Immunitaetsforsch.* **154**:357–359.

Ruitenberg, E.J., Elgersma, A., and Kruizinga, W., 1979, Intestinal mast cells and globule leucocytes: Role of the thymus on their presence and proliferation during a *Trichinella spiralis* infection in the rat, *Int. Arch. Allergy Appl. Immunol.* **60**:302–309.

Ruitenberg, E.J., Perrudet-Badoux, A., Boussac-Aron, Y., and Elgersma, A., 1980, *Trichinella spiralis* infection in animals genetically selected for high and low antibody production, *Int. Arch. Allergy Appl. Immunol.* **62**:104–110.

Russell, D.A., and Castro, G.A., 1979, Physiological characterisation of a biphasic immune response to *Trichinella spiralis* in the rat, *J. Infect. Dis.* **139**:304–312.

Smith, J.A., and Castro, G.A., 1978, Relation of peroxidase activity in gut mucosa to inflammation, *Am. J. Physiol.* **2341**:72–79.

Stefanski, W., and Kozar, M., 1969, Degree of resistance of some mouse strains to *Trichinella spiralis* infection, *Wiad. Parazytol.* **15:**571–575.

Tanner, C.E., 1978, The susceptibility to *Trichinella spiralis* of inbred lines of mice differing at the H-2 histocompatibility locus, *J. Parasitol.* **64:**956–957.

Tronchin, G., Dutoit, E., Vernes, A., and Biguet, J., 1979, Oral immunization of mice with metabolic antigens of *Trichinella spiralis* larvae: Effects on the kinetics of intestinal cell response including mast cells and polymorphonuclear eosinophils, *J. Parasitol.* **65:**685–691.

Wakelin, D., 1978, Genetic control of susceptibility and resistance to parasitic infection, *Adv. Parasitol.* **16:**219–308.

Wakelin, D., 1980a, Genetic control of immunity to parasites: Infection with *Trichinella spiralis* in inbred and congenic mice showing rapid and slow responses to infection, *Parasite Immunol.* **2:**85–98.

Wakelin, D., 1980b, Genetic control of immunologically mediated resistance to helminthic infections, in: *Genetic Control of Natural Resistance to Infection and Malignancy* (E. Skamene, P.A.L. Kongshavn, and M. Landy, eds.), Academic Press, New York, pp. 55–66.

Wakelin, D., and Donachie, A.M., 1980, Genetic control of immunity to parasites: Adoptive transfer of immunity between inbred strains of mice characterized by rapid and slow immune expulsion of *Trichinella spiralis, Parasite Immunol.* **2:**249–260.

Wakelin, D., and Donachie, A.M., 1981, Genetic control of immunity to *Trichinella spiralis*: Donor bone marrow cells determine responses to infection in radiation chimaeras, *Immunology* **43:**787–792.

Wakelin, D., Grencis, R.K., and Donachie, A.M., 1982, Short lived, dividing cells mediate adoptive transfer of immunity to *Trichinella spiralis* in mice. II. *In vivo* characteristics of the cells. *Immunology* **46:**451–457.

Wakelin, D., and Lloyd, M., 1976a, Immunity to primary and challenge infections of *Trichinella spiralis* in mice: A re-examination of conventional parameters, *Parasitology* **72:**173–182.

Wakelin, D., and Lloyd, M., 1976b, Accelerated expulsion of adult *Trichinella spiralis* in mice given lymphoid cells and serum from infected donors, *Parasitology* **72:**307–315.

Wakelin, D., and Wilson, M.M., 1977a, Transfer of immunity to *Trichinella spiralis* in the mouse with mesenteric lymph node cells: Time of appearance of effective cells in donors and expression of immunity in recipients, *Parasitology* **74:**215–224.

Wakelin, D., and Wilson, M.M., 1977b, Evidence for the involvement of a bone marrow-derived cell population in the immune expulsion of *Trichinella spiralis, Parasitology* **74:**225–234.

Wakelin, D., and Wilson, M.M., 1979a, T and B cells in the transfer of immunity against *Trichinella spiralis* in mice, *Immunology* **37:**103–109.

Wakelin, D., and Wilson, M.M., 1979b, *Trichinella spiralis*: Immunity and inflammation in the expulsion of transplanted adult worms from mice, *Exp. Parasitol.* **48:**305–312.

Wakelin, D., and Wilson, M.M., 1980, Immunity to *Trichinella spiralis* in irradiated mice, *Int. J. Parasitol.* **10:**37–41.

Walls, R.S., Carter, R.L., Leuchars, E., and Davies, A.J.S., 1973, The immunopathology of trichiniasis in T-cell deficient mice, *Clin. Exp. Immunol.* **13:**231–243.

Wassom, D.L., and Gleich, G.J., 1979, Damage to *Trichinella spiralis* newborn larvae by eosinophil major basic protein, *Am. J. Trop. Med. Hyg.* **28:**860–863.

Wassom, D.L., David, C.S., and Gleich, G.J., 1979, Genes within the major histocompatibility complex influence susceptibility to *Trichinella spiralis* in the mouse, *Immunogenetics* **9:**491–496.

Wassom, D.L., David, C.S., and Gleich, G.J., 1980, MHC-linked genetic control of the immune response to parasites: *Trichinella spiralis* in the mouse, in: *Genetic Control of Natural Resistance to Infection and Malignancy*, (E. Skamene, P.A.L. Kongshavn, and M. Landy, eds.), Academic Press, New York, pp. 75–82.

Williams, J.S., Gore, R.W., and Shoun, E.H., 1972, *Trichinella spiralis*: antigen-antibody interaction assayed by radioactive iodinated antigen, *Exp. Parasitol.* **31:**299–306.

9

Antigens

DAVID S. SILBERSTEIN

1. INTRODUCTION

There are four main goals of research regarding the purification and characterization of *Trichinella spiralis* antigens. The first and most important of these goals is the desire to understand the functions of the antigens for the parasite. While certain anatomical studies, which demonstrate the presence of antigens in specific worm tissues, have led to speculation concerning their functions, no experimental evidence of function has been reported.

The second aim is to use the antigens to explore further the mechanisms of protective immunity. In this respect, *Trichinella* serves as an excellent model for studying immunity to metazoan parasites. In essence, two mechanisms have been put forward to explain the immune effects against intestinal nematodes: (1) worm structures are damaged directly, at the point of contact, wherever antibody or effector cells are attracted by antigens; or (2) worms are damaged indirectly by the neutralization of function of one or more key antigenic molecules. Reports, which will be cited, of antibody deposits, complement components, and leukocyte adherence at the worm's pores or cuticle suggest immunity by blockade and bombardment, which would be consistent with model 1. On the other hand, work by Thorson (1956a,b) shows that immunity to *Ancylostoma caninum* is associated with neutralizing

DAVID S. SILBERSTEIN • Department of Microbiology, Columbia University, New York, New York 10032.

antibody against a secreted protease. Whether parallel effects exist for *Trichinella* is not known, but if they do, they would embody model 2.

Study of worms that are stunted, dying, or dead from immune mechanisms is generally unrevealing regarding the nature of the antigens involved. Examples of such studies follow. Adult *Trichinella* recovered at 11 and 14 days postinfection from immunocompetent hosts show the accumulation of lipid droplets and the degeneration of gametes at the electron-microscopic level (Love *et al.*, 1976), and such worms shed fewer larvae *in vitro* (Despommier *et al.*, 1977a). In the presence of immune serum and peritoneal cells, newborn larvae, infective larvae, and adults die. Infective larvae characteristically rupture at the cuticle and extrude internal organs (Mackenzie *et al.*, 1980). While these studies of worm pathology are informative, they cannot substitute for the isolation and characterization of the target antigens. One reason they cannot is that *Trichinella* is an intracellular parasite, except for brief migratory stages, and intracellular conditions cannot be duplicated *in vitro*. Furthermore, they do not identify clearly the structure that is the target of the immune attack. A particular pattern of damage could be the result of an apparent direct attack (model 1), but it could also be the result of an indirect attack on, for example, an enzyme critical to worm nutrition. Consider the case of the infective larva with the ruptured cuticle and extruding organs. If the cause of this lesion involves weakening of the cuticle by direct action of antibody and cells, then the newborn larvae and adults might also be expected to show a ruptured cuticle. But what is special about the infective larva is that it would normally be preparing to molt four times in its host. In this condition, an immune attack on nutrition might well interfere with the presumed cuticle synthesis in a manner to cause the observed rupture. One is reminded of the effect of penicillin on sensitive bacteria: cell-wall synthesis is inhibited, and as the time for cell division approaches, the wall ruptures, and cell contents are extruded. One way to investigate the mechanism that causes cuticular lesions would be to isolate cuticular antigens, prepare specific antisera against them, and use these antisera in the *in vitro* incubations.

Knowledge gleaned from the study of *Trichinella* antigens may be generalized to other parasitic nematodes, some of which infect nearly half the world's human population. As will be discussed later, many *Trichinella* antigens are presented to the host as secretions originating in the stichocyte cells of the stichosome (Despommier and Müller, 1976). All members of the order Trichurata possess this organ (Chitwood, 1930), and such secretions have been shown to be important in the host–parasite relationship for *Trichuris muris* (Wakelin and Selby, 1973) as well as for *Trichinella*. In addition, secretions from other organs of other nematodes have been shown to contain antigens. This was demonstrated for *Nippostrongylus muris* (Thorson, 1951, 1953, 1954), *A. caninum* (Thorson, 1956a,b), and *Ascaris suum* (Soulsby, 1963; Stromberg, 1979).

Other facets of the immune response are well studied with the *Trichinella* model. These include the role of eosinophils with immunoglobulin E (IgE) in resistance (Kazura and Grove, 1978; Dessein *et al.*, 1981) and the physiology of immune elimination from the gut (Love *et al.*, 1976; Wakelin and Lloyd, 1976; Despommier *et al.*, 1977; Wakelin and Wilson, 1979a; Castro *et al.*, 1980). It would be of great interest to identify the molecular targets of these immune attacks and to test whether certain antigens are likely to provoke restricted, specialized classes of immune response.

A third reason for studying *Trichinella* antigens is the desire to understand their adjuvant or mitogen effects on various populations of lymphocytes. It is known, for example, that products of many parasitic nematodes (Ogilvie and Jones, 1973; Ishizaka *et al.*, 1976) including *Trichinella* (Sadun *et al.*, 1968; Perrudet-Badoux and Binaghi, 1974) stimulate high levels of specific and nonspecific IgE synthesis in the host. Using unpurified products from *A. suum* and *N. brasiliensis*, Ishizaka and co-workers have shown that worm allergens influence immature bone-marrow-derived (B) lymphocytes to select the epsilon isotype for heavy-chain synthesis. This effect is achieved by means of both B-cell and thymus-derived (T)-cell regulatory pathways (Urban *et al.*, 1977a,b, 1978, 1980; Yodoi *et al.*, 1979; Yodoi and Ishizaka, 1980). All these experiments were conducted using crude worm extracts or experimental infections; the allergens themselves were never isolated. Because of this, it was impossible to study the allergen–lymphocyte encounter. It remains unknown, therefore, whether the antigens in question are acting as antigens or mitogens.

Trichinella infection or extracts exert other modulating effects on the immune system. One such effect is the depression of the antibody response to sheep erythrocytes (Faubert and Tanner, 1971; Barriga, 1975) and to cholera toxin (Ljungström *et al.*, 1980). It has been suggested that this is due to depressed or defective T-cell function (Barriga, 1975; Jones *et al.*, 1976; Tanner *et al.*, 1978; Ljungström, 1980) and to polyclonal B-cell activation (Tanner *et al.*, 1981). In contrast, *Trichinella* has been shown to potentiate resistance against certain tumors (Molinari and Ebersole, 1977). This effect is possibly mediated by a pathway involving mastocytosis, IgE–*Trichinella* antigen bridging, and T cells bearing histamine-2 receptors (Ruitenberg *et al.*, 1981).

Regarding IgE elevation, antibody depression, and tumor resistance, isolation of *Trichinella* antigens will illuminate regulatory pathways.

The fourth and most pragmatic purpose for the isolation of *Trichinella* antigens is the development of a sensitive, specific reagent for the serodiagnosis of human and swine trichinosis. The use of crude antigen preparations with any modern diagnostic system incurs an undesirably high level of false positives and false negatives [for discussion, see Despommier (1981b) and chapter 17]. However, the refinement of test antigen (i.e., removal of material that is not antigenic in a natural infection) improves diagnostic accuracy (Taylor *et al.*, 1980; Despommier, Seawright, and Isenstein, unpublished results).

2. SOURCE OF ANTIGENS

Inferences concerning *Trichinella* antigens have been derived from reports of immunity in response to challenge with various life-cycle stages of *Trichinella* (Oliver-Gonzalez, 1941; Chute, 1956; Despommier, 1971; James and Denham, 1975; Ruitenberg and Steerenberg, 1976; James *et al.*, 1977; Bell and McGregor, 1979a,b) or to serum or cell transfer (Love *et al.*, 1976; Crum *et al.*, 1977; Despommier *et al.*, 1977b; Wakelin and Wilson, 1979b; Wakelin and Donachie, 1980). The implications of these and other studies are discussed thoroughly in chapter 8. From this evidence, it is clear that successive stages of *Trichinella* possess unique antigenic molecules.

2.1. Cuticular Antigens

With the exception of the newborn larva, the enteral and parenteral stages of *Trichinella* live intracellularly (see chapter 3). It is not known how parasite antigens are exported from the host cell to stimulate the immune system. Nevertheless, because the cuticle is the most obvious point of contact between parasite and host, its potential antigenicity has attracted a great deal of attention.

Evidence has accumulated that the host does synthesize antibody to components of the cuticle. The cuticle preparation of Sulzer (1965) from infective first-stage (L_1) larvae was functional in the indirect fluorescent-antibody test. Moore (1965) found that a cuticle-enriched fraction derived from the same stage of the infection was a protective immunogen for mice. These preliminary indications were confirmed by a number of methods.

The ability to detect antibody on the cuticle by microscopy may depend on the sensitivity of the system used. For example, using a direct fluorescent-antibody stain, Jackson (1959) was unable to demonstrate antibody to the cuticle of infective L_1 larvae in immune rabbit serum. On the other hand, Crandall and Crandall (1972) found specific mouse antibody against the outer surface of the worm using an indirect fluorescence method. In view of other reports, it is unlikely that the difference was due to the species of host that was immunized. Despommier et al. (1967) were able, by electron microscopy, to detect rabbit antibody to the cuticle using a ferritin-conjugated antibody. Kim and Ledbetter (1981) used scanning electron microscopy to visualize presumed antibody precipitates distributed unevenly over the cuticles of infective L_1 larvae and adults. For this study, however, the immune sera were generated in guinea pigs by hyperimmunization with large quantities of an undefined antigen in adjuvant. It is not clear whether these results are relevant to antigenic presentation by the cuticle in a natural infection.

A second way of looking at cuticular antigens is by means of cell adherence. Gadea et al. (1967) found that globulin-coated erythrocytes would adhere to worms incubated in immune, but not normal, rabbit serum in the presence of antibody to rabbit immunoglobulin. Other investigators have taken advantage of active labeling by living cells. Stankiewicz and Jeska (1973) first demonstrated in vitro the adherence of peritoneal cells to the surface of the infective larva in the presence of fresh normal serum or heat-inactivated immune serum. The effect was reproduced by Vernes et al. (1974) and Perrudet-Badoux et al. (1978). McLaren et al. (1977) confirmed that rat eosinophils adhered to the infected larva when the culture contained antibody. Their electron micrographs of the cell–parasite interface showed that the eosinophils degranulated but did not damage the cuticle.

The phenomenon of cytoadherence to the surface of Trichinella was more carefully studied by Mackenzie et al. (1980), who used rat peritoneal cells under various culture conditions. The cuticle of infective L_1 larvae and adults and the midregion of newborn L_1 larvae in 3-day cultures activated complement by the alternative pathway. Anti-C3 immunofluorescence showed that complement was distributed evenly over the affected surfaces. Additionally, the three stages were each coated with cells in the presence of complement-depleted, stage-specific antisera. The conclusion that follows from this work is that either complement or antibody is sufficient to promote adherence.

Further work on cuticular antigens was reported by Phillip et al. (1980, 1981). They were able to label the worm's surface proteins with

^{125}I, dissolve the cuticle in buffer containing 2% deoxycholate, and precipitate the antigens with immune rat serum. Polyacrylamide gel electrophoresis (PAGE) of the precipitates in the presence of sodium dodecyl sulfate (SDS) followed by autoradiography revealed a number of stage-specific antigens. The newborn L_1 larva exhibited four antigens with apparent molecular weights of 28, 30, 58, and 64 kilodaltons (kd). Under these conditions of extraction, the infective L_1 larva also exhibited four antigens, but with molecular weights of 47, 55, 90, and 105 kd. Of these, the 55 and 105 kd antigens were shown to have carbohydrate moieties by binding to lentil lectin. Another set of antigens was identified in the cuticles of L_2 through L_4 larvae, with weights of 20, 33, 40, and 56 kd. This 56-kd antigen is known to be distinct from the 55-kd antigen of the L_1 larva. Only the three lightest of the antigens from L_4 larvae were found on the cuticle of the adult.

The authors also showed that labeled surface antigens were shed by worms into the culture medium. This occurred especially rapidly for the intestinal forms that were undergoing rapid growth and molting or when the culture included immune serum and neutrophils. The authors suggest that the preparation usually described as excretory–secretory (ES) products contains antigens shed from the surface. This hypothesis could be tested in two ways. The first of these would be to test whether ES products inhibit the capacity of immune serum to precipitate antigens. The second would be to collect ES products from labeled worms and calculate the ratio of labeled to unlabeled protein. A question that would be more difficult to test would be whether the reaction of iodination significantly affects the integrity of the surface.

2.2. Excretory–Secretory Antigens

The ES antigens will now be considered in detail. The first evidence that ES products of various stages of *Trichinella* contained antigens was obtained from experiments in which precipitates were observed at the oral, anal, and genital pores of worms incubated in immune serum. Taliaferro and Sarles (1939) first described this phenomenon for *N. muris*. Shortly afterward, it was also observed for *Trichinella* (Oliver-Gonzalez, 1940). In the latter study, it was noted that precipitates appeared at the mouths of infective L_1 larva and at the mouths, anuses, and vulvas of adult females. By light microscopy, the author was able to discern precipitates only in these parts of the worms. By direct fluorescent microscopy, Jackson (1959) also visualized the "oral cap" of the infective larva treated with antibody.

Direct evidence for the protective nature of ES antigens was obtained by Thorson (1951, 1953). He conducted a series of protection tests using ES products of *N. muris* that had been collected *in vitro* and showed that ES products injected into rats induced resistance to a challenge infection. Furthermore, Thorson (1954) was able to absorb the protective fraction from immune sera using these same ES products. Similar results were obtained using the ES products derived from *A. caninum* (Thorson, 1956a) or the infective L_1 larva of *Trichinella* (Campbell, 1955). In the latter study, immunity was manifested by the rapid loss of adults from the intestine, the stunted growth of adult females, and a reduction in the number of larvae maturing in the muscles. Chipman (1957) extended these studies to the adult worm. In this case, immunization resulted in a slight but statistically significant reduction in the number of adults and a substantial reduction in the number of muscle larvae.

The composition of *Trichinella* ES products has been partically characterized. Mills and Kent (1965) found that they comprised both proteins and glycoproteins, and were resolved into four fractions by ion-exchange chromatography and three fractions by electrophoresis on cellulose acetate strips. Most or all of the antigens were heat-stable at 56°C for 1 hr. Crandall and Zam (1968) resolved the ES products of the infective L_1 larva into a minimum of 12 components employing a combination of polyacrylamide-disk electrophoresis and immunodiffusion. A minimum of 7 precipitin arcs were observed, and in most instances it was possible to correlate the arcs with stained protein bands in the disk gel.

The ES antigens of stages other than the infective L_1 larva have been less well studied. Berntzen (1974) maintained *Trichinella* in a defined medium, throughout its development from L_1 to adult, with α_1- and β_1-globulins as the only protein supplements. He collected the ES products at 3, 12, and 20 hr and at 8 days. Immunoelectrophoresis of these samples, developed with serum from twice-infected rats, yielded from 3 to 9 precipitin arcs. When all fractions were pooled and analyzed, 17 arcs were distinguished, further suggesting the stage specificity of the antigens.

Figures 1 and 2 show substantial differences between the ES antigens of infective L_1 larvae and those of adults, but also some possible similarities. Figure 1 shows the immunoelectrophoresis of L_1 ES antigens collected from 1 to 12 hr following digestion from the muscle (upper well) and adult antigens collected at 3 days (lower well). The pattern obtained from the L_1 antigens is more complex and different from that of the adults. It is possible that the few adult antigens detected share

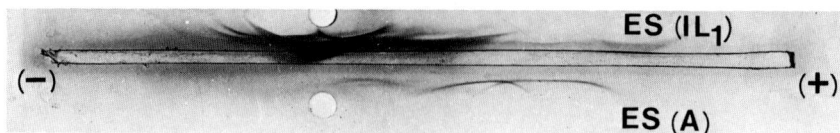

FIGURE 1. Immunoelectrophoresis comparing antigens in secretions from infective L_1 larvae [ES(IL1)] and adults [ES(A)].

identity with some of the L_1 antigens. A caveat must be issued, however, concerning the adult pattern. The antisera used to develop the pattern were raised in rabbits that were infected eight times. After the first infection, it is likely that few or no adults developed in the rabbit gut (see Wakelin and Lloyd, 1976). Therefore, most of the animals' exposure was to antigens from the larva. Of the antigens present in adult secretions, the ones most likely to be detected would be those, if any, that share identity with antigens of the larva. A more ideal immunization regimen for the study of adult antigens would be the repeated surgical

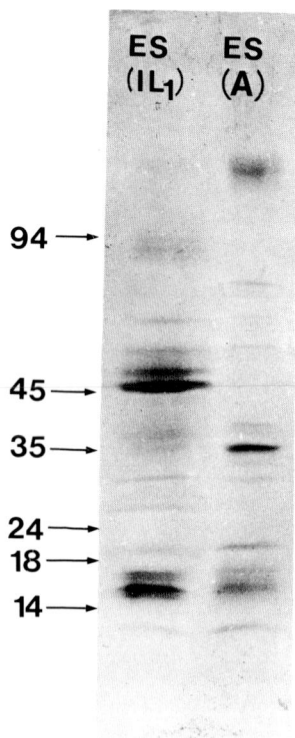

FIGURE 2. SDS-PAGE in a 7–20% gradient, comparing secretions from infective L_1 larvae [ES(IL$_1$)] and adults [ES(A)]. Arrows indicate molecular weights ($\times 10^{-3}$). From Despommier and Laccetti (unpublished).

implantation of adults in the host's gut with drug treatment before the beginning of larva production.

Figure 2 shows an analysis of the same ES samples in 7–20% gradient SDS-PAGE under nonreducing conditions. This system gives excellent resolution throughout the molecular-weight range of the antigens (see Despommier and Laccetti, 1981b). Several conclusions are suggested by this display. The ES products from both the infective L_1 larva and the adult worm have a complex protein composition. There are, however, pronounced differences between the two patterns in the higher-molecular-weight range. Of particular note is the absence of a band in the adult pattern equivalent to the 45-kd band in the larval pattern. Similarly, the pattern of the larva has no equivalent to the 33-kd band or the 120-kd band in the pattern of the adult. Other differences are also visible. In contrast, there are clear similarities between the patterns in the lower-molecular-weight range.

The anatomy of the infective L_1 larva, and to a lesser extent the adult, is dominated by the stichosome [for detailed structure of the stichosome, see Despommier (1974), Despommier and Müller (1976), and chapter 3]. That the stichosome is the source of the ES antigens from the infective larva is suggested by its structure (i.e., its dense granules and its secretory ducts leading to the esophagus). It is more strongly implicated as the source by its staining in tissue sections with fluorochrome- or enzyme-labeled antibody (Jackson, 1959; Crandall and Crandall, 1972; Despommier and Müller, 1976).

Studies on the isolation and characterization of stichocyte granules have been reported (Despommier and Müller, 1970, 1976). The study of antigens from these granules has three advantages over the study of ES products or extracts of crude homogenates. Substantial enrichment of the stichocyte antigens can be achieved, and the antigens can be collected in a brief time, at a low temperature. Moreover, if the antigens contain degradative enzymes, as Thorson found for *A. caninum*, isolation from the granules might capture them in the inactive form. This may very well contribute to the stability of the preparation, but at the same time might make it more difficult to discover the functions of the molecules. Differential centrifugation of homogenate of infective L_1 larvae resulted in a fraction (P_2) that was highly enriched in secretory granules, but also contained mitochondria and membrane fragments (Fig. 3). The P_2 fraction was washed and then treated with 2% Triton X100 to lyse the granules. The resulting soluble supernatant, designated the S_3 fraction, was shown by Ouchterlony analysis to contain all the antigens associated with an ES preparation from the same stage. There are two characteristic types of granules in the stichosome, designated

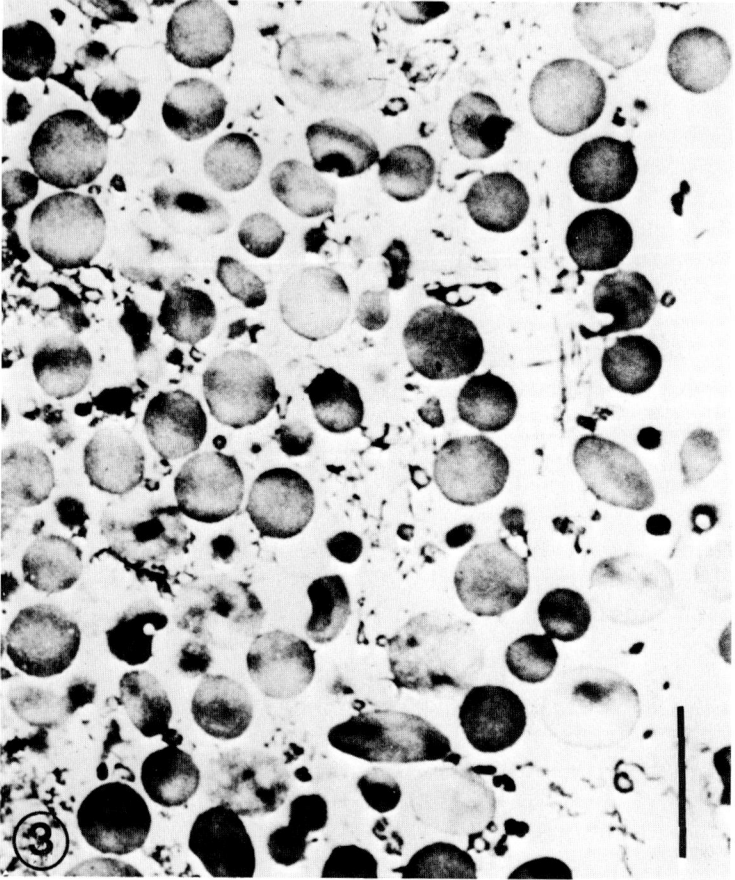

FIGURE 3. Electron micrograph of the P_2 fraction, showing prominent secretory granules. Scale bar: 1 μm. From Despommier (unpublished).

alpha and beta (see chapter 3). The authors described the features of each type in detail and were able to show that the antigens contained in each type do not cross-react.

The chemical composition of the S_3 fraction has been described by Despommier and Laccetti (1981a). It was resolved into six fractions by Sephacryl S-200 gel filtration. Electrophoresis in 10% SDS–polyacrylamide gels resolved a minimum of 28 proteins with molecular weights ranging from 11 to 200 kd. Analytical isoelectric focusing revealed 37 protein bands, 22 of which costained positive for carbohydrate. The glycoproteins were concentrated in the low end of the pH gradient. The S_3 fraction and several subfractions, which were prepared by isoelectric focusing in ionically neutral Sephadex, were shown to be strongly protective immunogens. The single most strongly protective subfraction was that with a *pI* of 4.3. This particular fraction was chosen for study because visible lines of focused material appeared in the Sephadex bed at this point, and therefore it was easy to cut the bands from the gel. Unfortunately, SDS-PAGE later showed this material to be heterogeneous with respect to protein composition.

Of the components in S_3, 20 were identified as antigens by immunoelectrophoresis and crossed immunoelectrophoresis. Despommier and Laccetti (1981b) were able to separate the antigens from nonantigens by immunoaffinity chromatography. The derived antigen preparation was designated pooled acid washes (PAW), and this fraction of S_3 was shown to contain strongly protective immunogens.

Immunoelectrophoresis (Fig. 4) showed that all antigens contained in a crude homogenate of larvae and in ES products of the infective L_1 larva are also contained in S_3 and PAW. Note, however, that the contaminating smear of protein cathodal to the crude antigen sample well is missing in the more refined preparations.

Figure 5 compares the same four preparations by electrophoresis in an SDS–polyacrylamide gradient gel. There are two points worth noting in Fig. 5. The first is the degree of the enrichment of antigens in the successive steps from crude homogenate to S_3 to PAW. The second is the similarity between ES products and PAW. A number of protein bands in the two preparations appear to have the same molecular

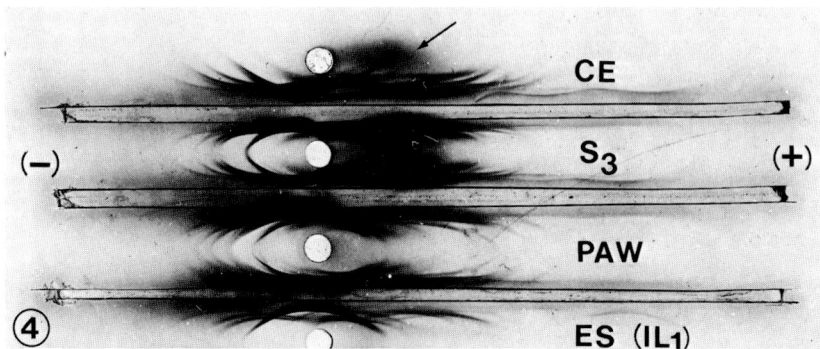

FIGURE 4. Immunoelectrophoresis comparing infective L_1 larva antigens contained in four preparations: crude extract (CE), S_3, PAW, and secretions [ES(IL)]. (←) Location in crude extract of contaminating nonantigen protein.

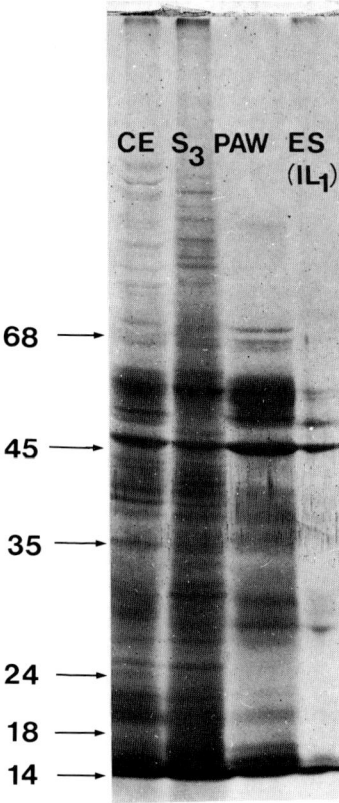

FIGURE 5. SDS-PAGE in a 7–20% gradient comparing proteins contained in four preparations from infective L_1 larvae: crude extract (CE), S_3, PAW, and secretions [ES(IL$_1$)]. Arrows indicate molecular weights ($\times 10^{-3}$).

weights and relative intensities. The latter piece of evidence argues in favor of the view that no substantial modification of antigens occurs as the result of secretion by the infective larva.

While the studies cited above demonstrate that antigens destined to be secreted can be derived via cell fractionation from a somatic source, they function in immunity as secretory products, and should be considered as such. Despommier and Müller (1976) made the point that the word "excretory" and the initial E should be dropped from the description of these antigens.

2.3. Somatic Antigens

In addition to specific immunofluorescence of the stichosome, Crandall and Crandall (1972) noted general staining of other internal structures, especially somatic cell membranes, by antibodies of the IgA and IgM classes. This finding is the only reported demonstration of internal somatic antigens. It remains unknown how these internal antigens reach the cells of the host's immune system.

3. ENUMERATION, ISOLATION, AND CHARACTERIZATION OF ANTIGENS

Accurate identification and enumeration of antigens depend on several facets of procedure. It is important to avoid preparative techniques that might degrade or denature antigens. While constraints of experimental design may require, for example, the use of organic solvents (Labzoffsky *et al.*, 1959) or prolonged incubations at warm temperature (e.g., for the collection of ES products), such procedures can interfere with analytical accuracy.

For the preparation of immune sera, animals should be hyperimmunized with the antigens that are relevant to the particular study. An inference available from the multitude of adult ES antigens in Fig. 2 and the dearth in Fig. 1 is that repeated oral infection does not generate strong antibodies against adult antigens. This is likely to be true for antigens of newborn larvae as well.

The third important procedural factor is the resolving power of the analytical technology. One way of increasing the resolving power is by the use of various configurations of two-dimensional electrophoresis. Figures 6 and 7 demonstrate this principle. In Fig. 6, it is possible to count, with some certainty, 20 *Trichinella* antigens. Figure 7 gives a clearer view of the antigens in the same sample, especially with regard to the identity or nonidentity of intersecting arcs (this figure does not show arcs for four antigens that are known to migrate cathodally).

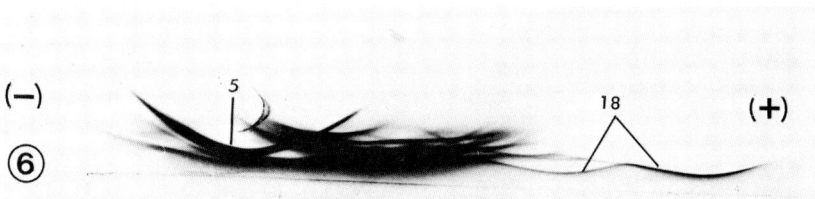

FIGURE 6. Immunoelectrophoresis showing antigens in S₃. Arcs 5 and 18 are numbered according to Despommier and Laccetti (1981a) and are described in the text. From Despommier (unpublished).

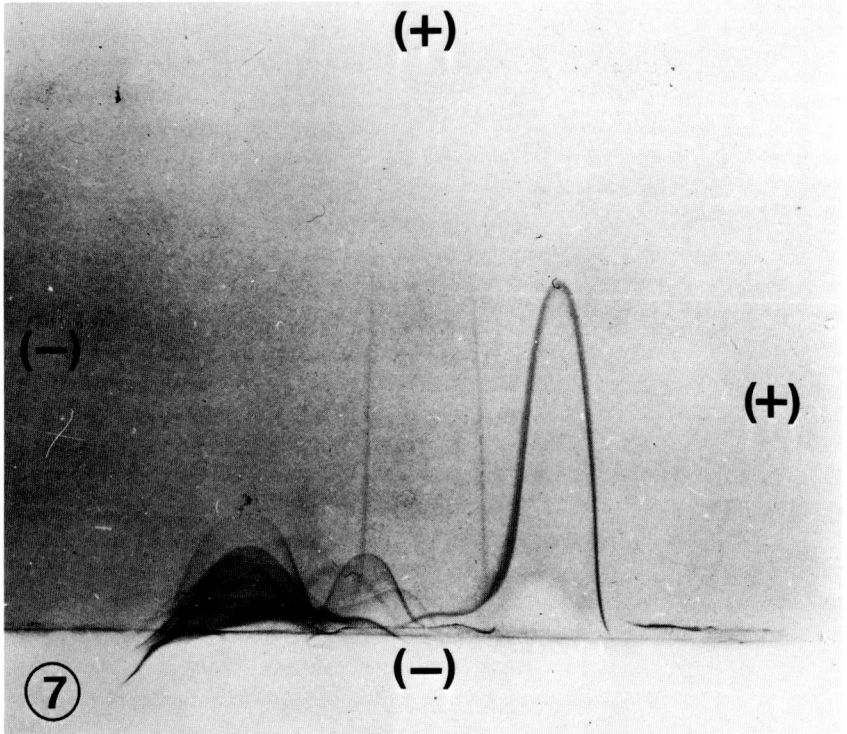

FIGURE 7. Crossed immunoelectrophoresis showing antigens in S_3. From Despommier (unpublished).

A more dramatic demonstration of the same principle is shown in Figs. 8 and 9. Figure 8 shows the resolution of more than 200 components from S_3 by two-dimensional electrophoresis (according to the method of O'Farrell *et al.*, 1977) where one-dimensional isoelectric focusing resolved only 37 components (Despommier and Laccetti, 1981a). Similarly, Fig. 9 demonstrates more than 50 components in PAW where one-dimensional SDS-PAGE resolved 20 (Despommier and Laccetti, 1981b).

It is likely that an even greater number of components could be detected in S_3 and PAW by more sensitive methods of staining. Ideally, one would like to incorporate radioactive label into all antigens and detect them in gels by autoradiography. To do this biosynthetically, by feeding labled nutrients to worms or infected hosts, would be difficult at best. To attach radioactive tags, such as ^{125}I, to all components in, for example, PAW incurs the risk of altering the physical and antigenic characteristics of the molecules beyond recognition. It might also be chemically difficult to do this for certain antigens, such as the *pI* 4.0 antigen, which is known to have little or no tryosine (Despommier, 1981a).

A simple way to increase the sensitivity of two-dimensional gel analysis would be to use the recently developed silver-based staining technique (Oakley *et al.*, 1980).

Many attempts have been made to characterize *T. spiralis* antigens biochemically. Some of these, not mentioned in the text, are described briefly in Table 1.

While many reports deal with complex antigens, there have been very few studies of single, purified antigens. Perrudet-Badoux and

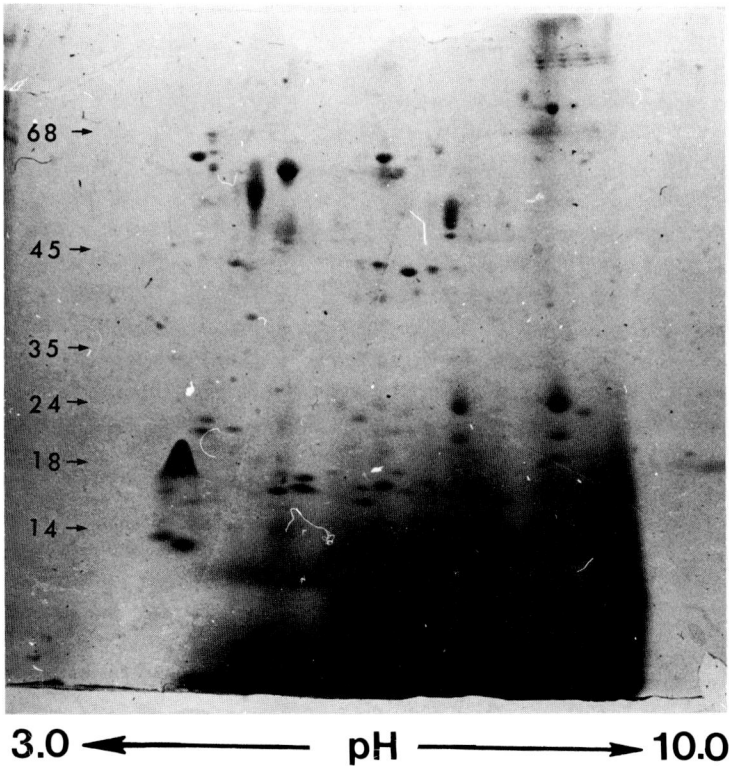

FIGURE 8. Two-dimensional display of components in S$_3$. Isoelectric focusing in a cylindrical gel in the horizontal dimension was followed by SDS-PAGE in a 7–20% gradient gel in the vertical dimension. Arrows indicate molecular weights ($\times 10^{-3}$). From Despommier and Laccetti (unpublished).

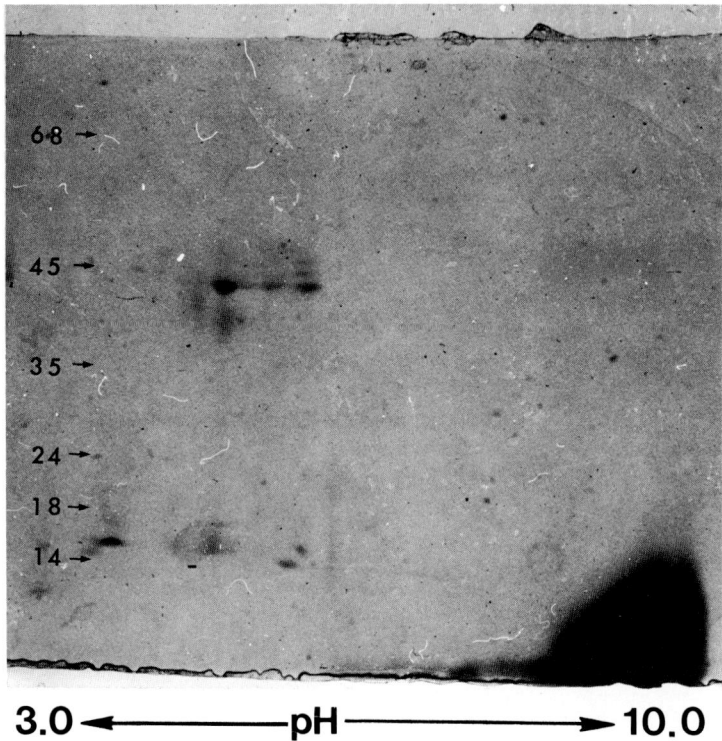

FIGURE 9. Two-dimensional display of components in PAW. Conditions were similar to those for Fig. 8. Arrows indicate molecular weights ($\times 10^{-3}$). From Despommier and Laccetti (unpublished).

Binaghi (1974) reported the isolation of a single *Trichinella* antigen with allergenic properties. They applied an extract of homogenized larvae to a diethylaminoethyl (DEAE)–Sephadex column at pH 8.0 in 0.005 M phosphate buffer. The fraction that did not adhere to the beads under these conditions yielded only one arc in immunoelectrophoresis and was designated protein A. Protein A was shown to stimulate IgE synthesis as determined by passive cutaneous anaphylaxis. This antigen had an apparent molecular weight of 12 kd as determined by G-100 Sephadex filtration. Its composition was measured as 70% protein and 30% carbohydrate. Unfortunately, the purity of this interesting antigen was not assessed by the conventional criteria.

Barriga and Segre (1974) used a sequence of ammonium sulfate precipitation, Sephadex filtration, and DEAE–cellulose chromatography to achieve a 45 fold enrichment of an antigen from the infective

L_1 larva. This antigen was designated antigen A. While no molecular characteristics of this antigen were measured, its electrophoretic mobility, prominent staining in immunoelectrophoresis, and elution from Sephadex suggest that it is the same as antigen 5 in Fig. 6, but different from the protein A isolated by Perrudet-Badoux and Binaghi. Barriga found his antigen to be rather sensitive and specific when used in immunodiagnosis.

Recently, Despommier and Laccetti (1981a,b) and Despommier (1981a) reported on the isolation and characterization of *Trichinella* antigens by physical and immunochemical methods. The rest of this section will be a summary of their results.

As noted earlier, fractionation of S_3 by Sephacryl S-200 gel filtration produced six peaks of material. Immunoelectrophoresis showed that most of the antigens were contained in peaks 3–5, while markers included with the chromatography and SDS-PAGE indicated that these peaks contained material ranging in molecular weight from 10 to 60 kd. Furthermore, the material in each peak was shown to be antigenically complex. Preparative isoelectric focusing of whole S_3 was not helpful in terms of absolute separation of antigens. On the other hand, focusing of the material in Sephacryl peak 4 led to the purification of two antigens. Analysis of the focused material in this gradient by fused-rocket immunoelectrophoresis indicated that large quantities of a single antigen were present in the pH 4.0 fraction. The antigen was collected and characterized in a number of ways. In immunoelectrophoresis, it is represented by arc 18 in Fig. 6. The shape of the arc suggests two components, moving with different mobilities, but sharing immunological identity. It was confirmed that this antigen exists in two forms by studying its elution profile in high-performance liquid chromatography. The antigen was applied to a column of silica gel to which an aliphatic (C = 18) side chain had been attached. It was then eluted isocratically with 65% acetonitrile in 0.1 N phosphoric acid. The elution profile showed two sharp peaks that exhibited total immunological identity, as judged by fused-rocket immunoelectrophoresis. Amino acid analysis showed no significant differences in the composition of the peaks. Since the antigens were not stained by periodic acid–Schiff's reagent, they probably do not contain carbohydrate. Therefore, the difference in the elution profile between the two peaks is unlikely to reflect microheterogeneity due to glycosylation. Moreover, dimerization or concatenation of peptide backbone cannot account for this difference, since both peaks elute in the same volume under gel filtration.

This antigen had a high content of aspartic acid (13%) and glutamic acid (18%) and a relatively low content of arginine (3%), lysine (3%), and histidine (3%). The ratio of acidic to basic amino acids accounts

TABLE 1
Biochemical Description of Some Antigen Preparations

References	Source	Components resolved	Characteristics
Bozicevich (1938)	Homogenized larvae	—	Stabile extracts, useful in immunodiagnosis.
Mauss (1941)	—	—	Forssman antigen present: elevated hemolysins in sera of infected rabbits.
Rose (1943)	—	—	Forssman antigen not present: normal titers of hemolysins in sera of 17 infected patients and 2 infected rabbits.
Melcher (1943)	Homogenized larvae	4	3 acid-soluble proteins and 1 carbohydrate; each induced precipitins in rabbits.
Aikawa et al. (1947)	Homogenized larvae	—	Sensitivity of skin test not destroyed by alkaline, tryptic digestion.
Wodehouse (1956)	Homogenized larvae	10	10 bands in two groups by double immunodiffusion; 5 nearest antigen source stable to 58°C for 1 hr and to tryptic digestion, unstable at 100°C; 5 nearest antibody source stable to 100°C, unstable to trypsin or autoclave.
Labzoffsky et al. (1959)	Lyophilized larvae	7	7 fractions isolated by differential solubility, all reactive in complement fixation.
Norman and Sadun (1959)	ES products of larvae	—	ES products of larvae useful in immunodiagnosis.

Reference	Material	Antigens	Notes
Sleeman and Mushel (1961), Sleeman (1961)	Homogenized larvae	2	Ethanol-soluble antigens (75% protein, 15% carbohydrate, all carbohydrate glucose units), ethanol-insoluble antigens (60% protein, 14% carbohydrate); both fractions function in complement fixation.
Tanner and Gregory (1961)	Intact larvae	11	Buffered saline extracts show 11 antigens by immunoelectrophoresis with immune rabbit serum.
Oliver-Gonzalez and de Sala (1963)	Homogenized larvae and adults	8–12 larvae 1–3 adults	Immunoelectrophoresis with immune rabbit serum.
Beltran-Hernandez et al. (1974)	Homogenized larvae	17	Acetone-insoluble, PBS-soluble extracts; 3 peaks by Sephadex G-100; 17 components by electrophoresis on cellulose strips.
Ermolin and Efremov (1974)	Sonicated larvae	19	19 components resolved by acrylamide-disk electrophoresis; a number of these react in double diffusion with immune sera from various animals.
Ermolin and Tarakanov (1974)	ES products of larvae, and homogenized larva	14 (ES) 17 (homog.)	14 (ES) or 17 (homogenate) protein components demonstrated by disk acrylamide electrophoresis and immunoelectrophoresis.
Barriga (1977)	Sonicated larvae	6	6 fractions by DEAE–cellulose chromatography of use in serodiagnosis.
Tronchin et al. (1979)	ES products of larvae	—	Immunization with ES products via oral route accelerates intestinal cellular response to challenge (inference: antigens resistant to gastric enzymes).

for the molecule's low isoelectric point. The antigen also had a very low content of aromatic amino acids (3% tyrosine and 1% phenylalanine) and, consequently, a very low absorbance at 280 nm.

Isoelectric focusing of peak 4 also permitted the isolation of a basic antigen, which has been less well characterized, with a *pI* of 9.0. This antigen was collected and tested in protective immunization experiments along with the *pI* 4.0 antigen. A third fraction, from *pI* 4.3 to 4.9, including seven antigens, was also tested. The results, summarized in Table 2, showed that all antigen preparations were effective immunogens to some degree, with the *pI* 4.0 antigen the least effective.

4. CONCLUDING REMARKS

The antigens from the infective L_1 larva have received much more attention than those from newborn larvae or adults. The reason is probably that the infective L_1 larva can be isolated from hosts in relatively large quantities. Twenty infected rats will yield a minimum of 20 ml of packed L_1 larvae, but less than 2 ml of adults, and a still smaller volume of newborns. Since the antigens represent only a small fraction of the protein present in *Trichinella*, and since any biochemical scheme of purification involves substantial losses of antigenic material, the high yield of infective L_1 larvae makes them attractive as a subject of study.

TABLE 2
Protective Immunization by Several Antigen Preparations[a]

Immunizing antigen	Reduction in muscle larvae (%)
CFA alone	0
S_3	88
PAW	86
Sephracryl peak 4 from S_3	88
pI 4.0 antigen	40
pI 4.3–4.9 fraction from peak 4 of S_3	64
pI 9.0 antigens	73

[a] Data from Despommier and Laccetti (1981a,b) and Despommier (1981a).

Very few antigens have been purified from the 50 or more components in the pooled acid washes and the others that may remain insoluble during extraction. Some of those that have been isolated have not been characterized in terms that permit their identification by other laboratories. The description of an isolated antigen should include the following minimum information: molecular weight, isoelectric point(s), protein and carbohydrate composition, and a detailed method for its purification. Any additional information on molecular characteristics would obviously also be helpful.

Because very few antigens have been described, it is difficult to draw any conclusions with respect to the four areas of investigation that were outlined in section 1. Of these four, the greatest difficulty may lie in the discovery of the antigen's function for the parasite. To evaluate function, certain preliminary information is necessary, but probably not sufficient. This includes the location of the antigen in the parasite, the time in development that the antigen appears, and any dimorphism or modification of the antigen that may occur during development (i.e., glycosylation or cleavage accompanying secretion). It would be a more difficult, but also informative, endeavor to screen purified antigens for enzyme activity.

For the same reason, i.e., the lack of characterized antigens, it is difficult to learn how antigens contribute to immunity. While support for a model of immunity will require more data than exist at present, the preliminary conclusion, from protection tests with the pI 4.0 and 9.0 antigens, is that some antigens are more effective immunogens than others. It remains unknown whether this has to do with the antigens' functions for the parasite, their presentation by the parasite, or the nature of the immune response they provoke.

Similarly, the lack of purified single antigens makes it difficult to study the modulating effects antigens have on the immune response, and whether they would be useful in immunodiagnosis. It is hoped that future studies will attend to these problems.

ACKNOWLEDGMENTS. The author gratefully acknowledges the helpful discussion and suggestions from Dr. Dickson D. Despommier, comments and assistance with the preparation of the manuscript from Ms. Mary M. MacLeod, and assistance with editing and typing the manuscript from Ms. Terri Terrilli. The author also wishes to thank Dr. Despommier and Mr. Anthony J. Laccetti for permission to cite unpublished data.

REFERENCES

Aikawa, J.K., Harrell, G.T., and Helsabeck, N.J., 1947, The effect of peptic and tryptic digestion on the antigenicity of *Trichinella spiralis, J. Clin. Invest.* **26**(1):73–76.

Barriga, O.O., 1975, Selective immunodepression in mice by *Trichinella spiralis* extracts and infections, *Cell. Immunol.* **17**:306–309.

Barriga, O.O., 1977, Reactivity and specificity of *Trichinella spiralis* fractions in cutaneous and serological tests, *J. Clin. Microbiol.* **6**(3):274–279.

Barriga, O.O., and Segre, D., 1974, Diagnosis of trichinellosis by hemagglutination with a purified larval antigen, in: *Trichinellosis* (C.W. Kim ed.), Intext, New York, pp. 421–441.

Bell, R.G., and McGregor, D.D., 1979a, *Trichinella spiralis*: Expression of rapid expulsion in rats exposed to abbreviated enteral infection, *Exp. Parasitol.* **48**:42–50.

Bell, R.G., and McGregor, D.D., 1979b, *Trichinella spiralis*: Role of different life cycle phases in induction, maintenance, and expression in rapid expulsion in rats, *Exp. Parasitol.* **48**:51–60.

Berntzen, A.K., 1974, Effects of environment on the growth and development of *Trichinella spiralis in vitro*, in: *Trichinellosis* (C.W. Kim, ed.), Intext, New York, pp. 25–30.

Bozicevich, J., 1938, Studies on trichinosis. XII. The preparation and use of an improved trichina antigen, *Public Health Rep.* **53**(48):2130–2138.

Campbell, C.H., 1955, The antigenic role of excretions and secretions of *Trichinella spiralis* in the production of immunity in mice, *J. Parasitol.* **51**:185–194.

Castro, G.A., Malon, C., and Smith, S., 1980, Systemic anti-inflammatory effect associated with enteric trichinellosis in the rat, *J. Parasitol.* **66**(3):407–412.

Chitwood, B.G., 1930, The structure of the esophagus in the Trichuroidea, *J. Parasitol.* **17**:35–42.

Chipman, P.B., 1957, The antigenic role of excretions and secretions of adult *Trichinella spiralis* in the production of immunity in mice, *J. Parasitol.* **43**(6):593–598.

Chute, R.M., 1956, The dual antibody response to experimental trichinosis, *Proc. Helminthol. Soc.* **23**(1):49–58.

Crandall, R.B., and Crandall, C.A., 1972, *Trichinella spiralis*: Immunologic response to infection in mice, *Exp. Parasitol.* **31**:378–398.

Crandall, R.B., and Zam, S.G., 1968, Analysis of excretory–secretory products of *Trichinella spiralis* by disc-electrophoresis and immunodiffusion, *Am. J. Trop. Med. Hyg.* **17**(5):747–751.

Crum, E.D., Despommier, D.D., and McGregor, D.D., 1977, Immunity to *Trichinella spiralis*. I. Transfer of resistance by two classes of lymphocytes, *Immunology* **33**:787–795.

Despommier, D.D., 1971, Immunogenicity of the newborn larva of *Trichinella spiralis, J. Parasitol.* **57**(3):531–535.

Despommier, D.D., 1974, The stichocyte of Trichinella spiralis during morphogenesis in the small intestine of the rat, in *Trichinellosis* (C.W. Kim, ed.), Intext Educational Publishers, New York, pp. 187–198.

Despommier, D.D., 1981a, Partial purification and characterization of protection-inducing antigens from the muscle larva of *Trichinella spiralis* by molecular sizing chromatography and preparative flatbed isoelectric focusing, *Parasite Immunol.* **3**:261–272.

Despommier, D.D., 1981b, Serodiagnosis of *Trichinella spiralis*, in: *Serodiagnosis of Parasitic Infections* (K. Walls, ed.), Marcel Dekker, New York (in press).

Despommier, D.D., and Laccetti, A., 1981a, *Trichinella spiralis*: Proteins and antigens isolated from a large-particle fraction derived from the muscle larva, *Exp. Parasitol.* **51**:279–295.

Despommier, D.D., and Laccetti, A., 1981b, *Trichinella spiralis*: Partial characterization of antigens isolated by immuno-affinity chromatography from the large-particle fraction of the muscle larva, *J. Parasitol.* **67**(3):332–339.

Despommier, D.D., and Müller, M., 1970, The stichosome of *Trichinella spiralis*: Its structure and function, *J. Parasitol.* **56**(Sect. II, Part I):76.

Despommier, D.D., and Müller, M., 1976, The stichosome and its secretion granules in the mature muscle larva of *Trichinella spiralis*, *J. Parasitol.* **62**(5):775–785.

Despommier, D.D., Kajima, M., and Wostman, S., 1967, Ferritin-conjugated antibody studies on the larva of *Trichinella spiralis*, *J. Parasitol.* **53**:618–624.

Despommier, D.D., Campbell, W.C., and Blair, L.S., 1977a, The *in vivo* and *in vitro* analysis of immunity to *Trichinella spiralis* in mice and rats, *Parasitology* **74**:109–119.

Despommier, D.D., McGregor, D.D., Crum, E.D., and Carter, P.B., 1977b, Immunity to *Trichinella spiralis*. II. Expression of immunity against adult worms, *Immunology* **33**:797–805.

Dessein, A.J., Parker, W.L., James, S.L., and David, J.R., 1981, IgE antibody and resistance to infection. I. Selective suppression of the IgE antibody response in rats diminishes the resistance and the eosinophil response to *Trichinella spiralis* infection, *J. Exp. Med.* **153**:423–436.

Ermolin, G.A., and Efremov, E.E., 1974, Isolation and purification of the main functional antigen from decapsulated Trichinella spiralis, in *Trichinellosis* (C.W. Kim, ed.), Intext, New York, pp. 187–198.

Ermolin, G.A., and Tarakanov, V.I., 1974, The antigens of *Trichinella spiralis* larvae incubated and cultivated under *in vitro* conditions, in: *Trichinellosis* (C. W. Kim, ed.), Intext, New York, pp. 199–206.

Faubert, G.M., and Tanner, C.E., 1971, *Trichinella spiralis*: Inhibition of sheep hemagglutinins in mice, *Exp. Parasitol.* **30**:120–123.

Gadea, D., Moore, L.L.A., and Oliver-Gonzalez, J., 1967, Adsorption of globulin to the cuticle of larvae and adults of *Trichinella spiralis*, *Am. J. Trop. Med. Hyg.* **16**(6):750–751.

Ishizaka, T., Urban, J.F., Takatsu, K., and Ishizaka, K., 1976, Immunoglobulin E synthesis in parasitic infection, *J. Allergy Clin. Immunol.* **58**:523–538.

Jackson, G.J., 1959, Fluorescent antibody studies of *Trichinella spiralis* infections, *J. Infect. Dis.* **105**(2):97–117.

James, E.R., and Denham, D.A., 1975, Antigenicity of the newborn larva of *Trichinella spiralis*, *J. Parasitol.* **61**(2):354.

James, E.R., Moloney, A., and Denham, D.A., 1977, Immunity to *Trichinella spiralis*. VII. Resistance stimulated by the parenteral stages of the infection, *J. Parasitol.* **63**(4):720–723.

Jones, J.F., Crandall, C.A., and Crandall, R.B., 1976, T-dependent suppression of the preliminary antibody response to sheep erythrocytes in mice infected with *Trichinella spiralis*, *Cell. Immunol.* **27**:102–110.

Kazura, J.W., and Grove, D.I., 1978, Stage-specific antibody-dependent eosinophil-mediated destruction of *Trichinella spiralis*, *Nature* (*London*) **274**(5671):588–589.

Kim, C.W., and Ledbetter, M.C., 1981, Detection of specific antigen–antibody precipitates on the surface of *Trichinella spiralis* by scanning electron microscopy, in: *Trichinellosis* (C.W. Kim, E.J. Ruitenberg, and J.S. Teppema, eds.), Reedbooks, Chertsey, England, pp. 65–69.

Labzoffsky, N.A., Kuitunen, E., Morrissey, L.P., and Hamvas, J.J., 1959, Studies on the antigenic structure of *Trichinella spiralis* larvae, *Can. J. Microbiol.* **5**:395–403.

Ljungström, I., 1980, Studies on the responsiveness of spleen cells to various T and B cell activators during *Trichinella spiralis* infection, *Parasite Immunol.* **2**:111–120.

Ljungström, I., Holmgren, J., Huldt, G., Lange, S., and Svennerbolm, A.M., 1981, Effect of *Trichinella spiralis* on the immune responsiveness to cholera toxin, in: *Trichinellosis* (C.W. Kim, E.J. Ruitenberg, and J.S. Teppema, eds.), Reedbooks, Chertsey, England, pp. 169–174.

Love, R.J., Ogilvie, B.M., and McLaren, D.J., 1976, The immune mechanism which expels the intestinal stage of *Trichinella spiralis* from rats, *Immunology* **30:**7–15.

Mackenzie, C.D., Jungery, M., Taylor, P.M., and Ogilvie, B.M., 1980, Activation of complement, the induction of antibodies to the surface of nematodes and the effect of these factors and cells on worm survival *in vitro*, *Eur. J. Immunol.* **10:**594–601.

Mauss, E.A., 1941, Occurence of Forssman heterogenetic antigen in the nematode *Trichinella spiralis*, *J. Immunol.* **16:**259–273.

McLaren, D.J., Mackenzie, C.D., and Ramalho-Pinto, F.J., 1977, Ultrastructural observations on the *in vitro* interaction between rat eosinophils and some parasitic helminths, *Clin. Exp. Immunol.* **30:**105–118.

Melcher, L.R., 1943, An antigenic analysis of *Trichinella spiralis*, *J. infect. Dis.* **73:**31–39.

Mills, C.K., and Kent, N.H., 1965, Excretions and secretions of *Trichinella spiralis* and their role in immunity, *Exp. Parasitol.* **16**(3):300–310.

Molinari, J.A., and Ebersole, J.L., 1977, Antineoplastic effects of long-term *Trichinella spiralis* infection on B-16 melanoma, *Int. Arch. Allergy Appl. Immunol.* **55:**444–448.

Moore, L.L.A., 1965, Studies in mice on the immunogenicity of cuticular antigens from larvae of *Trichinella spiralis*, *J. Elisha Mitchell Sci. Soc.* **81**(2):137–143.

Norman, L., and Sadun, E.H., 1959, The use of metabolic antigens in the flocculation tests for the serologic diagnosis of trichinosis, *J. Parasitol.* **45:**485–489.

Oakley, B.R., Kirsch, D.R., and Morris, N.R., 1980, A simplified ultrasensitive silver stain for detecting proteins in polyacrylamide gels, *Anal. Biochem.* **105:**361–363.

O'Farrell, P.Z., Goodman, H.M., and O'Farrell, P.H., 1977, High resolution two dimensional electrophoresis of basic as well as acidic proteins, *Cell* **12:**1133–1142.

Ogilvie, B.M., and Jones, V.E., 1973, Immunity in the parasitic relationship between helminth and hosts, *Prog. Allergy* **17:**93.

Oliver-Gonzalez, J., 1940, The *in vitro* action of immune serum on the larvae and adults of *Trichinella spiralis*, *J. Infect. Dis.* **67:**292–300.

Oliver-Gonzalez, J., 1941, The dual antibody basis of acquired immunity in trichinosis, *J. Infect. Dis.* **69:**254–270.

Oliver-Gonzalez, J., and de Sala, A.R., 1963, Immunoelectrophoretic analysis of adults and larvae of *Trichinella spiralis*, *Am. J. Trop. Med. Hyg.* **12**(4):539–540.

Perrudet-Badoux, A., and Binaghi, R.A., 1974, Isolation and properties of a soluble antigen of *Trichinella spiralis*, *Immunology* **26:**1217–1223.

Perrudet-Badoux, A., Anteunis, A., Dunitrescu, S.M., and Binaghi, R.A., 1978, Ultrastructural study of the immune interaction between peritoneal cells of larvae of *Trichinella spiralis*, *J. Reticuloendothel. Soc.* **24**(3):311–314.

Philipp, M., Parkhouse, R.M.E., and Ogilvie, B.M., 1980, Changing proteins on the surface of a parasitic nematode, *Nature (London)* **287:**538–540.

Philipp, M., Parkhouse, R.M.E., and Ogilvie, B.M., 1981, The molecular basis for stage specificity of the primary antibody response to the surface of *Trichinella spiralis*, in: *Trichinellosis* (C.W. Kim, E.J. Ruitenberg, and J.S. Teppema, eds.), Reedbooks, Chertsey, England, pp. 59–64.

Rose, H.M., 1943, On the occurrence of Forssman antigen in *Trichinella spiralis*, *J. Immunol.* **47**(1):53–57.

Ruitenberg, E.J., and Steerenberg, P.A., 1976, Immunogenicity of the parenteral stages of *Trichinella spiralis*, *J. Parasitol.* **62**(1):164–166.

Ruitenberg, E.J., Kruizinga, W., Steerenberg, P.A., Elgersma, A., and de Jong, W.H., 1981, The role of histamine-2-receptor bearing cells in the immuno-modulation caused by *Trichinella spiralis*, in: *Trichinellosis* (C.W. Kim, E. J. Ruitenberg, and J.S. Teppema, eds.), Reedbooks, Chertsey, England, pp. 147–152.

Sadun, E.H., Mota, I., and Gore, R.W., 1968, Demonstration of homocytotropic reagin-like antibodies in mice and rabbits infected with *Trichinella spiralis*, *J. Parasitol.* **54:**814–821.

Sleeman, H.K., 1961, Studies on complement fixing antigens isolated from *Trichinella spiralis* larvae. II. Chemical analysis, *Am. J. Trop. Med. Hyg.* **10**(6):834–838.

Sleeman, H.K., and Mushel, L.H., 1961, Studies on complement fixing antigens isolated from *Trichinella spiralis*. I. Isolation, purification and evaluation as diagnostic reagents, *Am. J. Trop. Med. Hyg.* **10**(6):821–823.

Soulsby, E.J.L., 1963, The nature and origin of the functional antigens in helminth infections, *Ann. N. Y. Acad. Sci.* **113:**492–509.

Stankiewicz, M., and Jeska, E.L., 1973, Leukocytes and *Trichinella spiralis, Immunology* **25:**827–834.

Stromberg, B.E., 1979, IgE and IgG1 antibody production by a soluble product of *Ascaris suum* in the guinea pig, *Immunology* **38:**489–495.

Sulzer, A.J., 1965, Indirect fluorescent antibody tests for parasitic diseases. I. Preparation of a stable antigen from larvae of *Trichinella spiralis, J. Parasitol.* **51**(5):717–721.

Taliaferro, W.H., and Sarles, M.P., 1939, The cellular reactions in the skin, lungs and intestine of normal and immune rats after infection with *Nippostrongylus muris, J. Infect. Dis.* **64:**157–192.

Tanner, C.E., Lim, H.C., and Faubert, G., 1978, *Trichinella spiralis*: Changes caused in the mouse's thymic, splenic, and lymph node cell populations, *Exp. Parasitol.* **45:**116–127.

Tanner, C.E., Ghadurian, E., Ulczak, O.M., and Lim, H.C., 1981, B-cell responses in experimental Trichinellosis, in: *Trichinellosis* (C.W. Kim, E.J. Ruitenberg, and J.S. Teppema, eds.), Reedbooks, Chertsey, England, pp. 159–162.

Taylor, S.M., Mallon, T., and Davidson, W.B., 1980, The micro-ELISA for antibodies to *Trichinella spiralis*: Elimination of false positive reactions by antigen fractionation and technical improvements, *Zentralbl. Vet. Med.* **27:**764–772.

Thorson, R.E., 1951, The relation of secretions and excretions of larvae of *Nippostrongylus muris* in the production of protective antibodies, *J. Parasitol.* **37**(Suppl.):18–19.

Thorson, R.E., 1953, Studies on the mechanism of immunity to the rat nematode *Nippostrongylus muris, Am. J. Hyg.* **58:**1–15.

Thorson, R.E., 1954, Absorption of the protective antibodies from the serum of rats immune to the nematode *Nippostrongylus muris, J. Parasitol.* **40:**300–303.

Thorson, R.E., 1956a, Proteolytic activity in extracts of the esophagus of adults of *Ancylostoma caninum* and the effect of immune serum on this activity, *J. Parasitol.* **42:**21–25.

Thorson, R.E., 1956b, The stimulation of acquired immunity in dogs by injections of extracts of the esophagus of adult hookworms, *J. Parasitol.* **42:**501–504.

Tronchin, G., Dutoit, E., Vernes, A., and Biguet, J., 1979, Oral immunization of mice with metabolic antigens of *Trichinella spiralis* larvae: Effects on the kinetics of intestinal cell response including mast cells and polymorphonuclear eosinophils, *J. Parasitol.* **65**(5):685–691.

Urban, J.F., Ishizaka, T., and Ishizaka, K., 1977a, IgE formation in the rat following infection with *Nippostrongylus brasiliensis*. II. Proliferation of IgE bearing cells in neo-natally thymectomized animals, *J. Immunol.* **118:**1982–1986.

Urban, J.F., Ishizaka, T., and Ishizaka, K., 1977b, Soluble factor for the generation of IgE bearing lymphocytes, *J. Immunol.* **119:**583–590.

Urban, J.F., Ishizaka, T., and Ishizaka, K., 1978, IgE B-cell generating factor from lymph node cells of rats infected with *Nippostrongylus brasiliensis*. I. Source of IgE B-cell generating factor, *J. Immunol.* **121:**192–198.

Urban, J.E., Ishizaka, K., and Bazin, H., 1980, IgE B-cell generating factor from lymph node cells of rats infected with *Nippostrongylus brasiliensis*. III. Regulation of factor formation by anti-immunoglobulin, *J. Immunol.* **124:**527–532.

Vernes, A., Poulain, D., Prensier, G., Deblock, S., Biguet, J., and Wattez, A., 1974, Trichinose experimentale. III. Action *in vitro* des cellules peritoneales sensibilisées sur les larves musculaires des premier stade: Étude préliminaire comparative en microscopie optique et electronique a transmission et balayage, *Biomedicine* **21:**140–145.

Wakelin, D., and Donachie, A.M., 1980, Genetic control of immunity to parasites: Adoptive transfer of immunity between inbred strains of mice characterized by rapid and slow immune expulsion of *Trichinella spiralis*, *Parasite Immunol.* **2(4):**249–260.

Wakelin, D., and Lloyd, M., 1976, Immunity to primary and challenge infections of *Trichinella spiralis*: A re-examination of conventional parameters, *Parasitology* **72:**173–182.

Wakelin, D., and Selby, G.R., 1973, Functional antigens of *Trichuris muris*: The stimulation of immunity by vaccination of mice with somatic antigen preparations, *Int. J. Parasitol.* **3:**711–715.

Wakelin, D., and Wilson, M.W., 1979a, *Trichinella spiralis*: Immunity and inflammation in the expulsion of transplanted adult worms from mice, *Exp. Parasitol.* **48:**305–312.

Wakelin, D., and Wilson, M.W., 1979b, T and B cells in the transfer of immunity against *Trichinella spiralis* in mice, *Immunology* **37(1):**103–109.

Wodehouse, R.P., 1956, Antigenic analysis and standardization of *Trichinella* extract by gel diffusion, *Ann. Allergy* **14(2):**121–138.

Yodoi, J., and Ishizaka, K., 1980, Lymphocytes bearing Fc receptors for IgE. IV. Formation of IgE-binding factor by rat T lymphocytes, *J. Immunol.* **124(3):**1322–1329.

Yodoi, J., Ishizaka, T., and Ishizaka, K., 1979, Lymphocytes bearing Fc receptors for IgE. II. Induction of Fc-epsilon receptor-bearing rat lymphocytes by IgE, *J. Immunol.* **124(1):**455–462.

10

Chemotherapy

WILLIAM C. CAMPBELL and DAVID A. DENHAM

1. INTRODUCTION

It is hardly surprising that soon after *Trichinella spiralis* was shown to be a human pathogen, assaults were made on it with all sorts of chemical weapons. For the most part, they were not deadly weapons (at least with respect to the parasite). Patients were treated with benzene, carbolic acid, garlic, arsenicals, mercurials, and many other natural and unnatural products. It is perhaps fortunate that the early exploratory trials were unsuccessful, or at best equivocal, so that these medications never became the drugs of choice for trichinosis.

In modern times, drugs with unequivocal, if not ideal, efficacy have been found. This chapter deals with these drugs and with methods for demonstrating efficacy against *Trichinella* in the laboratory. An earlier review (Campbell and Blair, 1974) dealt not only with active drugs, but also with inactive drugs and unacceptable drugs of doubtful efficacy. This review excludes such chemotherapeutic jetsam, but brief mention will be made of some compounds that offer no utility with respect to trichinosis but that are, for various reasons, of some interest in this context. The subject has also been reviewed in English by Zaiman (1970) and in Romanian by Lupascu *et al.* (1970).

Drugs are referred to herein by generic, nonproprietary names, although in some instances it has been considered helpful to provide

WILLIAM C. CAMPBELL • Merck Institute for Therapeutic Research, Rahway, New Jersey 07065. DAVID A. DENHAM • London School of Hygiene and Tropical Medicine, London WC1E 7HT, England.

proprietary names in addition, especially where a proprietary product is approved for use in man. The literature on trichinosis is replete with reports in which proprietary names are used without corresponding generic names, a practice greatly to be deplored.

2. EXPERIMENTAL CHEMOTHERAPY

Perhaps due as much to the ease with which *Trichinella* can be handled in the laboratory as to anything else, there is a large and expanding literature on the experimental chemotherapy of *Trichinella* infections in rodents. Because of the complications of having an intestinal and an extraintestinal phase, and two generations existing in the same individual and overlapping in time, much confusion can exist over the interpretation of the apparent effects of treatment on infection. This problem is considered later.

2.1. Methods

2.1.1. Primary Screening for Efficacy against Trichinella

Trichinella is occasionally used in anthelmintic screens as an experimental target representative of parasites dwelling in the extraintestinal tissues. Rarely is it used in primary screening programs as an example of an intestinal parasite, or as a chemotherapeutic target in its own right.

As discussed in Section 2.2.2, the immature and mature enteral stages are differentially susceptible to various classes of anthelmintics. As a generalization, compounds that affect the immature enteral stages are also active against the developing and even encysted parenteral phase. To circumvent the problem of differential susceptibility, compounds could be screened for activity against *Trichinella* by infecting the animals (presumably mice) with a moderate number of larvae and then treating them for the next 35 days. Activity against any stage of the parasite would then be indicated by a reduction in the number of larvae found in muscle digests on subsequent necropsy. However, this regime would be lengthy and very prodigal of labor and compound. Alternative strategies could be adopted depending on the objective of the screen. If, for example, activity against extraintestinal parasites were of only secondary interest, a reasonable compromise would be to treat from the time of infection until the 5th day and then count muscle larvae on day 28 or 35. This system would allow detection of lethal effects on all the preadult and adult stages, as well as chemosterilant effects on the adults, and, as will be seen later, is likely to select compounds that affect the extraintestinal stages, since compounds that kill juvenile intestinal worms are often active against the muscle stages.

All known anti-*Trichinella* compounds are active on oral administration, with the exception of methyridine, which has little or no activity when given by this route. In a primary screening program, oral administration (by gavage or dietary medication) would be a reasonable choice, but the selection of any one route will necessarily involve some risk of missing potentially active compounds.

An *in vitro* test, in which test compounds are added to a medium containing decapsulated muscle larvae, has recently been described (Jenkins and Carrington, 1981). It is designed to detect activity against the muscle stage of *T. spiralis* and is intended to be used for primary empirical screening. It was found capable of demonstrating not only activity against the muscle stage, but also the activity (albeit at rather high concentration) of compounds known only to have activity *in vivo* against the intestinal stages. This is hardly surprising, since larvae are incubated for 4 days at 37°C in a complex culture medium, which permits development of the worms to the point at which their movement becomes undulating rather than coiling. The test is done in plastic multichambered dishes, with each chamber containing 50 larvae in 2.0 ml medium. Any abnormal behavior of the larvae (usually paralysis or death) is indicative of drug efficacy. The test is highly successful in demonstrating the efficacy of known anti-*Trichinella* compounds (see Section 2.2.1).

2.1.2. Methods for Evaluating Efficacy against Intestinal Stages

The effect of a test compound on the enteral stages of *Trichinella* is easily determined. Mice have been used almost exclusively for this purpose, but Vanparijs *et al.* (1979) have used rats. Since there is such a profound difference in the response to treatment by the immature and mature enteral stages (see Section 2.2.2), the action of the compounds upon these stages must be differentiated. This can be done simply by infecting a group of mice, setting aside some untreated controls, and treating half the remaining mice when the infection is unequivocally immature (say, 2–6 hr after inoculation) and half when the infection is unequivocally mature (say, 5 days after inoculation). It is convenient to use single gavage treatment, with the drug being given in a range of dosages, using doubling dilutions of the drug preparation.

Depending on how much is previously known about the safety and biological activity of the test compound, such experiments can yield an acceptable dose–response curve with greater or lesser efficiency. In any case, additional experiments, using higher or lower dosages, may be required to obtain a good dose–response relationship.

Multiple treatment schedules will give acceptable results if treatment is started after day 3 of infection, when the worms are adult, since there can then be no confusion as to which stage of the parasite is affected. If treatment were given on, for example, days 1, 2, 3, and 4 of infection, one would not know whether any subsequent reduction in worm burden was due to drug action on the preadult or adult worms. It is possible that a drug would fail to act at either of the suggested treatment times (i.e., 2–6 hr and 5 days after infection) and yet be effective when given at other times or on several days. We do not know of any drug with this type of activity, and such a drug would in any case have little or no chemotherapeutic utility.

The third factor to be considered with respect to the enteral phase is the possible effect of a drug on worm fecundity. A reduction in fecundity can readily be demonstrated so long as precautions are taken to ensure that the effect is not confused with certain other anthelmintic effects. For example, mice may be treated during the enteral phase, and subsequent necropsy and digestion of host musculature may show an absence of larvae in the tissue. This, however, is not enough. It must also be shown, preferably in the same experiment, that the treatment in question does not reduce the number of adult worms and does not have a lethal effect on the newborn and developing larvae, and this requires sequential killing of treated and untreated mice until expulsion is complete. If these conditions have been met, the absence of larvae in the musculature can be attributed to a suppression of larviposition. In such experiments, some mice should be necropsied during the enteral phase and the females examined microscopically; in mice treated with certain drugs, the uterus of female worms from treated mice is conspicuously empty (Campbell and Cuckler, 1964), indicating a block-ade of the reproductive process. An alternative approach to the fe-cundity question would be to collect adult worms from treated mice, incubate them *in vitro*, and count the number of first-stage larvae produced. If there is an effect of the test compound on fecundity, there should be a lower (or conceivably a higher) production of newborn larvae per female worm in culture.

It is thus technically quite simple to evaluate and quantify the effects of a compound on the survival of immature and mature enteral stages and on worm fecundity.

2.1.3. Methods for Evaluating Efficacy against Extraintestinal Stages

Compounds can be tested directly against extraintestinal larvae *in vitro*, and in theory, newborn larvae, harvested from lymph, could be used as well as more developed larvae harvested from muscle. If infective muscle larvae are used, and if the test conditions permit even partial development *in vitro*, as in the test described by Jenkins and Carrington (Section 2.1.1), then the test organisms could be considered representative of intestinal rather than extraintestinal forms. It is simple to determine whether or not a compound is active *in vivo* against fully developed encysted larvae. Treatment is given when all larvae are known to have become infective and encysted—this would normally be 35 days after infection (although some larvae will have reached that stage much earlier). The host musculature is subsequently digested and the number of larvae counted. Lethal effects will be evidenced by reduced numbers of larvae. Light- and electron-microscopic studies can be used to document the disintegration of parasite and capsule, although such studies will not usually be undertaken until efficacy has been detected by larval counts. Sublethal effects may also be demonstrated; for example, larvae recovered from treated animals may be noninfective when inoculated into other animals.

Problems arise when one wishes to determine the effect of treatment on developing larvae, that is, muscle-dwelling larvae that have not yet attained their full size and that live in relatively thin-walled nurse cells. A popular way of doing this has been to treat infected animals during the period from 10 to 20 days after infection. If it has been shown that the test compound has absolutely no action on the survival or fecundity of adult worms (or that the female worms have been expelled prior to treatment), this is probably reasonable, but these criteria are rarely if ever satisfied. Treating while the larva-producing adults are in the gut means that treatment could affect adult survival or fecundity, the migrating newborn larvae, or early- to late-developing muscle larvae.

Fortunately, there are two methods of attacking this problem.

Methyridine is virtually 100% efficacious against enteral *Trichinella* (Denham, 1965), but appears to have no effect on developing muscle larvae. If animals are treated with methyridine after the start of larval production, the adult worms will be removed and the larvae produced by that time will go on to encyst and can be counted. Denham and Martinez (1970) used this technique to study the rate at which larvae were produced, and subsequently the method was used to study the effects of a number of benzimidazoles on developing *Trichinella* (Duckett and Denham, 1970; Fernando and Denham, 1976; Aboul-Atta and

Denham, 1978; Karunakaran and Denham, 1980). To test a drug against the early muscle phase, a large group of mice is infected with 400 *Trichinella* larvae and treated 7 days later with 2 × 500 mg/kg of methyridine by subcutaneous injection. A group of mice is left without further treatment and the remainder treated with different regimes of the test compound. The host musculature is digested 35 days after infection and larvae counted. If the test drug is effective against developing larvae, there will be fewer larvae in the mice treated with methyridine plus test drug than in the mice treated with methyridine alone. The larvae subjected to the test drug would have been born on days 5 and 6 of infection and would thus have been up to 2 days old when treated with methyridine. In this way, one can choose what age of worm to treat by leaving the required time between methyridine treatment and test-compound treatment.

An alternative approach is to collect newborn larvae produced by adult female *Trichinella* maintained *in vitro* (Denham, 1967; Dennis *et al.*, 1970) and inject them intravenously into mice. These will develop into normal muscle larvae, and again treatment can be directed against worms of a chosen age. It would even be possible to test the effect of a compound on migrating larvae by this method. We are not aware of any experiments done with anthelmintics using the technique of injecting newborn larvae.

From the preceding discussion, it can be seen that techniques are available for a complete dissection of the effects of anthelmintics on all stages of *Trichinella*, and it is to be hoped that standardized methods will be adopted in future work so that results from different laboratories can be compared in a meaningful way.

As a start, we would suggest (for the common laboratory strains of mouse and parasite) the following treatment regimens: for the immature intestinal phase, a single treatment at 4 hr after infection; for the mature intestinal phase, a single treatment on day 4 of infection; for the developing muscle phase, daily treatment on days 14–18 (following adulticidal medication); and for the fully developed and thoroughly encapsulated muscle larvae, daily treatment on days 35–40.

2.2. Drug Efficacy

2.2.1. Efficacy in Vitro

Until recently, no systematic study seems to have been made on the effect of drugs on *Trichinella in vitro*. Occasional observations, incidental to other studies, have been recorded. Piperazine, for example, was found to kill the adult worms *in vitro* (Spaldonova *et al.*, 1969). Decapsulated muscle larvae, when exposed *in vitro* to thiabendazole or its more soluble hydrochloride salt, lost neither their motility nor their infectivity (Campbell and Cuckler, 1964). Both motility and infectivity, however, were lost when decapsulated larvae were immersed in sublethal concentrations of ethanol (Campbell, 1977).

Recently, however, Jenkins and Carrington (1981) have tested a wide variety of anthelmintic agents against *Trichinella* under standardized *in vitro* conditions (see Section 2.1.1). The culture conditions permitted growth of the decapsulated larvae from a coiling to a "serpentine" state, but did not permit molting. The test lasted for 4 days, with the worms being in the serpentine condition for the final 2 days. Thus, although the test was designed to detect activity against the muscle stage, the test organisms were presumably in the early intestinal phase of development for part of the observation period. The test results correlated well with the relative potency of the compounds against the muscle stage, but since those compounds known to have such activity are also active against the early intestinal phase, the significance of this correlation is uncertain. Nevertheless, the report of Jenkins and Carrington gives a great deal of interesting information, with the following compounds being active at the minimum inhibitory concentration indicated (mg/liter): oxibendazole, 0.001; parbendazole, 0.005; cambendazole, 0.005; mebendazole, 0.005; albendazole, 0.005; fenbendazole, 0.01; oxfendazole, 0.01; thiabendazole, 0.05; thiophanate, 1.0; haloxon, 1.0; metrifonate, 1.0; levamisole hydrochloride, 10.0; methyridine, 20.0; and pyrantel tartrate, 50.0. The following compounds were inactive at a concentration of 100.0 mg/liter: amidantel, amoscanate, nitroscanate, phenothiazine, piperazine citrate, diethylcarbamazine citrate, suramin, and bephenium hydroxynaphthoate.

2.2.2. Efficacy against the Intestinal Phase

Some anthelmintics are more effective against immature *Trichinella* than against the mature worm, while others are more effective against the adult worm (Fig. 1). The biological significance of the difference is uncertain. It may reflect a metabolic difference associated with maturation or, less likely, a difference in microhabitat.

The difference in response of the different intestinal forms to drug treatment may be one of relative sensitivity only. For example, in mice, thiabendazole at 50 mg/kg is active at 2 hr of infection, but not at 16 hr, while a dosage of 150 mg/kg is fully active at 16 or 24 hr, but not at 36 or 48 hr; indeed, a dosage of 250 mg/kg had little effect at

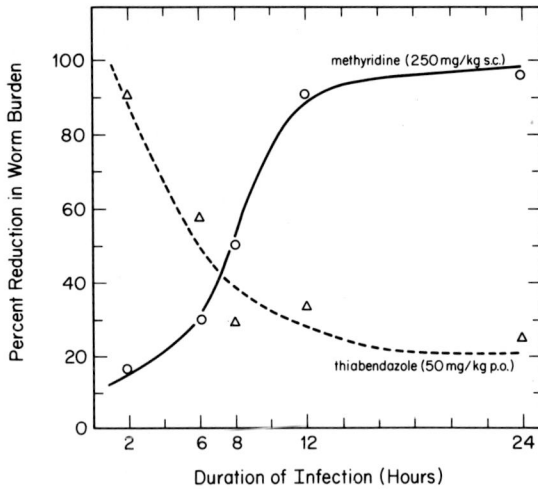

FIGURE 1. Change in efficacy of a given dosage of thiabendazole or methyridine with increasing maturation of the worm, in mice. Worms are susceptible to the benzimidazole at 24 hr but higher dosage is required. Adapted from Campbell and Hartman (1968).

the latter time, and a dosage of 500 mg/kg was ineffective at 72 hr after infection (Campbell and Cuckler, 1964). Even more extreme differences can be seen in mice treated with oxfendazole (Karunakaran and Denham, 1980). A single oral dose of 1.6 mg/kg eliminated 99% of 6-hr worms, whereas 800 mg/kg was only 91% effective against 5-day worms. With oxibendazole, 6.25 mg/kg was 99% effective against 6-hr worms, while 3200 mg/kg was only 69% effective against 5-day worms (Karunakaran and Denham, 1980). Again, caution must be exercised in drawing conclusions. It is tempting to conclude that benzimidazoles are active against immature and "adolescent" *T. spiralis*, but not against the sexually mature adult (i.e., 30 hr old). In fact, however, thiabendazole is fully effective in removing the mature adult when administered in the diet at a concentration of 1.0% (Campbell and Cuckler, 1964), and mebendazole removed 93% of adult worms when given at 7.5 mg/kg twice a day for 3 days (R.O. McCracken, unpublished data). The differential efficacy of benzimidazoles against various *Trichinella* stages can be used to study immune responses in chemically abbreviated infections (Campbell, 1965; Corba and Spaldonova, 1974; and others). Their activity against gut stages has also been demonstrated in swine (see Section 2.2.4).

Some drugs are more effective against one sex of *Trichinella* than against the other (Spaldonova *et al.*, 1974). Again, the difference is one of relative sensitivity, and no drug is known to be effective against one sex only.

Contrasting with the benzimidazoles is methyridine, which is more potent against the adult than against the immature worm (Fig. 1). Also in contrast to the benzimidazoles is the restriction of the efficacy of methyridine to the mature intestinal phase—an attribute that makes methyridine a quite useful biological tool (see Sections 2.1.2 and 2.2.3).

Apart from the killing or expulsion of worms from the host gut, some drugs can, if suitably administered, block the reproduction of *Trichinella* without eliminating the worms. This is of potential significance in both experimental and clinical chemotherapy. The inhibition of reproduction (chemosterilization) can be used to study the effects of adult worms, in the absence of their progeny, on such phenomena as immune protection and histamine sensitivity (Campbell, 1965; Campbell and Blair, 1978a).

All the individual compounds reviewed below are active against intestinal *T. spiralis*. No compound is known to have activity against *Trichinella* in muscle without also being active against the parasite in the gut (the converse is not true).

2.2.3. Drugs Active against Extraintestinal Stages

a. Dissemination Phase. Nothing is known of the effect of drugs on the dissemination phase, largely because the period during which *Trichinella* larvae are disseminated from the gut to the musculature is often confused with the early period of muscle invasion and encystation. In mice, for example, administration of drugs 14–21 days after inoculation is sometimes regarded as representing treatment of the "migratory" larvae. In most strains of mice, however, all the larvae would be expected to be lodged within muscle cells at that time. Since it is now generally believed that newborn larvae are transported rapidly and passively to the muscles, and that they quickly penetrate muscle cells, they would exist as "migratory larvae" for only a matter of seconds or minutes. There is no evidence that any drug is active, or indeed has been tested, against these fleeting chemotherapeutic targets. We have indicated in Section 2.1.3 how such studies could be carried out.

b. Intracellular Muscle Phase. Trichinosis is usually not diagnosed until larval invasion of muscle has occurred, and in most cases parasitization of the muscles is primarily responsible for the clinical illness. The muscle phase is therefore of particular interest with respect to chemotherapy. Indeed, the lack of drugs active in the muscle phase has historically been a major handicap for the physician faced with clinical trichinosis. Of several drug classes reported to have efficacy against the muscle-dwelling larvae of *T. spiralis* (organophosphates, benzimidazoles, tetramisole, and diethylcarbamazine, as well as certain immunomodulating and antimitotic agents), only the benzimidazoles have been shown to possess unequivocal efficacy at well-tolerated dosages (Campbell and Blair, 1974). In general, it can be said that drug efficacy in the muscle phase declines with duration of infection. Fortunately, this means that efficacy is greatest when the need for efficacy is likely to be greatest. Once the acute illness has abated, and the larvae have become fully encapsulated, chemotherapeutic intervention is generally less desirable as well as less feasible.

2.2.4. Review of Individual Drugs

a. Benzimidazoles

General. In the years that have elapsed since the first reports of the efficacy of the benzimidazole molecule against *T. spiralis* (Campbell, 1961; Campbell and Cuckler, 1962a), several dozen synthetic derivatives have been tested against the parasite in laboratory animals. Only a few of them have been examined closely, and the structure of the more significant compounds is shown in Table I. A few generalizations can

TABLE I
Structure of Benzimidazoles Mentioned in the Text

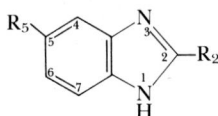

Name	R_2	R_5
Chlophasol	2-Chlorophenyl	H
Thiabendazole	4-Thiazolyl	H
Cambendazole	4-Thiazolyl	$-NHCOOCH(CH_3)_2$
5-Benzamidothiabendazole	4-Thiazolyl	$-NHCOC_6H_5$
Parbendazole	$-NHCOOCH_3$	$-nC_4H_9$
Albendazole	$-NHCOOCH_3$	$-SCH_2CH_2CH_3$
Mebendazole	$-NHCOOCH_3$	$-COC_6H_5$
Fenbendazole	$-NHCOOCH_3$	$-SC_6H_5$
Oxfendazole	$-NHCOOCH_3$	$-SOC_6H_5$
Oxibendazole	$-NHCOOCH_3$	$-OCH_2CH_2CH_3$
Flubendazole	$-NHCOOCH_3$	$-3-F-COC_6H_5$
Medamine	$-NHCOOCH_3$	H

TABLE II
Efficacy of Benzimidazoles against Intestinal *T.*
***spiralis* in Mice[a]**

| | Percent Reduction in Worm Burden | | | | | |
| | 12 hr | | 24 hr | | 48 hr | |
	F	M	F	M	F	M
Albendazole	100	76	100	55	38	0
Cambendazole	100	100	100	100	90	50
Fenbendazole	98	98	97	20	34	0
Mebendazole	100	100	100	50	95	52
Oxfendazole	100	100	72	1	68	6
Oxibendazole	100	100	100	42	93	11
Parbendazole	100	100	100	92	91	24
Thiabendazole	14	10	12	0	10	9

[a] For all compounds, a single oral dose of 15 mg/kg was used (for the non-carbamate compound thiabendazole, this dosage is well below the optimum). Note that the decrease in efficacy with increasing age of infection applies particularly to the male worms. F = female, M = male. Data from Spaldonova *et al.* (1978) and Spaldonova and Corba (1979).

be made about the group: they are effective against immature and mature intestinal stages, but are more effective against immature worms than against adults (the carbamate members of the series are more effective against female than against male worms) (Table II and Fig. 1); they suppress production of larvae at dosages not lethal to adult worms; they are active against preencystment larvae and encysted larvae in the host musculature, but relatively large dosages and continuous or frequent treatment may be needed to demonstrate efficacy against encysted larvae; they are used in the specific treatment of human trichinosis; at least some of them inhibit glucose uptake in *Trichinella*, but it is believed by many investigators that their general efficacy against helminths and fungi derives ultimately from their inhibition of tubulin polymerization and consequent blockade of microtubule assembly.

On the basis of studies in which several benzimidazoles were employed in each study, it has been reported that treatment suppressed oogenesis and spermatogenesis of *Trichinella* and caused degeneration of stichocytes (Veretennikova *et al.*, 1981) and that destruction of muscle larvae elicited an inflammatory response much more intense than that seen in the muscle of nontreated hosts (Pereverzeva *et al.*, 1981). In the case of mebendazole treatment, such inflammation could be suppressed by treatment of the host with niridazole, an inhibitor of cell-mediated immunity, but not by cyclophosphamide, an inhibitor of responses mediated by humoral antibody (Bolás-Fernández et al., 1981a).

Different species, subspecies, or geographic isolates of *Trichinella* may differ in response to benzimidazole therapy, but the differences observed thus far have been minor, and quantitative rather than qualitative (see Chapter 2).

Limited attempts have been made to explore structure–activity relationships with respect to the muscle phase of *Trichinella* infection. Gharizanova et al. (1972) found several 2-substituted benzimidazoles to be less active than thiabendazole and showed that if the 2-substituent is aryl, then *ortho* substitution enhances activity. Aboul-Atta and Denham (1978) made the surprising observation that 5-benzimidothiabendazole was more effective against the fully encysted larvae than against the developing muscle phase. From a study of structure–activity relationships among several dozen 2-substituted and 5-substituted benzimidazole carbamates (Ozeretskovskaya et al., 1971; Kolosova and Ozeretskovskaya, 1974; Bekish et al., 1979), it was concluded that the most potent compounds have 2-aryl or 2-alkylcarbamate substitution and that among the 2-arylbenzimidazoles the best activity is found in the *ortho*-substituted derivatives. The *ortho* substituent may be halogen or a heteroatom in the ring. Among the alkyl benzimidazole-2-carbamates, the best activity is found with the methyl carbamate; the ethyl carbamate is less active, and longer alkyl chains lead to virtually inactive compounds. For the most part, these compounds are not in general use, and they will not be considered individually. Medamine (methyl benzimidazole-2-carbamate) prevented muscle invasion when given to rats at 100 mg/kg on days 1–6, but was only moderately effective against larvae that had already invaded the muscle (Bekish et al., 1979). Chlophasol (*o*-chlorophenyl-benzimidazole) was considered sufficiently promising to warrant trial in man; a daily dosage of 25 mg/kg, given during the prepatent phase of infection, successfully prevented the appearance of symptoms (Ozeretskovskaya et al., 1978b). It does not seem to have been tried after the onset of clinical disease. For data on the comparative efficacy of seven 5-substituted benzimidazole carbamates, see Spaldonova and Corba (1979) and the discussion of individual drugs below.

We shall now review the commercially available benzimidazoles in alphabetical order.

Albendazole. McCracken (1978) showed albendazole to be 100% effective at 2 hr with a dosage of 12.5 mg/kg, in mice, but only 73% active at 72 hr with a dosage of 50 mg/kg. The same author reported that albendazole was 67% effective against the early muscle phase at 5

× 50 mg/kg. Spaldonova and Corba (1979) also reported the efficacy of albendazole against the intestinal phase and found that larvae encysted in the muscles could be reduced by a dosage of 100 mg/kg per day given orally on days 28–31.

Cambendazole. A single oral dose of cambendazole at 5 mg/kg was approximately 90% effective against the enteral stages of *Trichinella* when given to mice 2 hr after inoculation, but at 24 hr after inoculation, a dosage of 10 mg/kg was required for similar efficacy (Campbell and Yakstis, 1970). At 72 hr, a dosage of 400 mg/kg was required to give a 90% reduction in worm burden, but a dosage of 100 mg/kg caused a substantial decrease in the fecundity of the worms (Duckett and Denham, 1970). Spaldonova *et al.* (1978) showed that a single oral dose of cambendazole at 15 mg/kg was 100% effective against intestinal *Trichinella* in mice when given at 6, 12, or 24 hr after inoculation. At 60 hr after inoculation, the treatment was still highly effective (90%) against the female worms, but inactive against the males. Degenerative changes have been observed, by electron microscopy, in worms recovered from treated mice (Seniuta *et al.*, 1981).

Duckett and Denham (1970) claimed to have shown an effect on the dissemination phase (days 8–13), but this needs confirmation using the method described in Section 2.1.2. They also showed that larvae that survived treatment were still infective.

In mice, cambendazole was highly effective against the early muscle phase of *T. spiralis* when the drug was given at 0.025% in the diet on days 14–21 of infection (Campbell and Yakstis, 1970) or when given to guinea pigs at 20 mg/kg on days 14–23 of infection (Georgieva, 1972). It was effective against the later muscle phase when given to mice at 50 mg/kg on several occasions on days 28–38 (Duckett and Denham, 1970) or when given to guinea pigs at 20 mg/kg on days 40–50 (Georgieva, 1972). Spaldonova *et al.* (1978) found cambendazole highly effective against the muscle-dwelling larvae of *T. spiralis* or *T. pseudospiralis*, when given orally at 40 mg/kg on days 28–31; surprisingly, they found it only moderately effective against *T. spiralis* when given on days 22–25.

Even a single dose was highly effective against encysted larvae when a very high dosage was used. When given to mice on day 28 of infection, a single oral dose of the base compound at 250 mg/kg, or a single subcutaneous dose of the tartrate salt at the same dosage, gave reductions of 91% and 81%, respectively. The surviving larvae were fully infective to other mice (W.C. Campbell and L.S. Blair, unpublished data). In swine, the feeding of a diet containing 0.1% cambendazole, on days 28–35 of infection, was shown by the same investigators to give reductions of 75–89% in the number of larvae in the muscles sampled, and the remaining larvae were dead.

Fenbendazole. When given to mice as a single oral dose at 50 mg/kg, 7 hr after inoculation, fenbendazole was 99% effective, but at 72 hr, it was inactive (Fernando and Denham, 1976). Spaldonova *et al.* (1978) demonstrated the progressive decline in efficacy as the worms matured, with a dosage of 100 mg/kg being highly active against female and male worms up to 12 hr of infection, active only against females at 24 hr, and virtually inactive against either sex at 48 hr or more. Seniuta *et al.* (1981) have reported ultrastructural changes in worms from treated mice.

When given to mice at 50 mg/kg on days 8–14 (the adult worms having been chemotherapeutically removed on day 7), fenbendazole gave a reduction of 89% in the number of larvae subsequently recovered (Fernando and Denham, 1976); this indicates good activity against developing muscle larvae, but Spaldonova and Corba (1979) found little efficacy against that phase even with a dosage of 300 mg/kg. Both investigators found fenbendazole to be of low potency against the developed larvae (28 days old), with a dosage of 300 mg/kg being required for even moderate activity. Düwel (1981), however, showed that dietary medication with fenbendazole (0.05–0.1%) was highly effective against both the early and late muscle phases.

Flubendazole. When fed to infected rats at 0.0008% in the diet for 7 days, flubendazole was 100% effective against 7-day old *T. spiralis* (Vanparijs *et al.*, 1979). In the same study, flubendazole was highly active when fed to infected rats at 0.0125% in the diet on days 14–21 or 21–35 of infection. In an ultrastructural study of the effect of flubendazole in the encysted phase in rats, De Nollin and Borgers (1978) observed an effect, the disappearance of microtubules from the esophageal cells of the larvae, as early as 1 day after the beginning of treatment (0.05% in diet for 14 days, beginning on day 35). This was followed, from the 3rd day on, by vacuolization and degeneration of the larvae and disruption of the intracapsular matrix. These changes were accompanied by an inflammatory reaction in and around the infected muscle fibers, while muscle fibers in noninfected areas of muscle appeared normal. The remnants of larvae and capsules gradually disappeared, and the host tissue was essentially restored to normal within 3 months.

In swine, the efficacy of flubendazole against *T. spiralis* was similar to that in rats (Thienpont and Vanparijs, 1981). When fed in the diet at 0.0032% for 7 days, beginning on day 3 or day 7 of infection, the drug was fully effective against the adult worms. When flubendazole was fed at 0.0125% for 2 weeks, beginning on day 14 of infection, subsequent digestion of muscle tissue revealed no larvae—indicating complete efficacy against the early encystment phase. (Since the temporal limits of larval production in swine are uncertain, an effect against the dissemination phase cannot be excluded.) Against the encysted larvae, dietary concentrations of 0.0125% or higher were highly effective, with a concentration of 0.025% being 100% effective when treatment was begun 7 weeks after infection. Adverse reactions were not observed with the flubendazole treatment in any of these trials.

Flubendazole has been tried successfully against trichinosis in man and may supersede thiabendazole and mebendazole in clinical utility (Bouree et al., 1976).

Mebendazole—intestinal phase. The efficacy of mebendazole against intestinal *Trichinella* was reported by Thienpont et al. (1974), who found that the infection was eliminated from rats fed the drug at a concentration of 0.01% for 7 days, beginning 2 days before inoculation. The drug was 100% effective against 12-hr-old *T. spiralis* in mice, when given as a single oral dose at only 15 mg/kg (Spaldonova et al., 1978). These authors also reported that mebendazole is more effective against female worms than against males. Mebendazole at 50 mg/kg was 95% effective against 7-hr-old *T. spiralis* in mice, but only 67% effective at 72 hr (Fernando and Denham, 1976). When given on day 3 of infection at 7.5 mg/kg *bis in die* (b.i.d.) for one day, mebendazole was only 51% effective, but when this treatment was given on 3 successive days, it was 93% effective (R.O. McCracken, unpublished data)—again illustrating the value of frequent or continuous benzimidazole medication in some circumstances.

Mebendazole—muscle phase. Mebendazole was found highly active against the early muscle phase in rats, totally eliminating the larvae when fed at 0.01% on days 14–21 (Thienpont et al., 1974) and eliminating more than 95% of the larvae in mice when given orally at 50 mg/kg on days 8–14 of infection, after therapeutic elimination of adult worms (Fernando and Denham, 1976), or when given at 40 mg/kg on days 22–55 of infection (Spaldonova et al., 1978).

When given orally to mice at 50 mg/kg on days 14–18, mebendazole reduced by 96% the number of larvae subsequently recovered from the musculature (McCracken, 1978). When given twice daily on days 14–16, a dosage of 12.5 mg/kg was 90% effective (McCracken and Taylor, 1980).

Mebendazole is also remarkably active against the later muscle phase of trichinosis. In rats, a diet of 0.05% mebendazole was highly effective when fed on days 34–48 (Thienpont *et al.*, 1974), while in mice, more than 99% of the larvae were eliminated by an oral dose of 50 mg/kg on days 28–34 of infection (Fernando and Denham, 1976), and 85% were removed by a dosage of 40 mg/kg on days 28–31 (Spaldonova *et al.*, 1978). When given to mice twice daily on days 28–30, mebendazole at dosages of 3.125–12.5 mg/kg reduced by more than 80% the number of larvae subsequently recovered by digestion, and those that were recovered were patently dead (McCracken and Taylor, 1980). The extraordinary efficacy of mebendazole (Vermox) against encysted larvae has been put to good use in the prevention and treatment of human trichinosis (Sonnet and Thienpont, 1977; Klein *et al.*, 1981; Ozeretskovskaya *et al.*, 1978a,b, 1981). A dosage of 5.0 mg/kg per day for 5–10 days has given marked clinical improvement, and this compound is now the drug of choice in human trichinosis (see Chapter 11).

In ultrastructural studies on infected rats treated with mebendazole, the earliest discernible change was degeneration of the intracapsular matrix. This was followed by vacuolization, swelling, and loss of glycogen in the cells of the larvae. Damage to the larvae and surrounding matrix was followed by infiltration of the capsules by inflammatory cells, and calcification of larvae, with subsequent removal of the remnants within 50 days of treatment, and virtually complete restoration of the host tissue within 111 days (De Nollin *et al.*, 1974). According to Pereverzeva *et al.* (1981), the infiltrate in treated mice consisted mostly of lymphocytes, and there was no mast-cell reaction.

Although mebendazole is absorbed from the mammalian gut in only small amounts, the drug reaches larvae in the muscle and remains there longer than it remains in the surrounding host tissue. The drug inhibits the glucose uptake of the larvae in rats as it does also *in vitro*, and increases glycogen depletion—perhaps accounting thereby for the anthelmintic action of the drug (De Nollin and Van den Bossche, 1973). More recent studies, however, have suggested an alternative primary mode of action. Mebendazole binds to the embryonic tubulin of *Ascaris suum* with an affinity greater than that of its binding to mammalian tubulin, and it seems likely that this binding, with its resultant blocking of microtubule assembly, is responsible for the drug's anthelmintic action (Friedman and Platzer, 1980).

Oxfendazole. At 15 mg/kg, given to mice at 12 hr, oxfendazole was 100% effective against worms of either sex, but when given at 24 hr, the drug was only 72% effective against female worms and essentially inactive against males (Spaldonova and Corba, 1979). A dramatic decline in sensitivity was also recorded by Karunakaran and Denham (1981), who obtained a 99% reduction of 7-hr-old worms with a dosage of 1.6

mg/kg; against 5-day worms, however, dosages in excess of 100 mg/kg were needed for even moderate activity, and the extremely high dosage of 3200 mg/kg gave only 94% reduction. In the same study, excellent activity was obtained against developing larvae (98% at 7 × 25 mg/kg) and encysted larvae (98% at 7 × 50 mg/kg). In contrast, Spaldonova and Corba (1979) reported oxfendazole inactive against encysted larvae at an even higher dosage (4 × 200 mg/kg).

Oxibendazole. This compound was found to be extremely active against immature intestinal stages in mice, but activity declined as the worms matured. Dosages of 6.25–15.0 mg/kg were at least 99% effective at 6 hr after infection, but at 72 hr, 3200 mg/kg gave only 69% reduction in worm burden (Spaldonova *et al.*, 1978; Karunakaran and Denham, 1980).

In the treatment of the encysted phase in mice, there was a discrepancy between the results of Spaldonova *et al.* (1978) and those of Karunakaran and Denham (1981). The former authors found that 4 × 200 mg/kg was only 16% effective, whereas Karunakaran and Denham obtained an 82% reduction at this dosage and extremely good activity against developing larvae.

Parbendazole. A single oral dose of parbendazole was highly effective against *T. spiralis* in mice when given at 2 hr at a dosage of 6.25 mg/kg, or 24 hr at 12.5 mg/kg, or 36 hr at 50 mg/kg (Theodorides and Laderman, 1969). Spaldonova *et al.* (1978) confirmed the high activity of parbendazole against the early intestinal stages and the decline in efficacy (at least with respect to the female worms) associated with maturation (Table II). Theodorides and Laderman (1969) found parbendazole to be highly effective against the encysted larvae of *Trichinella* in mice. Even when treatment was started as late as 12 weeks after infection, administration of a diet of 0.05% parbendazole for 7 days gave a 91% reduction in the number of larvae. Spaldonova *et al.* (1978) reported that a dosage of 100 mg/kg given orally on days 28–31 reduced the number of larvae by 80%.

Thiabendazole—intestinal phase. In mice, a single oral dose of thiabendazole at 50 mg/kg was highly effective against 2-hr-old *Trichinella*, but not against 20-hr-old worms; however, a dosage of 150 mg/kg was highly effective against 24-hr-old worms. Loss of worms from the gut occurred more than 5 hr, but less than 24 hr, after the drug was administered. Against mature worms (i.e., 36 hr old or older), a dosage of 150 mg/kg was ineffective, and at 72 hr, even a dosage of 500 mg/kg failed to remove the worms (Campbell and Cuckler, 1964) (Fig. 1). The progressive loss of susceptibility with maturation of the worms was also shown by Spaldonova *et al.* (1978). Mature *Trichinella* (4 days old) can, however, be totally eliminated by feeding mice a diet containing 1.0% thiabendazole (Campbell and Cuckler, 1964). The same authors showed that although thiabendazole has very low aqueous solubility, it is effective against intestinal *Trichinella* when given by subcutaneous injection. A single subcutaneous injection of thiabendazole suspension at 250 mg/kg was highly effective, in mice, when given 24 hr after inoculation, but not at 72 hr.

When fed to mice at a concentration of 0.05% in the diet, beginning on day 4 of infection, thiabendazole blocked the production of larvae, while not removing the adult worms (Campbell and Cuckler, 1964). The effect was reversed when treatment was withdrawn (Blair and Campbell, 1971).

In rats, a single oral dose of thiabendazole at 250 mg/kg was 100% effective against a 24-hr-old infection, but a dosage of 2000 mg/kg was ineffective against a 6-day-old infection (Campbell and Cuckler, 1964).

In swine, thiabendazole was 100% effective when given as a single oral dose of 150 mg/kg, 16 hr after inoculation, but dosages of 150– 300 mg/kg were only moderately effective when given on day 7 of infection (Campbell and Cuckler, 1966). However, a very high degree of efficacy against mature worms was observed when thiabendazole was administered to swine at 25 mg/kg, given orally twice daily on days 7– 21 of infection.

Thiabendazole can be used prophylactically. When mice were given a single subcutaneous injection of thiabendazole (500 mg/kg in sesame oil) 1 day before inoculation with *Trichinella* larvae, no adult worms were recovered from the gut at necropsy 7 days after inoculation, and no larvae were recovered from the musculature 4 weeks after inoculation (Campbell and Cuckler, 1964). Even when the single injection was given 48 hr before inoculation, there was a 94% reduction in the number of worms recovered from the gut (as compared to untreated mice) and a 100% reduction in muscle invasion. A similar prophylactic effect was observed in swine (Campbell and Cuckler, 1966). Since thiabendazole has very low solubility in water or vegetable oils, it is likely that in these experiments the prophylaxis resulted from the anthelmintic effect of the drug as it leached from the site of injection. It is not clear whether *Trichinella* failed to become established under these circumstances, in which case the drug would have provided "causal prophylaxis," i.e., the prevention of disease by prevention of infection, as opposed to "clinical prophylaxis," or the prevention of disease by elimination of an infection in a prepathogenic phase. On the other hand, when treatment was given during, rather than before, the enteral phase, the vermicidal and chemosterilizing effect of thiabendazole prevented the parenteral phase of infection, and in this way clinical prophylaxis has been demonstrated in mice, swine (Campbell and Cuckler, 1964, 1966), and even man (Gerwel *et al.*, 1974).

Thiabendazole—muscle phase. In mice, dietary medication with thiabendazole was highly effective in reducing the number of larvae subsequently recovered by digestion of host muscle. The concentration of drug required for efficacy increased with increasing age of infection. When fed on days 7–14 (during which time newborn larvae would be disseminating and muscle invasion would occur), a concentration of 0.05% thiabendazole was highly effective. When treatment was given for 2 weeks, beginning at 3, 4, or 6 weeks (when the larvae would be encysted), a concentration of 0.5% was required for good efficacy. In older infections, a very high concentration of 1.0% was required (Campbell and Cuckler, 1964).

Ozeretskovskaya *et al.* (1974) reported that the efficacy of thiabendazole against encysted *Trichinella* was decreased by concurrent administration of methotrexate and increased by concurrent administration of phytohemagglutinin, but the evidence does not seem persuasive. It has also been reported that the efficacy of thiabendazole against encysted *T. spiralis* is antagonized by coadministration of corticosteroids (Ozeretskovskaya *et al.*, 1969), but again the evidence is not persuasive, and other workers have failed to confirm the antagonistic effect (Campbell and Blair, 1978b). Indeed, a combination of benzimidazole and steroid therapy has been advocated for severe human trichinosis (see Section 3.2.2).

Depending on the dosages and time intervals used, *Trichinella* larvae that survive sublethal thiabendazole treatments are noninfective for mice or have a reduced infectivity (Campbell and Cuckler, 1964; Tomasovicova *et al.*, 1972).

In rats, a dosage of 500 mg/kg was not effective when given on 5 consecutive days, beginning 11 or more days after inoculation (Ruitenberg and Steerenberg, 1974). This finding illustrates the importance of frequent dosing, or continuous medication, in the treatment of the muscle phase with thiabendazole. A "considerable" degree of efficacy was, however, reported for mice given a dosage of 500 mg/kg, provided that necropsy was delayed for 5 weeks after treatment (Tomasovicova *et al.*, 1974).

In swine, thiabendazole was administered by gavage at 50 mg/kg on days 14–19 or 14–24 of infection; this treatment resulted in reductions of 82 and 97%, respectively, in the number of larvae subsequently recovered by digestion, and many of the residual larvae were dead (Campbell and Cuckler, 1962a). When treatment was given at 25 mg/kg b.i.d., on days 14–27 of infection, the number of larvae recovered was reduced by approximately 90% in each of three experiments (Campbell and Cuckler, 1966). In these trials, the reduction in the number of larvae must be attributed to the drug's efficacy on the intestinal phase as well as its effect on the early muscle phase. In another study, treatment with thiabendazole at 0.3% in the diet on days 28–35 of infection resulted in a 94% reduction in the number of larvae recovered, and again many of the residual larvae were dead (Campbell and Cuckler, 1962b). Efficacy against intestinal worms may again have contributed to the final therapeutic effect, but could not have been a factor in other experiments, in which treatment was begun on day 35 or 56 of infection (Campbell and Cuckler, 1966). In these experiments, a dosage of 25 mg/kg b.i.d. on days 35–42 of infection did not result in a reduction in the number, viability, or infectivity of the larvae subsequently recovered. A dosage of 75 mg/kg b.i.d. on days 56–70 gave a reduction in larval burden of 76%, and more than half the remainder were dead. A dosage of 150 mg/kg on days 56–64 was toxic to the pigs and gave an apparent reduction of 74%—but 100% of the larvae recovered were dead; because of the toxicity of the regimen, the pigs were necropsied only 1 day after the end of treatment, and it may be assumed that the dead larvae would have disintegrated in the host tissue if necropsy had been performed a few weeks after the end of treatment.

In man, thiabendazole treatment has been followed by marked clinical improvement in some cases of trichinosis but not in others, and in many cases it has not been well tolerated (Zaiman, 1970; Campbell and Blair, 1974; Klein, 1978; Klein et al., 1981; Ozeretskovskaya et al., 1978b, 1981). Since the customary dosage of thiabendazole in man is 22 mg/kg b.i.d. for only a few days, the aforedescribed results with swine suggest that a typical clinical regimen would be unlikely to destroy Trichinella larvae in human patients. The clinical benefit observed in some cases of human trichinosis may derive from a reduction in the metabolism of the larvae and consequent reduction in allergenic metabolites. In at least two instances, however, dead larvae have been recovered from biopsy specimens of patients treated with thiabendazole (Hennekeuser et al., 1969; Casali and De Costa, 1977). The results in swine also point to the desirability of frequent treatment, over a prolonged period, in the use of thiabendazole against the muscle phase. It is unlikely, however, that thiabendazole would be sufficiently well tolerated to permit frequent and prolonged administration to human patients. Thiabendazole is no longer considered the drug of choice in human trichinosis (see below and Chapter 11).

Kozar *et al.* (1967) and Britov (1969) examined changes in *T. spiralis* larva and host tissue following subcutaneous injection of insoluble thiabendazole in large dosages. Kozar and colleagues concluded that a detrimental effect on the muscle led to the death of the larva. Britov, using infections in dogs, cats, guinea pigs, and rabbits, reported that all larvae were killed even when the infections were 3 years old. In early infections, treated before encapsulation, resorption of the parasites was completed in 1–2 weeks. In older infections, the larvae disintegrated, and the capsules became surrounded by infiltrates of neutrophils, eosinophils, and histiocytes. Granulomata formed around the remains of the capsules, and in most cases they disintegrated, leaving no trace of infection. In swine treated with thiabendazole by the more accepted oral route, histological examination showed some degenerate larvae, with granular, basophilic intracapsular matrix and a cellular infiltration between the disintegrating capsule wall and the surrounding muscle fibers (Campbell and Cuckler, 1966). As to whether the effect on the larva is primary or secondary, Gabryel *et al.* (1974) suggested that the destruction of the matrix was the cause of death of the larva, and it has also been proposed that thiabendazole blocks the role of histamine in the encapsulation process, resulting in the death of the larva (Kolosova and Ozeretskovskaya, 1974). In contrast, Jarczewska *et al.* (1974) proposed that the primary effect was on the larva and that the presence of inflammatory cells within the capsule was a consequent immunological event. Similarly, Pereverzeva *et al.* (1981) observed a mast-cell reaction and infiltration of plasma cells and lymphocytes and concluded that this effect was secondary to the anthelmintic effect on the larva. It has been suggested that thiabendazole acts on other helminths by inhibition of fumarate reductase (Prichard, 1970; Malkin and Camacho, 1972), but the observation that mebendazole disrupts the microtubular system of nematodes (see above) suggests that the whole question of the mode of action of the benzimidazoles on *Trichinella* should be reconsidered.

b. Other Drugs

Methyridine. In the early 1960s, the efficacy of methyridine against *T. spiralis* was shown by several workers—Janitschke, Denham, Khoschbin, Schanzel, Hegerova, and others (see Campbell and Blair, 1974). The efficacy of various dosages, given at various times of infection, was studied by Denham (1965), who showed that single doses of 200–500 mg/kg, subcutaneously, were highly effective against the intestinal worms 24 hr old, or older. *Trichinella* becomes highly susceptible to methyridine at approximately 12 hr of age, the drug having little effect at 6 hr after inoculation and essentially no effect at 2 hr (Campbell and Hartman, 1968) (Fig. 1). It is not active against the muscle phase.

Methyridine has proved of value as a research tool. By initiating treatment (500 mg/kg per day subcutaneously) in different groups of mice on each of the first 5 days of infection, it was shown that significant muscle invasion occurred only in mice in which treatment was begun on day 5—thus confirming unequivocally Gould's observation that the period of larviposition begins between day 4 and day 5 (Denham, 1965). Methyridine has also been of great utility in removing adult worms in order to test drugs against larvae in their intestinal phase, without the complication of having adult worms in the host gut (Denham, 1965) (see Section 2.1.3). It has been used to study the transplacental or transmammary transmission of infection (Denham, 1966a), the immunizing effect of chemically abbreviated infections (Denham, 1966b; and several other investigators), the rate of larval production by adult *Trichinella* (Denham and Martinez, 1970), and the biochemical effects of infection (Stewart and Read, 1973).

Organophosphates. Since the efficacy of trichlorfon against *Trichinella* was reported by Schoop and Lamina (1959), many organophosphates have been tested. They are especially active against the adult worm, but some are highly active against both the immature and mature enteral phases. For example, famophos, fed to mice at the very low concentration of 0.01% in the diet, gave 80% reduction in immature worms and 100% reduction in adults (Campbell and Cuckler, 1967). Rats fed a diet containing 0.1% haloxon on days 1–3 of infection were completely free of muscle-dwelling larvae at subsequent necropsy, reflecting activity against the adult worm (Martinez *et al.*, 1968a). As a tool for eliminating the enteral phase in experimental infections, naphthalofos (Maretin) can be used at 40 mg/kg on day 3 of infection (Martínez-Fernández *et al.*, 1981).

Although naphthalofos is very potent against intestinal *Trichinella*, it has little or no activity against the muscle phase. On the other hand, trichlorfon (metrifonate) is relatively weak against intestinal forms and is quite active against those in the muscle. Toxicity for both host and parasite is probably attributable to inhibition of cholinesterases (Ramisz *et al.*, 1967; Spaldonova, 1969). Nevertheless, there is a measure of differential toxicity, and the use of antidotes such as atropine has enabled investigators to achieve a high degree of efficacy. The narrow therapeutic index has, however, precluded the use of organophosphates in the treatment of clinical trichinosis. The efficacy and biochemical action of organophosphates in experimental trichinosis has been studied especially by Ramisz, whose more recent papers (Ramisz and Komorowski, 1975; Ramisz and Szankowska, 1978) may be consulted for further detail and references. The efficacy of selected organophosphates has also been summarized by Zaiman (1970) and Campbell and Blair (1974).

Pyrantel and oxantel. Howes and Lynch (1967) found a single oral dose of pyrantel tartrate at 50 mg/kg to be highly effective against the intestinal phase in mice when given 2 hr after inoculation and to be somewhat less effective if given when the worms were 24 hr old. A differential efficacy between young and old worms was also reported by Martinez *et al.* (1968b), who used dosages of 100–200 mg/kg and achieved 100% removal of immature worms. Only a slight age difference was observed by Campbell and Hartman (1968) using a dosage of 100 mg/kg at 2 and 24 hr after inoculation. Pyrantel pamoate (as Antiminth or Combantrin) is used in the treatment of other helminth infections in man. Oxantel is a derivative of pyrantel with exceptional activity against *Trichuris* spp. According to Howes (1972), oxantel is active against the intestinal phase in laboratory animals, with a potency similar to that of pyrantel. These compounds are not active against the muscle phase.

Tetramisole and levamisole. The efficacy of tetramisole against *T. spiralis* was reported by Thienpont *et al.* (1966). It is more potent against adult worms than against immature worms, with a single subcutaneous dose of 30 mg/kg giving 65% reduction in worm burden in mice at 7 hr postinfection and 95% at 24 hr (Campbell and Hartman, 1968). It has only slight activity against the muscle phase (Campbell and Cuckler, 1967). Tetramisole (racemic) has been superseded by levamisole (the levoisomer), which has been reported effective against the intestinal phase in rats by Zohdy and Gawish (1975). These authors, using a dosage of 2 mg/kg, concluded that the drug was effective against both immature and mature intestinal forms, but they did not apply treatment earlier than day 3 of infection, at which time the worms would have been mature. Levamisole hydrochloride, as Ketrax, is used for the treatment of other helminth infections in man.

Miscellany. Piperazine and its derivative diethylcarbamazine are important antinematode drugs in other clinical applications, but have given equivocal and mostly negative results when tested in experimental or clinical trichinosis. Other drugs with uncertain activity in experimental trichinosis include antimitotic agents such as methotrexate and immunomodulating agents such as phytohemagglutinin. Rotenone is active against adult worms, but too toxic to be useful. Cadmium oxide is active against immature and mature intestinal *Trichinella*, but is not in use as an anthelmintic. Dithiazanine iodide is highly active against the adult worm, but not against the immature intestinal or muscle stages; it is no longer used in human medicine. Further information on these drugs may be found in earlier reviews.

Ethanol warrants mention because of its widespread nonmedical usage coupled with historical claims of prophylactic efficacy against human trichinosis. It causes reversible paralysis of *T. spiralis in vitro* and under certain circumstances appears to provide protection against infection when given to laboratory animals and swine (Hovorka and Spaldonova, 1974; Campbell, 1977). It must be given immediately after infection, and small volumes of concentrated ethanol (30% by volume) are more effective than larger volumes of low concentration. The prophylactic action is probably due partly to inhibition of the release of larvae by digestive enzymes and partly to a direct action on the worms.

Omitted from a previous review (Campbell and Blair, 1974) and mentioned here for the record is the failure in clinical trichinosis of turpentine, opium, and lithium (Glazier, 1881). Drugs reported active against *Trichinella* since that review include the antitrematode drug hycanthone (Zohdy and Gawish, 1975) and the antinematode drug amidantel (Wollweber *et al.*, 1979); supporting data are not yet available. Febantel, believed to be metabolized in the host to form fenbendazole, had an activity similar to that of fenbendazole (Spaldonova, 1981; Bolás-Fernández *et al.*, 1981b). Tioxidazole, a benzothiazole carbamate with activity against a variety of nematodes, had very slight activity against *Trichinella* in mice (Bolás-Fernández *et al.*, 1981b). The anticestode drug niclosamide was moderately effective against intestinal *Trichinella* when given to mice at 200 mg/kg on day 3 of infection (Spaldonova and Vodrazka, 1969). The avermectins, which are active against nematode and arthropod parasites, have weak activity against *Trichinella* and are apparently inactive against the muscle phase (Campbell *et al.*, 1979; Taylor and Pearson, 1981).

3. CLINICAL CHEMOTHERAPY

The role of drugs in the prevention and treatment of human trichinosis is discussed briefly in this section. Information on the characteristics of particular drugs may be found in the preceding sections, while information on their clinical use may be found in Chapter 11.

3.1. Clinical Prophylaxis

On those rare occasions when it is known that a person has ingested infective larvae recently, several drugs would be of potential utility in preventing serious clinical consequences. Two approaches can be taken to the prevention of disease, depending on the time that has elapsed since ingestion of larvae.

3.1.1. Use of Drugs to Remove Preadult Worms

If the interval between ingestion of larvae and treatment is less than 24 hr, pyrantel, oxantel, or one of the benzimidazoles could be used, at least in theory, to remove the immature worms. This supposition is based entirely on studies in laboratory animals. Pyrantel pamoate (Antiminth, Combantrin), thiabendazole (Mintezole), and mebendazole (Vermox) are approved in many countries for clinical use and could be used at the dosages approved for use in other helminth infections. Albendazole may also become available for human use.

3.1.2. Use of Drugs to Remove or Sterilize Adult Worms in Prepatent Infections

If the interval between ingestion and treatment is greater than 1 day, but symptoms have not yet developed, pyrantel or levamisole hydrochloride (Ketrax) might be used to remove adult worms. Alternatively, however, a benzimidazole could be used to suppress the production of larvae and so prevent muscle invasion (see Section 3.2.2). Since the duration of the intestinal phase in man is unknown, it is not feasible to put a limit on the time period for which such medical intervention would be recommended. Gravid female worms have been found in man a couple of months after infection, but it is reasonable to assume that there is in man, as in swine, a major decline in the number of enteral worms about 3–5 weeks after ingestion of infective larvae.

3.2. Clinical Therapy (Treatment of Patent Infections)

Once signs or symptoms of intestinal trichinosis have appeared, treatment should be considered for two purposes: first, to alleviate the illness attributable to the presence of gut worms (which now could be presumed to be mature); and second, to prevent the onset of muscular trichinosis. When signs and symptoms can be attributed to the extraintestinal phase, treatment may be directed against the muscle-dwelling larvae, but unless there is reason to believe that there is no longer a significant number of worms in the gut, it would again be desirable to remove or sterilize the intestinal population. Fortunately, the same class of drug can be used against both phases of the disease.

3.2.1. Use of Drugs to Remove or Sterilize Adult Worms in Patent Infections

As indicated in Section 3.1.2, pyrantel or levamisole could be used to reduce the number of adult worms in the intestine. As an alternative to the elimination of worms, drugs could be used to suppress their reproduction and thus to prevent a parenteral phase of infection. For this purpose, a benzimidazole can be used, and although chemosterilization has been demonstrated primarily with thiabendazole, it would probably be preferable to use mebendazole because it is better tolerated. It is likely that other benzimidazoles, e.g., chlophasol, could also be used. The benzimidazole could be used at the recommended broadspectrum dosage, although smaller dosages may, by analogy with observations in laboratory animals, be sufficient. A more difficult question is the desired duration of treatment. As stated in Section 3.1.2, the duration of the enteral phase in man is unknown, but it would be prudent to continue chemosterilizing treatment for several weeks. The uncertainty about the duration of this treatment points to the desirability, in principle, of removing the adult worms rather than suppressing larviposition.

3.2.2. Use of Drugs to Kill or Inhibit Larvae in Muscles

As pointed out above, only a few drug types are known to be effective against the larvae of *Trichinella* in host muscle. Of these, only one class, the benzimidazoles, can currently be considered for use in the treatment of the muscle phase of trichinosis in man. Thiabendazole has been used for several years, but is now being supplanted by mebendazole, which appears to be more effective and better tolerated (see Section 2.2.4. and Chapter 11).

Benzimidazole treatment should be accompanied in many cases by corticosteroid treatment to alleviate inflammatory and allergic effects arising from the infection or from destruction of the larvae. Corticosteroids should not be used alone or in early infections (say, within 6 weeks after ingestion of larvae), because such treatment may prolong the presence of fecund adult worms in the gut and thereby lead to increased muscle parasitism.

ACKNOWLEDGMENT. We are indebted to Dr. M.H. Fisher for an assessment of the published studies on structure–activity relationships among benzimidazoles.

REFERENCES

Aboul-Atta, N., and Denham, D.A., 1978, The effect of 5-benzamido-2, 4-thiazolyl benzimidazole on Trichinella spiralis, Trans. R. Soc. Trop. Med. Hyg. 72:557–680.

Bekish, O.Y., Burak, I.I., and Kolosova, M.O., 1979, Search for active benzimidazole-2-carbamates for therapy of trichiniasis, Med. Parazitol. Parazit. Bolezni 48:32–35 (in Russian).

Blair, L.S., and Campbell, W.C., 1971, Reversibility of thiabendazole-induced sterilization of Trichinella spiralis, Wiad. Parazytol. 17:641–644.

Bolás-Fernández, F., Sanmartin Durán, M.L., and Martínez-Fernández, A.R., 1981a, The influence of immunomodulating drugs (niridazole and cyclophosphamide) on the effect of mebendazole on encysted larvae of Trichinella spiralis in: Trichinellosis (C.W. Kim, E. J. Ruitenberg, and J.S. Teppema, eds.), Reedbooks, Chertsey, England, pp. 337–342.

Bolás-Fernández, F., Martínez-Fernández, A.R., and Santos, M.C., 1981b, Anthelmintic effect of oxfendazole, febantel and tioxidazole on the various stages of Trichinella spp., in: Trichinellosis (C.W. Kim, E.J. Ruitenberg, and J.S. Teppema, eds.), Reedbooks, Chertsey, England, pp. 331–335.

Bouree, P., Kouchner, G., and Gascon, A., 1976, A propos d'une epidemie de trichinose dans la banlieue parisienne (note preliminaire), Bull. Soc. Pathol. Exot. 69:177–181.

Britov, B.A., 1969, Dynamics of death and resorption of larvae of Trichinella in animals as a result of the action of thiabendazole, Proceedings of the IV Interdisciplinary Scientific Methodology Conference of Veterinarians and Patho-anatomists, Kazan, pp. 12–13 (In Russian).

Campbell, W.C., 1961, Effect of thiabendazole upon infections of Trichinella spiralis in mice, and upon certain other helminthiases, J. Parasitol. 47(Suppl.):37.

Campbell, W.C., 1965, the immunizing effect of enteral and enteral–parenteral infections of Trichinella spiralis in mice, J. Parasitol. 51:185–194.

Campbell, W.C., 1977, Can alcoholic beverages provide protection against trichinosis?, Proc. Helminthol. Soc. Washington 44:120–125.

Campbell, W.C., and Blair, L.S., 1974, Chemotherapy of Trichinella spiralis infections (a review), Exp. Parasitol. 35:304–334.

Campbell, W.C., and Blair, L.S., 1978a, Role of enteral and parenteral stages of Trichinella spiralis in the induction of histamine sensitivity in mice, in: Trichinellosis (C.W. Kim and Z.S. Pawlowski, eds.), University Press of New England, Hanover, New Hampshire, pp. 263–269.

Campbell, W.C., and Blair, L.S., 1978b, Combined anthelmintic and corticosteroid therapy of trichinellosis in mice, in: Trichinellosis (C.W. Kim and Z.S. Pawlowski, eds.), University Press of New England, Hanover, New Hampshire, pp. 409–417.

Campbell, W.C., and Cuckler, A.C., 1962a, Effect of thiabendazole upon experimental trichinosis in swine, *Proc. Soc. Exp. Biol. Med.* **110:**124–128.

Campbell, W.C., and Cuckler, A.C., 1962b, Thiabendazole treatment of the invasive phase of experimental trichinosis in swine, *Ann. Trop. Med. Parasitol.* **56:**500–505.

Campbell, W.C., and Cuckler, A.C., 1964, Effect of thiabendazole upon the enteral and parenteral phases of trichinosis in mice, *J. Parasitol.* **50:**481–488.

Campbell, W.C., and Cuckler, A.C., 1966, Further studies on the effect of thiabendazole on trichinosis in swine, with notes on the biology of the infection, *J. Parasitol.* **52:**260–279.

Campbell, W.C., and Cuckler, A.C., 1967, Comparative studies on the chemotherapy of experimental trichinosis in mice, *Z. Tropenmed. Parasitol.* **18:**408–417.

Campbell, W.C., and Hartman, R.K., 1968, Changes in the efficacy of three anthelmintics during the maturation of a nematode (*Trichinella spiralis*), *J. Parasitol.* **54:**112–116.

Campbell, W.C., and Yakstis, J.J., 1970, Efficacy of cambendazole against *Trichinella spiralis* in mice, *J. Parasitol.* **56:**839–840.

Campbell, W.C., Hartman, R.K., and Cuckler, A.C., 1963, The effect of certain antihistamine and antiserotonin agents upon experimental trichinosis in mice, *Exp. Parasitol.* **14:**29–36.

Campbell, W.C., Blair, L.S., and Lotti, V.J., 1979, Efficacy of avermectins against *Trichinella spiralis* in mice, *J. Helminthol.* **53:**254–256.

Casali, A.J., and De Costa, E.A., 1977, Investigacion clinica y anatomopatologica del tratamiento de la triquinosis aguda con tiabendazol. *Bol. Chil. Parasitol.* **32:**66–70.

Corba, J., and Spaldonova, R., 1974, Immunity in mice against *Trichinella spiralis* after administration of benzimidazoles: Development of immunity during the intestinal and early migration stages of infection, in: *Trichinellosis* (C.W. Kim, ed.), Intext, New York, pp. 213–219.

Denham, D.A., 1965, Studies with methyridine and *Trichinella spiralis*. 1. Effect upon the intestinal phase in mice, *Exp. Parasitol.* **17:**10–14.

Denham, D.A., 1966a, Infections with *Trichinella spiralis* passing from mother to filial mice pre- and post-natally, *J. Helminthology* **40:**291–296.

Denham, D.A., 1966b, Immunity to *Trichinella spiralis*. I. The immunity produced by mice to the first four days of the intestinal phase of the infection, *Parasitology* **56:**323–327.

Denham, D.A., 1967, Applications of the *in vitro* culture of nematodes especially *Trichinella spiralis*, in: *Problems of in vitro culture* (A.E.R. Taylor, ed.) Blackwell Scientific Publications, Oxford, pp. 49–60.

Denham, D.A., and Martinez, A.R., 1970, Studies with methyridine and *Trichinella spiralis*. 2. The use of the drug to study the rate of larval production in mice, *J. Helminthol.* **44:**357–363.

Dennis, D., Despommier, D.D., and Davis, N., 1970, The infectivity of the newborn larvae of *Trichinella spiralis* in the rat, *J. Parasitol.* **56:**974–977.

De Nollin, S., and Borgers, M., 1978, An ultrastructural study on the effects of flubendazole on the encysted phase of *Trichinella spiralis* in the rat, in: *Trichinellosis* (C.W. Kim and Z.S. Pawlowski, eds.), University Press of New England, Hanover, New Hampshire, pp. 445–462.

De Nollin, S., and Van den Bossche, H., 1973, Biochemical effects of mebendazole on *Trichinella spiralis* larvae, *J. Parasitol.* **59:**970–976.

De Nollin, S., Borgers, M., Vanparijs, O., and Van den Bossche, H., 1974, Effects of mebendazole on the encysted phase of *Trichinella spiralis* in the rat: An electron-microscope study, *Parasitology* **69:**55–62.

Duckett, M.G., and Denham, D.A., 1970, The effect of cambendazole on *Trichinella spiralis* infections in mice, *J. Helminthol.* **44:**211–218.

Düwel, D., 1981, Trichinellosis: Successful treatment with fenbendazole, in: *Trichinellosis* (C.W. Kim, E.J. Ruitenberg, and J.S. Teppema, eds.), Reedbooks, Chertsey, England, pp. 299–303.

Fernando, S.S.E., and Denham, D.A., 1976, The effects of mebendazole and fenbendazole on *Trichinella spiralis* in mice, *J. Parasitol.* **62**:874–876.

Friedman, P.A., and Platzer, E.G., 1980, Interaction of anthelmintic benzimidazoles with *Ascaris suum* embryonic tubulin, *Biochim. Biophys. Acta* **630**:271–278.

Gabryel, P., Gustowska, L., and Blotna, M., 1974, Morphology and histochemistry of muscle in *Trichinella*-infected rats treated with thiabendazole, in: *Trichinellosis* (C.W. Kim, ed.), Intext, New York, pp. 135–144.

Georgieva, D., 1972, Chemotherapeutic activity of cambendazole in experimental *Trichinella spiralis* infection, *Vet.-Med. Nauki (Sofia)* **9**:85–92 (in Bulgarian) abstract in *Vet. Bull.* **42**:785 (1972).

Gerwel, C., Pawlowski, Z., Mochecka, W., and Chodera, L., 1974, Probable sterilization of *Trichinella spiralis* by thiabendazole: Further clinical observations of human infections, in: *Trichinellosis* (C.W. Kim, ed.), Intext, New York, pp. 471–475.

Gharizanova, T., Torlakov, I., Zhelyaskov, N., Todorova, N., and Sheikov, N. 1972, Antinematodic activity of 2-substituted benzimidazoles, in: *Advances in Antimicrobial and Antineoplastic Chemotherapy* (M. Hejzlar, M. Semonsky and S. Masak, eds.) University Park Press, Baltimore, pp. 449–451.

Glazier, W.C.W., 1881, *Report on Trichinae and Trichinosis*, U.S. Public Health Service, Government Printing Office, Washington, D.C., 212 pp.

Hennekeuser, H.H., Pabst, K., Peoplan, W., and Gerok, W., 1969, Thiabendazole for the treatment of trichinosis in humans, *Tex. Rep. Biol. Med.* **27**:(Suppl. 2):581–596.

Hovorka, J., and Spaldonova, R., 1974, The influence of alcohol on larvae of *Trichinella spiralis, Acta Parasitol. Litu.* **12**:153–157.

Howes, H.L., 1972, Trans-1,4,5,6-tetrahydro-2-(3-hydroxystyryl)-1-methyl pyrimidine (CP-14,445), a new antiwhipworm agent, *Proc. Soc. Exp. Biol. Med.* **139**:394–398.

Howes, H.L., and Lynch, J.E., 1967, Anthelmintic studies with pyrantel. 1. Therapeutic and prophylactic efficacy against the enteral stages of various helminths in mice and dogs, *J. Parasitol.* **53**:1085–1091.

Jarczewska, K., Gorny, M., and Zeromski, J., 1974, Immunological studies of rat skeletal muscles in the course of *Trichinella spiralis* infection treated with thiabendazole, in: *Trichinellosis* (C.W. Kim, ed.), Intext, New York, pp. 221–229.

Jenkins, D.C., and Carrington, T.S., 1981, An *in vitro* screening test for compounds active against the parenteral stages of *Trichinella spiralis, Tropenmed. Parasitol.* **32**:31–34.

Karunakaran, C.S., and Denham, D.A., 1980, A comparison of the anthelmintic effects of oxfendazole and oxibendazole on *Trichinella spiralis* in mice, *J. Parasitol.* **66**:929–932.

Klein, J.S., 1978, Treatment of severe trichinellosis in: *Trichinellosis* (C.W. Kim and Z.S. Pawlowski, eds.), University Press of New England, Hanover, New Hampshire, pp. 395–406.

Klein, J. Zakharenko, D.F., Dolgina, L.E., Braginetz, W.R., and Linko, I.A., 1981, Etiotropic therapy and prophylaxis of trichinellosis, in: *Trichinellosis* (C.W. Kim, E.J. Ruitenberg, and J.S. Teppema, eds.), Reedbooks, Chertsey, England, pp. 291–296.

Kolosova, M.O., and Ozeretskovskaya, N.N., 1974, Search for trichinellocides: The relationship between the structure and activity of benzimidazoles, in: *Trichinellosis* (C.W. Kim, ed.), Intext, New York, pp. 477–481.

Kozar, Z., Zarzycki, J., Seniuta, R., and Martynowicz, T., 1967, Histochemical study of drug effects on mice infected with *Trichinella spiralis, Exp. Parasitol.* **21**:173–185.

Lupascu, G., Cironeanu, I., Hacig, Z., Pambuccian, G., Simionescu, O., Solomon, P., and

Tintareanu, J., 1970, *Trichineloza*, Editura Academici Republicii Socialiste Romania, Bucharest, 246 pp.

Malkin, M.F., and Camacho, R.M., 1972, The effect of thiabendazole on fumarate reductase from thiabendazole-sensitive and resistant *Haemonchus contortus, J. Parasitol.* **58**:845–846.

Martinez, A.R., Cordero, M.C., and Aller, B., 1968a, The prophylactic effect of haloxon against experimental *Trichinella spiralis* infections in rats, *Ann. Trop. Med. Parasitol.* **62**:63–66.

Martinez, A., Cordero, M., and Aller, B., 1968b, Versuche über die Wirksamkeit von Pyrantel-tartrat gegen *Trichinella spiralis, Tieraerztl. Wochenschr.* **81**:223–225.

Martínez-Fernández, A.R., Sanmartin Durán, M.L., Ortega, M.G., and Garate, T., 1981, Cross immunity levels among sibling species of *Trichinella*, in: *Trichinellosis* (C.W. Kim, E.J. Ruitenberg, and J.S. Teppema, eds.), Reedbooks, Chertsey, England, pp. 129–133.

McCracken, R.O., 1978, Efficacy of mebendazole and albendazole against *Trichinella spiralis* in mice, *J. Parasitol.* **64**:214–219.

McCracken, R.O., and Taylor, D.D., 1980, Mebendazole therapy of parenteral trichinellosis, *Science* **207**:1220–1222.

Ozeretskovskaya, N.N., Kolosova, M.O., Tchernyaeva, A.I., Pereverzeva, E.V., Tumolskaya, N.I., and Bekish, O.Y.L., 1969, Benzimidazoles and steroid hormones in the therapy of experimental trichinellosis, Abstracts of Papers, Second International Conference on Trichinellosis, Wroclaw, 1969, pp. 77–80.

Ozeretskovskaya, N.N., Chernyaeva, A.I., Kolosova, M.O., and Kriventsova, T.D., 1971, Search for the specific therapy for trichinellosis in white mice. V. Chlorophenyl derivatives of benzimidazole in experimental trichinellosis in white mice, *Med. Parazitol. Parazit. Bolezni* **40**:411–414 (in Russian).

Ozeretskovskaya, N.N., Pereverzeva, E.V., and Veretennikova, N.L., 1974, The effect of thiabendazole and methotrexate or phytohemagglutinin on the experimental trichinellosis, in: *Trichinellosis* (C.W. Kim, ed.), Intext, New York, pp. 499–514.

Ozeretskovskaya, N.N., Morenets, T.M., and Grigorenko, T.A., 1978a, Mebendazole in the treatment of acute and chronic stages of helminthiases. Communication I. Mebendazole treatment of acute and chronic trichinelliasis caused by *Trichinella* strains from wild animals, *Med. Parazitol. Parazit. Bolezni* **47**:43–51.

Ozeretskovskaya, N.N., Pereverzeva, E.V., Tumolskaya, N.I., Bronshtein, A.M., Morenets, T.M., and Imumkuliev, K.D., 1978b, Benzimidazoles in the treatment and prophylaxis of synanthropic and sylvatic trichinellosis, in: *Trichinellosis* (C.W. Kim and Z.S. Pawlowski, eds.), University Press of New England, Hanover, New Hampshire, pp. 381–393.

Ozeretskovskaya, N.N., Morenets, T.M., Pereverzeva, E.V., Bronstein, A.M., Veretennikova, N.L., Kolosova, M.O., Poverenny, A.M., Podgorodnichenko, V.K., and Kagorodin, D.A., 1981, Therapeutical properties of benzimidazoles in trichinellosis and the side effects of the treatment, in: *Trichinellosis* (C.W. Kim, E.J. Ruitenberg, and J.S. Teppema, eds.), Reedbooks, Chertsey, England, pp. 287–290.

Pereverzeva, E.V., Veretennikova, N.L., and Ozeretskovskaya, N.N., 1981, The effect of benzimidazoles on inflammatory cell reactions in mice in experimental trichinellosis, in: *Trichinellosis* (C.W. Kim, E.J. Ruitenberg, and J.S. Teppema, eds.), Reedbooks, Chertsey, England, pp. 311–315.

Prichard, R.K., 1970, Mode of action of the anthelminthic thiabendazole in *Haemonchus contortus, Nature (London)* **228**:684–685.

Ramisz, A., and Komorowski, A., 1975, Histochemical study of the effect of phospho-roorganic esters Z-50 (Fenchlorfos) and Z-51 (Bromofos) on the cholinesterase activity in the course of muscle phase of experimental trichinellosis, *Pol. Arch. Weter.* **17:**623–631.

Ramisz, A., and Szankowska, Z., 1978, The effect of lethal dose of E 600 under the cover of antidote (Toxobidin, Polfa) on the course of muscle phase of experimental trichinellosis in mice, in: *Trichinellosis* (C.W. Kim and Z.S. Pawlowski, eds.), University Press of New England, Hanover, New Hampshire, pp. 477–483.

Ramisz, A., Lamina, J., and Schoop, G., 1967, Die Beeinflussing von Cholinesterase und Acetylcholinesterase durch das Phosphorsäureesterpräparat Tiguvon (Bayer) bei künstlich mit Trichinen infizierten Mäusen, *Zentralbl. Bakteriol. Parasitenkd. Abt. 1: Orig.* **204:**289–293.

Ruitenberg, E.J., and Steerenberg, P.A., 1974, Influence of thiabendazole on a *Trichinella spiralis* infection, *Tijdschr. Diergeneeskd.* **99:**347–351 (in Dutch).

Schoop, G., and Lamina, J., 1959, Uber die Wirkung von Neguvon auf *Trichinella spiralis* in experimentell infizierten Mäusen, *Monatsh. Tierheilkd.* **11:**167–171.

Seniuta, R., Dlugiewicz-Bulla, N., Piotrowski, R., and Grzywinski, L., 1981, The influence of fenbendazole and cambendazole on the course of experimental trichinellosis in mice. I. Intestinal phase, in: *Trichinellosis* (C.W. Kim, E.J. Ruitenberg, and J.S. Teppema, eds.). Reedbooks, Chertsey, England, pp. 317–321.

Sonnet, J.J., and Thienpont, D., 1977, The treatment of trichinosis with mebendazole, *Acta Clin. Belg.* **32:**297–302.

Spaldonova, R., 1969, Über den Mechanismus der Wirkung der Anthelminthika aus der Reihe der Alkylphosphate, *Helminthologia* **11:**279–283.

Spaldonova, R., 1981, Efficacy of febantel on *Trichinella spiralis* larvae in white mice, in: *Trichinellosis* (C.W. Kim, E.J. Ruitenberg, and J.S. Teppema, (eds.), Reedbooks, Chertsey, England, pp. 323–325.

Spaldonova, R., and Corba, J., 1979, Relationship between the antitrichinellous effect of seven derivatives of benzimidazole carbamates and their clinical structures, *Folia Parasitol.* **26:**145–149.

Spaldonova, R., and Vodrazka, J., 1969, The effect of niclosamide in experimental trichinellosis of mice, *Folia Parasitol.* **16:**375–377.

Spaldonova, R., Hovorka, J., and Tomasovicova, O., 1969, Effect of eustydil in experimental trichinellosis, *Vet. Cas.* **12:**85–87.

Spaldonova, R., Corba, J., and Tomasovicova, O., 1974, The influence of mebendazole on the course of *Trichinella* infection in mice, *Proc. Third Int. Congr. Parasitol., Munich* (Facta Publications) **2:**675–676.

Spaldonova, R., Corba, J., and Tomasovicova, O., 1978, Comparison of the efficacy of different benzimidazole anthelmintics against *Trichinella spiralis* and *Trichinella pseudospiralis*, in: *Trichinellosis* (C.W. Kim and Z.S. Pawlowski, eds.), University Press of New England, Hanover, New Hampshire, pp. 437–443.

Stewart, G.L., and Read, C.P., 1973, Changes in RNA in mouse trichinosis, *J. Parasitol.* **59:**997–1005.

Taylor, S.M., and Pearson, G.K., 1981, The effect of a single injection of ivermectin on encysted muscle larvae of *Trichinella spiralis* in experimentally infected pigs, in: *Trichinellosis* (C.W. Kim, E.J. Ruitenberg, and J.S. Teppema, eds.), Reedbooks, Chertsey, England, pp. 353–367.

Theodorides, V.J., and Laderman, M., 1969, Activity of parbendazole upon *Trichinella spiralis* in mice, *J. Parasitol.* **55:**678.

Thienpont, D., and Vanparijs, O., 1981, Prophylactic and curative action of flubendazole against experimental trichinellosis in pigs, in: *Trichinellosis* (C.W. Kim, E.J. Ruitenberg, and J.S. Teppema, eds.), Reedbooks, Chertsey, England, pp. 343–346.

Thienpont, D., Vanparijs, O.F.J., Raeymaekers, A.H.M., Vandenberk, J., Demoen, P.J.A., Allewijn, F.T.N., Marsboom, R.P.H., Niemgeers, C.J.E., Schellekens, K.H.L., and Janssen, P.A.J., 1966, Tetramisole (R8299), a new potent broad spectrum anthelmintic, *Nature (London)* **209:**1084–1086.

Thienpont, D., Vanparijs, O.F., and Vandesteene, R., 1974, Anthelmintic and histopathological effects of mebendazole on *Trichinella spiralis* in the rat, in: *Trichinellosis* (C.W. Kim, ed.), Intext, New York, pp. 515–527.

Tomasovica, O., Podhajecky, R., and Spaldonova, R., 1972, Die Wirkung des Thiabendazols auf die Ontogenese von *Trichinella spiralis, Folia Vet.* **16:**139–154.

Vanparijs, O., Hermans, L., and Thienpont, D., 1979, Anthelmintic activity of flubendazole against *Trichinella spiralis* in rats, *Vet. Parasitol.* **5:**237–242.

Veretennikova, N.L., Pereverzeva, E.V., and Timonov, E.V., 1981, On the mechanism of the action of benzimidazoles on intestinal *Trichinella*, in: *Trichinellosis* (C.W. Kim, E.J. Ruitenberg, and J.S. Teppema, eds.), Reedbooks, Chertsey, England, pp. 305–310.

Wollweber, H., Niemers, E., Flucke, W., Andrews, P., Schulz, H.-P., and Thomas, H., 1979, Amidantel, a potent anthelminthic from a new chemical class, *Arzneim.-Forsch.* **29:**31–32.

Zaiman, H., 1970, Drug treatment of trichinosis, in: *Trichinosis in Man and Animals* (S.E. Gould, ed.), Charles C. Thomas, Springfield, Illinois, pp. 329–347.

Zohdy, A., and Gawish, N., 1975, Studies on *Trichinella spiralis* chemotherapy, *J. Drug Res. (Egypt)* **7:**177–182.

11

Clinical Aspects in Man

ZBIGNIEW S. PAWŁOWSKI

1. INTRODUCTION

The other chapters in this book present knowledge based mainly on experimental work; in contrast, this chapter dealing with the clinical aspects of trichinosis is based primarily on clinical observations and experience. Here I wish to quote Dr. C.C. Booth (1980), who said that "those who decry the observational aspect of clinical research should recall that astronomy, whose scientific credentials have never been questioned, is an entirely observational science." In trichinosis, the links between clinical research and basic science are strong. Much of the modern knowledge and techniques used in parasitology, immunology, and clinical pathology have been introduced for better understanding of trichinosis as a disease. On the other hand, clinical studies of human trichinosis have promoted interest in the basic biological problems such as differences in various *Trichinella spiralis* strains. In the last two decades, great progress has been made in understanding the pathological mechanisms, symptoms, and signs of human trichinosis as well as in more rational treatment of the infection. However, many aspects of clinical trichinosis still remain unknown or vague, due in part to the limited possibilities for studying trichinosis in man.

There are two sources of information on clinical problems of trichinosis: publications from clinical centers working on trichinosis and reports from hospitals and clinics where cases of trichinosis have been

ZBIGNIEW S. PAWŁOWSKI • Clinic of Parasitic and Tropical Diseases, Medical Academy of Poznań, Poznań, Poland and Parasitic Diseases Programme, World Health Organization, Geneva 27, Switzerland.

treated sporadically. The latter often describe only some selected aspects of the clinical problems or deal with unusual cases and are rarely accompanied by satisfactory parasitological documentation. On the other hand, there are a few clinics situated in the areas endemic for trichinosis that are doing, or have already done, some more systematic clinical studies and that have published their experience in several reviews (Gould, 1970; Gerwel and Pawłowski, 1975; Kassur *et al.*, 1978; Ozeretskovskaya, 1978).

This chapter is intended, not to compete with other reviews in an exhaustive presentation of clinical aspects of trichinosis, but rather to provide an overview of the present status and approaches to the clinical aspects of *T. spiralis* infection and disease.

2. INFECTION AND DISEASE

The term trichinosis (trichinellosis) implies both the infection with *Trichinella spiralis* and the disease caused by *T. spiralis*. For clinical and epidemiological needs, as well as for research and didactic purposes, more precise classifications of the clinical course and the severity of the disease may be useful and are outlined in Sections 2.2 and 2.3. Both parasite and host factors have some influence on the severity of clinical trichinosis; with the parasite, both the qualitative factors (degree of invasiveness, strain of parasite) and the quantitative factors (number of larvae) play a role. The parasite factors seem to be responsible for the various clinical expressions found in different epidemics. The host reaction is very individualized, and as a rule, the clinical course of trichinosis therefore varies considerably in different groups of individuals.

2.1. Proportion of Symptomatic and Asymptomatic Cases in Trichinosis

Trichinosis is no exception to the general helminthological rule that only some of the infections present in man are symptomatic and cause a disease.

The prevalence of *T. spiralis* infections, including those that are asymptomatic, can be evaluated only by seroepidemiological study or by post-mortem examination for *T. spiralis* muscle larvae. Serological tests have not been widely used for epidemiological studies in trichinosis, mainly because of the difficulties in obtaining blood and doing intradermal tests and in evaluating the results. Postmortem examination also has some limitations: the cases examined do not constitute a true sample of the population; the parasites found may have been acquired several years before the examination. However, some useful epidemiological data can be obtained when enough examinations are carried out.

In a study in the United States in 1966–1970, of 8071 human diaphragms examined, 4.2% were found to be infected with *T. spiralis* (Zimmermann *et al.*, 1973). Since older age groups were more widely examined and more frequently found to be infected, the correct prevalence, weighted for age of the population in the United States, was calculated as being 2.2%. Taking into account that the prevalence of infections with living *T. spiralis* larvae was only 0.73%, the number of human infections in the United States contracted every year was estimated at between 149,000 and 298,000. There were 110 clinical cases reported annually, which means that apart from some misdiagnosed or nondiagnosed cases, the majority of infections were mild or asymptomatic. In fact, 37.9% of the positive muscle samples had fewer than 1 *T. spiralis* larva per gram, and as many as 51.9% of the samples had 1–10 larvae per gram of diaphragm; only 0.9% of the positive samples had more than 101 larvae per gram and would therefore be expected to have had a symptomatic infection.

Similar data were reported from Poland (Kozar and Kozar, 1965). In 1961–1964, 3.3% of 3065 cases examined postmortem had *T. spiralis* larvae in the diaphragm. Only 0.8% of the positive samples had more than 100 larvae per gram, and 36% had fewer than 1 larva per gram.

The high proportion of light, asymptomatic infections is the result of the *T. spiralis* larvae being diluted during industrialized meat-production processes. On the other hand, in epidemics confined to a few families or a group of hunters, most of the cases are found to be symptomatic, since the number of infective larvae is usually high in these cases (Ciszewska-Olczak *et al.*, 1974; Barrett-Connor *et al.*, 1976; Bura and Willett, 1977).

2.2. Course of Trichinosis

As with most acute infectious diseases, trichinosis has an incubation period, an acute stage of disease, and a recovery period, as well as its consequences.

The incubation period of trichinosis reported in man varies widely from 1 to 51 days, depending on what has been accepted as the end of incubation: the first day of gastrointestinal symptoms or the first day of fever, myalgia, and periorbital edema. Gastrointestinal symptoms occur only in fewer than one seventh of trichinosis cases and many depend on other concomitant infections [e.g., sarcocystosis (Sapunar *et al.*, 1965)], intoxication (alcohol), or simply indigestion, since the trichinosis dish is often only a part of the feast. The gastrointestinal symptoms do not present a picture specific for trichinosis and may occur within several hours, days, or weeks after ingestion of the infected meat. Since the occurrence of gastrointestinal symptoms is a rather uncertain criterion, most frequently nonexistent and nonspecific even if present, it is better to accept that the incubation period in trichinosis ends with the appearance of the typical complex of symptoms, including fever. This complex occurs not earlier than 5 days after ingestion of infected meat, when a new generation of *T. spiralis* larvae starts to invade the muscle tissue.

It is generally thought that the duration of the incubation period is related to the severity of the clinical course: the earlier the complex of pathognomonic symptoms, the more severe is the clinical course of the trichinosis. This was well demonstrated by Januszkiewicz (1969) in 147 cases of trichinosis: 29 severe cases had a mean incubation period of 7.6 (± 3.2) days, 58 moderate cases had 16 (± 5.9) days, 53 light cases 21 (± 9.1) days, and 7 abortive cases 30 (± 7.3) days. According to this rule, the first cases that occur in an epidemic are usually the most severe ones. But there are also some exceptions to the rule in cases where the severity of the clinical course is related not so much to the intensity of the infection as to the serious complications that may occur in less intensive infections. Death from trichinosis was also observed in those cases that had a longer incubation period.

The incubation period is followed by acute or subacute symptomatic trichinosis, which slowly transmutes into a convalescence stage. Trichinosis has some analogies with acute viral or bacterial infections in which recovery from the infection, recovery from the acute disease, and recovery from persistent symptoms can be observed (Pawłowski, 1978). A classification of the clinical course in human trichinosis is proposed in Fig. 1. Recovery from the infection, i.e., by destruction of the *T. spiralis* larvae in the muscle tissue, takes several years and may remain incomplete. Recovery from the acute disease, much accelerated by modern therapy, takes 1–8 weeks; very rarely is it incomplete due, for example, to mechanical injuries caused by aberrant larvae or to an extremely heavy invasion. Recovery from persistent symptoms in trichinosis is a far slower process. In some patients, the muscle pains and feeling of weakness and fatigue may persist for months or even years, although these symptoms usually become less pronounced with time. It has been suggested that in influenza, weakness and fatigue, the most commonly persistent symptoms, are closely correlated with the depres-

Timing   Manifestations

0   Infection by ingestion of invasive *T. spiralis* larvae

5–51 days | Incubation period |

Appearance of the trichinosis syndrome (fever, myalgia, periorbital edema, eosinophilia)

1–8 weeks | Acute trichinosis |

Recovery from the disease (disappearance of the acute syndrome and complications, if any)

Few months to a | Convalescence stage |
few years

Complete recovery from the illness (disappearance of any signs and symptoms related to trichinosis)

Several years | Asymptomatic infection |

Recovery from the infection (no more *T. spiralis* larvae alive in the muscle tissue)

FIGURE 1. Clinical course in trichinosis.

sive propensity of the afflicted patients and the increased awareness of the disease. There have been no similar studies in human trichinosis as to whether or not the depressive inclination of these patients is responsible for the protracted recovery or whether the lower biological potential is responsible for both the depressive propensity and the delayed recovery (Pawłowski, 1978).

The protracted recovery from illness that occurred in some cases of human trichinosis stimulated the establishment of the theory of "chronic trichinosis" (Kozar *et al.*, 1964), which is supposed to be a chronic allergic phase of infection following the sensitization phase (incubation period) and the hyperergic phase (acute trichinosis). The common occurrence of the syndrome of chronic trichinosis has not been confirmed in better-controlled studies (Cox *et al.*, 1969; Kassur and Januszkiewicz, 1970; Chodera *et al.*, 1974). This does not exclude the possibility that trichinosis, like some other infections, may cause permanent, irreparable damage, e.g., to the retina, the nervous system, or the myocardium, or that it may alter an individual's reactivity in the future.

2.3. Severity of Trichinosis

The clinical course of symptomatic trichinosis varies greatly from abortive cases, through mild, moderate, and severe, to fatal ones. There has been much controversy regarding the criteria for the classification of cases, which is necessary for research, clinical, epidemiological, and didactic purposes. By analyzing the many different factors that influence the severity of the disease (see Section 2.4), one may easily conclude that the classification cannot be based on a single criterion such as the number of *T. spiralis* larvae in the muscle, or the titers of serological tests, or the degree of eosinophilia. The classification must be based on the presence and intensity of several clinical signs and symptoms (fever, myalgia, periorbital edema), laboratory measurements (eosinophilia, hypoalbuminemia), evaluation of the complications, and the timing of recovery, as well as on the epidemiological data and serological tests.

Table I presents the classification based on the proposals of Kassur and Januszkiewicz (1968). As with all other classifications of biological phenomena, this one is not perfect; for example, it may happen that a case is moderate in the early stages of the disease and finally becomes mild, or vice versa. Nevertheless, the practicability of this classification has been proved by several years of experience with it in some clinical centers in Poland.

The occurrence ratios of various forms of clinical trichinosis differ widely according to the epidemiological situation; in general, the severity of trichinosis is negatively proportional to the number of people involved in an epidemic. In the large-town type of epidemic, the trichinosis usually has a relatively light clinical course. In an outbreak of trichinosis in Liverpool in 1953, 60 of 82 cases diagnosed were treated at home and 22 were hospitalized; 1 patient died (Semple *et al.*, 1954). During an epidemic in Mosina, Poland, in 1960, of 2678 persons examined, 1122 were diagnosed as having symptomatic trichinosis, 286 were hospitalized, and 2 died (Neyman and Talarczyk, 1961). In an outbreak at Diez/Lahn (West Germany) in 1967, 24 of 486 infected cases were hospitalized, and 1 patient died (Hennekeuser *et al.*, 1968).

TABLE I
Classification of the Severity of the Clinical Course in Trichinosis[a]

Findings	Asymptomatic	Abortive	Mild	Moderate	Severe
History of exposure	Positive	Positive	Positive	Positive	Positive
Serological tests (4–8 weeks)	Positive	Positive	Positive	Positive	Positive
Eosinophilia > 500/mm³	Usually transient	Nearly always	Almost always	Always	May be absent
Symptoms and signs (fever, myalgia, periorbital edema)	—	Few signs, transient (1–2 days)	Usually a complex of signs, mildly expressed	Full complex of signs, well expressed	Full complex of signs, intensively expressed
Fever	—	—	Below 38°C for less than 1 week[b]	Over 38°C for up to 2 weeks[b]	Over 39°C for more than 2 weeks[b]
Recovery from disease	—	—	Within 3 weeks	Within 5–7 weeks	in more than 7 weeks
Hypoalbuminemia in 3–4 weeks	—	—	—	<3 g[c]	<2.5 g[c]
Complications	—	—	—	Rare, transient	Common
Number of larvae per gram of muscle tissue	Usually <10		Usually >100		
Hospitalization	Possible treatment as outpatient			Hospitalization	

[a] Based on Kassur and Januszkiewicz (1968).

[b] If not treated with steroids.   [c] If not prevented by treatment.

In the smaller, family-type epidemics of trichinosis, the severity of cases is usually greater. For example, in an epidemic in Opatowek, Poland, there were 15 persons suspected to having contracted *T. spiralis* infection; all were confirmed, and 13 were hospitalized because of severe (4 cases), moderate (4), or light (5) infection. There were no deaths. The intensity of infection varied from 4 to 1130 *T. spiralis* larvae per gram of deltoid muscle (Ciszewska-Olczak *et al.*, 1974).

2.4. Factors That Influence the Severity of Trichinosis

The severity of clinical trichinosis depends both on the parasite and on the host. Among the parasite factors, the most important are the number and invasiveness, and the strain of *T. spiralis* ingested.

For a long time, the intensity of the infection, as measured by the number of *T. spiralis* larvae per gram of muscle tissue in man, was thought to be the most important factor. Hall and Collins (1937) suggested that infections with fewer than 1 *T. spiralis* larva per gram of muscle tissue are asymptomatic, those with more than 100 larvae per gram produce pronounced clinical symptoms, and those with over 1000 larvae per gram are critical. However, it is not generally accepted that the relationship between the intensity and the severity of infection is directly proportional: infections with fewer than 1 larva per gram may be either asymptomatic or symptomatic; fewer than 10 larvae per gram may even be severe (Kershaw *et al.*, 1956); infections with more than 100 larvae per gram are usually moderate or severe, but infections with over 1000 larvae per gram are not necessarily fatal (Forrester *et al.*, 1961).

The correlation between the clinical picture and the intensity of infection in man may be negatively influenced by inaccurate methods of measurement. If only a small quantity of muscle tissue is biopsied, one can obtain only a rough estimate of the intensity of infection; the more accurate measurements obtained from postmortem examination are rarely compared with the detailed clinical data.

The number of invasive larvae is more difficult to calculate, even when the intensity of infection in the meat ingested and the amount of meat eaten are known, since the invasiveness of the larvae depends on the way in which the food is stored and processed. In an outbreak in Alaska, it was found that individuals who ate only boiled bear meat did not contract trichinosis, whereas the incidence rate was 78% in those who ate meat that had been cooked in a "bul koki pan" (a Korean utensil) and 88% in those who ate charcoal-grilled bear meat. The bear meat, which had up to 1200 larvae per gram, was stored at approximately −18°C for several weeks, but it still contained invasive larvae; the *T.*

spiralis Alaska strain seems to be less sensitive to freezing (Centers for Disease Control, 1979). Data on the number of *T. spiralis* larvae in ingested meat, plus information on the storage and processing of the meat, have more epidemiological than clinical importance; however, an estimate of the low or high invasive dose expected provides useful, though not decisive, information for the clinician.

An epidemic among Kikuyu males, described by Forrester *et al.* (1961), not only was the first report on human trichinosis south of the Sahara, but also drew attention to the fact that the so-called "African" strain might be less pathogenic to man than the northern-hemisphere strains. During this epidemic, eight males aged from 7 to 22 years survived though they had from 420 to 2800 (with an average of 1829) *T. spiralis* larvae per gram of muscle tissue.

On the other hand, infections in man caused by an Arctic strain have been described as being more severe and having a more protracted clinical course (Ozeretskovskaya *et al.*, 1970).

Nowadays, there is enough evidence to show that the clinical course of trichinosis is one of the biological characteristics of *T. spiralis* that differ from strain to strain, e.g., *T. spiralis domestica, nativa,* and *nelsoni* (Ozeretskovskaya, 1978).

Any investigator involved in the study of trichinosis in animals has observed that despite using the same strain of *T. spiralis* and closely adjusted infective doses for inoculation, the final intensity of infection differs widely; this illustrates the influence of the host factors and is evident even in carefully selected groups of animals. In natural epidemics, the host factors have a much more decisive influence both on the number of *T. spiralis* larvae developed and on the clinical course, which is a very individual reaction to the infection.

Among the host factors, there are the classic ones such as age, sex, and ethnic group that are easy to determine and there are the more difficult ones such as the genetic background, the general health status, including immune status, previous infections, concomitant diseases, and individual reactivity. There have been few observations on the host factors in man; most of those reported have dealt with the factors that influence the number of invasive larvae ingested and excysted (including the effect of alcohol, digestive potential, and intestinal passage).

3. SYMPTOMS, SIGNS, AND CLINICAL PATHOLOGY

Trichinosis belongs to the group of diseases characterized by a remarkable variety of symptoms and signs. In the tabulation prepared by Gould (1970), there are 34 symptoms and 33 signs listed as being frequently encountered and 26 symptoms and 48 signs reported as infrequently observed in trichinosis—141 different symptoms and signs altogether. The best way to represent the symptomatology of trichinosis and its relationship to the clinical pathology is by grouping the symptoms and signs into categories of early and late, those that occur in uncomplicated infections and those due to complications.

Clinical trichinosis has traditionally been divided into the intestinal stage, the muscle-invasion stage, and the convalescent stage, with an unjustified tendency for all these stages to be regarded as separate. In fact, the intestinal invasion overlaps the muscle invasion, which is by no means terminated in the convalescent stage.

The symptoms and signs will be considered here under the following headings: (1) the abdominal syndrome, which is the first to appear; (2) the general syndrome, which starts at the end of the incubation period, but is unspecific; (3) signs of allergic vasculitis, which are common and characteristic for trichinosis; (4) symptoms and signs associated with muscle tissue; (5) metabolic signs, which may occur in the later stages; (6) complications of trichinosis: cardiac, respiratory, neurological, ocular, and others; and (7) pathology in laboratory tests.

3.1. Abdominal Syndrome

The abdominal syndrome, consisting mostly of abdominal pain and diarrhea, may occur early in the course of trichinosis or in the later periods of the disease. The early abdominal syndrome is related to trichinous enteritis due to an inflammatory reaction of the mucosa of the small intestine to the adult worms parasitizing there for 1–2 months (if the patient has not been treated).

This syndrome is frequently related to the intensity of infection; for example, in an epidemic in Tanzania in which the mean number of larvae was 3390 per gram of muscle tissue, diarrhea was one of the most prominent symptoms (Bura and Willett, 1977). It was suggested that the diarrhea was either of the "exudative type" due to the inflammatory reaction of the mucosa or of the "osmotic type" due to secondary lactase deficiency caused by damage to the villi brush borders.

The abdominal syndrome may also occur in the later stages of trichinosis and may be of a recurrent nature. A late abdominal syndrome, occurring between the 3rd and 5th weeks of the disease, has been described as being characteristic for infections with the Arctic strain of *T. spiralis* (Ozeretskovskaya and Tumolskaya, 1974). The same authors suggested that a delayed hypersensitivity reaction might be responsible for the late occurrence or recurrence of the abdominal syndrome.

Abdominal symptoms and signs have been reported with a frequency varying from a few to 42% of the cases, but, as mentioned in Section 2.2, some of the abdominal symptoms may be due to causes other than trichinosis (Sapunar *et al.*, 1965).

3.2. General Trichinosis Syndrome

The general trichinosis syndrome consists of fever, myalgia, and malaise. It comes at the end of the incubation period, and the fever usually comes first, followed by myalgia and malaise.

Although fever is one of the most common signs in symptomatic trichinosis (in over 90% of the cases), it differs as to onset, degree, type, and duration. The fever usually reaches its peaks in a few days. It may not be higher than 38°C in mild cases, but in severe cases it may exceed 40°C. The fever is mostly of a remittent type, but can also be continuous or intermittent. In untreated cases, it can last from a few days to a few weeks; steroid treatment normally reduces the fever within a few days.

The pathological mechanism of the fever remains unclear, since it is difficult to study this in experimental animals. The stimuli that activate the endogenous pyrogens may use both a nonspecific pathway, e.g., a reaction to antigen–antibody complexes or changes in protein metabolism, and an immunologically specific pathway through the activated host target cells, i.e., segmented neutrophils, eosinophils, and monocytes as well as bone-marrow-derived phagocytic cells, including Kupffer cells. The human host's tolerance to endotoxin may determine the amount of time (1 or more weeks) before the occurrence of the fever, which may arise abruptly as soon as the tolerance is broken.

Myalgia usually occurs at the same time as, or shortly after, the onset of fever; it, too, is one of the better established but uncharacteristic symptoms of trichinosis and is discussed in Section 3.4.

Malaise occurs more in moderate or severe cases of trichinosis and depends much on the individual reaction of the patient; it has been reported in as many as 56% of cases (Kassur *et al.*, 1978). The malaise is due to fever, marked muscular exhaustion, and generalized disease. The feeling of weakness or fatigue or both may last for a long time and does not respond well to steroid therapy.

3.3. Signs of Allergic Vasculitis

In moderate and severe trichinosis, vasculitis is often present. Although the details of its mechanism are not very clear, it is generally believed to be a result of the hyperergic processes typical of the early stage of the disease (Ozeretskovskaya and Vikhert, 1960; Ozeretskovskaya, 1978).

Signs of allergic vasculitis usually appear together with the general symptoms including fever, i.e., from 7 to 21 days after ingestion of the invasive *T. spiralis* larvae. There are two basic consequences of allergic vasculitis: leakage of fluid from the vascular to the interstitial compartment and hemorrhage.

In cases of trichinosis, the leakage of fluid is most visible as a periorbital edema (Fig. 2). Most often, it starts with edema of the upper and lower eyelids, and frequently extends to the whole periorbital area and sometimes to the whole face. In some cases, an early edema of the subcutaneous tissue of the legs also occurs. The edema usually disappears at the same time as the fever.

Early hemorrhage usually occurs together with the periorbital edema and fever, but dissipates more slowly. Hemorrhage of the bulbar conjunctiva (Fig. 3) and in the fingernail beds is characteristic of trichinosis.

Hemorrhages are usually found on both eyes, localized on the bulbar conjunctiva between the two lids; they are more intense at the medial angle of eye and close to the cornea and, being deep red in color, contrast well against the rest of the bulbar conjunctiva even when it is congested. The hemorrhage subsides slowly, changing from a deep red color to a waxy yellow, and it is sometimes still visible near the cornea in the 2nd week of the disease.

In severe cases, small hemorrhages can sometimes be seen in the retina at fundoscopy. Hemorrhagic changes in the brain are thought to be responsible for the general or focal neurological symptoms. Hemorrhagic extravasations are occasionally found at postmortem

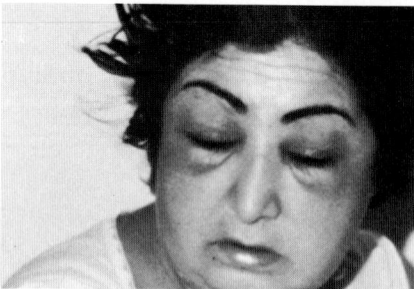

FIGURE 2. Trichinosis patient in acute stage, with fever and malaise, showing characteristic periorbital edema. Photograph by Prof. R.M. Matossian; published by permission.

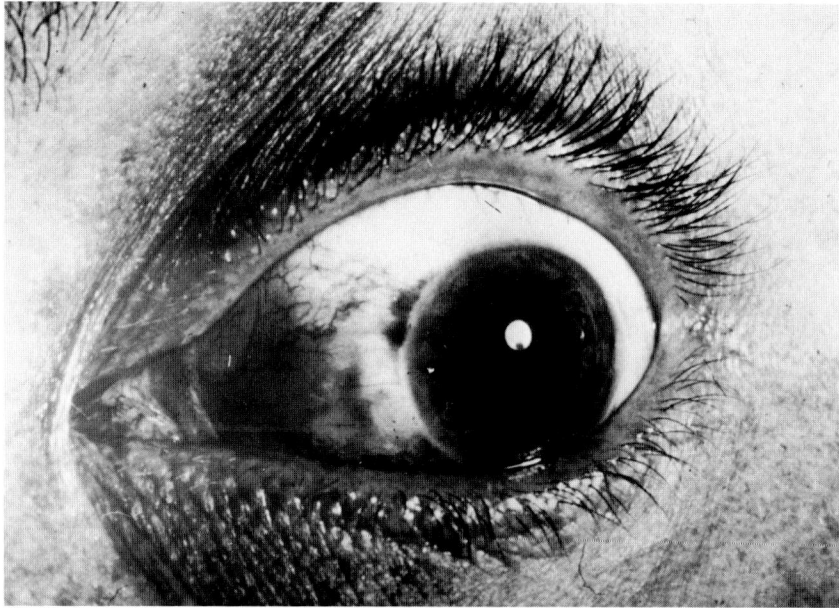

FIGURE 3. Eye of trichinosis patient, showing conjunctival hemorrhage.

examination in the pericardium, the endocardium, the pleura and the lung tissue and brain.

Splinter hemorrhages of the nailbeds on the fingers and toes are not infrequent in trichinosis; the possible embolic character of these hemorrhages cannot be excluded, since they are similar to the changes observed in bacterial endocarditis.

3.4. Symptoms and Signs Associated with Muscle Tissue

Myalgia usually accompanies the fever and signs of allergic vasculitis, which are the early symptoms of trichinosis, but in rare cases it occurs a few days later. The pain is referred to the muscle most frequently used, such as the extraocular muscles, masseters, tongue, respiratory muscles, neck muscles, and flexor muscles of the extremities. There is some spontaneous pain, but the intensity normally increases greatly with movement; therefore, heavily infected patients try to immobilize their bodies as far as possible, breathe superficially, and find it more comfortable to keep their elbow, hip, and knee joints flexed. Fixed contractures can be observed in untreated patients.

On examination, the muscles of the extremities are tender at palpation and painful with deeper pressure or induced movement. The strength of the hands, arms, and legs is diminished. Flexor contractions may induce tetanic rigidity; rigidity of the masseters is not uncommon in intensive infections.

The muscle pain is not helped much by steroid therapy, but reacts better to salicylates; it is diminished gradually as the inflammatory process in the muscle tissue subsides.

Complete recovery may take several months or even years. The myalgia usually disappears faster than the feeling of weakness; a pseudomyasthenic form of trichinosis has been reported.

Electromyographic (EMG) studies may give evidence of acute myositis and, in later stages, of diffuse myopathic dysfunction. Profuse spontaneous fibrillation, being an indication of muscle fiber denervation, probably reflects a disconnection of the muscle fibers from their endplate regions due to focal muscle fiber necrosis rather than primary involvement of the intramuscular nerve endings (Gross and Ochoa, 1979). In general, the EMG pathological findings are related to the intensity of infection and may not be apparent in cases with fewer than 10 T. spiralis larvae per gram of muscle. During experimental infection in monkeys, the EMG pathological changes at first preceded the histopathological changes, but in the later period of infection, they correlated well with the histopathological changes examined in the biopsy material (Kocięcka et al., 1974). In human trichinosis, the correlation is evident only in the acute stage of intensive infections; some EMG changes may be present 1–8 years after the acute trichinosis, but are not correlated to the intensity of infection or the clinical course (Kocięcka et al., 1975). Since EMG changes are not characteristic for trichinosis, great care should be taken in interpreting the EMG tracings of patients.

Evaluation of the muscle tissue involvement should be based on clinical examination and observations, as well as on laboratory findings, including leukocytosis and muscle enzyme activity in the serum. EMG tracings and muscle biopsy should be done whenever the signs are unusual or persistent.

3.5. Signs of Metabolic Disorders

Our knowledge of exactly how T. spiralis infection affects the human host metabolism is limited to those aspects that can be either clinically observed or measured in the laboratory. i.e., hypoalbuminemia, hypokalemia, and hypoglycemia, changes in the activity of various enzymes, and corticosteroids examined in the blood serum (Buşilă et al., 1968).

Hypoalbuminemia is in some way related to the intensity of infection and the severity of the clinical course of trichinosis. It is not usually found in mild cases of trichinosis. In severe cases, it may occur early, i.e., in the 2nd week of disease, but in other cases it is not manifest before the 3rd week of disease. Hypoalbuminemia reaches its lowest value between the 5th and 6th weeks of infection and slowly becomes normal over the following few weeks, independent of the severity of the clinical course. This observation (Rachoń et al., 1967) suggests that hypoalbuminemia is related to the growing process of the T. spiralis larvae and their encystation. An increased demand for protein at the site of the growing parasite and a change in the metabolism of the muscle tissue are probably the main causes of the hypoalbuminemia. However, a decrease in albumin synthesis during the disease or leakage of albumin and fluid from the intravascular compartment to the interstitial space or both, may also play a role. A substantial loss of albumin through the urinary tract may occur in some cases, but does not constitute a main cause of albuminuria.

Hypoalbuminemia is clinically expressed by the presence of hydrostatic edema that can readily be observed on the legs and back and in more severe cases by ascites and effusions in the pleural cavities.

The serum hypoproteinemia usually reflects the degree of hypoalbuminemia, since the decrease in albumin is not compensated by the increase in serum gammaglobulins.

Hypokalemia in the serum and muscle cells is usually linked with hypoalbuminemia. Hypokalemia can be expressed clinically by muscle weakness, but this has not been confirmed. The effect of hypokalemia is more evident in ECG tracings and signs of various heart arrhythmias. Depletion of the K^+ ions at the myocardial cell membrane level leads to disturbances of the repolarization or depolarization processes, or both, of the myocardium. It has been shown that infusion of potassium ions immediately normalizes the ECG signs of hypokalemia in T. spiralis-infected rabbits (Chodera and Pawłowski, 1974). The beneficial effect of the normalization of K^+ ion serum level on the cardiovascular system of human patients has been observed.

Although a moderate enlargement of the liver is observed in some cases of trichinosis, the serum level of specific liver enzymes such as ornithine-carbamoyl transferase and 1-monophosphofructoaldolase remains unchanged. Therefore, it is reasonable to accept that the main source of increased activity of some of the serum enzymes is the muscle tissue (Januszkiewicz et al., 1970). The increased metabolism of some muscle fibers and damage to others, together with increased permeation through the muscle fiber membranes, cause a leakage of enzymes into the serum. The most common and marked increase is that of creatine phosphokinase (CPK) and 1,6-diphosphofructoaldolase; less common and less pronounced is the increase of the aminotransferases (Asp AT and Ala AT). The increase in CPK activity varied in individual patients from 2 to 105 times above the normal value and was observed as early on as the 18th day after ingestion of invasive *T. spiralis* larvae (Wiśniewska, 1970).

Impaired adrenocortical function has been found in some patients with trichinosis, expressed as a transient deficiency in 17-hydroxy- and 17-ketosteroids and lowered urine excretion of 17-hydroxy- and 17-ketosteroids after ACTH stimulation. An insufficient functional reserve of the adrenal cortex has been observed more frequently in severe cases of trichinosis (Dziubek, 1969).

3.6. Complications of Trichinosis

Trichinosis not only affects the intestinal tract and muscle tissue, where the parasite completes its life cycle, but also may provoke several complications due either to the ectopic migration of the larvae, as in the case of some ocular and cerebral manifestations, or to a hypersensitive reaction of the host, as in the case of some cardiac and lung manifestations. It is often not easy to differentiate the manifestations that result from pathological mechanisms typical for trichinosis from complications of a secondary character.

3.6.1. Ocular Manifestations and Complications

Periorbital edema and conjunctival hemorrhages, as described in Section 3.3, are the first ocular signs of trichinosis; they appear early and are characteristic enough to be helpful in establishing an early clinical diagnosis, which is not infrequently first suggested by an ophthalmologist. In addition to these signs, there are often various other ocular symptoms such as photophobia, blurring, disturbed vision, and pain in the eyeball. The variability of the ocular symptoms and signs is related to their different mechanisms and localization. The eyeball can be affected not only by vascular changes but also by any or a combination of an ectopic migration of the larvae, intensive invasion of the eyeball muscles, increased intracranial pressure, and affected cranial nerves or visual centers. Experiments in animals have shown that most ocular pathology is caused by the *T. spiralis* larva itself either straying to the different parts of the eyeball or invading the ocular muscles (Schoop *et al.*, 1961).

The ocular muscles are usually invaded more intensively than the skeletal muscles, and their impaired function causes more visible symptoms and signs. Painful movement of the eyeballs and easy tiredness from reading, strabismus, and exophthalmos are sometimes present for several weeks.

3.6.2. Neurological Manifestations and Complications

Neurological manifestations occur in 10–24% of cases of trichinosis, mainly in the severe ones. They may appear early or late; they may be of a diffuse or focal character and may be caused by the migration of ectopic *T. spiralis* larvae or by a hypersensitive host reaction to the infection.

At the end of the 2nd week of infection (i.e., the 1st week of disease), early and diffuse manifestations are caused by meningitis and encephalitis. At that time, the larval migration is at its peak and also the vascular changes are most pronounced. As seen from the results of postmortem examination, hyperemia, edema, hemorrhage, emboli, and perivascular cellular infiltrates are quite common in fatal cases with neurological manifestations or because of early neurological complications. Strong headache, insomnia, delirium, apathy, or psychosis, contemporaneous with high fever and malaise, are the most common symptoms. The level of consciousness usually remains undisturbed even in critically ill patients.

Focal manifestations may develop at any period of the disease, but they are most common during and after the 3rd week of infection when the host cellular reaction to the straying *T. spiralis* larvae becomes intensive. The manifestations reported include hemianopsia, aphasia, cranial nerve deficits, anisocoria, tinnitus, decreased hearing and deafness, ataxia, seizures, and various types of paralysis, paresis, and neuropathies (Gould, 1970; Kramer and Aita, 1978).

3.6.3. Cardiovascular Manifestations and Complications

Cardiovascular manifestations and complications of trichinosis are the most frequent and the most serious. With *T. spiralis* infection, at least some of the newborn larvae have to migrate through the myocardium and are either destroyed there or escape back into the circulation. As a rule, *T. spiralis* larvae do not encyst in the myocardium, but they do stay there for some time before being destroyed. A focal cellular infiltration, composed mostly of eosinophils and mononuclear cells, and necrosis of some myocardial fibers have been observed in rabbits as early as the 6th day after infection. In the latter stages of trichinosis, the infiltration may become more diffuse, causing an eosinophilic myocarditis. Granulomas are formed, and connective tissue fibers may replace myocardial fibers causing an interstitial myocarditis with fine fibrosis; the latter is rare, but it may cause permanent cardiac damage. Most patients recover fully from the myocarditis caused by trichinosis. The cardiovascular complications are related to the intensity of infection and are clinically manifest in about 20% of hospitalized patients; however, it is not rare to find that the few clinical signs are not in proportion to the severe myocardial changes.

It is not only the myocardial changes in trichinosis that are responsible for the cardiovascular complications, but also arrhythmias caused by hypokalemia, adrenal gland insufficiency, and functional changes in the blood vessel circulation.

A review of 41 fatal cases of acute trichinosis examined postmortem disclosed three major causes of death: (1) myocarditis, (2) encephalitis, and (3) pneumonitis; myocarditis was the most common cause of death, being diagnosed in 32 cases (Andy *et al.*, 1977). Acute cardiac failure may occur at any time in trichinosis, but it is most frequent between the 4th and 8th weeks of infection (i.e., 3rd to 6th week of disease). Sudden death without premonitory cardiac symptoms may occur in the 1st week of disease, but has more often been reported later, when the acute general syndrome is over, the muscle symptoms have begun to subside, and the patient is about to leave his bed; pulmonary embolism or bouts of paroxysmal tachycardia have then been reported as a cause of sudden death. Frequently, even intensive therapy cannot improve the chances of survival of patients who have advanced myocardial lesions in the course of intensive trichinosis improperly treated or diagnosed too late.

The recovery of patients with cardiovascular complications may be slow, especially in cases of thrombosis, hypoalbuminemic edema, extreme hypotension, or pulmonary complications.

3.6.4. Pulmonary Manifestations and Complications

In trichinosis, pulmonary complications occur rather infrequently, in less than 5% of hospitalized patients. They may have an immunological or circulatory background (Januszkiewicz, 1967).

There are some similarities between antigenic pneumonitis and the pulmonary changes in trichinosis, which may appear as infiltrations at the base of the lungs, disappearing quickly even without steroid therapy; as migrating focal infiltrations with a pleural reaction that becomes protracted if not treated with steroids; or, finally, as a severe, frequently fatal pulmonary syndrome with disseminated foci of infiltration, caused by vasculitis, small emboli, or infarcts, and refractory to the steroid therapy (Ozeretskovskaya, 1978). Spastic bronchitis can be included as a lung complication of immunological origin. These changes are likely to occur in the first 2 weeks of the disease.

In the later stages of trichinosis (3–7 weeks), bacterial lung infections are more likely, due either to the immobility of the severely ill patients or to the immunosuppressive effects of the trichinosis or its cardiovascular complications; as in many other severe diseases, bronchopneumonia may occur a few days before death. Hypoalbuminemia or circulatory complications may cause effusions in the pleural cavities. The possibility of pulmonary embolism due to cardiovascular changes has already been mentioned (Section 3.6.3).

3.6.5. Other Manifestations and Complications

Skin eruptions are sometimes seen in human trichinosis and may appear as a fine macular rash a few days after the start of the fever or may emerge later in the 2nd week of the disease as a maculopapular exanthema. The skin lesions may be transient, persistent, even for a few weeks, or recurrent. The underlying cause of the skin eruption is probably immunological.

Any urinary problems that arise are usually secondary, except in rare cases of mild immune-complex glomerulonephritis (Sitprija et al., 1980).

3.7. Pathology in Laboratory Tests

The most common and characteristic changes found in the laboratory tests for human trichinosis are concerned with eosinophilia, leukocytosis, and enzymatic and serological tests. As in many other infectious or parasitic diseases, the other tests may yield abnormal values for secondary reasons.

3.7.1. Eosinophilia

Eosinophilia is one of the earliest, most stable, and characteristic signs of human trichinosis. It is found in many subclinical cases and all symptomatic cases except for very severe ones a few days before death, and in those cases complicated by a concomitant bacterial infection (e.g., bronchopneumonia, peritonitis). Eosinophilia is proportionally related to the intensity of infection. It can be slight (500 cells/mm^3) and transient in light infections, but more usually is well pronounced (over 1000 cells/mm^3) and protracted for many weeks. Eosinophilia is diminished by steroid therapy.

In experiments in animals, eosinophilia has been observed as early as 5 days after inoculation, but in man it is already the 2nd or 3rd week of infection before the eosinophilia is detected. It is at its height during the next few weeks and slowly declines thereafter. The usual values are between 1000 and 3000/mm^3 (i.e., 15–45% of all white blood cells), but in sporadic cases as much as 70–89% eosinophils has been reported. Eosinophilia can be better expressed by the number of eosinophils per cubic millimeter than by the percentage of all white blood cells; it is easier to measure the number of eosinophils per cubic millimeter by a chamber technique than by counting them in proportion to hundreds of other white blood cells.

The eosinophils circulating in the blood are usually in proportion to those present in the muscle tissue or inner organs. Recently, a significant correlation was found between the peripheral eosinophil count and the antibody-dependent, eosinophil-mediated death of *Schistosoma mansoni* schistosomulae tested *in vitro* (David *et al.*, 1980).

There are two mechanisms that increase the number of eosinophils. First, eosinophilia may be a response to chemotactic agents released from degranulating mast cells or other mediators released as a result of other immunological reactions; such mediators include split products of complement (C5, C6, C7, and C5a) and products of activated lymphocytes (eosinophil-stimulation promoter and eosinophil chemotactic factor). Second, eosinophilia may be due to the antibody-dependent or complement-dependent ability of eosinophils to damage *T. spiralis* tissue larvae, not only those present in the muscle tissue but also those that have strayed to other organs. It has recently been suggested that the major basic protein of the eosinophils when released intravascularly may exert nonspecific toxic effects, e.g., damage to the endothelial cells.

Although the role of the eosinophils is still not clear, eosinophilia is a sign that should be carefully observed during human trichinosis, since it expresses some of the pathological processes occurring during the disease.

3.7.2. Leukocytosis

Many clinical data on leukocytosis in human trichinosis are available in case reports, but they have rarely been analyzed in relation to the severity and course of the disease. Leukocytosis is somewhat less consistent, evident, and persistent than eosinophilia. It is probably related to the intensity of the inflammatory reaction in the muscles, myocardium, and other organs. Leukocytosis is present in most hospitalized patients; the number of leukocytes is usually around 15,000/mm^3, but it may be as high as 50,000/mm^3. Both leukocytosis and eosinophilia occur early, at the same time as the general trichinosis syndrome, but the leukocytosis subsides earlier, usually with recovery from the disease. Lymphocytes, which are less abundant initially, may be more common in the later stages of trichinosis.

3.7.3. Other Pathological Changes

Despite rather frequent changes in serum protein levels and albumim/globulin ratios, the blood sedimentation rate is rarely high.

Changes in serum enzyme activity, especially CPK, were discussed in Section 3.5. A high creatinine level and creatinuria are usually present. The possibility of hypokalemia was also mentioned in Section 3.5; the levels of other electrolytes do not seem to be affected as much.

An elevated level of immunoglobulin E (IgE) was observed at the onset of the disease, but elevated levels of IgG and IgM occurred only in the later stage of trichinosis (Matossian et al., 1977).

Some pathological changes that may be seen by EMG, ECG, or X-ray examination of the chest are not characteristic of trichinosis. The EMG abnormalities are myogenic in origin and are not pathognomonic for trichinosis (see Section 3.4). The ECG changes most frequently observed are flattening or inversion of the T wave, low amplitude of the QRS complex, intraventricular or atrial ventricular blocks, and conduction disturbances. The chest X-ray may show some infiltrates in the lung tissue or effusion in the pleura.

4. DIAGNOSIS

Human trichinosis is a difficult parasitic infection to diagnose, for several reasons. It is usually found as a group infection, but can also be seen in sporadic cases or as the first index case of an epidemic. Trichinosis is most likely to be diagnosed in patients living in Europe or North America, but it may also occur in Egypt, Kenya, Tanzania, and Thailand, or be contracted there by tourists or by eating imported infected meat (Pawłowski, 1981b). Patients with trichinosis may be first seen shortly after ingestion of the infected meat, because of the resulting abdominal syndrome, but before the general trichinosis syndrome has

TABLE II
Steps in the Diagnosis of Trichinosis

Steps in diagnosis	Source of information			
	Epidemiological data	Clinical data	Results of laboratory tests	Parasitological examination
1. Trichinosis suggested (one positive finding)	Exposure to infected *or* meat	Symptoms and signs *or*	Eosinophilia	—
2. Trichinosis probable (all three positive)	Exposure to infected *and* meat	Symptoms and signs *and*	Eosinophilia	—
3. Trichinosis confirmed	—	Clinical course (including positive response to treatment)	Enzymatic tests Serological tests	—
4. Definite diagnosis of trichinosis	—	—	—	Finding the parasite

developed, or during the acute stage of the disease, or a few weeks afterward if the trichinosis has not been diagnosed and has led to cardiac failure or muscle contracture, or even several months or years after acute trichinosis if the patient has still not fully recovered from the illness. Few of the symptoms of trichinosis are pathognomonic. The disease may have various degrees of severity from abortive to fatal and may be accompanied by a great many different complications that sometimes overshadow the basic disease. A definite diagnosis can be made by finding the parasite, a process that requires muscle biopsy; serological and other laboratory tests are usually positive only when the acute stage of the disease is almost over. Finally, since trichinosis is not a common disease, it may not always be even considered as a possible diagnosis.

The clinical diagnosis of trichinosis is based on: (1) clinical history-taking (including the results of epidemiological surveillance); (2) physical examination; (3) paraclinical testing (including serology); (4) finding the parasite; and (5) differential diagnosis.

Trichinosis may be suggested by (1) exposure to infected meat; (2) symptoms and signs, or (3) high eosinophilia. It might be further confirmed by enzymatic or serological tests and by the clinical course, but a definite diagnosis can be made only by finding the parasite (Table II).

4.1. Clinical History-Taking

Clinical history-taking should concentrate on three questions: Is trichinosis likely? What is the history of exposure? What are the past or present symptoms?

Trichinosis can be a prime suspect when one is faced with a group infection in people who have eaten meat from the same source. Examples of this are the inhabitants of a small village in Mosina, Poland (Neyman and Talarczyk, 1961), four families in the Mbulu district in Tanzania (Bura and Willett, 1977), a group of campers in Hawaii (Barrett-Connor et al., 1976), an ethnic group of Thais in New York City (Imperato et al., 1974), and the members of a youth gathering in West Germany (Bommer et al., 1980).

It is more difficult to consider trichinosis as a diagnosis when it appears as the first, and usually the most severe, case in an epidemic; or as an isolated case; or as one of several widespread cases occurring when the infected meat was served to travelers or distributed to several distant places; or as an unlucky case where an individual has eaten a portion of a beef hamburger that was accidentally adulterated with infected pork.

With trichinosis, close cooperation between clinicians and epidemiologists is essential. Early case notification might enable rapid examination of the suspected meat for *T. spiralis* larvae and prevent further consumption of any infected meat that is still being kept, e.g., as a delicacy (bear meat) or as preserved food (smoked ham). In an epidemic in 1978, the infected bear meat had been served at seven meals attended by 65 people in two states (Alaska and California) over a period of 24 months (Centers for Disease Control, 1979).

When meat is suspect, large samples of it (20 g) should be examined for *T. spiralis* by the digestion technique and small samples (1 g) by trichinoscopy, since the digestion technique is not the best one for examining fatty pork products or for finding young or calcified larvae. Knowing how many *T. spiralis* larvae there are per gram of consumed meat, the way in which the meat was prepared prior to consumption, and the amount of meat eaten may be helpful in establishing the extent of exposure for therapeutic and prognostic purposes. For clinical and research reasons, it is important to examine the strain of the invasive *T. spiralis* larvae and to determine whether it is *nativa, nelsoni,* or a classic domestic strain.

Trichinosis may occur in anyone who has eaten infected meat, regardless of age, sex, or any previous exposure to the infection. What may play an important role are the eating habits: trichinosis is more likely to occur or be more intensive in those individuals who prefer raw meat, or raw or semiraw meat products, and also in those who tend to eat unusual dishes such as bear or walrus meat. In 1979, in the United States, 93 cases of human trichinosis were caused by pork, or pork products, from domestic pigs, and 26 cases were due to the consumption of walrus meat, 2 to bear meat, and 5 to ground beef that had probably been adulterated with pork. The source of infection was unknown in 9 cases (Centers for Disease Control, 1980). Butchers and cooks are more exposed than other people. Some degree of immunity probably already exists in those who are repeatedly exposed to the infection, but it is not a protective immunity; for example, a butcher examined in Poland was found to have calcified *T. spiralis* larvae next to new uncapsulated ones in the deltoid muscle, biopsied because of acute trichinosis (author's unpublished observation).

Ascertaining the history of exposure may not be easy because of the time lapse between the ingestion of infected meat and the first symptoms and because some individuals are reluctant to tell the truth in order to avoid any responsibility or blame for exposing other people to infection.

Taking the history of past signs and symptoms may not be as

important for diagnosis as is the history of exposure; it is necessary, however, for establishing the duration of the incubation period and determining the current stage of the disease. When asking about past or present symptoms, one should bear in mind the changing pattern of symptomatology, as described in Section 3. There may be no abdominal symptoms, but it is rare that there is no general trichinosis syndrome in the history of a patient first seen because of the complications or recurrent muscle problems.

4.2. Physical Examination

In trichinosis, there are nearly as many subjective symptoms of the disease reported as there are objective signs (Gould, 1970). Therefore, when examining patients, subjective feelings such as myalgia, malaise, and visual disturbances should be made objective as far as possible by comparing them with the existing signs of trichinosis. On the other hand, in the later stages of the disease, any cardiac, neurological, or pulmonary symptoms deserve thorough analysis, since they may precede signs of complications.

The first signs suggestive of trichinosis are periorbital edema and hemorrhagic lesions in the eyeballs associated with fever, myalgia, and malaise, all of which have been described in the sections on the general trichinosis syndrome (Section 3.2) and allergic vasculitis (Section 3.3).

However, for the diagnosis of trichinosis, the value of the physical examination itself is limited in most cases, especially isolated ones; one may conclude only that the diagnosis is highly probable but needs confirmation by laboratory tests. This statement does not diminish the role of the physical medical examination in severe or complicated cases of the disease.

4.3. Paraclinical Tests

Examinations for eosinophilia and serum enzymes, and immuno-serological tests, are the most valuable ones for confirming the diagnosis of trichinosis (Table II).

It was mentioned in Section 3.7.1 that eosinophilia (500 cells/mm^3 or more) is the earliest and the most stable laboratory sign of human trichinosis; it occurs in the 2nd or 3rd week of infection, i.e., in the 1 week of disease, and usually persists as long as the symptoms exist.

An increased level of serum CPK, 1,6-diphosphofructoaldolase, and lactic dehydrogenase is usually first observed in the 2nd week of disease and is present for the next 2–5 weeks (Gentilini et al., 1976;

Kassur *et al.*, 1978). These tests are not, however, as universally useful as the test for eosinophilia because in some individuals the changes in serum enzyme levels are negligible.

Contrary to the eosinophilia and enzymatic tests, which are non-specific but characteristic, several serological tests are highly specific and sensitive. For clinical purposes, the most sensitive serological tests are passive hemagglutination (PHA) and enzyme-linked immunosorbent assay (ELISA); indirect immunofluorescence (IF) is less sensitive (Engvall and Ljungström, 1975; Gancarz and Jędrzejewska, 1978) (see Chapter 12). All these tests become positive in the 2nd week of the disease, which is the 3rd or 4th week of infection; the PHA and ELISA tests may remain positive for a few years. The indirect IF test becomes negative after 1 year. Flocculation of agglutination techniques (with bentonite, latex, and cholesterol) have a low sensitivity, but are highly specific; they become positive in the 3rd week of the disease and remain so for several years; they are widely used because of the simplicity of the test, which is available in kits. Counterelectrophoresis and double diffusion techniques have also been developed (Despommier *et al.*, 1974) and are available in kit form. Their applicability is similar to that for the bentonite-flocculation technique. The complement-fixation text, ring precipitation, and microprecipitation with living *T. spiralis* larvae are now rarely used for clinical purposes. At present, it is good clinical practice in trichinosis to use two different immunoserological tests at the same time and to repeat the examinations to observe a positive conversion and changes in their titers. In 1978, in the United States, 11 of 19 notified cases of human trichinosis were positive, both serologically and by muscle biopsy; 2 were serologically positive and negative by biopsy; and 6 were negative serologically and positive by biopsy (Centers for Disease Control, 1979). The test most frequently used was bentonite flocculation.

4.4. Finding the Parasite

A definite diagnosis of trichinosis can be made only by finding the parasite. Attempts to find adult *T. spiralis* worms in the duodenal juices or in the feces are fruitless. It is somewhat easier to find the female worms in the small intestine during postmortem examination; this was shown by Zenker in 1860 (see Chapter 1) and by the author in the first fatal case of an epidemic in Mosina, Poland, in 1960 (unpublished data).

It is much easier to determine the larval stages of *T. spiralis* in the muscle tissue; unfortunately, this requires the biopsy of 0.5–1 g of muscle tissue. Muscle biopsy confirms the presence (or absence) of trichinosis, gives an idea of the intensity of infection, enables identification of the *Trichinella* strain, and shows the pathological changes in the muscle tissue, and may also be helpful for decisions regarding therapy. For these reasons, muscle biopsy is justified for some selected cases in epidemics of trichinosis and for sporadic cases in which the diagnosis or the course of the disease is not clear.

The following procedures can be used to find *T. spiralis* larvae in the muscle tissue: classic trichinoscopy, digestion, mincing or squeezing procedures, and xenodiagnosis, as well as histological and histochemical techniques. Trichinoscopy after compression of thin pieces of muscle and subsequent digestion in artificial digestive fluid are techniques that are described in many publications (Gould, 1970). These two techniques complement each other and should be used in all cases of muscle biopsy together with histopathological techniques. In the early stage of infection, when the larvae are not coiled and are easily recognized but susceptible to digestion, mincing techniques or simple squeezing of the very small cuts of muscle tissue and examination for young larvae are suggested. Xenodiagnosis (the easiest way is by feeding mice with the suspected muscle tissue) is a technique that is useful more for further taxonomic studies than for diagnostic purposes. Histopathology is more valuable in intensive infections; it may not show the larvae in light infections, but even then the characteristic basophilic changes of the muscle fibers are already present from the 5th day after ingestion of the infected meat. Thus, contrary to general opinion, it is not necessary to wait to take the diagnostic muscle biopsy until the later stages of infection; the results might already be positive in the 2nd week of infection (Gabryel *et al.*, 1974; Gerwel *et al.*, 1970).

Trichinella spiralis larvae can sometimes be found in the blood, the cerebrospinal fluid, or the mother's milk (Gould, 1970).

4.5. Differential Diagnosis of Trichinosis

Because of the diversity of symptoms, signs, and pathological mechanisms and the difficulties in establishing a definite diagnosis, especially in sporadic or index cases, as discussed in Section 3, human trichinosis frequently remains undiagnosed or is incorrectly diagnosed. Some tens of diseases to be considered for differential diagnosis have been mentioned in various publications (Gould, 1970; Kassur *et al.*, 1978). These could be grouped as discussed below.

In the incubation period of trichinosis, food intoxication, food allergy, and nonspecific gastroenterocolitis were most commonly misdiagnosed. The general trichinosis syndrome (fever, myalgia, malaise) is similar to several viral infections (influenza or prodromal viral hepatitis, mumps, and infectious mononucleosis) and to typhoid fever, leptospirosis, rheumatic fever, and septicemia. Allergic components, when they dominate trichinosis, may also be confused with dermato-myositis, periarteritis nodosa, angioneurotic edema, serum sickness, and drug allergy (Altus *et al.*, 1980). In the case of manifestations from other organs or complications, the range of diseases for differential diagnosis increases greatly. Neurological complications may suggest poliomyelitis, meningitis, encephalitis, cerebral hemorrhage, or multiple (intercostal) neuritis. Pulmonary or cardiac symptoms and signs domi-nating the clinical picture may be misdiagnosed as pneumonia, bron-chopneumonia, pleurisy, and spastic bronchitis, as well as endocarditis, myocarditis, cardiac failure, or nephritis.

Some laboratory results such as the lack of eosinophilia, or a highly positive nonspecific serological test for typhoid, that occasionally occur in trichinosis (Rodriguez-Osorio and Gomez-Garcia, 1978) may be misleading unless interpreted in relation to other symptoms and signs and the course of disease.

5. MANAGEMENT AND TREATMENT

The diversity of the clinical picture of trichinosis, the wide range of severity of the clinical course, and possible complications mean that there is no single rule for the management and treatment of *T. spiralis* infections. In some cases, the first imperative is to save life by intensive care for shock, toxemia, and circulatory failure, the main causes of death. In any case of recent infection, chemotherapeutic action against the adult intestinal worms is obligatory to prevent further production of newborn *T. spiralis* larvae. In many light cases, there is no need for treatment other than symptomatic treatment and therapy directed against intestinal worms.

The treatment of human trichinosis depends much on the intensity of infection, the strain of *T. spiralis* involved, the duration of infection, and the character and intensity of the host response, including compli-cations (Pawłowski, 1981a). The treatment of intestinal infection, acute severe trichinosis, and moderate and mild infections, as well as the late phase of trichinosis, are discussed separately below.

5.1. Treatment of the Intestinal Infection

The production of newborn *T. spiralis* larvae, migrating to the muscle tissue and other organs, is stopped by ridding the small intestine of *T. spiralis* adult female worms. Therefore, treatment for intestinal infection is mandatory in all cases, irrespective of whether or not they are symptomatic, severe or mild, early or late (up to 6 weeks after ingestion of infected meat). At present, two drugs are widely used; pyrantel (10 mg/kg body weight daily for 4 days) and mebendazole (in adults, 200 mg daily for 4 days); mebendazole is not given to pregnant women. Other anthelmintics, old or new, might be equally effective, but their efficacy has not been satisfactorily proven in man (see also Chapter 10, Sections 2 and 3).

From time to time, *T. spiralis* larvae are identified in animal flesh a short time after the infected meat has been eaten raw. When it was only a question of a few hours, and the benzimidazoles had not yet been introduced, measures such as inducing vomiting or washing out the stomach, and administration of alcoholic drinks or purgatives, were employed to reduce the infective dose. In the few days following ingestion of infected meat, thiabendazole, given orally in a daily dose of 50 mg/kg body weight for 5 days, has been reported to prevent symptomatic trichinosis (Gerwel *et al.*, 1974). It has been suggested that the course of treatment should be repeated after a week in intensive infections. Mebendazole was found to be even better than thiabendazole for preventing symptomatic trichinosis (Ozeretskovskaya, 1978; Ozeretskovskaya *et al.*, 1978). It is probable that pyrantel and piperazine would have a similar effect, but this has not been reported in man.

5.2. Acute Severe Trichinosis

Corticosteroids are the drugs of choice in acute severe *T. spiralis* trichinosis because of their antiinflammatory, antiallergic, and antishock action. The usual dose is 40–60 mg prednisolone per day, given until the fever and allergic signs disappear. More severe cases may require higher doses of corticosteroids as well as supportive drugs. Any cardiac, circulatory, neurological, or pulmonary complications may need additional intensive, specific treatment, such as cardiac glucosides, diuretics, anticoagulants, and antihistamines. In infections with *T. spiralis* var. *nativa* (sylvatic strain), corticosteroids may exert a much less beneficial effect and even delay the convalescence from trichinosis (Ozeretskovskaya, 1978). Bed rest is always necessary.

As far as specific treatment is concerned, thiabendazole has been used in severe trichinosis, but with very controversial results; a dramatic clinical improvement was observed by some authors (Hennekeuser *et al.*, 1968) and no beneficial action by others (Łapszewicz *et al.*, 1969). By destroying muscle larvae and liberating antigenic substances, thiabendazole can provoke additional systemic hypersensitivity responses, such as allergic myocarditis, dermatitis, and pneumonitis (Kean and

Koskins, 1964; Klein, 1978b). Thiabendazole is now no longer recommended for the treatment of acute trichinosis, having been replaced by mebendazole.

Treatment with mebendazole is usually given in a daily dose of 5 mg/kg body weight. The use of mebendazole in severe trichinosis should be individualized; the need to remove adult intestinal worms and diminish the load of migrating or nonencapsulated muscle larvae, as well as the risk of side effects, should be carefully considered. The action of benzimidazoles against muscle larvae may cause side effects of a hypersensitivity nature, such as higher fever, increased periorbital swelling, and myalgia, and higher eosinophilia; allergic myocarditis or pneumonitis sometimes develops. Therefore, benzimidazole therapy should be combined with corticosteroids and discontinued whenever serious side effects appear. It should be mentioned that several severe cases of trichinosis have recovered without being treated with benzimidazoles but only with other anthelmintics active against intestinal worms and with corticosteroids. In cases of severe trichinosis caused by *T. spiralis var. nativa*, which do not respond to corticosteroids, mebendazole is the drug of choice. However, it is still better to use corticosteroids together with mebendazole to avoid any side effects of a hypersensitive nature (Ozeretskovskaya, 1978; Ozeretskovskaya *et al.*, 1978) (see also Chapter 10, Sections 2 and 3).

5.3. Moderate or Mild Trichinosis

The use of corticosteroids is justified only in patients with fever, allergic vasculitis, high leukocytosis, and eosinophilia. Others can be successfully treated with antipyretic and analgesic drugs. Any patients with moderate trichinosis should be kept in bed and be regularly examined to diagnose any possible complications as early as possible.

5.4. Late and Convalescent Phases of Trichinosis

From the 3rd week of the disease onward, metabolic and circulatory disorders dominate the clinical picture of trichinosis. Profound hypoalbuminemia responds best to replacement human-serum therapy (Rachoń *et al.*, 1967). Restoring the electrolyte balance may easily control the cardiac symptoms caused by hypokalemia.

Trichinosis is a self-limiting disease in both the intestinal and the muscular phases, and complete recovery usually occurs within a few months. In sporadic cases, some symptoms have been reported to persist for several years; those cases should be carefully examined to find the reasons for the delay in complete recovery (immunosuppression, impaired detoxification ability, hypersensitivity) or other concomitant diseases. There is no justification for the use of larvicidal drugs, such as mebendazole, when the infection has already been present for several months, unless there is evidence of an unusual host response, with the patient being in either a hypersensitive or a suppressed condition. Muscle biopsy and immunological tests are useful for diagnosis in these cases. Treatment with mebendazole in the late stage of trichinosis should be given only in hospitalized patients.

Proper mental and physical rehabilitation is important in trichinosis; the patients should be convinced that many people become perfectly well despite having some *T. spiralis* larvae encapsulated in their muscles.

5.5. Trichinosis in Children, Pregnant and Lactating Women, and Immunosuppressed Patients

Trichinosis in children is, in general, considered to be less severe than in adults. This is not necessarily true, however, and cannot be explained simply by the assumption that the number of *T. spiralis* larvae consumed is usually smaller; severity of disease is often not correlated to the body weight. The symptoms and signs of trichinosis are frequently more intense in children than in adult patients, but there are usually fewer complications from the other organs, and the recovery starts earlier and is more rapid. The process of destruction of the *T. spiralis* larvae and regeneration of the muscle fibers seems to be more active in children; muscle biopsy usually reveals fewer *T. spiralis* larvae and less pathological change in the muscles in comparison with adults who have a similar clinical picture (author's unpublished observations). The management and treatment of trichinosis in children need special care in the early acute stage of the disease, but do not cause many problems in the later stages.

Trichinosis occurs not infrequently in pregnant and lactating women, but reports on this aspect are few. Studies carried out in ten pregnant and ten lactating patients by Klein (1978a) showed that the course of trichinosis was milder in pregnancy but more severe in lactating women in comparison with ten infected patients who were neither pregnant nor lactating. It was suggested that the naturally increased level of steroids in pregnancy alleviates the course of trichinosis and makes the use of corticosteroids unnecessary; corticosteroid therapy may also be deleterious for the fetus. The life of the fetus seems to be endangered more by the *T. spiralis* infection than does the life of the mother. There are many reports of a healthy child being born to a mother with trichinosis, but there are also reports of abortions and stillbirths. In the study group reported by Klein (1978a), there was one natural abortion on the 11th day of the disease and in the 7th week of pregnancy and one fetal death on the 21st day of the disease in the 38–39th week of pregnancy. *Trichinella spiralis* larvae have been described in the human maternal placenta (Draghici *et al.*, 1976) and in children a few weeks old (Bourns, 1952). *Trichinella spiralis* infection is not considered a cause of congenital defects in newborn children.

The clinical course of trichinosis in ten lactating women reported by Klein (1978a) was described as severe in five cases, moderate in four, and mild in one case; in the most severe case, the birth occurred on the 11th day of acute trichinosis. The treatment of trichinosis in lactating patients usually requires higher doses of corticosteroids. Lactation decreases and often stops completely during trichinosis.

Trichinosis itself leads to suppression of specific immune and nonspecific inflammatory reactions, which may be clinically expressed in secondary complications such as pneumonia. On the other hand, *T. spiralis* infection in immunosuppressed patients may have a more dramatic course; a fatal case of acute myelomonocytic leukemia and trichinosis with a serum-sickness-like syndrome and shock has been observed (Jacobson and Jacobson, 1977). In immunosuppressed patients, the prevention of trichinosis, as well as of other infections, is of primary importance, since the host may not respond well to specific treatment.

REFERENCES

Altus, P., Blanco, R., and Chazal, R., 1980, Trichinosis masquerading as a penicillin allergy, *J. Am. Med. Assoc.* **243:**767–768.

Andy, J.J., O'Connell, J.P., Daddario, R.C., and Roberts, W.C., 1977, Trichinosis causing extensive ventricular mural endocarditis with superimposed thrombosis, *Am. J. Med.* **63:**824–829.

Barrett-Connor, E., Davis, C.F., Hamburger, R.N., and Kagan, I., 1976, An epidemic of trichinosis after ingestion of wild pig in Hawaii, *J. Infect. Dis.* **133:**473–477.

Bommer, W., Kaiser, H., Mergerian, H., and Pottkamer, G., 1980, An outbreak of trichinellosis in a youth center of northern Germany caused by imported air-dried camel meat, Abstracts of the Xth International Congress on Tropical Medicine and Malaria, Manila, 1980, p. 156.

Booth, C.C., 1980, Clinical science in the 1980s, *Lancet* **2:**904–907.

Bourns, T.K.T., 1952, The discovery of trichina cysts in the diaphragm of a six week-old child, *J. Parasitol.* **38:**367.

Bura, M.W.T., and Willett, W.C., 1977, An outbreak of trichinosis in Tanzania, *East Afr. Med. J.* **54:**185–193.

Buşilá, V.T., Dragomirescu, M., Dragomirescu, L., and Maager, P., 1968, Functional and metabolic alterations in human trichinellosis, *Wiad. Parazytol.* **14:**195–199.

Centers for Disease Control, 1979, Trichinosis Surveillance, Annual Summary for 1978, U.S. Department of Health, Education and Welfare.

Centers for Disease Control, 1980, Trichinosis Surveillance, Annual Summary 1979, U.S. Department of Health, Education and Welfare.

Chodera, L., and Pawłowski, Z., 1974, Electrocardiographic changes in trichinellosis: Experimental studies in rabbits, in: *Trichinellosis* (C.W. Kim, ed.), Intext, New York, pp. 413–420.

Chodera, L., Gerwel, C., Kocięcka, W., and Pawłowski, Z., 1974, On the problem of late clinical sequelae of human trichinellosis, *Wiad. Parazytol.* **20:**125–131.

Ciszewska-Olczak, B., Kocięcka, W., Kozakiewicz, B., and Olczak, S., 1974, Endemic foci of trichinellosis in the Kalisz district in the years 1953–1972, *Wiad. Parazytol.* **20:**147–151 (in Polish).

Cox, P.M., Schultz, M.G., Kagan, I.G., and Preizler, J., 1969, Trichinosis—five-year serologic and clinical follow-up, *Am. J. Epidemiol.* **89:**651–657.

David, J.R., Vadas, M.A., Butterworth, A.E., Azevedo de Brito, P., Carvalho, E.M., David, R.A., Bina, J.C., and Andrade, Z.A., 1980, Enhanced helminthotoxic capacity of eosinophils from patients with eosinophilia, *N. Engl. J. Med.* **303:**1147–1152.

Despommier, D., Müller, M., Jenks, B., and Fruitstone, M., 1974, Immunodiagnosis of human trichinosis using counterelectrophoresis and agar gel diffusion techniques, *Am. J. Trop. Med. Hyg.* **23:**41–44.

Draghici, O., Va Sadi, T., Drachci, G., Codrea, A., Mihuta, A., Dragan, S., Biro, S., Mocuta, D., and Mihuta, S., 1976, Observations on a trichinellosis focus, *Rev. Ig.* (*Bacteriol.*) **21:**99–104 (in Romanian).

Dziubek, Z., 1969, Adrenal cortex efficiency in human trichinosis, *Wiad. Parazytol.* **15:**714–719.

Engvall, E., and Ljungström, I., 1975, Detection of human antibodies to *Trichinella spiralis* by enzyme-linked immunosorbent assay, ELISA, *Acta Pathol. Microbiol. Scand. Sect. C* **83:**231–237.

Forrester, A.T.T., Nelson, G.S., and Sander, G., 1961, The first record of an outbreak of trichinosis in Africa south of the Sahara, *Trans. R. Soc. Trop. Med. Hyg.* **55:**503–517.

Gabryel, P., Gerwel, C., Gustowska, L., Kocięcka, W., and Pawłowski, Z., 1974, Muscle biopsy in human trichinellosis, *Proceedings of the VIth International Congress of Infectious and Parasitic Diseases*, Warsaw, 1974, Vol. II, pp. 388–393.

Gancarz, Z., and Jędrzejewska, B., 1978, The dynamics of passive haemagglutination and indirect immunofluorescence tests in cases of human trichinosis, *Przegl. Epidemiol.* **32:**357–362 (in Polish).

Gentilini, M., Vernes, A., Gentilini, J.L., Richard-Lenoble, D., Bourée, P., and Wattez, A., 1976, Etude enzymatique et sérologique de la trichinose humaine: A propos d'une récente épidémie de la banlieue sud de Paris, *Bull. Soc. Pathol. Exot.* **69:**525–531.

Gerwel, C., and Pawłowski, Z., 1975, Studies on the epidemiology and biology of trichinellosis in Poland (1964–1974), *Wiad. Parazytol.* **21:**513–540.

Gerwel, C., Kocięcka, W., and Pawłowski, Z., 1970, Parasitologic examination of muscles several years after trichinosis, *Epidemiol. Rev.* **24:**262–269.

Gerwel, C., Pawłowski, Z., Kocięcka, W., and Chodera, L., 1974, Probable sterilization of *Trichinella spiralis* by thiabendazole: Further clinical observation of human infections, in: *Trichinellosis* (C.W. Kim, ed.), Intext, New York, pp. 471–475.

Gould, S.E., 1970, *Trichinosis in Man and Animals*, Charles C. Thomas, Springfield, Illinois.

Gross, B., and Ochoa, J., 1979, Trichinosis: Clinical report and histochemistry of muscle, *Muscle Nerve* **2:**394–398.

Hall, M.C., and Collins, B.J., 1937, Studies on trichinosis. II. Some correlations and implications in connection with incidence of trichinae found in 300 diaphragms, *Public Health Rep.* **52:**512–527.

Hennekeuser, H.H., Pabst, K., Poeplau, W., and Gerok, W., 1968, Zur Klinik und Therapie der Trichinose: Beobachtungen an 47 Patienten während einer Epidemie, *Dtsch. Med. Wochenschr.* **93:**867–873.

Imperato, P.J., Harvey, R.P., Shookhoff, H.B., and Chaves, A.D., 1974, Trichinosis among Thais living in New York City, *J. Am. Med. Assoc.* **227:**526–529.

Jacobson, E.S., and Jacobson, H.G., 1977, Trichinosis in an immunosuppressed human host, *Am. J. Clin. Pathol.* **68:**791–794.

Januszkiewicz, J., 1967, Participation of the respiratory system in trichinosis, *Epidemiol. Rev.* **21:**169–178.

Januszkiewicz, J., 1969, The incubation period of trichinosis, *Przegl. Epidemiol.* **23:**35–42 (in Polish).

Januszkiewicz, J., Kowalczyk, M., Poznańska, H., and Wehr, H., 1970, Evaluation of liver involvement in trichinosis, *Epidemiol. Rev.* **24:**270–278.

Kassur, B., and Januszkiewicz, J., 1968, Clinical classification of trichinosis, *Epidemiol. Rev.* **22:**134–139.

Kassur, B., and Januszkiewicz, J., 1970, On the inappropriateness of the idea of chronic trichinellosis, *Epidemiol. Rev.* **24:**68–75.

Kassur, B., Januszkiewicz, J., and Poznańska, H., 1978, Clinic of trichinellosis, in: *Trichinellosis* (C.W. Kim and Z.S. Pawłowski, eds.), University Press of New England, Hanover, New Hampshire, pp. 27–44.

Kean, B.H., and Hoskins, D.W., 1964, Treatment of trichinosis with thiabendazole: A preliminary report, *J. Am. Med. Assoc.* **190:**852–853.

Kershaw, W.E., Hill, C.A.St., Semple, A.B., and Davies, J.B.M., 1956, The distribution of the larvae of *Trichinella spiralis* in the muscle, viscera and central nervous system in cases of trichinosis at Liverpool in 1953, and the relation of the severity of the illness to the intensity of infection, *Ann. Trop. Med. Parasitol.* **50:**355–361.

Klein, J.S., 1978a, Trichinellosis during pregnancy and laction, *Med. Parasitol.* (*Moscow*) **47**(5):51–54 (in Russian).

Klein, J.S., 1978b, Treatment of severe trichinellosis, in: *Trichinellosis* (C.W. Kim and Z.S. Pawłowski, eds.), University Press of New England, Hanover, New Hampshire, pp. 395–406.

Kocięcka, W., Gerwel, C., Pawłowski, Z., Kaczmarek, J., Stachowski, B., Gabryel, P., and Gustowska, L., 1974, Experimental trichinellosis and thiabendazole treatment in *Macaca mulatta*: Clinical and electromyographic observations, in: *Trichinellosis* (C.W. Kim, ed.), Intext, New York, pp. 123–133.

Kocięcka, W., Kaczmarek, J., and Stachowski, B., 1975, Electromyographic studies in persons with trichinellosis history, *Wiad. Parazytol.* **21:**721–730.

Kozar, Z., and Kozar, M., 1965, Incidence of *Trichinella spiralis* in the Polish population on the basis of post-mortem examinations. *Wiad. Parazytol.* **11:**233–243.

Kozar, Z., Sładki, E., and Żołnierkowa, D., 1964, Clinical aspects of chronic trichinellosis in people, Part I–III, *Wiad. Parazytol.* **10:**651–690.

Kramer, M.D., and Aita, J.F., 1978, Trichinosis, in: *Infections of the Nervous System*, Part III (P.J. Vinken and G.W. Bruyn, eds.), North-Holland, Amsterdam, pp. 267–290.

Łapszewicz, A., Pawłowski, Z., and Gabryel, P., 1969, Thiabendazole in human trichinellosis, *Wiad. Parazytol.* **15:**759–760.

Matossian, R.M., Salti, I., and Stephan, E., 1977, Variation in serum immunoglobulin levels in acute trichinosis, *J. Helminthol.* **51:**1–4.

Neyman, K., and Talarczyk, Z., 1961, An epidemic of trichinosis at Mosina, *Przegl. Epidemiol.* **15**:279–283 (in Polish).

Ozeretskovskaya, N.N., 1978, Pathogenesis, pathomorphology and clinics of trichinellosis: Treatment of trichinellosis, in: *Trichinelly i Trichinelliez* (S.N. Boev, V.I. Bondareva, and I.B. Sokolova, eds.), Akademija Nauk Kazahskoj SSR, pp. 165–213 (in Russian).

Ozeretskovskaya, N.N., and Tumolskaya, N.I., 1974, Clinical pattern and pathogenesis of the abdominal syndrome in trichinellosis, in: *Trichinellosis* (C.W. Kim, ed.), Intext, New York, pp. 389–398.

Ozeretskovskaya, N.N., and Vikhert, A.M., 1960, Systemic vasculitis in trichinosis, *Klin. Med. (Moscow)* **38**:67–76 (in Russian).

Ozeretskovskaya, N.N., Romanova, V.I., Alekseeva, M.I., Pereverzeva, E.V., and Uspenskii, S.M., 1970, Human trichinosis in the Soviet Arctic and the characteristics of the strain of Arctic *Trichinella*, Proceedings of the Conference on Productivity and Conservation in Northern Circumpolar Lands, Edmonton, 1969, pp. 133–142.

Ozeretskovskaya, N.N., Pereverzeva, E.V., Tumolskaya, N.I., Bronshstein, A.M., Morenez, T.M. and Imamkuliev, K.D., 1978, Benzimidazoles in the treatment and prophylaxis of synanthropic and sylvatic trichinellosis, in: *Trichinellosis* (C.W. Kim and Z.S. Pawłowski, eds.), University Press of New England, Hanover, New Hampshire, pp. 381–393.

Pawłowski, Z., 1978, Reflexions on late sequelae of human trichinellosis, in: *Trichinellosis* (C.W. Kim and Z.S. Pawłowski, eds.), University Press of New England, Hanover, New Hampshire, pp. 359–361.

Pawłowski, Z., 1981a, Trichinellosis, in: *Current Therapy* (H.S. Conn, ed.), W.B. Saunders, Philadelphia, p. 84.

Pawłowski, Z., 1981b, Control of trichinellosis, in: *Trichinellosis* (C.W. Kim, E.J. Ruitenberg, and J.S. Teppema, eds.), Reedbooks, Chertsey, England, pp. 7–20.

Rachoń, K., Januszkiewicz, J., and Wehr, H., 1967, Serum proteins in human trichinosis, *Am. J. Med.* **26**:934–938.

Rodriguez-Osorio, M., and Gomez-Garcia, V., 1978, Nonspecificity of the immunofluorescent antibody test for trichinellosis in sera from patients with typhoid fever, in: *Trichinellosis* (C.W. Kim and Z.S. Pawłowski, eds.), University Press of New England, Hanover, New Hampshire, pp. 371–374.

Sapunar, J., Palma, R., Palma, J., and Munoz, A., 1965, Un caso de isosporosis asociada con triquinosis, *Bol. Chil. Parasitol.* **20**:18–20.

Schoop, G., Lieb, W.A., Lamina, J., and Hiemisch, I., 1961, Die Parasiten des Auges: Tierexperimentelle Untersuchungen über die Trichinose des Auges, *Klin. Monatsbl. Augenheilkd.* **139**:433–465.

Semple, A.B., Davies, J.B.M., Kershaw, W.E., and Hill, C.A.St., 1954, An outbreak of trichinosis in Liverpool in 1953, *Br. Med. J.*, May 1, pp. 1002–1006.

Sitprija, V., Keoplung, M., Boonpucknavig, V., and Boonpucknavig, S., 1980, Renal involvement in human trichinosis, *Arch. Intern. Med.* **140**:544–546.

Wiśniewska, M., 1970, *Trichinella spiralis*: Diagnostic value of creatine kinase levels in rat and man, *Exp. Parasitol.* **28**:577–584.

Zimmermann, W.J., Steele, J.H., and Kagan, I.G., 1973, Trichiniasis in the U.S. population, 1966–70, *Health Serv. Rep.* **88**:606–623.

12

Immunodiagnosis in Man

INGER LJUNGSTRÖM

1. INTRODUCTION

The parasite *Trichinella spiralis* has its whole life cycle in one host. Definite proof of infection resides in the demonstration of muscle larvae. The contact between the host and the parasite during the infection results in a variety of host–parasite interactions including stimulation of specific humoral and cellular immune responses. Protective immunity is developed, but as in many other parasitic infections, immune protection is not complete. It is clearly T-cell-dependent (reviewed by Wakelin, 1978), and a number of observations indicate that antibody-dependent cell cytotoxicity may be involved. It has been shown that specific circulating antibodies belong to various immunoglobulin classes, predominantly IgG but also IgM and IgA. In man, a high level of total IgE has occasionally been demonstrated (Rosenberg *et al.*, 1971; Ljungström, 1974; Pattersson *et al.*, 1975; Barrett-Connor *et al.*, 1976; Matossian *et al.*, 1977) and, in a few cases, specific IgE antibodies (Stumpf *et al.*, 1981). Data on specific cell-mediated immunity provoked by *T. spiralis* in human are very limited. A few workers (Sladki, 1960; Chicoine *et al.*, 1966) have reported delayed-type hypersensitivity using skin tests in the diagnosis of trichinosis in epidemiological studies, but the significance of the delayed reaction is not known. In experimentally infected animals or animals immunized with *T. spiralis* antigen, delayed hypersensitivity including macrophage inhibition has been

INGER LJUNGSTRÖM • Department of Parasitology, National Bacteriological Laboratory, S-105 21 Stockholm, Sweden.

demonstrated (Larsh and Weatherly, 1974; Grove *et al.*, 1977; Vernes *et al.*, 1975). A few studies have also demonstrated specific cellular reactions, assessed by the lymphocyte-transformation response to *Trichinella* antigen (Ottesen *et al.*, 1975; Ljungström, unpublished data).

Immunological diagnosis of trichinosis started with Ströbel (1911), who used the complement-fixation test, and this was followed by precipitin and intradermal tests (Bachman, 1928a,b). Since 1940, a great variety of serological methods have been applied, such as microprecipitin tests, flocculation tests, the latex-agglutination test, the indirect hemagglutination test, indirect immunofluorescence (IF), crossed electrophoresis, and the enzyme-linked immunosorbent assay (ELISA). In general, these methods have shown an increased sensitivity, resulting in a demand for greater quality and specificity of the antigens employed. However, the soluble antigens that have been utilized in most of the tests are crude extracts of muscle larvae. Particulate antigens have been used in IF.

The aim of this review is to describe briefly the immunological methods generally used in the diagnosis of trichinosis, to evaluate these methods comparatively, and to recommend the most suitable techniques for different diagnostic purposes. Finally, detailed protocols for indirect IF and ELISA are presented in Section 5.

2. IMMUNODIAGNOSTIC METHODS

2.1. Parasite Antigens

In 1911, Ströbel (1911) demonstrated antigenic activity in extracts from *T. spiralis* muscle larvae. Since then, a number of reports on antigens in such extracts have been published and reviewed, most recently by Kagan and Norman (1970). Using immunodiffusion in gel, at least 16 precipitating systems have been detected in such extracts, but the nature and immunological relevance of these antigens are largely unknown.

Interest has been focused on metabolic antigens of *T. spiralis*. The existence of such antigens was demonstrated by Campbell (1955) and by Mills and Kent (1965). In 1976, Despommier and Müller (1976) showed that the stichocytes contain two major types of granules that differ in morphology. Each of these types contains different antigens, some of which seem to be identical with those previously described from the excretion–secretion products of muscle larvae. It has been shown that some of the metabolic antigens, when injected into a host, can elicit protective immunity (Campbell, 1955; Mills and Kent, 1965; Despommier and Laccetti, 1981), and it has been suggested that the corresponding antibodies in some way inhibit adult worm fecundity (Denham and Martinez, 1970; Despommier, 1974; Despommier et al., 1977).

The cuticle of T. spiralis is also known to be antigenic (for a review, see Ogilvie et al., 1980). With radioactive iodine, molecules located on the surface of the larvae can be labeled, and these labeled molecules are immunogenic (Parkhouse et al., 1981). The labeled components can be reduced to only two basic subunits, a glycoprotein and a protein. Both the glycoprotein and the protein failed to react with rabbit antibodies against the stichosome antigen prepared by Despommier (Parkhouse et al., 1981), indicating at least two different antigen–antibody sytems in the muscle larvae.

Immune sera from naturally infected hosts give a distinct fluorescent pattern, if used in IF with cryostat sections of muscle larvae as antigen. Strong fluorescence is observed in the stichosome and in the intestinal tract (Jackson, 1959; Brzosko et al., 1965; Crandall and Crandall, 1972; Kozeck and Crandall, 1974). Marked fluorescence is also seen in the cuticle (Sadun et al., 1962; Baratawidjaja et al., 1963; Sultzer, 1965, Engelbrecht, 1966; Kozar et al., 1966; Chroust et al., 1966). By the aid of histochemical and IF techniques, Brzosko et al. (1965) showed that a considerable part of the stichosome antigens contains neutral polysaccharides.

While the majority of the studies on T. spiralis antigens have been performed on the most easily accessible developmental form, the muscle larave, recent studies by Mackenzie et al. (1978) included other forms. They found that serum factors, presumably antibodies, from immune rats react specifically with each one of the developmental stages and that this reaction mediates lytic attacks by various inflammatory cell types on the nematode surface. The existence of stage-specific surface antigens has also been demonstrated by the aid of conventional radiolabeling techniques (Philipp et al., 1980).

However, despite continued interest in the production of antigenic preparations for use in immunodiagnosis, no reliable standards have been created for Trichinella antigens.

2.2. Indirect Immunofluorescence

The common methods in which fluorescent-labeled antibody is utilized are the direct, inhibition, and indirect staining techniques. In the *direct method*, the antibody is labeled with a fluorescent compound and is used to detect the presence of antigen in tissue fixed to a slide. The *inhibition method* is often employed as a control for testing the specificity of the antibodies in the direct fluorescent procedure. The *indirect method* is utilized for detection of either unknown antigen in tissue sections or unknown antibody in the patient's serum. This is based on the principle that a specific antigen–antibody reaction may be visualized by addition of a labeled second antibody directed against the antibody in the specific immune reaction.

Jackson (1959) was the first to apply the IF technique in *T. spiralis* studies. With the aid of direct IF, he demonstrated antigen–antibody reactions as brightly stained precipitates formed around the orifices of living muscle larvae. By using paraffin and cryostat sections of the muscle larvae, he showed internal antigenic sites in the muscle larvae. The indirect method confirmed the results obtained with the direct method on fixed antigens. In 1962, Sadun *et al.* (1962) applied the indirect IF technique for serological diagnosis of trichinosis, by employing killed intact *T. spiralis* muscle larvae as antigen. This whole-larvae antigen has a shelf life of only a few weeks. Sultzer (1965) showed that the cuticle of *T. spiralis* larvae with their internal organs removed by pepsin digestion could be used as antigen. This antigen was relatively stable on storage. The test as described by Sadun *et al.* (1962) and modified by Sultzer (1965) was performed in test tubes. Baratawidjaja *et al.* (1963) fixed cuticle antigen to slides with gentle heating or used frozen sections of rat diaphragm infected with *T. spiralis*. From this study, they concluded that the fluorescence of both the internal antigens and the cuticle was specific. Z. Kozar *et al.* (1966) also fixed the cuticle antigen to slides by heat, but they found that this antigen gave false-positive reactions. The advantages of antigen particles fixed to slides were obvious, and Chroust and Dubansky (1970) employed frozen sections of muscle larvae as antigen, while Wegesa *et al.* (1971) converted Sultzer's tube test to a slide test by sectioning fixed cuticles of larvae embedded in a freezing compound.

Cryostat sections of rat muscle larvae were used as antigen to follow the development and the persistence of antibody response to *T. spiralis* infection during two small outbreaks of trichinosis in Sweden in 1969 (Ljungström, 1974). This study showed that the IF could detect specific antibodies from day 6 after the onset of illness. The staining pattern of the sectioned muscle larvae was pronounced, and both cuticle and stichosome–gut staining were observed when sera from the acute and chronic stages of the infection were tested. However, the cuticle staining disappeared at lower serum dilution compared to that of stichosome–gut. Another variation of antigen was obtained by preparing cryostat sections of isolated muscle larvae embedded in a freezing compound (Ljungström and Ruitenberg, 1976).

A comparison between the sensitivity of the tube test (the cuticle of whole larvae as the antigen) and the cryostat method (both cuticle and internal structures as the antigenic sites) revealed that the cryostat method was more sensitive than the tube test (Ruitenberg et al., 1975a). Additionally, the slide test was easier and quicker to perform and also appeared to be more specific than the tube test.

Indirect IF can be used to detect antibodies of single antibody classes, which can provide valuable diagnostic information. The presence of IgM, IgA, and IgG antibodies in sera from patients with a range of parasitic infections was studied by Kane et al. (1971). Specific IgM antibodies were detectable only during recent infections, and IgA antibodies were also commonly found in sera taken at this time. Long-term follow-up studies of class-specific immunoglobulin response during trichinosis revealed that in most cases, all three antibody classes were present in the first sample taken within 20 days after the onset of the illness (Ljungström, 1974). IgM antibodies were in some cases demonstrated as late as 5 months and IgA antibodies as late as 4 months after the onset of illness. After 2 years, about 50% of the sera had a low IgG titer, with no IgM or IgA.

Indirect IF shows high reproducibility if performed under optimal conditions. However, it seems to be of critical importance that chessboard titrations of conjugates against antisera be performed in each antigen–antibody system (Huldt et al., 1975). There is reason to believe that the difference in plateau end points obtained with the same conjugate is due to the presence of different amounts of reactive antigen in the various systems.

2.3. Passive Hemagglutination

The attraction of agglutination is that it can so readily be observed. Passive hemagglutination (PHA) was first employed in 1956 for serodiagnosis of trichinosis by Price and Weiner (1956) and by Kagan and Bargai (1956). The antigens used in these two studies were isolated by methods described by Witebsky et al. (1942) (a boiling extract of muscle larvae) and by Melcher (1943) (an acid-soluble larval protein fraction).

PHA is a very sensitive method, more sensitive than the complement-fixation test, precipitin test (Price and Weiner, 1956; Kagan and Bargai, 1956), or bentonite-flocculation test (Barriga, 1977), and comparable to ELISA using the same crude antigen preparation (Engvall and Ljungström, 1975).

The specificity of PHA seems to be lower than that of indirect IF. The reactivity of sera from 467 healthy Swedes and 550 healthy Finnish Lapps was tested in PHA and indirect IF (Ljungström, 1974, 1979). For PHA, a crude saline extract of muscle larvae, prepared according to Bozicevich *et al.* (1951), was used. The test was carried out in principle as described by Boyden (1951) with the micromodification of Takatsy (1955). For indirect IF, frozen sections of rat muscle larvae were used as antigen. It was found that 23% of these sera were reactive in PHA and 6% in indirect IF. However, reactivity was demonstrated only in low titers. Since trichinosis exists in Scandinavia and occasionally produces clinical disease, it cannot be excluded that some of the serological reactions in the two Scandinavian populations represent specific antibodies. But it is more likely that the majority of the reactive sera contain heterophilic antibodies most easily detected by PHA. It is well known that PHA, like other agglutination reactions, strongly favors IgM antibodies (Greenbury *et al.*, 1963) and that heterophilic antibodies often belong to this immunoglobulin class (Svehag, 1964). By using a semipurified antigenic preparation coupled to sheep erythrocytes by the glutaraldehyde method, Barriga (1977) seems to have increased the specificity of the test.

A number of false-negative tests may be produced due to the prozone phenomena, unless the sera are fully titrated; agglutination occurs in the presence of higher dilutions of antiserum, but not in lower dilutions.

One drawback of PHA is that red cells must be freshly tanned and sensitized, which is very time-consuming and requires access to sheep blood. The use of sheep erythrocytes sensitized with antigen by glutaraldehyde is an obvious improvement, because the sensitized cells retain the specific *Trichinella* activity for over 6 months at 4°C (Ali-Khan, 1974) or cells may be lyophilized and stored at 4°C for at least 3 months (Barriga, 1977).

To increase the reliability of PHA in the serodiagnosis of trichinosis, further work is needed to purify and characterize the antigens used to sensitize the red cells. In itself, the orientation of the antigen on the cell support can play a major part in determining its serological behavior.

2.4. Enzyme-Linked Immunosorbent Assay

Primary binding reactions between antigen and antibody form the basis for very sensitive and quantitative methods such as radioimmunoassays (RIAs) and the enzyme-linked immunosorbent assay (ELISA). However, RIAs have certain disadvantages, such as the instability of labeled preparations, which can be overcome if radioactive isotope is substituted by an enzyme (Engvall and Perlmann, 1971, 1972; Engvall *et al.*, 1971; Van Weemen and Schuurs, 1971, 1972). ELISA in which the coated-plastic techniques were introduced (Engvall *et al.*, 1971; Engvall and Perlmann, 1972) has become well established and fulfills the requirements of objectivity, simplicity, and sensitivity previously provided only by RIAs. Furthermore, in comparison with RIAs, the ELISA requires less expensive equipment and is more suitable for automation.

Variants of ELISA can be used, such as *competitive ELISA* for measuring antigen. This test requires pure antigen in quantities sufficient for enzyme labeling. *Sandwich ELISA* is an assay of antigen with labeled antibody, which has to be specific for the antigen. Quantitation of specific antibody classes can be performed by *indirect ELISA*, in which the enzyme is linked to an antiimmunoglobulin.

As solid phase, almost any plastic surface can be used. Most plastics have the capacity to adsorb proteins, glycoproteins, and lipopolysaccharides. Polystyrene has been most popular, but polypropylene and polyvinyl also work well. Most molecules adsorb physically to the hydrophobic surface, but some of the antigen desorbs during incubation with antibody. In general, this desorption of antigen is the same in every tube or well and has no influence on the final results. However, some antigens adsorb more easily to one type of plastic than to another. To determine which plastic surface gives the best reproducibility, the various antigens may be tested with different plastic surfaces. The sensitivity and perhaps the nonspecificity of the test may also increase due to the plastic. Polyvinyl, for instance, adsorbs almost twice as much protein per unit surface area as polystyrene (Engvall and Rouslahti, 1979).

ELISA exhibits, as already mentioned, a high degree of sensitivity, and to achieve quantitative and reproducible results, the reagents need to be of high quality. Purified antigens and standardized conjugates are desirable. To facilitate the standardization, defined enzyme–immunoglobulin complexes of small size are preferable. A new heterobifunctional agent, *N*-succinimidyl 3-(2-pyridyldithio)propionate (Carlsson *et al.*, 1978), proposed for coupling the enzyme to the immunoglobulin, seems very promising (P. Nilsson *et al.*, 1981). Many different enzymes can be employed in ELISA, but they have to fulfill the requirements of being stable, reactive, readily available, cheap, and safe. The most common enzymes have been alkaline phosphatase, horseradish peroxidase, glucose oxidase, and β-galactosidase. In diagnosis of trichinosis, alkaline phosphatase and horseradish peroxidase have been used.

Ljungström *et al.* (1974) were the first first to employ ELISA for serodiagnosis of trichinosis in man. The test was performed in polystyrene tubes coated with a crude saline extract of muscle larvae. To reduce the quantity of necessary reagents and to simplify the handling of the samples, Ruitenberg *et al.* (1975b) introduced micro-ELISA in the serodiagnosis of *Trichinella* infection. The microtiter plates are particularly convenient for mass processing, since they enable hundreds of samples to be processed simultaneously. Since ELISA is preferable to all other techniques applied for seroepidemiological surveys, an improvement of the antigen is urgently needed. ELISA is a very sensitive test, and with the use of the crude *Trichinella* antigen, the negative controls sometimes give unacceptably high values. Crude antigen may also desorb more readily and unequally than purified antigen.

The specificity of ELISA is comparable to that of PHA in that cross-reactions with filaria antigen are seen when a crude saline extract of muscle larvae is used as antigen (Engvall and Ljungström, 1975). However, preliminary data, using stichocyte antigen (Despommier and Laccetti, 1981), indicate very few cross-reacting sera from patients infected with different filarial worms. The reactivity was observed only at low serum dilutions (Despommier and Ljungström, unpublished data).

ELISA can be used to detect antibodies of single antibody classes (Engvall and Ljungström, 1975; Stumpf *et al.*, 1981). It is of important diagnostic value because the demonstration of specific IgM or IgA antibodies or both most probably indicates recent infection. To avoid competition between antibodies of different affinities or avidities or both, the class-specific antibody must be determined in the presence of antigen excess.

2.5. Counterimmunoelectrophoresis

For rapid screening of sera, counterimmunoelectrophoresis (CIE) is the method of choice, (Gocke and Howe, 1970), since the results are obtained within 1 hr. The technique requires anodically migrating antigens to meet cathodically migrating antibodies at a zone of equivalence during electrophoresis to form visible precipitin lines. To enhance the visibility of the precipitin pattern, they may be stained. As a neutral support matrix, agarose or agar is usually employed. However, CIE can detect only antigens and antibodies with appropriately opposing electrophoretic properties.

CIE, like other techniques, must be adjusted to the specific analysis, and Despommier *et al.* (1974) have applied the test for diagnosis of trichinosis in man. The antigen used was a semipurified antigen obtained from muscle larvae, mainly consisting of stichocyte secretory granules (Despommier and Müller, 1970). In diagnosis of trichinosis, few studies have been performed to evaluate the sensitivity of CIE. It has been concluded that CIE is equivalent to the bentonite-flocculation test (Despommier et al., 1974) and the latex-agglutination test (Barrett-Connor et al., 1976). However, the latter authors claimed that CIE is more sensitive than the bentonite-flocculation test, whereas another study (Norman and Kagan, 1975) showed that CIE was less sensitive than the bentonite-flocculation test, double diffusion, and PHA. Since CIE is based on the capacity of antigen–antibody reactions to give visible precipitates, the divergent results may be due to the antigens used in the studies. Unfortunately, the antigens employed are not adequately described except in the original paper (Despommier et al., 1974).

Autoradiography combined with CIE (Tsotsos and Corbitt, 1973) increases the sensitivity of CIE in the diagnosis of trichinosis (Dzbinski et al., 1974). However, employing autoradiography eliminates one of the advantages of CIE, namely, rapidity, since the developing of the autoradiography takes about 1 week.

2.6. Other Serological Methods

The complement-fixation (CF) test was one of the first serological techniques introduced for diagnosis of trichinosis (Ströbel, 1911) and has been one of the most widely used methods. Only certain kinds of antibodies can be detected by the CF assay, since not all antibodies fix complement. The test is rather complicated, and the sensitivity and specificity vary greatly from laboratory to laboratory (Kagan and Norman, 1970). The CF test is time-consuming and requires highly trained technicians.

Two types of precipitin tests have been used for the diagnosis of trichinosis, the ring precipitin test (Bachman, 1928a) and the microprecipitin test, in which precipitates are formed around the orifices of both adult and larval worms immersed in immune serum (Mauss, 1940; Oliver-González, 1940; Roth, 1941). The ring precipitin test is performed by layering the antigen over the serum. After incubation, the interface between the antigen and serum is examined for the presence of a precipitate. The ring precipitin test is relatively insensitive (Kagan and Bargai, 1956) and the specificity questionable (Kagan and Norman, 1970). The microprecipitin test is reasonably sensitive. Of 14 sera from T. spiralis-infected patients, 10 were positive (Ljungström, 1979). In 5 cases, a positive reaction was obtained 3–4 weeks after the onset of the illness, and in 5 cases, after 7–10 weeks. Roth (1941) also reported positive reactions in convalescent sera. However, the microprecipitin test requires a supply of living larvae and is a procedure too specialized for most laboratories.

Several flocculation tests have been applied for the diagnosis of trichinosis such as the cholesterol-flocculation test (Suessenguth and Kline, 1944), the bentonite-flocculation test (Bozicevich *et al.*, 1951), and the card charcoal-flocculation test (Anderson *et al.*, 1963). In these tests, different particles serve as inert carriers for the *Trichinella* antigen, such as cholesterol crystals, bentonite particles (a mineral colloid), and cholesterol–lecithin particles mixed with charcoal. When these antigen-coated particles are mixed with antiserum, aggregates are formed, and the degree of aggregation is estimated with the aid of a microscope at low magnification, or when charcoal is incorporated, the floccules are visible on white plastic-coated cards. The tests are rapidly performed, but the preparation of the coated particles is laborious. It can generally be concluded that the methods are reasonably specific and relatively sensitive (Kagan and Norman, 1970). The bentonite-flocculation test is widely used in the United States.

The latex agglutination test is a rapid slide test (Innella and Redner, 1959; Muraschi *et al.*, 1962). However, it has been found that this test is less sensitive than other agglutination or flocculation methods (Norman and Kagan, 1963; M. Kozar *et al.*, 1964).

2.7. Skin Tests

Skin tests have been widely used in the diagnosis of parasitic infections. Following injection of antigens, inflammatory reactions may be observed, caused by immediate-type hypersensitivity within 10–20 min, Arthus or immune-complex reaction within 4–8 hr, or delayed-type hypersensitivity after 12–48 hr. The immediate-type hypersensitivity is evoked by reaction between IgE antibodies fixed to mast cells or basophil cells and the antigen. This reaction results in the release of biologically active substances. The Arthus reaction is evoked by complement-activating IgG antibodies, which form complexes with the locally injected antigen, resulting in the release of chemotactic factors and cell infiltration. Finally, the delayed-type hypersensitivity is evoked by the reaction between activated T lymphocytes and the corresponding antigen.

Augustine and Theiler (1932) found that skin tests used by Bachman (1928b) were of diagnostic value in human trichinosis. Since then, the skin test has been used for many years as an aid in the diagnosis of trichinosis, and the reports have been reviewed by Gould (1945), Kagan (1960), and Kagan and Norman (1970). Both immediate- and delayed-type hypersensitivity have been reported in infections with *T. spiralis*. However, the published reports indicate that much work remains to be done before skin tests can be properly employed for diagnostic or epidemiological purposes. It is likely that the specificity and sensitivity of the skin test will improve with the isolation of the antigen or antigens that specifically stimulate the IgE response. The obvious disadvantage of the test is the requirement to inject substances of unknown complexity into human subjects.

3. EVALUATION AND RECOMMENDATION

Immunodiagnosis of trichinosis is of importance in three different circumstances: to identify the infection during the acute stage, to confirm the disease retrospectively, and to be used in epidemiological studies. To fulfill these requirements, the methods selected should provide specificity, sensitivity, and reproducibility. Occasionally, it is necessary to give a rapid diagnosis. The methods should also be safe for the personnel handling the investigations. It is an advantage if the test is cheap and if untrained or minimally trained personnel can perform the assays. The last two requirements are particularly important for the developing countries.

The heterogeneity of the *Trichinella* antigens affects the specificity of the tests. Further characterization and standardization of the antigens are needed; otherwise, the specificity of the tests, at low serum dilutions, will be a problem. Another problem is the occurrence of the same antigenic determinants on otherwise unrelated macromolecules. This is true for many polysaccharide antigens and may cause cross-reactivity, which will complicate the evaluation of the test results.

The selection of diagnostic methods also involves the properties of antibodies. There is quite a considerable difference in the ways in which classes and subclasses produce secondary manifestations, such as precipitation, agglutination, and binding of complement. The ability to agglutinate is in general much higher for the multivalent IgM antibodies compared to the bivalent IgG antibodies of the same specificity.

The serodiagnostic methods used in the diagnosis of trichinosis vary in sensitivity. Most of the techniques used in the past are based on secondary manifestations following the reaction between antigen and antibody. The most sensitive techniques, e.g., enzyme immunoassay, which is a primary antigen–antibody binding test, are 10^5–10^6 times more sensitive than techniques based on precipitation.

Given the heterogeneity of the *Trichinella* antigens and the antibodies in the test serum, it is evident that the serodiagnosis of trichinosis must be carried out by at least two independent methods, e.g., one utilizing soluble antigens and the other particulate antigens.

In indirect IF, particulate antigens are employed. The test is sensitive, and since the test is based on primary antigen–antibody reactions, the ability of the antibodies to cause secondary manifestations is of no importance. The indirect IF technique seems to be specific, and the distinct staining pattern, consisting of a bright staining of the cuticle and stichosome–gut, is simple to distinguish from nonspecific staining. The ability of indirect IF to detect specific IgM and IgA antibodies is of great importance, since the presence of these antibody classes gives an indication of a recent or fairly recent infection. The reproducibility of indirect IF is high if the test is performed under optimal conditions. For seroepidemiological surveys or for screening purposes, indirect IF is tedious compared to ELISA and PHA, although the use of multitest slides has increased the capacity.

ELISA, a primary antigen–antibody binding test, is sensitive and employs soluble antigens, which in the diagnosis of trichinosis have been crude extracts of muscle larvae. By the aid of class-specific conjugates, specific antibodies of various classes can be detected, which is of importance for the diagnosis of acute trichinosis. The assay can also be used as a screening test to practically rule out the possibility that a significant level of antibody is present in the sera investigated. For seroepidemiological surveys, micro-ELISA is preferable, since the assay allows the simultaneous examination of hundreds of sera when the equipment specifically developed for the microsystem is employed. However, a lot of work still remains to be done before ELISA is fully standardized for the diagnosis of trichinosis. Increased specificity and reproducibility seem to be obtained by the use of immunoaffinity-column-purified antigens and defined conjugates. As a complement to the indirect IF technique, ELISA can be a good choice.

PHA is an assay that depends on the ability of the antibodies to produce agglutination. In specificity, sensitivity, or reproducibility, PHA seems to have no advantages over ELISA and to be less specific than indirect IF. To diagnosis acute trichinosis by PHA, the changes in the specific antibody level have to be determined, which always gives valuable information, but consecutive serum samples are not always available. As a supplementary test to the indirect IF technique, PHA may be a matter of choice, but should not be the only laboratory test for the diagnosis of trichinosis. The same evaluation and recommendation as for PHA are also valid for all the other agglutination or flocculation methods.

CIE is a method that depends on a secondary manifestation—precipitation. For rapid analysis of sera, CIE is recommended, since the results are obtained within 1 hr. However, further studies are needed before the specificity, sensitivity, and reproducibility can be evaluated.

The antigens used in skin tests for immunodiagnosis of trichinosis are still substances of unknown complexity. Not until the knowledge of these antigens has improved can skin tests be recommended for diagnosis of trichinosis in man.

There are some promising methods for the future: thin-layer immunoassay (TIA) (Elwing et al., 1976, 1977; Elwing and Nilsson, 1980) and diffusion-in-gel ELISA (DIG-ELISA) (Elwing and Nygren, 1979). The chief advantage of TIA is its techniqual simplicity. No sophisticated equipment is required, and the test may be performed with material that is available in any laboratory. The antigen–antibody reaction takes place on a flat polystyrene surface, e.g., a petri dish. Visualization of the antigen–antibody reaction is performed through condensation of water on the surface. TIA has been applied to the demonstration of antibodies against various parasites, such as *Schistosoma* and *Entamoeba* (Ismail et al., 1979; L.-Å. Nilsson et al., 1980a,b). In DIG-ELISA, the serum sample to be analyzed is applied to an agar gel on top of the antigen-coated surface. During diffusion, antibodies will bind to the fixed antigen on the surface. After removal of the gel, the surface is treated with enzyme-labeled antiimmunoglobulin. A second gel containing the enzyme substrate is applied as a layer on top of the surface. Antigen–antibody reactions on the surface are revealed as circular areas with changed color. Compared with ELISA, the evaluation of DIG-ELISA results is simpler, since only the diameter of the area reacted is recorded.

4. CONCLUSIONS

At present, there is no single test that meets all the requirements for the immunodiagnosis of *Trichinella* infection. A combination of indirect IF and ELISA seems to offer the best compromise, although these tests may not always be applicable for work in developing countries.

Further work is required in the preparation and purification of antigens, and collaborative studies, perhaps under the aegis of the

World Health Organization, should be undertaken in an effort to create international standards.

One final point to be borne in mind relates to the immune status of different population groups. For example, individuals in developing countries, subjected to multiple parasitic infections, may behave differently in diagnostic tests than those from developed countries.

5. PROTOCOLS FOR INDIRECT IMMUNOFLUORESCENCE AND ENZYME-LINKED IMMUNOSORBENT ASSAY

5.1. Indirect Immunofluorescence

A. *Preparation of Antigen*

1. Excise the diaphragms from *T. spiralis*-infected rats 6–8 weeks after infection. The rats have to be heavily infected.
2. Cut the diaphragm into 5-mm-wide strips.
3. Roll the strips and put them into small test tubes.
4. Store the tubes containing the diaphragm rolls at $-70°C$.

B. *Preparation of Sections*

1. Fix one roll of diaphragm with the aid of 1 or 2 drops of a freezing compound (e.g, Tissue Tek) onto the holder used for cryostat sectioning.
2. Prepare frozen sections ($\approx$5 mm) with the aid of the cryostat.
3. Put 2 or 3 sections per circle on a microscope multitest slide at room temperature and preferentially use slides with 3 circles.
4. Fix the sections in acetone (p.a.-grade) for 10 min at room temperature.
5. Store the slides at $+4°C$.

C. *Serum Dilution*

Dilute the patient sera in phosphate-buffered saline (PBS), pH 7.4. A dilution of 1:10 is recommended to be the first serum dilution. From this serial dilutions can be prepared. Two-step dilution is recommended for human routine serology.

D. *Chessboard Titration of the Conjugate*

For each batch of fluorescein-conjugated antihuman antibody (conjugates), end-point titrations of antisera against serial dilutions of conjugates (Huldt *et al.*, 1975) have to be done. The working dilution should be one next to the plateau end point.

E. *Counter staining*

To avoid nonspecific staining, immerse the slides in Evan's Blue, diluted 1:500 in PBS, pH 7.4 [see G(12)].

F. *Controls*

Positive serum with known titer.
Negative serum (sera).
Buffer, when testing the specificity of the second layer or the third layer or both in the staining procedure.

G. *Staining Procedure*

1. Make a test protocol.
2. Place the number of slides to be used at room temperature and allow to dry before the staining procedure.
3. Mark the slides according to the test protocol.
4. Place the slides horizontally in a moist chamber.
5. Pipette the serum dilutions onto the slides, according to the test protocol, so that the antigen sections are completely covered.
6. Incubate the slides in a moist chamber for 30 min at room temperature.
7. a. Wash the slides one at a time by dipping them into PBS.
   b. Remove the excess of PBS by touching the edge of the slide against filter paper.
   c. Place the slides together in a washing basin containing PBS and let stand for 5 min. Repeat (b) and (c) twice with fresh PBS in the basin.
8. Remove all buffer from the slides with filter paper and place the slides in the moist chamber [see (4)]. DO NOT ALLOW THE SECTIONS TO DRY!
9. Pipette the conjugate, suitably diluted in PBS (see D), onto the sections, so that the sections are completely covered.
10. Incubate [see (6)].
11. Wash [see (7)].
12. Place the slides in a basin containing Evan's Blue, diluted 1:500 in PBS.
13. Incubate for 13 min at room temperature.
14. Wash [see (7)].

15. Remove all buffer on both sides of the slide with filter paper. DO NOT ALLOW THE SECTIONS TO DRY during the procedure.
16. Add 1 drop of glycerine buffer (1 part PBS, pH 7.8–7.9, to 9 parts of glycerine) to each dot on the slide and place a coverglass on the top.
17. Examine the sections under a fluorescence microscope equipped for fluorescein isothiocyanate (FITC) fluorescence.

Comments: Class-specific conjugates can be used instead of anti-Ig.

Sera from various species can be examined. In this case, a conjugated antispecies has to be used. If a conjugated antispecies is not available, a third layer can be used, e.g., mouse antibody, goat antimouse antibody, and antigoat antibody–FITC.

In some antibody–antigen systems, the muscle tissue around the encysted larvae may complicate the evaluation of the results. In this case, use cryostat sections of free-prepared muscle larvae embedded in a freezing compound.

5.2. Enzyme-Linked Immunosorbent Assay

A. Antigen

Soluble antigen, as well characterized as possible, is used. To achieve the highest possible diagnostic specificity, especially when crude antigens are employed, determination of the optimal concentration of the antigen used for coating is important. This may be performed by chessboard titration using both positive and negative sera. In general, the optimal concentration is between 1 and 5 µg protein/ml.

B. Serum Dilution

Dilute the patient sera in incubation buffer (PBS, pH 7.4, with 0.05% Tween 20). A dilution of 1 : 100 is recommended as the first serum dilution. From this, serial dilutions can be prepared. Three-step dilution is recommended for human routine serology.

C. Chessboard Titration of the Conjugate

For each batch of horseradish peroxidase (or alkaline phosphatase)-conjugated antihuman antibody (conjugate), end-point titrations of antisera against serial dilutions of conjugates have to be done. The working dilution should be one next to the plateau end point.

D. Controls

Positive serum with known titer.
Negative serum (sera).
Incubation buffer.

E. Staining Procedure

1. Make a test protocol.
2. Dissolve the antigen to suitable concentration in coating buffer (0.05 M carbonate buffer, pH 9.6).
3. Coat the microtiter plate with 0.2 ml/well (or 0.1 ml/well) of the antigen.
4. Incubate the plate overnight at room temperature.
5. Wash the plate three times in washing solution (PBS, pH 7.4 with 0.05% Tween 20). Make sure that the plate is empty after the last washing by shaking the plate against a filter paper.
6. Dilute the serum samples to a suitable concentration in the incubation buffer.
7. Pipette 0.2 ml/well (or 0.1 ml/well) of the dilutions into the wells according to the test protocol.
8. Incubate the plate 1 hr at 37°C.
9. Wash [see (5)].
10. Incubate with 0.2 ml/well (or 0.1 ml/well) of the conjugate diluted in incubation buffer (see C) for 2 hr at 37°C.
11. Wash [see (5)].
12. Add 0.2 ml/well of enzyme substrate.
13. Stop the reaction by adding 0.025 ml/well of NaOH after a suitable time, approximately 10 min for horseradish peroxidase conjugate.
14. Measure the optical density in a spectrophotometer.

Comments: Recrystallized 5-amino-2-hydroxybenzoic acid (Ellens and Gielkens, 1980) or *p*-phenylenediamine in combination with H_2O_2 are the most widely used substrates to horseradish peroxidase. The optical density is measured at 449 nm.

p-Nitrophenylphosphate is employed as substrate for alkaline phosphatase, and the optical density is measured at 400 nm.

There does not at present seem to be general agreement as to how the results should be expressed. Two different principles have usually been applied: (1) The titer is determined from a dose–response curve at the serum dilution that gives an extinction value that exceeds, by a defined amount, that given by a negative sample. (2) The results can be expressed as the extinction value given by a single defined dilution of a serum. In seroepidemiological surveys, the quantitative aspects may be of minor importance, while a qualitative answer, as obtained by this procedure, may be sufficient.

REFERENCES

Ali-Khan, Z., 1974, Glutaraldehyde fixed–antigen sensitized stable cells in indirect hemagglutination test for rapid diagnosis of hydatid disease, trichinosis and amoebiasis, *Int. J. Parasitol.* **4**:549–554.

Anderson, R.I., Sadun, E.H., and Schoenbechler, M.J., 1963, Cholesterol–lecithin slide (TsSF) and charcoal card (TsCC) flocculation tests using an acid-soluble fraction of *Trichinella spiralis* larvae, *J. Parasitol.* **49**:642–647.

Augustine, D.L., and Theiler, H., 1932, Precipitin and skin tests as aids in diagnosing trichinosis, *Parasitology* **24**:60–82.

Bachman, G.W., 1928a, A precipitin test in experimental trichiniasis, *J. Prev. Med.* **2**:35–48.

Bachman, G.W., 1928b, An intradermal reaction in experimental trichiniasis, *J. Prev. Med.* **2**:169–173.

Baratawidjaja, R.K., Hewson, A., and Labzoffsky, N.A., 1963, Fluorescent antibody staining in the serodiagnosis of trichinosis, *Can. J. Microbiol.* **9**:625–628.

Barrett-Connor, E., Davis, C.F., Hamburger, R.N., and Kagan, I., 1976, An epidemic of trichinosis after injestion of wild pig in Hawaii, *J. Infect. Dis.* **133**:473–477.

Barriga, O., 1977, Reactivity and specificity of *Trichinella spiralis* fractions in cutaneous and serological tests, *J. Clin. Microbiol.* **6**:274–279.

Boyden, S.V., 1951, The adsorption of proteins on erythrocytes treated with tannic acid and subsequent hemagglutination by antiprotein sera, *J. Exp. Med.* **93**:107–200.

Bozicevich, J., Tobie, J.E., Thomas, E.H., Hoyem, H.M., and Ward, S.B., 1951, A rapid flocculation test for the diagnosis of trichinosis, *Public Health Rep.* **66**:806–814.

Brzosko, W., Gracarz, Z., and Nowoslawski, A., 1965, Immunofluorescence in the serological diagnosis of *Trichinella spiralis* infection, *Exp. Med. Microbiol.* **17**:355–365.

Campbell, C.H., 1955, The antigenic role of the excretions and secretions of *Trichinella spiralis* in the production of immunity in mice, *J. Parasitol.* **41**:483–491.

Carlsson, J., Drevin, H., and Axén, R., 1978, Protein thiolation and reversible protein-protein conjugation: N-Succinimidyl 3-(2-pyridyldithio)propionate, a new heterobifunctional reagent, *Biochem. J.* **173**:723–737.

Chicoine, L., Proulx, C., Lafleur, L., and Tanner, C.E., 1966, Trichinosis: An epidemiological study in children using five immunological methods, *Can. J. Public Health* **57**:357–365.

Chroust, K., and Dubansky, V., 1970, The indirect fluorescent antibody method in experimental trichinosis diagnostics, *Acta Vet. (Brno)* **39**:157–163.

Chroust, K., Dubansky, V., and Piskac, A., 1966, Fluorescent antibody studies of muscle larvae *Trichinella spiralis* (Owen, 1835), *Sb. Vys. Sk. Zemed. Brne*, **14**:505–514.

Crandall, R.B., and Crandall, A.C., 1972, *Trichinella spiralis*: Immunologic response to infection in mice, *Exp. Parasitol.* **31**:378–398.

Denham, D.A., and Martinez, A.R., 1970, Studies with methyridine and *Trichinella spiralis*. 2. The use of the drug to study the rate of larval production in mice, *J. Helminthol.* **44**:357–363.

Despommier, D.D., 1974, The stichocyte of *Trichinella spiralis* during morphogenesis in the small intestine of the rat, in: *Trichinellosis* (C.W. Kim, ed.), Intext, New York, pp. 239–254.

Despommier, D.D., and Laccetti, A., 1981, *Trichinella spiralis*: Proteins and antigens isolated from a large-particle fraction derived from the muscle larva, *Exp. Parasitol.* **51**:279–295.

Despommier, D.D., and Müller, M., 1970, Functional antigens of *Trichinella spiralis*, *J. Parasitol.* **56**(Sect. II, Part 1):76.

Despommier, D.D., and Müller, M., 1976, The stichosome and its secretion granules in the mature muscle larva of *Trichinella spiralis*, *J. Parasitol.* **62**:775–785.

Despommier, D.D., Müller, M., Jenks, B., and Fruitstone, M., 1974, Immunodiagnosis of human trichinosis using counterelectrophoresis and agar gel diffusion techniques, *Am. J. Trop. Med. Hyg.* **23**:41–44.

Despommier, D.D., Campbell, W.C., and Blair, L.S., 1977, The *in vivo* and *in vitro* analysis of immunity to *Trichinella spiralis* in mice and rats, *Parasitology* **74**:109–119.

Dzbinski, T.H., Plonka, W.S., and Jedrzejewska, B., 1974, Use of radioimmunoelectro-osmophoresis for the diagnosis of human trichinosis, *Experientia* **30**:1269–1270.

Ellens, D.J., and Gielkens, L.J., 1980, A simple method for the purification of 5-aminosalicylic acid: Application of the product as substrate in enzyme-linked immunosorbent assay (ELISA), *J. Immunol. Methods* **37**:325–332.

Elwing, H., and Nilsson, L.-Å., 1980, Diffusion-in-gel thin layer immunoassay (DIG-TIA): Optimal conditions for quantification of antibodies, *J. Immunol. Methods* **38**:257–268.

Elwing, H., and Nygren, H., 1979, Diffusion-in-gel-enzyme-linked immunosorbent assay (DIG-ELISA): A simple method for quantitation of class-specific antibodies, *J. Immunol. Methods* **31**:101–107.

Elwing, H., Nilsson, L.-Å., and Ouchterlony, Ö., 1976, Visualization principles in thin-layer immunoassays (TIA) on plastic surfaces, *Int. Arch. Allergy Appl. Immunol.* **51**:757–762.

Elwing, H., Nilsson, L.-Å., and Ouchterlony, Ö., 1977, A simple spot technique for thin layer immunoassays (TIA) on plastic surfaces, *J. Immunol. Methods* **17**:131–145.

Engelbrecht, E., 1966, Diagnosis of recent and long standing *Trichinella spiralis* infections by means of immunofluorescence tests, *Arch. Roum. Pathol. Exp. Microbiol.* **25**:831–848.

Engvall, E., and Ljungström, I., 1975, Detection of human antibodies to *Trichinella spiralis* by enzyme-linked immunosorbent assay, ELISA, *Acta Pathol. Microbiol. Scand. Sect C* **83**:231–237.

Engvall, E., and Perlmann, P., 1971, Enzyme-linked immunosorbent assay, ELISA: Quantitative assay of immunoglobulin G, *Immunochemistry* **8**:871–874.

Engvall, E., and Perlmann, P., 1972, Enzyme-linked immunosorbent assay, ELISA. III. Quantitation of specific antibodies by enzyme-labeled anti-immunoglobulin in antigen-coated tubes, *J. Immunol.* **109**:129–135.

Engvall, E., and Rouslahti, E., 1979, Principles of ELISA and recent applications to the study of molecular interactions, in: *Laboratory and Research Methods in Biology and*

Medicine, Vol. 3 (R.M. Nakamura, W.R. Dito, and E.S. Tucker III, eds.), Alan R. Liss, New York, pp. 89–97.

Engvall, E., Jonsson, K., and Perlmann, P., 1971, Enzyme-linked immunosorbent assay. II. Quantitative assay of protein antigen, immunoglobulin G, by means of enzyme-labeled antigen and antibody-coated tubes, *Biochim. Biophys. Acta* **251**:427–434.

Gocke, D.J., and Howe, C., 1970, Rapid detection of Australia antigen by counterimmunoelectrophoresis, *J. Immunol.* **104**:1031–1032.

Gould, S.E. (ed.), 1945, *Trichinosis*, Charles C. Thomas, Springfield, Illinois.

Greenbury, C.L., Moore, D.H., and Nunn, L.A.C., 1963, Reaction of 7S and 19S components of immune rabbit antisera with human group A and AB red cells, *Immunology* **8**:421–433.

Grove, D.I., Hamburger, J., and Warren, K.S., 1977, Kinetics of immunological responses, resistance to reinfection and pathological reactions to infection with *Trichinella spiralis*, *J. Infect. Dis.* **136**:562–570.

Huldt, G., Ljungström, I., and Aust-Kettis, A., 1975, Detection by immunofluorescence of antibodies to parasitic agents: Use of class-specific conjugates, *Ann. N.Y. Acad. Sci.* **254**:304–314.

Innella, F., and Redner, W. J., 1959, Latex agglutination serologic test for trichinosis, *J. Am. Med. Assoc.* **171**:885–887.

Ismail, M., Draper, C., Ouchterlony, Ö., Nilsson, L.-Å., and Terry, R., 1979, A comparison between a new serological method, thin-layer immunoassay (TIA), and the enzyme-linked immunosorbent assay (ELISA) for the detection of antibodies in schistosomiasis, *Parasite Immunol.* **1**:251–258.

Jackson, G.J., 1959, Fluorescent antibody studies of *Trichinella spiralis* infections, *J. Infect. Dis.* **105**:97–117.

Kagan, I.G., 1960, Trichinosis: A review of biologic, serologic, and immunologic aspects, *J. Infect. Dis.* **107**:65–93.

Kagan, I.G., and Bargai, U., 1956, Studies on the serology of trichinosis with hemagglutination, agar diffusion tests and precipitin ring tests, *J. Parasitol.* **42**:237–245.

Kagan, I.G., and Norman, L.G., 1970, The serology of trichinosis, in: *Trichinosis in Man and Animals* (S.E. Gould, ed.), Charles C. Thomas, Springfield, Illinois, pp. 222–268.

Kane, G.J., Matossian, R., and Batty, I., 1971, Fluorochrome-labeled anti-immunoglobulin fractions used with stabilized antigen preparations for the assessment of parasitic diseases, *Ann. N. Y. Acad. Sci.* **177**:134–145.

Kozar, M., Kozar, Z., and Karmanska, K., 1964, The comparative evaluation of some agglutination tests in the diagnosis of trichinellosis, *Wiad. Parazytol.* **10**:717–737.

Kozar, Z., Karmanska, K., and Kozar, M., 1966, Indirect fluorescent antibody test with isolated *Trichinella spiralis* larvae, *Wiad. Parazytol.* **12**:637–642.

Kozek, W.J., and Crandall, C.A., 1974, Immunogenicity of the stichosome of *Trichinella spiralis* in mice, in: *Trichinellosis* (C.W. Kim, ed.), Intext, New York, pp. 231–237.

Larsh, J.E., and Weatherly, N.F., 1974, Studies on delayed (cellular) hypersensitivity in mice infected with *Trichinella spiralis*. IX. Delayed dermal sensitivity in artificly sensitized donors, *J. Parasitol.* **60**:93–98.

Ljungström, I., 1974, Antibody response to *Trichinella spiralis*, in: *Trichinellosis* (C.W. Kim, ed.), Intext, New York, pp. 449–459.

Ljungström, I., 1979, *Trichinella spiralis*: Formation of specific antibodies and modulation of the immune response, Ph.D. thesis, University of Stockholm, Sweden, 17 pp.

Ljungström, I., and Ruitenberg, E.J., 1976, A comparative study of the immunohistological and serological response of intact and T cell-deprived mice to *Trichinella spiralis*, *Clin. Exp. Immunol.* **24**:146–156.

Ljungström, I., Engvall, E., and Ruitenberg, E.J., 1974, ELISA, enzyme linked immunosorbent assay—a new technique for serodiagnosis of trichinosis, *Parasitology* **69**:xxiv.

Mackenzie, C.D., Preston, P.M., and Ogilvie, B.M., 1978, Immunological properties of the surface of parasitic nematodes, *Nature (London)* **276**:826–828.

Matossian, R.M., Salti, I., and Stephan, E., 1977, Variation in serum immunoglobulin levels in acute trichinosis, *J. Helminthol.* **51**:1–4.

Mauss, E.A., 1940, The *in vitro* effect of immune serum upon *Trichinella spiralis* larvae, *Am. J. Hyg.* **32**(Sect. D):80–83.

Melcher, L.R., 1943, An antigenic analysis of *Trichinella spiralis*, *J. Infect. Dis.* **73**:31–39.

Mills, C.K., and Kent, N.H., 1965, Excretions and secretions of *Trichinella spiralis* and their role in immunity, *Exp. Parasitol.* **16**:300–310.

Muraschi, T.F., Bloomfield, N., and Newman, R.B., 1962, A slide latex–particle agglutination test for trichinosis, *Am. J. Clin. Pathol.* **37**:227–231.

Nilsson, L.-Å., Björck, L., Capron, A., Elwing, H., and Ouchterlony, Ö., 1980a, Application of thin layer immunoassay (TIA) as a serodiagnostic tool in schistosomiasis: A preliminary report, *Trans. R. Soc. Trop. Med. Hyg.* **74**:201–204.

Nilsson, L.-Å., Petchclai, B., and Elwing, H., 1980b, Application of thin layer immunoassay (TIA) for demonstration of antibodies against *Entamoeba histolytica*, *Am. J. Trop. Med. Hyg.* **29**:524–529.

Nilsson, P., Bergquist, N.R., and Grundy, M.S., 1981, A technique for preparing defined conjugates of horseradish peroxidase and immunoglobulin, *J. Immunol. Methods* **41**:81–93.

Norman, L., and Kagan, I., 1963, Bentonite latex and cholesterol flocculation tests for the diagnosis of trichinosis, *Public Health Rep.* **78**:227–239.

Norman, L., and Kagan, I., 1975, An evaluation of crude and fractionated trichina antigens in the diagnosis of trichinosis, *Bol. Chil. Parasitol.* **30**:58–64.

Ogilvie, B.M., Philipp, M., Jungery, M., Maizels, R.M., Worms, M.J., and Parkhouse, R.M.E., 1980, The surface of nematodes and the immune response of the host, in: *The Host-Invader Interplay* (H. Van den Bossche, ed.), Elsevier, Amsterdam, pp. 99–104.

Oliver-González, J., 1940, The *in vitro* action of immune serum on the larvae and adults of *Trichinella spiralis*, *J. Infect. Dis.* **67**:292–300.

Ottesen, E.A., Smith, T.K., and Kirkpatrick, C.H., 1975, Immune response to *Trichinella spiralis* in the rat. I. Development of cellular and humoral responses during chronic infection, *Int. Arch. Allergy Appl. Immunol.* **49**:396–410.

Parkhouse, R.M.E., Philipp, M., and Ogilvie, B.M., 1981, Characterization of surface antigens of *Trichinella spiralis* infective larvae, *Parasite Immunol.* **3**:339–352.

Pattersson, R., Robert, M., Slonka, G., and McAninch, J., 1975, Studies on immunoglobulins, bentonite flocculation and IgE, IgG and IgM antibodies in serum from patients with trichinosis, *Am. J. Med.* **58**:787–793.

Phillip, M., Parkhouse, R.M.E., and Ogilvie, B.M., 1980, Changing proteins on the surface of a parasitic nematode, *Nature (London)* **287**:538–540.

Price, S.G., and Weiner, L.M., 1956, Use of hemagglutination in the diagnosis of trichinosis, *Am. J. Clin. Pathol.* **26**:1261–1269.

Rosenberg, E.B., Polman, S.H., and Whalen, G.E., 1971, Increased circulating IgE in trichinosis, *Ann. Intern. Med.* **75**:575–578.

Roth, H., 1941, The *in vitro* action of trichina larvae in immune serum—a new precipitin test in trichinosis, *Acta pathol. Microbiol. Scand.* **18**:160–167.

Ruitenberg, E.J., Ljungström, I., Steerenberg, P.A., and Buys, J., 1975a, Application of immunofluorescence and immunoenzyme methods in the serodiagnosis of *Trichinella spiralis* infection, *Ann. N.Y. Acad. Sci.* **254**:296–303.

Ruitenberg, E.J., Steerenberg, P.A., and Brosi, B.J.M., 1975b, Microsystem for the application of ELISA (enzyme linked immunosorbent assay) in the serodiagnosis of *Trichinella spiralis* infections, *Medicon Nederl.* **4**:30–31.

Sadun, E.H., Anderson, R.I., and Williams, J.S., 1962, Fluorescent antibody test for the serological diagnosis of trichinosis, *Exp. Parasitol.* **12**:423–433.

Sladki, E., 1960, The importance of intradermal test to diagnose the hidden and protracted forms of trichinellosis in the light of focal infection, *Wiad. Parazytol.* **6**:346–347.

Ströbel, H., 1911, Die Serodiagnositic der Trichinosis, *Muench. Med. Wochenschr.* **58**:672–674.

Stumpf, J., Undeutsch, K., and Landcraf, H., 1981, Results of the clinical and serological diagnosis of an epidemic of *Trichinella spiralis*, in: *Trichinellosis* (C.W. Kim, E.J. Ruitenberg, and J.S. Teppema, eds.), Reedbooks, Chertsey, England, pp. 279–282.

Suessenguth, H., and Kline, B.A., 1944, A simple rapid flocculation slide test for trichinosis in man and in swine, *Am. J. Clin. Pathol.* **14**:471–484.

Sultzer, A.J., 1965, Indirect fluorescent antibody tests for parasitic diseases. 1. Preparation of a stable antigen from larvae of *Trichinella spiralis*, *J. Parasitol.* **51**:717–721.

Svehag, S.-E., 1964, The formation and properties of poliovirus-neutralizing antibody. IV. Normal antibody and early immune antibody of rabbit origin: A comparison of biological and physicochemical properties, *J. Exp. Med.* **119**:517–535.

Takatsy, G., 1955, The use of spiral loops in serological and virological micromethods, *Acta Microbiol. Acad. Sci. Hung.* **3**:191–202.

Tsotsos, A.S., and Corbitt, G., 1973, Radioimmunoelectroosmophoresis, a technique combining immunoelectrophoresis with autoradiography; applications to virology, *J. Immunol. Methods* **3**:53–62.

Van Weemen, B.K., and Schuurs, A.H.W.M., 1971, Immunoassay using antigen–enzyme conjugates, *FEBS Lett.* **15**:232–236.

Van Weemen, B.K., and Schuurs, A.H.W.M., 1972, Immunoassay using hapten–enzyme conjugates, *FEBS Lett.* **24**:77–81.

Vernes, A., Floc'h, F., Biguet, J., and Tailliez, R., 1975, Experimental trichinosis. I. The course of delayed hypersensitivity in the CBA mouse and Wistar rat, *Int. J. Parasitol.* **5**:63–70.

Wakelin, D., 1978, Immunity to intestinal parasites, *Nature (London)* **273**:617–620.

Wegesa, P., Sulzer, A.J., and van Orden, A., 1971, A slide antigen in the indirect fluorescent antibody test for *Trichinella spiralis*, *Immunology* **21**:805–808.

Witebsky, E., Wels, P., and Heide, A., 1942, Serodiagnosis of trichinosis by means of complement fixation, *N. Y. State J. Med.* **42**:431–435.

13

Epidemiology I

Modes of Transmission

WILLIAM C. CAMPBELL

1. INTRODUCTION

Trichinosis is a zoonosis, a disease of nonhuman animals transmissible to man. Because of the direct life cycle of *Trichinella*, and the parasite's lack of host specificity and wide geographic distribution, there are many opportunities for interspecific transmission. As more of these transmission possibilities have been recognized, the epidemiological concept of trichinosis has been modified, and what had appeared to be a simple epidemiological pattern has tended to give way to a picture of considerable complexity (Kozar, 1962; Madsen, 1976; Steele and Schultz, 1978; Stoimenov and Gradinarski, 1981; Pawlowski, 1981). The situation has been aggravated in recent years by the discovery of regional variants of the parasite having greater or lesser infectivity for synanthropic animals (e.g., rats, mice, swine) as compared to their infectivity for feral animals. These interrelationships have been analyzed recently by Pawlowski (1981) and Dick (Chapter 2).

There is some evidence that one of the newly discovered *Trichinella* variants, given the specific or subspecific name *pseudospiralis*, is a natural parasite of birds (see Chapter 2). The modes of transmission of this organism, however, are unknown, and this chapter is limited to the

WILLIAM C. CAMPBELL • Merck Institute for Therapeutic Research, Rahway, New Jersey 07065.

well-known mammalian species *T. spiralis* (including the variants designated *nativa* and *nelsoni*). It would seem helpful to reduce the epidemiological complexity associated with this parasite to two simple transmission cycles—the sylvatic and the domestic—and to recognize that some forms of transmission may represent departures from these basic cycles.

2. SYLVATIC CYCLE

Trichinosis was known as a zoonosis, transmitted from pig to man, for many years before there was any real appreciation of its existence in wildlife. For the past century, there have been sporadic reports of *Trichinella* larvae in various wild animals, but only in the past 40 years has it become clear that the parasite is widespread among wildlife and is transmitted in a sylvatic cycle that is independent of man or domestic animals. This transmission cycle is illustrated in Fig. 1.

The sylvatic cycle is widely regarded as an exchange between predator and prey. Carnivorous animals devour infected animals, and it is postulated that animals weakened by muscle parasitism would be preferentially captured, and so parasite propagation would be ensured. The postulate is not fundamentally teleological, but it probably arises from our sense of the fitness of things rather than being derived from scientific data. Predation probably accounts for transmission of *Trichinella* in some instances, but it has been argued persuasively that the eating of carrion is of greater epidemiological significance (Madsen, 1976; Cameron, 1970; Rausch, 1970; Zimmermann, 1971). Many epidemiological surveys have been based on examination of the small rodents that constitute so much of the prey of wild carnivores. Where the number of rodents examined is small, the absence of *Trichinella* is of little significance, because the pyramidal nature of the food chain means that the infection in carnivores could be maintained by a low infection rate in rodents (Schad and Chowdhury, 1967). Some surveys, however, have involved many hundreds of rodents, and the relative rarity of *Trichinella* larvae in these animals is puzzling within the context of the predator–prey hypothesis but readily explicable in terms of carnivore–carrion transmission. The distinction should thus be kept in mind in interpreting past surveys and planning future surveys.

The distinction is also important in relation to the evolution and comparative biology of helminth life cycles. *Trichinella* does not have an intermediate host, but the proponents of the predation hypothesis have tended to regard the muscle phase as analogous to the infection

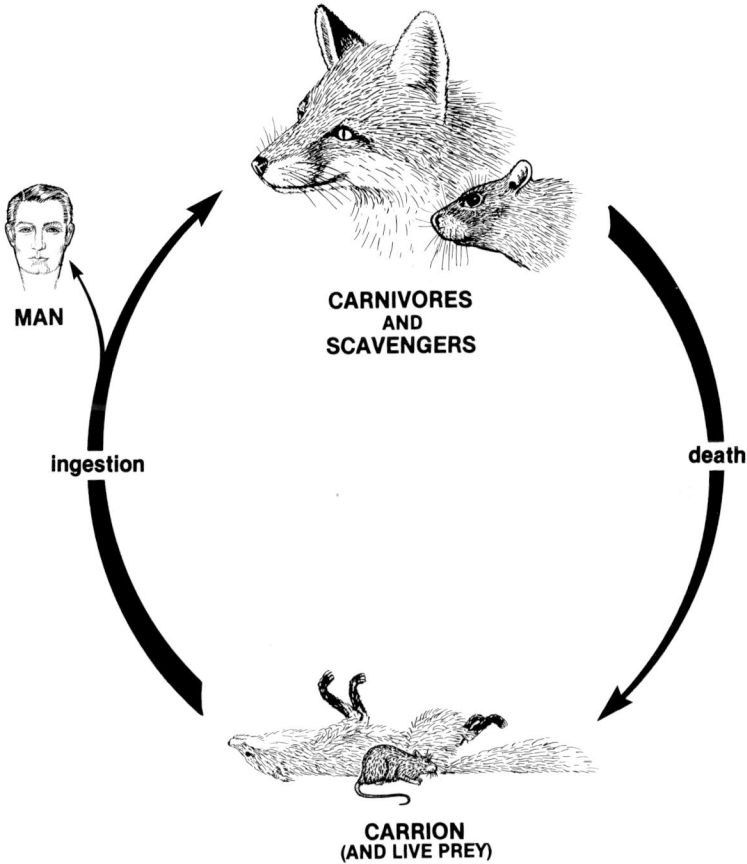

FIGURE 1. Sylvatic cycle, representing the transmission of trichinosis in nature, independent of man. "Carnivores and scavengers" include fox, bear, rat, walrus, hyena, wildcats, and many others. In the case of human infection, the source would be called game meat, rather than carrion, and the infection would represent an offshoot of the cycle. Original diagram.

of an intermediate host (the difference being simply that *Trichinella*, instead of infecting another species as intermediate host, invades another anatomical part of the definitive host). When viewed from the perspective of the carrion hypothesis, however, the muscle phase of *Trichinella* becomes on the death of the host, analogous to the free-living phase of other nematodes; larvae in decaying flesh are nonparasitic, presumably metabolically quiescent, and protected from a hostile environment until another host is reached.

Wild animals that are infected with *Trichinella* are carnivorous or omnivorous, and on the present evidence it seems reasonable to accept the proposition that they become infected by eating the carrion of dead carnivores. Large, long-lived carnivores probably play a particularly important role, because they have several years in which to accumulate significant numbers of larvae in their musculature and because their carcasses provide copious infective material. A prime example is the polar bear, in which the prevalence of infection is very high and which is often hunted for its pelt alone, with the result that hundreds of kilograms of infective flesh are left to be eaten by carrion feeders. It is also of evident epidemiological significance that the parasite, like the host, enjoys remarkable longevity; infective larvae have been recovered from a black bear (*Ursus americanus*) 10 years after experimental infection (Rausch, 1970).

We tend to think of carnivores devouring their prey freshly killed, but many of them will feed on carrion, and indeed the Kodiak bear (*U. arctos middendorffi*) is said to prefer flesh softened by autolysis. Transmission of *Trichinella* through carrion would not be effective if the death of the host were quickly followed by decay of the Nurse cell or "capsule" and death of the larva within. In fact, the resistance of the larvae to putrefaction of the host muscle has been well known since the last century, and more recent studies have shown considerable resistance to salinity and cold (Madsen, 1974). The modern concept of the host capsule as a living, transformed muscle cell or "Nurse cell" takes on a new and puzzling aspect in the context of nonliving flesh. Presumably the cell is no longer a "nurse" when the host is no longer alive. Perhaps the larva then draws on endogenous food reserves, while being protected more or less mechanically inside the capsule.

Nowhere is the sylvatic cycle more in evidence than in the Arctic and sub-Arctic, where *Trichinella* occurs commonly in both terrestrial mammals (polar bear, brown bear, arctic fox, wolf, lynx) and marine mammals (walrus, seal). Rates of infection can be very high (see Chapter 14). The parasite may have undergone evolutionary adaptation toward higher resistance to low temperatures, since viable larvae have been recovered from carcasses that have remained frozen in the Arctic for long periods. In some instances, such larvae, when transferred to laboratory animals, have lost their elevated resistance to freezing, suggesting that the resistance may have been dependent on the characteristics of the muscle tissue of the original Arctic host, and not on the parasite.

The resistance of *Trichinella* to cold has been of interest to investigators since the discovery of the worm. The pioneering work of

Leuckart and others gave an impression of considerable resistance to freezing. The early studies were reviewed by Ransom (1916), who concluded that the impression was founded on very weak evidence. Having carried out an extensive study on the ability of larvae to survive in meat held at various temperatures for various periods, Ransom found that the viability of the larvae was severely curtailed at a temperature of 15°F (-4°C), but that total suppression of infectivity required cooling to 5°F (-12°C), or lower, for 10–20 days. Such findings will need to be reevaluated in the light of recent evidence of regional differences in the attributes of *Trichinella*. Larvae encysted in Arctic mammals sometimes show little calcification even after many years (Rausch, 1970), perhaps constituting further evidence of adaptation in the regional strain. It has been suggested that the predominant strain of high latitudes is an isolated population, deserving subspecific or even specific rank (*Trichinella nativa*). This question is examined in Chapter 2.

Polar bears become infected by eating the flesh of seals as well as the flesh of land animals, including their own species (Fay, 1960; Manning, 1961). Other terrestrial Arctic mammals probably become infected in similar fashion. The infections in Arctic marine mammals, however, are something of an enigma, especially in terms of the predator–prey hypothesis. Walruses usually feed on mollusks and other invertebrates, but some individuals adopt a diet of mammalian flesh, especially when food is scarce. It is uncertain whether such "carnivorous" walruses prey on live seals, but there is evidence that they eat dead seals, and they probably eat flesh of any kind available. Given *Trichinella* infection in seals and terrestrial mammals, therefore, it is not difficult to account for infection in walruses by means of carrion and possibly by prey (Fay, 1960; Manning, 1961). The infection in seals is more difficult to explain. The prevalence of infection is low (and essentially confined to the bearded seal, *Erignathus barbatus*, and the ringed seal, *Pusa hispida*), and the seal is not considered a major component of the sylvatic cycle (Rausch, 1970). It has been speculated that seals, which feed primarily on fish and invertebrates, may become infected by ingesting small crustacea that feed on carrion in the sea. Indeed, amphipod crustaceans have been shown by Britov [cited by Rausch (1970) and Kozlov (1971)] to ingest encysted *Trichinella* in fragments of flesh and to be capable of transmitting the infection mechanically to an experimental mammalian host; that is, the amphipods do not become infected with *Trichinella*, but simply convey the larvae to a susceptible host. The larvae may be retained in the gut of crustacea for up to 28 hr (Hulebak, 1980). The available carrion would include the carcasses of polar bear and arctic fox, which roam the Arctic sea ice, and perhaps carcasses of dogs thrown into the sea by man (Madsen, 1974). Transmission by carrion, employing crustacean transport, is thus quite plausible, but the natural mode of infection in seals is not known with certainty.

Rodents are more commonly infected in the Arctic than in temperate or tropical regions, and probably become infected by scavenging carrion when food is scarce. Presumably, Arctic carnivores can become infected by eating infected rodents either as carrion or as prey.

While trichinosis has long been known as a disease of temperate and Arctic regions, it has only recently been shown to be endemic in tropical lands. Wildlife hosts that may be significant in the perpetuation of the tropical and subtropical sylvatic cycle include various hyenids, canids, and felids in East Africa (Nelson, 1970), the civet cat in India (Schad and Chowdhury, 1967), and the jackal in Iran (Massoud, 1978). In these regions, and in Thailand (Khamboonruang et al., 1978), wild pigs are important as sources of infection for man, but wild rodents are, as in most other regions, noticeably free of *Trichinella* except in the vicinity of towns. In the tropics, as in the Arctic, there is some evidence of regional adaptation, with the East African variant [sometimes called *Trichinella nelsoni* (see Chapter 2)] having an unusually low infectivity for rats and mice.

The relevance of the sylvatic cycle is not restricted to wildlife, for man can become infected by eating the flesh of infected wild animals. There is thus an offshoot of the sylvatic cycle that, while not important to the perpetuation of the cycle, is of special significance for *Homo sapiens*. Many outbreaks of clinical trichinosis among indigenous Arctic people have been attributed to the eating of infected polar bear and walrus (Madsen, 1961; Rausch, 1970; Margolis et al., 1979). In temperate and tropical regions, too, sylvatic trichinosis leads to human disease. In Germany, where clinical trichinosis is now almost unknown, an outbreak of 60 cases occurred in 1976 and was attributed to wild pig meat (Lamina, 1978). Infected bear meat has been implicated in several outbreaks of trichinosis in the United States, while the first outbreak recorded in Africa was attributed to consumption of wild bush pig (Forrester et al., 1961). These are just a few examples of the threat posed to human populations by the sylvatic cycle. The magnitude of the problem varies greatly, depending on cultural as well as biological factors. In the North American Arctic, where the flesh of terrestrial and marine animals is commonly eaten, the threat is large. This is especially true for indigenous people leading a traditional way of life; according to Cameron (1970), "trichinosis is probably the most important disease among native Eskimos who have not moved to settlements." On the other hand, the incidence of trichinosis may be very high in animals such as the red fox (35% in Bulgaria, 20% in Sweden) without exposing man to a significant hazard. The degree of risk may change in time, as illustrated by a Kenyan outbreak in which infection was attributed to a departure from a cultural norm (Nelson, 1972).

3. DOMESTIC CYCLE

The first element in the domestic cycle of trichinosis (transmission of the infection to man) has been known for more than a century: man becomes infected by eating the flesh of infected domestic pigs. The other half of the cycle, the source of infection for pigs, has been more difficult to resolve. Indeed, considering the long-standing interest in the subject, our knowledge of the domestic cycle is remarkably poor. Thus, the concept outlined below, and illustrated in Fig. 2, must be regarded as tentative.

On one mode of infection of swine there has long been agreement: pigs become infected by eating pig flesh—usually in the form of uncooked scraps from the dining room, the kitchen, and the slaughterhouse. Between 1874 and 1890, several investigators in the United States found the incidence of *Trichinella* in garbage-fed pigs to be much higher than in grain-fed or pasture-raised pigs. Furthermore, investigations on hog cholera at that time established the high prevalence of uncooked pork scraps in household garbage and especially in hotel garbage and the offal of slaughterhouses. Subsequent curtailment of the feeding of uncooked garbage and offal to swine (usually imposed for the control of bacterial and viral infections) was followed by marked reduction in the incidence of *Trichinella* in swine, thus adding strong circumstantial evidence for the role of pork scraps in the transmission of trichinosis to swine (Hall, 1937).

There may be other ways in which *Trichinella* is transmitted from pig to pig, and these are of particular interest with respect to grain-fed swine, in which infection can hardly be attributed to the consumption of pork scraps. When infected pigs are housed with noninfected pigs, tail-biting can result in the ingestion of sufficient flesh to transmit the infection from infected to noninfected animals (Zimmermann *et al.*, 1962). It is not known whether this mode of transmission is of practical importance. Nor is it known whether pigs become infected in practice by eating the feces of other pigs that have been recently infected, although this is a theoretical possibility (see Section 4).

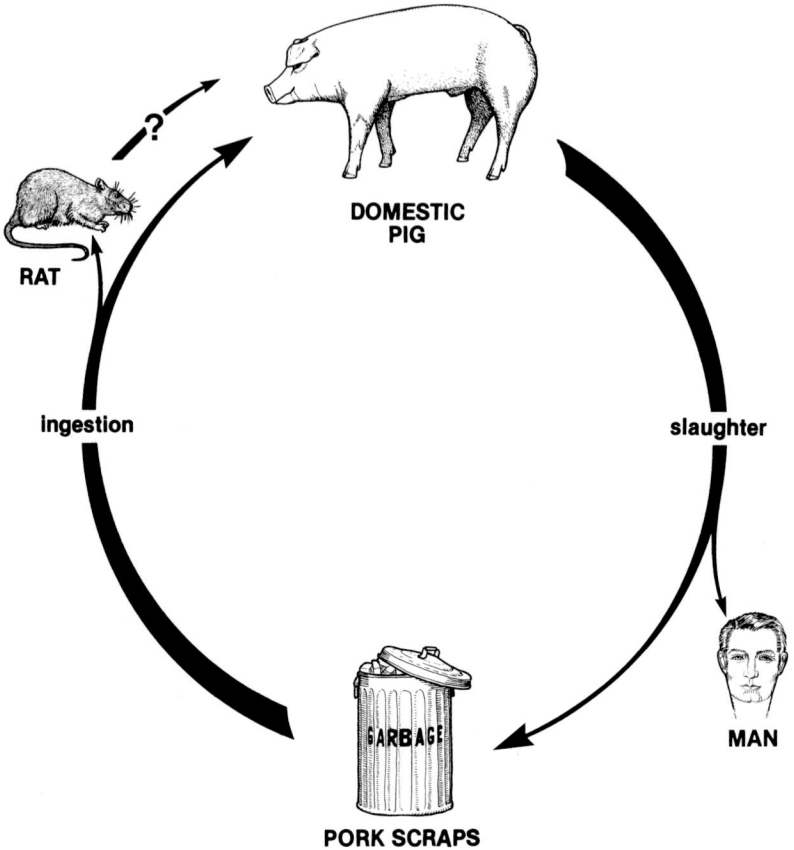

FIGURE 2. Domestic cycle, the predominant source of human trichinosis. Man, however, is an offshoot—not a participant in the cycle. The rat may be either an offshoot or a component of the cycle. A key feature of the cycle is that the porcine flesh is uncooked. Original diagram.

The perennial controversy concerning the source of infection in swine is the question of whether the rat plays a significant role. *Trichinella* is relatively common in rats, especially in those living near city dumps, and no doubt rats can, at least in theory, transmit it to other rats, to wild carnivores, and to domestic swine. But do they, in practice, transmit it to domestic swine?

The dispute goes back to the contrasting views of Leuckart and Zenker, who contributed much to the early studies on *Trichinella* infection (see Chapter 1). Leuckart believed that the ingestion of rats represented a significant source of infection for swine, but Zenker regarded the infected rats merely as *indicators* of the existence of infection in the local swine. Billings (1884) observed that "whenever rats have opportunity to get at the trimmings or refuse of slaughtered hogs, there the rats will be found to be most profusely trichinous; while in other localities it will not be so." The point also emerges from modern surveys; in Iowa, for example, *Trichinella* was found in 7% of dump-dwelling rats, but in none of the farm rats examined (Zimmermann, 1972). Billings could not accept the proposition (which he attributed to Leisering) that swine usually become infected by eating trichinous rats, and stated: "I am strongly inclined to think that quite the contrary is the case; though I willingly admit that an occasional hog may become invaded in this manner."

Calvin and Mark, each investigating trichinosis in the United States in the latter part of the 19th century, reached opposite conclusions, the former believing that rats were major vectors of the infection and the latter disagreeing (Hall, 1937). Hall made much of the fact that swine raisers and workers in garbage-feeding plants had rarely if ever seen a pig eat a rat. (One wonders how much of their observation had been nocturnal.) He acknowledged that pigs might eat rats under special conditions, such as that of protein deficiency. In Canada, *Trichinella* is common in dump-dwelling rats and in rats in piggeries lacking proper disposal of offal; but Cameron (1970) doubted whether rats play even a minor role in infecting pigs, pointing out that "our experiments and observations have shown that not only is it difficult for a pig to catch a rat, but that pigs show a great reluctance to eat a dead one". On the other hand, in an experiment in 1982, pigs which were given access to dead infected rats (not skinned or eviscerated) ate enough of the head portion of the rats to acquire *Trichinella* infection (K.D. Murrell, unpublished data). Furthermore, a high incidence of *Trichinella* has been found, in the United States, in a herd of hogs ostensibly fed only on grain, but raised on premises that would not have excluded rats (R.S. Isenstein, unpublished data). The arguments against the "rat theory" have been vigorously expounded by Madsen (1974); but the theory has become deeply entrenched, and the rat continues to be prominently featured in almost all epidemiological diagrams of trichinosis.

What, then, are we to make of these conflicting views on the significance of the rat in the epidemiology of trichinosis? Clearly the high incidence of trichinosis in dump-dwelling rats is an indication that the rat (like man) becomes infected by ingestion of uncooked pork scraps and offal—transmission in rats probably being reinforced by cannibalism. Thus infected rats represent an offshoot of the domestic cycle, being *recipients* of infection from that cycle. As to whether rats also *donate* infection significantly to the domestic cycle, it would seem that there is insufficient evidence to permit an unequivocal answer. It would be prudent, however, to acknowledge that there are some epidemiological circumstances in which infection in pigs is very difficult to explain in terms other than the ingestion of rats.

4. SPECIAL EPIDEMIOLOGICAL CIRCUMSTANCES

The domestic and sylvatic cycles are not wholly independent. It was pointed out above that the sylvatic cycle may be the source of some *Trichinella* infections in man, but in those circumstances, the parasite usually has reached a dead end without entering the domestic cycle. It is of course possible that man would feed uncooked flesh of bear, for example, to domestic swine and thereby transmit the infection from the sylvatic to the domestic cycle. There are some cultures in which human bodies can provide meals for scavenging animals, and so it is possible for *Trichinella* to be transferred in that way from man to wildlife. Dump-dwelling rats, as already stated, may maintain the infection through cannibalism, and the rats can provide a link between the domestic and sylvatic cycle with the exchange, theoretically at least, going in either direction. Bears, like rats, may feed at city dumps, and so acquire infection from pork scraps. The important thing here is that any given epidemiological enigma should be examined in its own right and should be regarded, if necessary, as an exceptional case.

While *Trichinella* infection is ubiquitous, it is not uniformly distributed. Many observers have pointed out that the sylvatic or synanthropic animals in certain regions have much higher prevalence rates than in other regions of the same geographic area. In Poland, for example, the prevalence in swine slaughtered in a village was more than 100 times higher than in swine slaughtered in a nearby city (Pawlowski, 1981). This focality or nidality of infection can generally be understood once the local modes of transmission have been identified, and the concept is of evident importance in control measures.

In addition to the sporadic transfer of infection between sylvatic and domestic cycles, there exist other modes of infection that might be considered minor transmission cycles. Through human intervention, they perpetuate the infection in a regular way, but again they must be regarded as special cases and not be allowed to distort our concept of natural transmission. In the commercial rearing of fur-producing animals, especially mink, uncooked flesh of these animals may be fed to other individual animals in the production cycle. *Trichinella*, once introduced, is thus likely to be propagated. Similarly, sledge dogs in the Arctic are often fed the flesh of other sledge dogs, and so trichinosis may be transmitted from dog to dog in a man-made variant of the natural carnivore–carrion cycle. These "cycles" are almost as artificial as laboratory propagation of *Trichinella*, but are of significance because of the potential for crossover of the parasite from these cycles to other feral or domestic animals, or even man.

Among the epidemiological enigmas mentioned in Section 3 is *Trichinella* infection in grain-fed swine. It is possible that grain-fed swine become infected through tail-biting or ingestion of the feces of infected rats or other wildlife (or other swine). When recently infected foxes were housed in cages over the feeding troughs of swine, the swine became infected (Zimmerman *et al.*, 1959). However, the foxes had been given overwhelming numbers of infective larvae (causing death in a few days); only a very small proportion of the larvae passed through the gut to become a source of infection for swine; and the passage of infective larvae in feces of foxes or rats was particularly low except during the first 4 hr of infection (and was higher in immune than in nonimmune animals). Concrete-floored pens, simulating commercial swine facilities, were used in a study in which freshly inoculated swine were housed under conditions that allowed their feces to be eaten by a group of noninoculated swine, while a third group of swine did not have access to the feces of the inoculated swine (Schnurrenberger *et al.*, 1964). Infection developed in 5 of 26 noninoculated pigs given access to feces passed by experimentally inoculated pigs within 5 days of the experimental inoculation. However, infection was not acquired in any of 15 pigs given access to feces passed 5 days or more after experimental inoculation. These studies, and similar studies by earlier workers, show that fecal transmission of *Trichinella* is possible; whether it plays a role in either the domestic or the sylvatic cycle remains to be determined.

Herbivorous animals are, by virtue of their diet, outside either of the major transmission cycles. Yet even herbivores cannot be ruled out as occasional agents of transmission. Sheep, cattle, and horses have been infected experimentally, and natural infection has been found in the horse (Beck, 1970). Horses have been shown to eat proferred meat, and have been circumstantially implicated in outbreaks of human trichinosis (Bellani *et al.*, 1978; Pawlowski, 1981). It has been suggested that these herbivores may ingest dead mice or rats contained in feed; if the rodents are infected, consumption of horse flesh may result in human trichinosis.

Intrauterine or transmammary transmission of *T. spiralis* has been reported for mice (Denham, 1966) and man (see Chapter 14), but is not known to be of epidemiological significance.

5. SUSCEPTIBLE HOST SPECIES

To appreciate the variety of circumstances that can give rise to *Trichinella* infection, it is only necessary to consider the variety of animals that are inherently susceptible to infection. There are wide differences in degree of susceptibility [the Chinese hamster, *Cricetulus griseus*, is exceptional in restricting infection to the intestinal phase (see Chapter 5)], but it would be rash to allege that any mammalian species is fully refractory to infection. Indeed, susceptibility extends even beyond the class Mammalia, although special circumstances (elevated environmental temperature) may be necessary for successful infection. For a discussion of the susceptibility of fish, amphibia, reptiles, and birds, see Beck (1970) and Tomasovicova (1981). The occurrence of *Trichinella* in the mammalian order Insectivora has been reported, but is the subject of controversy. It has been suggested that insectivores may become infected by eating insects that have fed on carrion, with the insects serving merely as transport hosts, by virtue of *Trichinella* larvae carried temporarily in their gut (Rausch 1970). It has also been suggested that larvae in insectivores have been ascaridoid or spiruroid larvae incorrectly identified as *Trichinella* (Madsen, 1974). Misidentification may also account for some of the reports of natural infection in nonmammalian hosts.

Table I presents a list of mammalian hosts for which *T. spiralis* infection has been reported. The reports of infection in nonmammalian hosts (above), being of doubtful significance, have been excluded from the table [the reported avian infections may have been *T. pseudospiralis* infections (see Section 1 and Chapter 2)]. It would have been more conservative to have also excluded *mammalian* species in which the diagnosis of *Trichinella* has not been unequivocally confirmed, but such a principle would exclude not only the species of particularly doubtful status (e.g., insectivores) but also many other species for which there is no reason to be skeptical of the diagnosis. It is important to note that the references in Table I are not intended to represent the earliest or

TABLE I
Mammalian Hosts of *Trichinella spiralis*

	Scientific name	English name	Reference
Order Family	MARSUPIALIA Didelphidae		
	Didelphis marsupialis	Northern opossum	Zimmermann and Hubbard (1969)
	Didelphis virginiana	Opossum	Beck (1970)
Order Family	INSECTIVORA Soricidae		
	Neomys fodiens	Water shrew	Rausch (1970)
	Sorex araneus	Common shrew	Rausch (1970)
	Sorex caecutiens	Laxmann's shrew	Rausch (1970)
	Sorex hawkeri	Pygmy shrew	Zimmermann (1971)
	Sorex minutus	Lesser shrew	Rausch (1970)
	Sorex vagrans	Shrew	Kim (Chapter 14)
Family	Talpidae		
	Talpa europaea	Common mole	Rausch (1970)
Family	Erinaceidae		
	Erinaceus europaeus	Hedgehog	Merkushev (1970)
	Hemiechinus auritus	Long-eared hedgehog	Zimmermann (1971)
	Hemiechinus megalotis	Afghan hedgehog	Kim (Chapter 14)
Order	CHIROPTERA		
	Unspecified[a]	Bat	Beck (1970)
Order Family	EDENTATA Dasypodidae		
	Chaetophractus villosus	Armadillo	Neghme and Schenone (1970)
Order Family	PRIMATES Callithricidae		
	Leontocebus geoffroyi[a]	Marmoset	McCoy (1932)
Family	Cebidae		
	Alouatta palliata[a]	Howler monkey	McCoy (1932)
	Aotus zonalis[a]	Night monkey	McCoy (1932)
	Ateles dariensis[a]	Spider monkey	McCoy (1932)
	Ateles geoffroyi[a]	Spider monkey	McCoy (1932)
	Cebus capucinus[a]	White-throated monkey	McCoy (1932)
	Saimiri örstedii[a]	Yellow titi	McCoy (1932)
Family	Cercopithecidae		
	Papio dognera[a]	Baboon	Beck (1970)
	Cercopithecus aethiops[a]	Grass monkey	Beck (1970)
	Macaca mulatta[a]	Rhesus monkey	Beck (1970)
	Macaca fasciolaris[a]	Monkey	Kociecka *et al.* (1981)
Family	Hominidae		
	Homo sapiens	Man	Many authors

continued

TABLE 1   (*Continued*)

Scientific name	English name	Reference
Order LAGOMORPHA		
Family Leporidae		
Lepus europaeus	European hare	Zimmermann (1971)
Lepus americanus	Varying hare	Rausch (1970)
Oryctolagus cuniculus	Old World rabbit	Beck (1970)
Order RODENTIA		
Family Castoridae		
Castor canadensis	Beaver	Rausch (1970)
Family Caviidae		
Cavia aperea porcellus[a]	Guinea pig	Beck (1970)
Family Cricetidae		
Arvicola terrestris[b]	Water rat	Merkushev (1970)
Clethrionomys glareolus	Bank vole	Rausch (1970)
Clethrionomys rufocanus	Red-backed vole	Bessonov (1981)
Clethrionomys rutilus	Northern red-backed vole	Rausch (1970)
Cricetulus griseus[a]	Chinese hamster	Beck (1970)
Lemmus sibiricus	Lemming	Rausch (1970)
Meriones persicus	None	Kim (Chapter 14)
Meriones unguiculatus	Jird	Panitz (1974)
Mesocricetus auratus[a]	Golden hamster	Beck (1970)
Microtus arvalis	Common vole	Gerwel and Rauhut (1969)
Microtus gregalis	Vole	Rausch (1970)
Microtus miurus	Narrow-skulled vole	Zimmermann (1971)
Microtus oeconomus[a]	Tundra vole	Rausch (1970)
Microtus pennsylvanicus	Meadow vole	Holliman and Meade (1980)
Ondatra zibethica	Muskrat	Rausch (1970)
Peromyscus leucopus	White-footed mouse	Holliman and Meade (1980)
Pitymys subterraneus	European pine vole	Zimmermann (1971)
Pitymys pinetorum	American pine vole	Zimmermann (1971)
Sigmodon hispidus	Cotton rat	Holliman and Meade (1980)
Family Muridae		
Apodemus agrarius	Striped field mouse	Rausch (1970)
Apodemus flavicollis	Field mouse	Rausch (1970)
Mastomys natalensis	Multimammate rat	Nelson (1970)
Mus musculus	Mouse	Rausch (1970)
Micromys minutus	Harvest mouse	Rausch (1970)
Rattus exulans	Field rat	Alicata (1970)
Rattus norvegicus	Brown rat	Many authors
Rattus rattus	Black rat	Many authors
Family Sciuridae		
Citellus undulatus	Ground squirrel	Rausch (1970)

TABLE 1 (Continued)

	Scientific name	English name	Reference
	Citellus richardsonii	Gopher	Beck (1970)
	Marmota marmota	Marmot	Zimmermann (1971)
	Sciurus niger	Fox squirrel	Zimmermann and Hubbard (1969)
	Sciurus vulgaris	Red squirrel	Merkushev (1970)
	Spermophilus columbianus	Ground squirrel	Kim (Chapter 14)
	Tamiasciurus hudsonicus	Red squirrel	Rausch (1970)
Family	Gliridae		
	Glis glis	Dormouse	Bessonov (1981)
Order	CETACEA		
Family	Monodontidae		
	Delphinapterus leucas	White whale	Rausch (1970)
	Monodon monocerus	Narwhal	Zimmermann (1971)
Order	CARNIVORA		
Family	Canidae		
	Alopex corsac	Corsac fox	Zimmermann (1971)
	Alopex lagopus	Polar fox	Merkushev (1970)
	Canis aureus	Golden jackal	Merkushev (1970)
	Canis adustus	Side-striped jackal	Nelson (1970)
	Canis familiaris	Domestic dog	Yamashita (1970)
	Canis latrans	Coyote	Rausch (1970)
	Canis lupus	Wolf	Merkushev (1970)
	Canis mesomelas	Black-backed jackal	Nelson (1970)
	Lycaon pictus	Wild dog	Kim (Chapter 14)
	Nyctereutes procyonides	Raccoon-dog	Merkushev (1970)
	Urocyon cinereoargenteus	Gray fox	Zimmermann and Hubbard (1969)
	Pseudolopex gracilis	Fox	Neghme and Schenone (1970)
	Vulpes vulpes fulva	Red fox	Zimmermann and Hubbard (1969)
	Vulpes vulpes	Red fox	Merkushev (1970)
Family	Felidae		
	Felis chaus	Jungle cat	Yamashita (1970)
	Felis concolor	Puma, mountain lion	Worley *et al.* (1974)
	Felis domestica	Domestic cat	Beck (1970)
	Felis (Lynx) lynx	Lynx	Merkushev (1970)
	Felix serval	Serval	Nelson (1970)
	Felix silvestris	Wildcat	Merkushev (1970)
	Lynx rufus	Bobcat	Worley *et al.* (1974)
	Panthera leo	Lion	Nelson (1970)
	Panthera onca	Jaguar	Zimmermann (1971)
	Panthera pardus	Leopard	Nelson (1970)
	Panthera tigris	Tiger	Merkushev (1970)
	Prionailurus bengalensis	Leopard cat	Zimmermann (1971)

continued

TABLE 1 *(Continued)*

	Scientific name	English name	Reference
Family	Hyaenidae		
	Crocuta crocuta	Spotted hyena	Nelson (1970)
	Crocuta mesomelas	Black-backed hyena	Kim (Chapter 14)
	Hyaena hyaena	Striped hyena	Nelson (1970)
Family	Mustelidae		
	Gulo gulo	Wolverine	Merkushev (1970)
	Gulo luscus	Wolverine	Zimmermann and Hubbard (1969)
	Lutra lutra	River otter	Zimmermann (1971)
	Martes foina	Stone marten	Bessonov (1974)
	Martes flavigula	Yellow-throated marten	Zimmermann (1971)
	Martes martes	Marten	Merkushev (1970)
	Martes pennanti	Fisher	Worley *et al.* (1974)
	Martes zibellina	Sable	Merkushev (1970)
	Meles meles	European badger	Merkushev (1970)
	Mephitis mephitis	Skunk	Zimmermann and Hubbard (1969)
	Mustela altaica	Altai weasel	Zimmermann (1971)
	Mustela erminae	Ermine	Merkushev (1970)
	Mustela frenata	Long-tailed weasel	Kim (Chapter 14)
	Mustela lutreola	European mink	Merkushev (1970)
	Mustela minuta	Dwarf weasel	Zimmermann (1971)
	Mustela nivalis	Weasel	Merkushev (1970)
	Mustela putorius	Polecat	Merkushev (1970)
	Mustela putorius furo[a]	Ferret	Campbell *et al.* (1982)
	Mustela rixosa	Least weasel	Zimmermann and Hubbard (1969)
	Mustela sibiricus	Siberian ferret	Merkushev (1970)
	Mustela vison	American mink	Zimmermann (1971)
	Spilogale interrupta	Skunk	Zimmermann and Hubbard (1969)
	Taxidae taxus	American badger	Zimmermann and Hubbard (1969)
	Vormela peregusna	Marbled polecat	Bessonov (1981)
Family	Procyonidae		
	Procyon lotor	Racoon	Zimmermann and Hubbard (1969)
Family	Ursidae		
	Ursus americanus	Black bear	Rausch (1970)
	Ursus arctos	Brown bear	Merkushev (1970)
	Ursus arctos horribilis	Grizzly bear	Worley *et al.* (1974)
	Thalarctos maritimus	Polar bear	Merkushev (1970)
Family	Viverridae		
	Atilax paludinosus[b]	Marsh mongoose	Nelson (1970)
	Genetta genetta[a]	Common genet	Nelson (1970)

TABLE 1 *(Continued)*

	Scientific name	English name	Reference
	Genetta tigrina[a]	Large-spotted genet	Nelson (1970)
	Herpestes ichneumon	African ichneumon	Yamashita (1970)
	Herpestes javanicus	Javan mongoose	Alicata (1970)
	Myonax sanguineus[a]	Slender mongoose	Nelson (1970)
	Paradoxurus hermaphroditus	Palm civet	Kim (Chapter 14)
	Viverricula indica	Small Indian civet	Schad and Chowdhury (1967)
Family	Phocidae		
	Erignathus barbatus	Bearded seal	Rausch (1970)
	Pusa hispida	Ringed seal	Rausch (1970)
	Phoca groenlandica	Greenland seal	Bessonov (1974)
Family	Otariidae		
	Eumetopias jubatus	Eared seal	Bessonov (1981)
Family	Odobenidae		
	Odobenus rosmarus	Walrus	Rausch (1970)
Order	PERISSODACTYLA		
Family	Equidae		
	Equus caballus	Horse	Bellani *et al.* (1978)
Order	ARTIODACTYLA		
Family	Suidae		
	Phacochoerus aethiopicus	Warthog	Nelson (1970)
	Potamochoerus porcus	Bush pig	Nelson (1970)
	Sus scrofa	Domestic pig	Many authors
	Sus scrofa ferus	Wild boar	Many authors
Family	Bovidae		
	Bos taurus[a]	Cow	Billings (1884)
	Capra hircus[a]	Goat	Beck (1970)
	Ovis aries[a]	Sheep	Ducas (1921)
Family	Cervidae		
	Rangifer tarandus	Reindeer	Bessonov (1981)
Family	Hippopotamidae		
	Hippopotamus amphibius[b]	Hippopotamus	Nelson (1970)
Order	TYLOPODA		
Family	Camelidae		
	Camelus sp.[c]	Camel	Bommer *et al.*, cited by Pawlowski (Chapter 11)

[a] Experimental infection.   [b] Infection in captive individuals.   [c] Circumstantial evidence only.

most persuasive host records, but rather are intended to provide minimal documentation in support of the host list. Scientific names, being subject to revision, are not necessarily those used by the authors cited.

REFERENCES

Alicata, J., 1970, Trichinosis in the Pacific Islands and adjacent areas, in: *Trichinosis in Man and Animals* (S.E. Gould, ed.), Charles C. Thomas, Springfield, Illinois, pp. 465–472.

Beck, J.W., 1970, Trichinosis in domesticated and experimental animals, in: *Trichinosis in Man and Animals* (S.E. Gould, ed.), Charles C. Thomas, Springfield, Illinois, pp. 61–80.

Bellani, L., Mantovani, A., Pampiglione, S., and Filippini, I., 1978, Observations on an outbreak of human trichinellosis in northern Italy, in: *Trichinellosis* (C.W. Kim and Z.S. Pawlowski, eds.), University Press of New England, Hanover, New Hampshire, pp. 535–539.

Bessonov, A.S., 1974, Epizoology and epidemiology of trichinellosis in the U.S.S.R.: Prospects for eradication of the infection, in: *Trichinellosis* (C.W. Kim, ed.), Intext, New York, pp. 557–562.

Bessonov, A.S., 1981, Changes in the epizootic and epidemic situation of trichinellosis in the U.S.S.R., in: *Trichinellosis* (C.W. Kim, E.J. Ruitenberg, and J.S. Teppema, eds.), Reedbooks, Chertsey, England, pp. 365–368.

Billings, F.S., 1884, *The Relation of Animal Diseases to the Public Health and Their Prevention*, Appleton, New York, pp. 2–41.

Cameron, T.W.M., 1970, Trichinosis in Canada, in: *Trichinosis in Man and Animals* (S.E. Gould, ed.), Charles C. Thomas, Springfield, Illinois, pp. 374–377.

Campbell, W.C., Blair, L.S., Kung, F., and Ewanciw, D.V., 1982, Experimental *Trichinella spiralis* infection in the ferret, *Mustela putorius furo*, *J. Helminthol.* **56:**55–58.

Denham, D.A., 1966, Infections with *Trichinella spiralis* passing from mother to filial mice pre- and post-natally, *J. Helminthol.* **40:**291–296.

Ducas, R., 1921, L'immunité dans la trichinose, M.D. thesis, Jouve, Paris, 47 pp.

Fay, F.H., 1960, Carnivorous walrus and some Arctic zoonoses, *Arctic* **13:**111–122.

Forrester, A.T.T., Nelson, G.S., and Sander, G., 1961, The first record of an outbreak of trichinosis in Africa south of the Sahara, *Trans. R. Soc. Trop. Med. Hyg.* **55:**503–513.

Gerwel, M., and Rauhut, W., 1969, Course of *Trichinella spiralis* intestinal phase in common vole (*Microtus arvalis Pallas*) and house mouse (*Mus musculus* L.), *Wiad. Parazytol.* **15:**576–577.

Hall, M.C., 1937, Studies on trichinosis. IV. The role of the garbage-fed hog in the production of human trichinosis, *Public Health Rep.* **52:**873–886.

Holliman, R.B., and Meade, B.J., 1980, Native trichinosis in wild rodents in Henrico County, Virginia, *J. Wildl. Dis.* **16:**205–207.

Hulebak, K.L., 1980, Mechanical transmission of larval *Trichinella* by Arctic crustacea, *Can. J. Zool.* **58:**1388–1390.

Khamboonruang, C., Thitasut, P., and Pan-In, S., 1978, The role of pigs and rats in the transmission of trichinellosis in northern Thailand, in: *Trichinellosis* (C.W. Kim and

Z.S. Pawlowski, eds.), University Press of New England, Hanover, New Hampshire, pp. 545–550.

Kociecka, W., van Knapen, F., and Ruitenberg, E.J., 1981, *Trichinella pseudospiralis* and *T. spiralis* infections in monkeys. I. Parasitological aspects, in: *Trichinellosis* (C.W. Kim, E.J. Ruitenberg, and J.S. Teppema, eds.), Reedbooks, Chertsey, England, pp. 199–203.

Kozar, Z., 1962, Incidence of *Trichinella spiralis* in the world and actual problems connected with trichinellosis, in: *Trichinellosis* (Z. Kozar, ed.), Polish Scientific Publishers, Warsaw, pp. 15–67.

Kozlov, D.P., 1971, Sources of *Trichinella* infection in pinnipeds, *Trudy Gel'mintol. Lab. Akad. Nauk SSSR* **21:**36–40 (in Russian); English translation by Z. Kabata and L. Margolis, *Fish. Res. Board Can. Transl. Ser.,* No. 3010.

Lamina, J., 1978, Report on *Trichinella spiralis* in the Federal Republic of Germany (1975–1976), *Wiad. Parazytol.* **24:**111–112.

Madsen, H., 1961, The distribution of *Trichinella spiralis* in sledge dogs and wild animals in Greenland under a global aspect, *Medd. Groenl.* **159:**1–124.

Madsen, H., 1974, The principles of the epidemiology of trichinelliasis with a new view on the life cycle, in: *Trichinellosis* (C.W. Kim, ed.), Intext, New York, pp. 615–638.

Madsen, H., 1976, The life cycle of *Trichinella spiralis* (Owen, 1835) Railliet, 1896 (Syns: *T. nativa* Britov et Boev, 1972, *T. nelsoni* Britov et Boev, 1972, *T. pseudospiralis* Garkavi, 1972), with remarks on epidemiology, and a new diagram, *Acta Parasitol. Pol.* **24:**143–158.

Manning, T.H., 1961, Comments on "Carnivorous walrus and some Arctic zoonoses," *Arctic* **14:**76–77.

Margolis, H.S., Middaugh, J.P., and Burgess, R.D., 1979, Arctic trichinosis: Two Alaskan outbreaks from walrus meat, *J. Infect. Dis.* **139:**102–105.

Massoud, J., 1978, Trichinellosis in carnivores in Iran, in: *Trichinellosis* (C.W. Kim and Z.S. Pawlowski, eds.), University Press of New England, Hanover, New Hampshire, pp. 551–554.

McCoy, O.R., 1932, Experimental trichiniasis infections in monkeys, *Proc. Soc. Biol. Med.* **30:**85–86.

Merkushev, A.V., 1970, Trichinosis in the Union of Soviet Socialist Republics, in: *Trichinosis in Man and Animals* (S.E. Gould, ed.), Charles C. Thomas, Springfield, Illinois, pp. 449–456.

Neghme, A., and Schenone, H., 1970, Trichinosis in Latin America, in: *Trichinosis in Man and Animals* (S.E. Gould, ed.), Charles C. Thomas, Springfield, Illinois, pp. 407–422.

Nelson, G.S., 1970, Trichinosis in Africa, in: *Trichinosis in Man and Animals* (S.E. Gould, ed.), Charles C. Thomas, Springfield, Illinois, pp. 473–492.

Nelson, G.S., 1972, Human behaviour in the transmission of parasitic diseases, in: *Behavioural Aspects of Parasite Transmission* (E.U. Canning and C.A. Wright, eds.), Academic Press, New York, pp. 109–122.

Panitz, E., 1974, Immunosuppressive effect of betamethasone and the distribution of adult *Trichinella spiralis* in the intestine of the jird (*Meriones unguiculatus*), *Proc. Helminthol. Soc. Washington* **41:**257–259.

Pawlowski, Z.S., 1981, Control of trichinellosis, in: *Trichinellosis* (C.W. Kim, E.J. Ruitenberg, and J.S. Teppema, eds.), Reedbooks, Chertsey, England, pp. 7–20.

Ransom, B.H., 1916, Effects of refrigeration upon the larvae of *Trichinella spiralis, J. Agric. Res.* **5:**819–854.

Rausch, R.L., 1970, Trichinosis in the Arctic, in: *Trichinosis in Man and Animals* (S.E. Gould, ed.), Charles C. Thomas, Springfield, Illinois, pp. 348–373.

Schad, G.A., and Chowdhury, A.B., 1967, *Trichinella spiralis* in India. I. Its history in India, rediscovery in Calcutta, and the ecology of its maintenance in nature, *Trans. R. Soc. Trop. Med. Hyg.* **61:**244–248.

Schnurrenberger, P.R., Masterson, R.A., Suessenguth, H., and Bashe, W.J., Jr., 1964, Swine trichinosis. I. Fecal transmission under simulated field conditions, *Am. J. Vet. Res.* **25:**174–178.

Steele, J.H., and Schultz, M.G., 1978, Trichinellosis: A review of the current problem, in: *Trichinellosis* (C.W. Kim and Z.S. Pawlowski, eds.), University Press of New England, Hanover, New Hampshire, pp. 45–75.

Stoimenov, K., and Gradinarski, I., 1981, On the epizootiology of *Trichinella spiralis*, in: *Trichinellosis* (C.W. Kim, E.J. Ruitenberg, and J.S. Teppema, eds.), Reedbooks, Chertsey, England, pp. 373–376.

Tomasovicova, O., 1981, The role of fresh water fish in transfer and maintenance of trichinellae under natural conditions, *Biologia (Bratislava)* **36:**115–125.

Worley, D.E., Fox, J.C., Winters, J.B., and Greer, K.R., 1974, Prevalence and distribution of *Trichinella spiralis* in carnivorous mammals in the United States northern Rocky Mountain region, in: *Trichinellosis* (C.W. Kim, ed.), Intext, New York, pp. 597–602.

Yamashita, J., 1970, Trichinosis in Asia, in: *Trichinosis in Man and Animals* (S.E. Gould, ed.), Charles C. Thomas, Springfield, Illinois, pp. 457–464.

Zimmermann, W.J., 1971, Trichinosis, in: *Parasitic Diseases of Wild Mammals* (J.W. Davis and R.C. Anderson, eds.), Iowa State University Press, Ames, pp. 127–139.

Zimmermann, W.J., 1972, Prevalence and control of *Trichinella spiralis* in swine and pork products, *Public Health Rep.* **1:**72–90.

Zimmermann, W.J., and Hubbard, E.D., 1969, Trichiniasis in wildlife in Iowa, *Am. J. Epidemiol.* **90:**84–92.

Zimmermann, W.J., Hubbard, E.D., and Matthews, J., 1959, Studies on fecal transmission of *Trichinella spiralis*, *J. Parasitol.* **45:**441–445.

Zimmermann, W.J., Hubbard, E.D., Schwarte, L.H., and Biester, H.E., 1962, Trichiniasis in Iowa swine with further studies on modes of transmission, *Cornell Vet.* **52:**156–163.

14

Epidemiology II

Geographic Distribution and Prevalence

CHARLES W. KIM

1. INTRODUCTION

It is probably correct to assume that trichinosis was present, and quite extensive in its geographic distribution, long before *Trichinella spiralis* was identified as the causative agent. There have been numerous comprehensive reviews on the epidemiology of trichinosis (Steele, 1970; Steele and Arambulo, 1975; Steele and Schultz, 1978; and others). This chapter is devoted to a survey of old and new findings on the distribution and prevalence of trichinosis throughout the world. For each geographic region, the information is presented, where available, with respect to the infection first in wildlife, then in domestic animals, and finally in man.

Heretofore, much of the data has been on the prevalence of the infection in the domestic pig because it is the best known and most important source of infection for man. Also, the infection was reported usually from urban centers or from countries with large ethnic groups whose eating habits included consumption of either raw or poorly

---

CHARLES W. KIM • State University of New York at Stony Brook, Stony Brook, Long Island, New York 11794.

cooked pork. More recently, however, there have been more reports of the infection from rural areas and countries where the infection was merely sporadic or even unknown and where the source of infection proved to be an animal other than the domestic pig. These findings have suggested a reevaluation of the epidemiology of trichinosis with respect to the sources of infection and geographic distribution.

2. NORTH AMERICA

2.1. Canada and Alaska

2.1.1. Wildlife

Trichinella infection appears to occur frequently throughout northern Canada, especially the Canadian Arctic, where carnivore eats carnivore out of necessity. Although the most important source of human trichinosis in northern Canada seems to be the polar bear, several other animals are also involved, including the walrus (Cameron, 1970). Rausch (1970) reported different infection rates for the walrus from various regions. He suggested that since *T. spiralis* was found in both ringed and bearded seals, although very uncommonly, it might be transmitted to the walrus by these animals. The incidence of trichinosis in polar bears in the Arctic seems to be high, varying considerably depending on the region (Cameron, 1970). *Trichinella spiralis* has been reported once in the white whale (*Delphinapterus leucas*) from the arctic coast of Alaska (Rausch *et al.*, 1956).

Trichinella spiralis appears to be a common parasite among the terrestrial mammals of the Arctic and sub-Arctic (Rausch, 1970). Nearly all species of carnivores appear to have the infection, including the arctic fox (*Alopex lagopus*), the wolf, and the red fox. Earlier, it was reported that the overall rate of infection among mammals in Alaska was 11.7% based on tissue samples taken from 2433 mammals representing 42 species (Rausch *et al.*, 1956). The domestic dog appears to be an important synanthropic host of *T. spiralis* at high latitudes. An overall infection rate of 45.3% was recorded from all localities in Alaska (Rausch *et al.*, 1956). High rates were also observed in dogs used for transportation in the Arctic (Rausch, 1970).

A study of the incidence of trichinosis in wild animals in the Atlantic provinces of Canada in 1971–1976 (Smith, 1978) showed that of the 73 black bears (*Ursus americanus*) and 1 polar bear (*Thalarctos maritimus*) examined, only the polar bear was infected.

Of 96 black bears examined in Quebec Province in 1971–1973, only one was infected (Fréchette and Panisset, 1973). In addition, *Trichinella* was found in 3 of 33 raccoons, 2 of 21 coyotes, 1 of 5 wolves, 3 of 17 foxes, and 1 of 2 lynxes. All these animals originated from northern, northwestern, and southeastern woodlands of Quebec.

In a study in the Kootenay District of British Columbia in 1972–1973, 5 of 62 black bears (*U. americanus*) were infected, as well as the 1 grizzly bear (*U. arctos horribilis*) that was examined (Schmitt *et al.*, 1976). A high percentage of coyotes (*Canis latrans*) (25 of 104 examined) and martens (*Martes americana*) (22 of 36 examined) were infected. *Trichinella* was also found in the lynx (*Lynx canadensis*), skunk (*Mephitis mephitis*), cougar (*Felis concolor*), bobcat (*Lynx rufus*), weasel (*Mustela frenata*), and wolverine (*Gulo luscus*), as well as in various species of small mammal, e.g., shrew (*Sorex vagrans*), white-footed deer mouse (*Peromyscus maniculatus*), ground squirrel (*Spermophilus columbianus*), and red squirrel (*Tamiasciurus hudsonicus*). Further investigation showed that trichinosis is widespread in wild mammals in the southern and central parts of British Columbia (Schmitt *et al.*, 1978). The demonstration of *Trichinella* in 15 wildlife species in the absence of the infection in domestic pigs (attributed to sanitary and garbage feeding regulations) seems to confirm that sylvatic trichinosis exists as an independent cycle.

2.1.2. *Domestic Animals*

Numerous surveys have been carried out to determine the prevalence of trichinosis in pigs by digesting portions of the diaphragm or intercostal muscles. Cameron (1970) reported that the infection rate in pigs was 4–4.5% in Vancouver, 6.5% at Kamloops, 2% in Montreal, and 0.4% in the Maritime provinces. Most of the infections were in garbage-fed hogs. In 1949, a high incidence (7.1%) of trichinosis was recorded for swine in British Columbia, with the infection being confined to garbage-fed hogs (Moynihan and Musfeldt, 1949). A few years later, the incidence fell to zero, the change being attributed to moving the swine to locations that provided rigid rat control (Tailyour and Hampton, 1954). A later survey of 390 swine from eight piggeries in Vancouver reported only 2 carcasses from two establishments that were positive (Tailyour and Steele, 1960). A long-standing regulation of the Canadian Department of Agriculture requires that garbage containing animal refuse, especially of porcine origin, shall not be fed to hogs without a license from the Federal government, requiring the licensee to cook such material, but there is no assurance that everyone adheres to the regulation.

A study (Smith *et al.*, 1976) conducted in the Atlantic provinces from 1968 to 1975, in which 68,451 porcine carcasses were examined by trichinoscopy and more than 9000 by the digestion method, revealed an infection rate of 0.13%. Infection was attributed to rats, garbage feeding, and tail-chewing. However, Cameron (1970) reported earlier that although the infection rate in rats was about 1.5% in Toronto, 2% in Montreal, and 4% in the Maritime provinces, there was no evidence that rats played a major role in infecting pigs.

2.1.3. Man

Despite the wide distribution of *T. spiralis* in wild and domestic animals in northern latitudes, human infection has been sporadic in Canada (Cameron, 1970), and there has not been any accurate assessment of the infection rate. Recently, cases of human trichinosis have been reported in rural and urban areas in all provinces, as indicated by 31 cases reported in 1976, 23 in 1977, and 32 in 1978 (Tanner, 1979).

A prevalence rate as high as 95% has been reported among Eskimos in the central Arctic region (Cape Dorset) (Davies and Cameron, 1961). However, in the more populated urban centers such as Toronto, the incidence of trichinosis in humans has been reported to be low (Kuitunen-Ekbaum, 1941); only 7 cases were found following postmortem examination of 420 diaphragms from adults and children in 1939 and 1940. In 1963, four acute cases of trichinosis at the Ottawa Civic Hospital were attributed to eating infected pork; in addition, examination of 500 diaphragms from cadavers in Ottawa revealed an infection rate of 0.8% (Barr, 1966).

Human incidence of trichinosis in Montreal was reported to be 1.5%, based on 539 samples of diaphragm (Cameron, 1943). A study in 1966 (Chicoine *et al.*, 1966) indicated that the incidence of "nonclinical trichinosis" in the population of Quebec was considerably higher than had been suspected. Human infections have been traced to specialty meat stores preparing pork products in the European manner. A recent outbreak, which occurred in the province of Quebec, involved 28 persons who became infected from eating raw or undercooked pork (Faubert *et al.*, 1981). Another outbreak in Montreal was attributed to salami made from pork (Viens and Auger, 1981).

Trichinosis is believed to be transmissible *in utero*, since it was reported in Vancouver in a 6-week-old infant who was born 5 weeks prematurely and died 6 weeks later; a heavily infected fetus has also been reported (Bourns, 1952).

Outbreaks of trichinosis at high latitude frequently follow consumption of the meat of polar bear and brown bear. In Alaska, outbreaks attributable to bear meat have been reported by Rausch *et al.* (1956), Maynard and Pauls (1962), Wilson (1967), and Clark *et al.* (1972).

In 1971, a large outbreak of trichinosis in British Columbia was traced to the consumption of inadequately smoked bear meat (*U. americanus*) (Schmitt *et al.*, 1972). Eight trichinosis incidents reported from British Columbia between 1949 and 1971 involved a total of 59 clinical cases, mostly acquired by consumption of bear meat or pork (Bowmer, 1974).

While the incidence of trichinosis in the more populated regions of Canada has declined with improved feeding and inspection of hogs, outbreaks in humans in the Canadian North still persist. An outbreak in northern Saskatchewan resulted from the consumption of undercooked bear meat, presumably from the black bear (*U. americanus*) (Emson *et al.*, 1972).

In 1975–1976, the first two well-documented epidemics due to the consumption of walrus meat occurred in Barrow, Alaska (Margolis *et al.*, 1979). In the first epidemic, 64% of those eating the meat became ill, and the infection rate of those who ate meat prepared with little or no cooking was 4 times as great as that of persons eating cooked meat. A year later, a second outbreak occurred in a family whose members ate partially cooked walrus meat. Two cases of trichinosis in Canadian Eskimo siblings were attributed to bearded seal and black bear meat, which are usually eaten raw or half-cooked (Coffey and Wiglesworth, 1956).

As long as the population of wild carnivores remains unchanged, and man continues to eat not only the meat of carnivores but also that of marine mammals such as the walrus, the possibility of human infection in these regions will remain.

2.2. Greenland

Although it had been presumed that trichinosis was present in Greenland in mammals, it was not discovered there until 1948, when Thorborg *et al.* (1948) found the parasite in 2 of 3 polar bears (*T. maritimus*) from the Thule district and 4 of 13 polar bears from the east Greenland coast. A high incidence was found in sledge dogs (*C. familiaris*); 41 of 54 dogs from west Greenland districts were infected. The infection was also reported in the bearded seal (*Erignathus barbatus*), which has the same living habits as the walrus. The infection in the bearded seal was the first observation of the parasite in a marine mammal. Further investigation by Roth (1949) showed that arctic foxes (*A. lagopus*) were also infected, but to a much lesser degree than sledge dogs or polar bears. Of 101 arctic foxes examined, 3 were infected. The infection rate in dogs was extremely high; i.e., 46 of 66 examined were infected. The infection rate for polar bears was 30%. On examination of 24 walruses (*Odobenus rosmarus*) from the Thule district, *T. spiralis* was detected in 1 adult male (Thing *et al.*, 1976). With the use of the digestion method, 1–2 larvae per gram of muscle tissue were found.

The first report of human trichinosis in Greenland was that of Thorborg *et al.* (1948). The outbreak occurred in the spring of 1947 in the district around Disco Bay and Holsteinberg, western Greenland. Approximately 300 native Greenlanders showed signs and symptoms, and 33 deaths were attributed to the disease. The cases were equally distributed between the two sexes. The youngest patient was 2 years of age, the oldest 63. The evidence pointed to the consumption of walrus meat and dog meat as the source of infection. Because of the similarity of this outbreak to outbreaks at Holsteinberg in the past, previously thought to be typhoid, the authors suggested that the earlier cases may also have been trichinosis. They also felt that the outbreak of meat poisoning in Nugssuak on Disco Bay in 1933 was undoubtedly trichinosis.

During the winter of 1959–1960, an epidemic of trichinosis occurred in Upernavik, Greenland, that affected 56 persons, of whom 24 required hospitalization, but none died (Holgersen, 1961). In the spring of 1975, a Dane was taken to the hospital with trichinosis after having eaten walrus meat in the Thule district (Thing *et al.*, 1976). *Trichinella spiralis* had been reported previously in the walrus population throughout the Arctic, but not in the Thule district, where the temperature is below freezing for many months of the year. Trichinosis has been reported to be more common in south Greenland.

2.3. United States

The epidemiology of trichinosis in the United States has been studied extensively and is the subject of excellent reviews (Zimmerman, 1970a, 1974; Steele, 1970; Zimmermann *et al.*, 1973; and others).

2.3.1. Wildlife

Although the infection in man and swine has been well studied, its existence in wildlife and its relationship to the infection in humans and

swine have been poorly understood. The importance of wildlife trichinosis, however, is becoming increasingly evident, since the parasite
seems to be ubiquitous and to lack host specificity. In the state of New
York, of 45 black bears (*U. americanus*) examined, 3 were found to be
infected (King *et al.*, 1960). In six northeastern states, 5 of 372 bears
(1.3%) were infected, including 2 of 158 from New York, 1 of 77 from
Pennsylvania, 1 of 60 from Vermont, and 1 of 28 from West Virginia
(Zimmermann, 1970b). Schultz (1970) found that approximately 1.6%
of New England black bears were infected. A study (Worley *et al.*, 1974)
designed to determine the prevalence of *T. spiralis* in carnivores from
rural or wilderness areas in Montana, Idaho, and Wyoming revealed
that the grizzly bear (*U. arctos horribilis*) was the most commonly infected
host of 15 species examined. The black bear (*U. americanus*) was also
infected, but to a lesser degree.

Mountain lions (*F. concolor*) have been shown to be infected in the
wilderness regions of western Montana; Winters (1969) found that 3
of 6 mountain lions were infected. In Montana, Idaho, and Wyoming,
the mountain lion was the second most infected host of 15 species
examined (Worley *et al.*, 1974). A mountain lion in a Washington, D.C.,
zoo was found to be infected (Kluge, 1967). These findings suggested
that trichinosis in mountain lions may be more widespread than
previously recognized. The bobcat (*L. rufus*) from Colorado (Olsen,
1960) and from Montana, Idaho, and Wyoming (Worley *et al.*, 1974)
has been shown to be infected.

The first natural infection of trichinosis in the skunk (*M. mephitis*)
was reported in 3 of 4 adult skunks captured in Beltsville, Maryland
(Spindler and Permenter, 1951), and it was later reported in skunks in
Louisiana (Babero, 1960). Trichinosis in the American badger (*Taxidea
taxus taxus*) was first recorded in a female badger from the New York
Zoological Park (Herman and Goss, 1940).

Significant wildlife reservoirs have been found in Iowa. During the
1953–1961 period, *Trichinella* was found in 14 species of wildlife in
Iowa, namely, rat (*Rattus norvegicus*), 6.4%; mink (*Mustela vison*), 5.1%;
red fox (*Vulpes fulva*) and gray fox (*Urocyon cinereoargenteus*), 7.3%;
opossum (*Didelphis marsupialis*), 0.9%; raccoon (*Procyon lotor*), 0.7%;
striped skunk (*M. mephitis*), 2.0%; spotted skunk (*Spilogale interrupta*),
1.7%; coyote (*C. latrans*), 11.4%; badger (*T. taxus*), 5.3%; beaver (*Castor
canadensia*), 0.5%; weasel (*M. rixosa*), 33.3% or 1 of 3; wolverine (*G.
luscus*), 1 of 1; fox squirrel (*Sciurus niger*), 4.8%; and owl (*Bubo virgini-
anus*), 0.5%, the last being perhaps a spurious finding (Zimmermann *et
al.*, 1962a). During the 1953–1968 period, Zimmermann and Hubbard
(1969) detected *T. spiralis* larvae in the same 14 species and in another

wildlife species, the muskrat (*Ondatra zibethica*). The infection rate of the fox, rat, and mink was greater than 5%. They found that about 84% of the infected mink and 78% of the pasture rats had infective levels of more than one larva per gram. The maximum larval count for mink was 3451 per gram, while that for the rats was 18,890. Earlier, Olsen (1960) had reported the infection in the coyote (*C. latrans*) and fox (*V. fulva*). More recently the wolverine (*Gulo gulo*), as well as the coyote (*C. latrans*) and the fox (*V. vulpes*), from Montana, Idaho, and Wyoming have been reported to be hosts for *Trichinella* (Worley *et al.*, 1974).

Trichinella spiralis has been found in spotted skunk, opossum, and long-tailed weasel in Mount Lake, Virginia (Solomon and Warner, 1969); in a muskrat (*O. zibethica*) in Ohio (Beckett and Gallichio, 1967); in striped skunks (*M. mephitis*) in North Dakota (Dyer, 1970) and in Montana, Idaho, and Wyoming (Worley *et al.*, 1974); and in Norway rats (*R. norvegicus*) *and white-footed mouse (Peromyscus leucopus)* in Illinois (Martin *et al.*, 1968). The latter is believed to be the first report of natural *T. spiralis* infection in *P. leucopus*. Other hosts for *Trichinella* include the fisher (*Martes pennanti*) and the marten (*M. americana*) from the rural regions of Montana, Idaho, and Wyoming (Worley *et al.*, 1974).

The widespread distribution of trichinosis in such varied mammalian species would suggest that the infection may be more prevalent in the wild than previously presumed. This has great public-health significance in terms of the role of scavenging in the epidemiology of the infection and the difficulty of eradicating the etiological agent from the environment.

2.3.2. Domestic Animals

Although many dogs and cats in the United States are fed on commercially prepared foods, some are still fed scraps from the meat market or table. In rural areas, they may consume various species of wildlife. A survey was conducted to ascertain the prevalence of *T. spiralis* in dogs and cats in the New Orleans area (Sawitz, 1939). The diaphragms of 300 dogs were examined by the digestion method, and the larvae were recovered in 4, an incidence of 1.3%. The incidence was higher (10%) in cats; 9 cats of 90 examined were positive, and in 5 the infection was heavy. In the Detroit area, *T. spiralis* larvae were recovered in 4.5% of 180 dogs and 5% of 20 cats examined (DeGiusti and Field, 1952).

In 1954–1957, a survey of dogs and cats in Iowa showed that 10% of the 521 dogs examined were infected (Zimmermann and Schwarte, 1958). Although the number of cats in this study was comparatively small (50), 3 (6%) were found to be infected, and the highest number of larvae (2437 per 45 g) was observed in a stray captured in a wooded area.

It is interesting to note that when portions of diaphragms from 100 dogs from dealers whose sources ranged as far west and south as Texas were fed to mice, the subsequent presence of larvae in mouse diaphragms indicated that 9 of the 100 dogs had been infected with *T. spiralis* (Geller and Zaiman, 1965). A 2.6% infection rate for dogs and 3.2% for cats in New Jersey seemed to indicate that the infection rates may be declining in dogs and cats, as in swine and man, in the United States (Hunt, 1967).

Of the many mammalian hosts of *T. spiralis*, the domestic swine is still the most important source of human infection. The infection in swine has long been a major problem from the standpoint of both economics and public health. In 1940, McNaught and Zapata (1940) reported a 4% infection rate of the 495 garbage-fed pigs examined in San Francisco, which was much lower than for humans (24%) in this area. Schwartz (1953) reported that of more than 3000 hogs in several corn-belt states, *Trichinella* was found in 0.6%, using the digestion method. In contrast to this, 11.5% of the garbage-fed hogs on the eastern seaboard were found to be infected using the digestion method and nearly 5% when examined in press preparation. These data emphasized the role of garbage in the transmission of the parasite to hogs and to humans who eat raw or inadequately cooked or cured pork.

Zimmermann *et al.* (1962b) reported the incidence in hogs in Iowa, in 1953–1957, to be 0.17% (6 of 3597 hog diaphragm samples contained *T. spiralis* larvae). The number of larvae recovered from the 45-g diaphragm samples varied, with a maximum of 58,000. Rothrock (1965) reported one of the heaviest naturally occurring infections known in hogs. Of the 3 positive diaphragm samples examined by the digestion method, of 482 Iowa hogs killed for export, 1 sample contained 4361 larvae per gram of tissue. Although it was not possible to establish a definite source of infection for this swine herd, the most likely source appeared to be infected swine carcasses that were left to be eaten by the remainder of the herd.

A study was conducted in 1961–1965 to determine the incidence of *T. spiralis* in United States swine by examining a total of 21,417 diaphragms of farm-raised butcher hogs, farm-raised breeder hogs, and garbage-fed hogs (Zimmermann and Brandly, 1965). Of the 9495 farm-raised butcher hogs, only 11 (0.12%) were infected, and of the 6881 farm-raised breeder hogs, 15 (0.22%) were infected. In contrast to these low incidence rates of trichinosis in farm-raised hogs, a significantly higher incidence (2.6%) was observed among the 5041 garbage-fed hogs. The concentration of larvae per gram of diaphragm of garbage-fed hogs was higher than that in farm-raised hogs. There were indications, however, during the 4-year period of study that the role of garbage-fed swine in the perpetuation of the infection was declining as a result of the declining number of pigs being fed garbage.

A nationwide outbreak of vesicular exanthema in 1952 resulted in legislation that required the cooking of garbage before it was fed to swine. This resulted in a dramatic decrease in the prevalence of *Trichinella* infection in garbage-fed swine. However, after eradication of vesicular exanthema, there was an increase in prevalence (Zimmermann and Brandly, 1965). Fortunately, a national hog cholera eradication program initiated in 1962 again emphasized the importance of cooking garbage.

A prevalence of 0.5% in 5955 swine examined in 1964–1966 (Jefferies *et al.*, 1967) indicated a marked improvement in the control of garbage feeding. Diaphragm samples of 700 grain-fed and garbage-fed hogs were examined by artificial digestion, and 5 were found to be infected—an incidence of 0.71% (Bair and Etges, 1969). The density of infection in each case was fewer than 10 larvae per gram. A study by Zimmermann and Zinter (1971) of farm-raised butcher hogs for the period 1966–1970 showed a prevalence of only 0.125%, but indicated increased intensity of infection, greater herd involvement, and increased concentration of the problem in the major hog-producing regions.

According to Zimmermann (1974), an estimated 111,000 swine are infected each year in the United States, resulting in at least 40 million potential meal exposures. Therefore, although there has been a decline in the infection rate of swine, indicated by a prevalence rate of 0.194% in sows slaughtered at a Federally inspected abattoir in Kentucky (Pullen *et al.*, 1977), and 0.1% in grain-fed pigs (which constitute 98.5% of the United States pork supply) and 0.5% in garbage-fed pigs (Juranek and Schultz, 1978), swine remain a major source of infection for humans.

2.3.3. Man

Trichinosis in humans in the United States has been reviewed by Zimmermann (1970a) and others. Some 40 years ago, the National Institutes of Health carried out a study to determine the prevalence of trichinosis in humans (Wright *et al.*, 1943, 1944). They examined 5313 diaphragm samples from cadavers in hospitals from 37 states and the District of Columbia and reported an overall prevalence of 16.1%. There were some interesting epidemiological findings including the following: (1) the peak incidence of 19.1% was in persons in the 65- to 74-year age group and (2) the infection rate was very high in certain ethnic groups, being, for example, 28.7% for those of Italian and German extraction. The infection rate was low (2.1%) in the Jewish population, reflecting the practice of general abstinence from eating pork and its products. An earlier study had shown a high rate of 36.0% for the Cleveland area (Evans, 1938) by postmortem examination of diaphragms and skeletal muscles from 100 consecutive autopsies. A low prevalence of 2.8% was reported in North Carolina in autopsy material (Harrell and Johnston, 1939). There were additional autopsy reports from other cities, including Minneapolis with a prevalence of 17.9% (Riley and Scheifley, 1934), San Francisco with 24.0% (McNaught and Anderson, 1936), and New York City with 22.0% (Most and Helpern, 1941).

The epidemiology of trichinosis in the United States in humans has changed considerably since those surveys were made. Beard (1951) reported a prevalence of 8.0% from 161 unselected autopsies done in San Francisco. A prevalence of 3.5% in New York City was reported by Most (1965). More important, there was a reduction in the degree of infection. Of 22 compressed, sectioned, and digested diaphragms, only 1 contained more than 10 larvae/50 g (0.2/gram), and none contained more than 100/50 g (2/gram); this may be compared to findings in 1941 that showed that about one half had more than 100 larvae/50 g (2/gram) of diaphragm. Zimmermann (1967) reported a similarly low infection rate of 2.8% from Iowa. A reduction in prevalence was reported by Zimmermann *et al.*, (1968) on the basis of a 1966–1968 study of 5000 diaphragms, revealing a prevalence of 4.2%. The Pacific area had the highest prevalence rate; the Middle Atlantic and New England areas had rates somewhat higher than the national rate, while the lowest regional rate of 1.8% was obtained from the west south central region. For persons 44 years and under, the prevalence was 1.6%, but it was 4.7% for persons 45 years and older. However, the infections were generally light; i.e., 80 of the 210 positive samples yielded fewer than 1 *Trichinella* larva per gram. Extending the survey to cover the period 1966–1970, Zimmermann *et al.* (1973) again showed that 4.2% (335 of 8071) of the diaphragms contained *Trichinella* larvae or cysts or both. Infected diaphragm samples were obtained from 130 hospitals in 42 states and the District of Columbia. States with a prevalence rate of more than 6% were Oregon, 8.3%; New Jersey, 7.7%; Main, 6.9%; Washington, 6.1%; and Nevada, 20.0% (but Nevada was represented by only 5 samples).

In addition to the prevalence rates based on autopsy findings, there are considerable data based on clinical findings. Data collected by the U.S. Public Health Service show that clinical cases may occur throughout the United States, with an overall incidence of 0.6 case per one million population (Centers for Disease Control, 1968, 1980). There has been a downward trend in the number of reported cases since 1947 (Fig. 1), and in 1967 there were only 67 reported cases and no deaths. Since that time, the incidence has leveled off or even shown some increase. The 284 cases reported in 1975 represent the highest annual incidence since 1961 (Schantz et al., 1977). Despite fluctuation in the number of clinical cases, the number of fatalities has remained low, with only 10 deaths reported in the decade following 1967 (Juranek and Schultz, 1978).

The epidemiological aspects of trichinosis in wildlife have become increasingly important since humans have become infected directly by ingesting improperly prepared flesh of infected wildlife or indirectly through consumption of swine that have fed on wildlife carcasses (Zimmermann, 1970c). In an epidemic reported by Roselle et al. (1965), all 6 cases had eaten bear meat that had been purchased at one country store in Vermont. In fact, bear meat (45 cases) and walrus meat (28 cases) accounted for 6.0% of the cases reported to the Centers for Disease Control in the past 9 years (Juranek and Schultz, 1978).

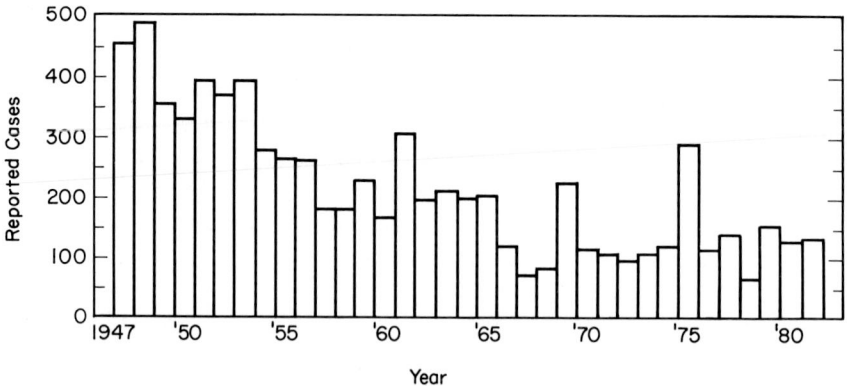

FIGURE 1. Numbers of clinical cases of human trichinosis in the United States. Data for 1947–1975 from Centers for Disease Control (1976); data for 1976–1980 from Centers for Disease Control (1981); data for 1981 from Centers for Disease Control (1982).

Although the role of the bear in the transmission of human trichinosis may be major in some locales, such as California (Lyman, 1974), in general it is minor compared to the role of swine (Schultz and Juranek, 1974).

Analysis of trichinosis surveillance data on 1212 cases revealed no seasonal patterns in the occurrence of cases (Juranek and Schultz, 1978), although an earlier report from California (Lyman, 1974) showed that the infection had a spring–summer predominance among individuals in their 30s. The mean age of 1119 patients was 33.7 years, and there was no difference in the sex distribution of cases.

The general decline in trichinosis in the United States has occurred without the benefit of specific control measures aimed at the detection or elimination of *Trichinella*-infected swine carcasses from consumer markets (Zimmermann, 1974). Improvements in swine husbandry, such as the discontinuation of feeding raw garbage, and the widespread use of household freezers, have helped to reduce human exposure to *Trichinella* in pork. Such measures, however, have by no means eradicated the infection in swine or man.

2.4. Latin America

In their view of trichinosis in Latin America, Neghme and Schenone (1970) suggested that *T. spiralis* may have been introduced to Central or South America or the West Indies from Europe or other regions where it was enzootic. They stated that adequate research on the infection in the southern half of the western hemisphere has been conducted chiefly in Argentina and Chile.

2.4.1. Wildlife

Trichinosis in Argentina has been reported in 1 of 4 foxes (*Pseudolopex gracilis gracilis*), in 1 of 8 edentates (*Chaetophractus villosus*), and in 1 of 8 rodents (*Graomis griseoflavus centralis*) (Neghme and Schenone, 1970). In Chile, however, not a single infection was found after examination of 2063 specimens of mammals from the central region of Chile, including 5 species of carnivores and 9 species of rodents (Alvarez *et al.*, 1970). Also, none of 80 whales caught in Chilean waters was infected.

Neghme and associates showed a very high infection rate (72%) in 36 dogs caught inside the Santiago municipal abattoir, where there was availability of *Trichinella*-infected meat or meat products (Neghme and

Schenone, 1970). Elsewhere in the city, the rate was only 4.0% in dogs. Other studies in Santiago showed infection rates of 1.6 and 2.0%. A study of stray dogs in Santiago, Chile, revealed an infection rate of 5.4% based on encysted larvae found in 6 of 111 dogs' diaphragms (Letonja and Ernst, 1974). Neghme and Schenone (1970) cited a study showing an infection rate of 2.0% among cats in Santiago.

Synanthropic rodents of the genus *Rattus*, naturally infected with *T. spiralis*, have been reported to be present in Argentina, Chile, Peru, Uruguay, and Mexico (Neghme and Schenone, 1970). The high infection rate in these animals has been attributed to scavenging cannibalism, and is higher among those living in or near slaughterhouses. Of 100 *R. norvegicus* caught in the sewage system and in some building of the municipal abattoir in Santiago, 25% were found to be infected as determined by trichinoscopy and artificial digestion (Schenone *et al.*, 1967). This infection rate was much higher than the previous 10% detected in a similar study done in 1951.

Examination of 38 rats (*R. rattus*) and 107 mongooses (*Herpestes auropunctatus*) trapped from various parts of Jamaica failed to reveal any *Trichinella* larvae (Alicata and Amiel, 1971). No *Trichinella* larvae were observed in the following species of rats in Puerto Rico (Jeffery and Oliver-Gonzalez, 1948): 179 *R. norvegicus*, 106 *R. rattus rattus*, 58 *R. rattus alexandrinus*, and 75 *R. rattus frugivorus*. A few cases of trichinosis have been reported in animals in British Guiana, but were believed to have originated outside the country (Guilbride, 1953).

2.4.2. Domestic Animals

The frequency of the infection in pigs appeared to be low (from 0.14 to 0.33%) in countries where trichinoscopy is routinely performed, on the basis of data from various sources (Neghme and Schenone, 1970). During 1962–1963, examinations in 31 slaughterhouses in Chile revealed that of 454,016 pigs, 1490 (0.33%) were infected (Barriga, 1966). The breeding of pigs in dumping grounds was believed to have contributed to the maintenance of infection, since the infection rate (5.2%) for pigs raised in dumping grounds was 25 times greater than the rate for hogs raised elsewhere in Chile. In a study conducted at the Valdivia slaughterhouse in Chile during 1970–1976, the average infection rate for swine was found to be 0.27% (Ernst and Aguilar, 1978). The infection rate in slaughter swine in Chile for 1976 was 0.16% and for 1977 0.2% (Neghme, 1979). Neghme also reported that in one place in Chile, 13 of 14 pigs were found to be infected; the pigs belonged to a piggery that was near a garbage lot and were probably fed on garbage.

2.4.3. Man

Trichinosis in humans has been reported to be most prevalent in the southern regions of South America (Neghme, 1979). Sporadic human cases of trichinosis have been reported from Argentina and Chile, and a few cases have been reported from Mexico and Venezuela; however, cases have not been reported from Uruguay since 1948. Different eating habits seemed to determine the prevalence of the infection. Due to the sizable German immigrant population, the custom of eating raw, salted, or smoked pork was introduced to Chile, which accounted for several epidemics; the native population was accustomed to eating well-cooked sausages. Autopsy surveys between 1942 and 1967 in Chile indicated a decline in incidence in the population of Santiago from 13.0% in 1942 to only 2.2% in 1967 (Neghme and Schenone, 1970). Over the years, many sporadic outbreaks in Chile have been reported, including a fatal case in 1967 in which 1600 *T. spiralis* larvae per gram of muscle were found. In July 1963, an outbreak of trichinosis in Antofogasta, Chile, involved 36 cases (Schenone *et al.*, 1968). It was assumed that infected pork derived from clandestinely slaughtered pigs from farms located in the vicinity of refuse dumps was responsible for the infection. To determine the frequency of human trichinosis in Santiago, samples of diaphragm and temporal muscles were obtained from 1000 cadavers and examined by trichinoscopy and artificial digestion (Schenone *et al.*, 1969). A total of 22 (2.2%) were found to be infected, indicating a decline of human trichinosis that was attributed to better systems of pig-breeding and improvement of the sanitary measures in slaughterhouses. During the period 1961–1971, there were 1005 cases of trichinosis with 22 (2.2%) fatalities (Schenone *et al.*, 1972). The annual mean attack rate of the infection per 100,000 population before 1965 was 1.2 and after 1965 was 1.6. Moreover, the prevalence of infection in cadavers increased from 2.2% in 1967 to 3.4% in 1972. The increased infection rates were attributed to greater pork consumption, especially from swine that were slaughtered without the knowledge or control of the health authorities. A trichinosis outbreak in Santiago during August–October 1975, involving 76 cases, was reported by Sapunar and Székely (1977). The diagnosis was based on clinical findings. The average incubation period was 15.8 days, but it was shorter in severe cases.

Trichinosis is not widespread in Argentina, although outbreaks have been reported from several provinces. The Andean regions bordering Chile are believed to be endemic areas (Neghme and Schenone, 1970). These authors have tabulated the morbidity and mortality from trichinosis in Argentina since the earliest report in 1897. Bilbao (1965) reported 48 human cases that occurred in Coronel Pringles, south of Buenos Aires. Outbreaks had been reported from the same locality in 1960 (38 cases) and in 1964 (1 case). An outbreak of trichinosis in the city of Mercedes, Argentina, in July 1967, involved 31 cases (Ossola *et al.*, 1969), the source of infection for 24 patients being traced to an infected pig.

Trichinosis is endemic in Uruguay (Neghme and Schenone, 1970). In Brazil, although there is a large German population that supposedly consumes raw or poorly cooked pork products, trichinosis has not been reported to be indigenous. The few recorded cases are believed to have been acquired abroad. Likewise, trichinosis appears not to be endemic in Venezuela and Peru. The infection is unknown in Colombia and in both British and French Guiana (Guilbride, 1953). It is believed to be fairly common in the Bahama Islands; however, it is unknown in other islands of the West Indies (Guilbride, 1953). Trichinosis in humans has not been reported from Puerto Rico (Jeffery and Oliver-Gonzalez, 1948; Guilbride, 1953).

Information for Central America is sparse, but negative findings have been reported from Guatemala, Honduras, Costa Rica, and Panama. Guilbride (1953) felt that since trichinosis was a disease of garbage-fed pigs, this accounted for the fact that it was very uncommon in the tropics, where pigs are usually left to forage for themselves and rarely have the opportunity to feed on other animal protein. In addition, most people in these areas subject their food to prolonged cooking.

There are historical accounts of the presence of trichinosis in Mexico, but most infections have been mild (Neghme and Schenone, 1970). Diaphragms of 100 human cadavers from two hospitals in Mexico City were examined to determine the prevalence and degree of trichinosis. Direct microscopic examination of samples weighing 50 g or more revealed a high incidence (15%) of low-grade infections. Of the 15 positive cases, 12 showed fewer than 1 cyst per gram of tissue, while 9 showed fewer than 0.1 cyst per gram of tissue (Beck, 1953).

3. EUROPE

3.1. British Isles

Even though trichinosis in man was first described and identified by Paget in England, there is very little information on the infection in England or other parts of the British Isles.

The only account of *T. spiralis* in wildlife in England was reported in a single red fox in Cornwall during press-preparation examination of portions of diaphragms of several carcasses of wild red foxes (Oldham and Beresford-Jones, 1957).

In an effort to find a wild carnivore reservoir in Ireland, 70 fresh specimens of the red fox (*V. vulpes*) from Counties Cork, Waterford, and Tipperary were examined by the compression method (Corridan *et al.*, 1969). Of these, 3 (4.3%) were infected, and after digestion the numbers of larvae per gram of thigh muscle were 1, 2, and 6.

A survey of human trichinosis, based on 200 autopsies at four hospitals in London (including representative locations and population classes in the vicinity of London), showed that only 1% were infected (Van Someren, 1937). A decade later, M.R. Young (1947) reported that although outbreaks of trichinosis in Great Britain have been sporadic, the incidence in southern England was between 7.9 and 13.7%, with an average of 10.8%, on the basis of digestion of 472 human diaphragms from Wolverhampton, Birmingham, Cambridge, Bristol, Cardiff, Llandough, and Leeds. Kozar (1970) pointed out the rarity of clinical trichinosis in Great Britain up to 1940, with only 59 reported cases, of which 47 originated in southern Wales. It was not until World War II and thereafter that epidemics in England were reported. In early 1941, an epidemic occurred in Wolverhampton in which at least 500 people were affected, but there were no deaths (Sheldon, 1941; Todd, 1979). The infection was confined to the industrial working class, with most cases being in females—both features being consistent with a relatively high consumption of uncooked pork sausage.

An epidemic that occurred in Liverpool in 1953 involved 82 cases with 2 deaths (Semple *et al.*, 1954; Kershaw *et al.*, 1956). The source of the epidemic was sausages in most cases, and many of the patients had eaten them raw. According to Harvey and Kershaw (1964), outbreaks of trichinosis in England and Wales are rare compared to continental Europe and the United States. They believed that for each outbreak, there were many latent (subclinical) cases associated with those that were diagnosed. A survey was begun in 1958 and completed in 1963. The incidence of latent trichinosis in 512 cadavers examined by digestion was 0.4% in an area near Blackpool.

The first cases of trichinosis in the population of Ireland were reported in 1957 and again in 1966, although there had been a severe outbreak among confined German prisoners of war in 1946 (see Chapter 1). In 1967, 26 cases of trichinosis were diagnosed in Cork based on positive bentonite-flocculation and latex-agglutination tests or muscle biopsy (Corridan and O'Meara, 1968). There was a preponderance of females, 17 being females and 9 males. The source of the outbreak was believed to be sausages and/or a pork product consisting of sausage meat and scraps of raw pork. Another outbreak of 50 cases of trichinosis was reported in Kerry in which all 50 patients had positive latex-agglutination tests (Corridan and Gray, 1969). An addendum to this report cited a sporadic case in Waterford as well as other cases in another area of Ireland. The authors feared that the disease may become endemic.

3.2. Germany

The first studies of sylvatic trichinosis were inaugurated in Germany in the 1930s by investigators who were the first to report the prevalence of the infection among foxes and other wildlife. During the years 1919–1943, 1620 foxes were examined, of which 87 (5.4%) were found to be infected; in the period 1958–1965, the following rates of infection were observed: 24 of 1259 foxes (1.9%), 2 of 72 badgers (2.8%), 1 of 16 wild boars (6.3%), and none of 396 mice (Lehmensick, 1970).

Small house pets, dogs, and cats play only a minor role in the transmission of trichinosis in Germany, since their flesh is seldom eaten by man or other animals. The few reports available have shown the incidence of infection to be very low.

At the time of the initial introduction of regulatory measures for the inspection of pork for human consumption in 1878, the rate of infection among hogs was 0.05% (Lehmensick, 1970). In 1907, 30 years later, the rate was 0.005%, or one tenth of the rate in 1878. The rate declined progressively to 0.001% in 1926, and to 0.0007% in 1936 (Lehmensick, 1970) (see also Chapter 1). Measures for the safe disposition of wildlife carcasses and measures to control contagious diseases in animals helped to maintain the low prevalence of trichinosis among swine. The rate has steadily declined since World War II, so that in 1966, of approximately 3 million pigs slaughtered in the Federal Republic of Germany, only 1, or 0.000028%, was found to be infected. The distribution of infected swine varies for different German states. It is highest in Bavaria, and this is probably related, at least in part, to the method of hog-raising used in this densely wooded region (Lehmensick, 1970).

Germany has had an interesting history of outbreaks of human trichinosis (see Chapter 1). During the 30 years from 1860 to 1890, 13,557 cases of human trichinosis were reported in Germany (an average of 450 cases per year), of which approximately 5% were fatal (Lehmensick, 1970). The number of infections became significantly less after the institution of inspection of slaughtered swine. Since the end of World War II, the Federal Republic of Germany has been remarkably free of clinical trichinosis. For periods as long as 17 years, no clinical cases have been reported. The scattered outbreaks that have occurred have usually been attributable to factors other than defective trichinoscopy (e.g., consumption of noninspected meat, especially that of wild boar). However, a large outbreak in 1950 (436 cases and 0 deaths) and another in 1967 (250 cases and 2 deaths) were probably due to improper inspection of swine carcasses.

3.3. Austria

In 1970, Hinaidy (1970) reported that *T. spiralis* was found in 10 of 71 foxes examined during studies on the parasite fauna of the red fox (*V. vulpes*) in Austria. The tail muscles were found to be one of the predilection sites. In a more recent review, Hinaidy (1978) reported that of a total of 204 foxes from eight different districts examined trichinoscopically in 1969–1976, only 21 were infected. Other animals, including badgers (*Meles meles*), polecats (*Mustela putorius*), weasels (*M. nivalis*), martens (*Martes martes*), and stoats (*Mustela erminea*) were examined, but all were negative. Thus, the fox (*V. vulpes*) appears to be the only reservoir in Austria.

In the years 1952–1968, *T. spiralis* was found in 47 slaughtered domestic pigs, only 12 of which were native (Hinaidy, 1978).

In 1970, a small epidemic occurred in Austria, involving 12 persons who had eaten smoked bacon from a pig that had been fed the flesh of an apparently infected fox (Hinaidy, 1978).

3.4. Switzerland

There is evidence for the existence of trichinosis in wildlife in Switzerland. During 1942–1949, systematic examination of red foxes (*V. vulpes*) was performed in east Switzerland. *Trichinella* was detected in animals from Zurich, Argona, Saint-Gall, and Grisons cantons (Bouvier, 1966). Subsequently, the infection was found in 35 of 245 foxes (*V. vulpes*) and in 1 of 34 badgers (*M. meles*), 1 of 21 stone martens (*M. foina*), and 1 of 3 pine martens (*M. martes*) (Hörning, 1977, 1978).

Trichinoscopy is not required by law for swine slaughtered in Switzerland, it is required only for imported pork and bear meat and for wild boars shot in Switzerland or imported.

Human cases of trichinosis are extremely rare in Switzerland (Hörning, 1978). On the basis of a personal communication from Hörning in 1967, Kozar (1970) reported that a few autochthonous outbreaks occurred during the past century, and since then there have been outbreaks in 1936, 1938, 1954, and 1955. The more recent outbreaks were reported to have been caused not by infected pork but by infected mink and dog meat.

3.5. The Netherlands

On the basis of investigations by various individuals, using both trichinoscopy and artificial digestion, trichinosis apparently had not occurred in man or animals in the Netherlands for more than 40 years. However, a more recent investigation of pooled samples of porcine flesh by means of the digestion method led to the conclusion that trichinosis occurred throughout the Netherlands (Ruitenberg and Sluiters, 1974). The authors felt that this was not a sudden reappearance of trichinosis, but rather a redetection of the infection, since it was very likely that a low level of infection had always been present. Although the infection rate was very low, trichinosis was found in both pigs and wildlife (Ruitenberg, 1974).

Of 96 foxes (*V. vulpes*) that were examined in 1969–1971, 3 were infected (Ruitenberg and Sluiters, 1974). Wild rats (*R. norvegicus*) were also found to be infected and were believed to play a role as a wildlife reservoir of *T. spiralis*. The level of infection was low, however, as was the case in other wildlife. The black rat (*R. rattus*) was also infected. Later, Ruitenberg and van Knapen (1978) reported that *T. spiralis* was found occasionally in wildlife, including foxes (*V. vulpes*), polecats (*P. putorius*), and wild rats (*R. norvegicus*). During 1977–1978, wild boars (*Sus scrofa*) were examined, and although anti-*Trichinella* antibodies were found in the serum of some, larvae were not found (Ruitenberg, 1979).

Since 1967, sera from healthy pigs have been examined annually for antibodies against *Trichinella*, using the immunofluorescence test (Ruitenberg and Sluiters, 1974). After examination of 10,000 sera, 1 serum showed a titer of 1:4. Further investigations were carried out on the farm where the positive pig originated, with pigs being examined by means of trichinoscopy, immunofluorescence test, and the digestion method. Of 44 pigs examined, 11 were positive with the digestion method, while all the animals were negative with trichinoscopy and the immunofluorescence test. Of 9 sera from sows, 3 were positive with the immunofluorescence test. Of 29 rats examined by the digestion method, only 3 yielded larvae. These findings necessitated reevaluation of trichinosis in the Netherlands. With the use of a modified digestion method, 337 lots of at least 10 animals were examined in 1969–1971, of which 23 lots were positive; in 1971, of 501 lots examined, 23 were positive. In the majority of the lots, only 0.0025–0.025 larvae per gram were present. The farms from which the positive lots originated were mainly in the southern and eastern parts of the Netherlands. Ruitenberg and van Knapen (1978) reported that during 1975–1976, 5 of 10,000 (0.05%) slaughtered pigs were positive based on the pooled-sample digestion method. The number of larvae found was very low (0.05–0.1 per gram diaphragm tissue). In 1973, the infection rate for slaughter pigs had been reported to be 0.01%, with very low numbers of larvae (Ruitenberg, 1975).

Examination of 1104 human diaphragms, by trichinoscopy and the digestion method, did not reveal any *Trichinella* larvae (Kampelmacher *et al.*, 1968). However, 2 cases of human trichinosis were diagnosed in 1975 and 2 in 1976 (Ruitenberg and van Knapen, 1978). The authors felt almost certain that the patients had become infected during a stay in Yugoslavia. A later report revealed 4 cases of human trichinosis in 1977, but none in 1978 (Ruitenberg, 1979). The first 2 cases were infected while in the United States, the 3rd patient came from Poland, and the 4th patient was infected from an unknown source.

These data on man and animals have shown that trichinosis is indeed present in the Netherlands.

3.6. Belgium

A recent epidemiological study carried out in Belgium has revealed that trichinosis occurs among wild boars and rodents (Famerée *et al.*, 1981). Of 45 indigenous wild boars, 3 (6.7%) were infected. Of 550 rodents examined, the following were found to be infected: 9 of 403 (2.2%) muskrats (*O. zibethica*), 7 of 108 (6.5%) rats (*R. norvegicus*), and 2 of 18 (11.1%) domestic rats (*R. rattus*). None of 21 voles was infected. Except for one heavily infected wild boar, the other animals were only mildly infected.

Although there is no information on trichinosis in humans, there is concern for possible human infection, inasmuch as in certain provinces in Belgium the muskrat is relished as game.

3.7. France

Trichinosis in wildlife in France was first reported in 1978 by Artois (1978). An investigation for the period 1976–1977 revealed that of the various species of wildlife animals examined by artificial digestion,

Trichinella was detected in 8 of 201 red foxes captured in the east and southeast of France. The other animals examined were negative.

There is no information on the prevalence of trichinosis in swine or other domestic animals in France.

France had a severe outbreak of human trichinosis in 1878 and a mild one in the north of the country in 1952, according to a personal communication from Guilhon (Kozar, 1970). In both instances, boar meat was the source of infection. In 1976, an outbreak occurred in the southern suburbs of Paris (Bouree *et al.*, 1977, 1979). The outbreak involved 125 cases, of whom 95 were adults and 30 were children. They were diagnosed clinically and confirmed immunologically. The parasite was found in only 3 of 32 muscle biopsies, but this investigation was made relatively early in the disease. There were no deaths, and all patients recovered quickly. The outbreak was attributed to the consumption of horse meat, although the meat was not available for examination. Since the horse is herbivorous, the tentative explanation given was that the horses may have become infected by hay contaminated with the carcasses of infected rodents.

3.8. Spain

Trichinosis is considered to be an important zoonosis in Spain because of its existence in sylvatic and domestic hosts.

A survey of the incidence of trichinosis in wild animals from the Cantabrian Mountains between 1960–1969 (Cordero del Campillo *et al.*, 1970) showed a widespread infection involving many host species, with the following infection rates: badger (*M. meles*), 40.0%; genet (*Genetta genetta*), 38.8%; fox (*V. vulpes*), 31.6%; wildcat (*F. sylvestris*), 31.5%; ferret (*M. putorius furo*), 25.0%; wolf (*C. lupus*), 20.0%; and marten (*M. martes*), 5.5%. In the period 1975–1978, *T. spiralis* was detected in wild boar, wildcat, fox, genet (*G. genetta*), and wolf (*C. lupus*) (Martinez-Gomez, 1979).

The high incidence of rat trichinosis in Spain is well known. The infection rate varied from 7.0% in various parts of Madrid to 42.2% in the province of Ciudad-Real (Cordero del Campillo *et al.*, 1970). It is believed that the rat plays a role in maintaining the infection in swine. Dogs have also been found to be infected in Spain.

The infection rate in pigs has varied according to region (Cordero del Campillo *et al.*, 1970). The rate ranged from 0.02% in Leon for the period 1948–1968 to 0.43% in Pola de Lena for the period 1959–1961. The infection rate in 1965 for all of Spain was 0.0007%. This was not presumed to be accurate, since official reports were not always made.

From 1971 to 1975, Cordoba had no positive cases in swine (Martinez *et al.*, 1978). Martinez-Gomez (1978) reported 13 cases of swine trichinosis in 1975 and 58 in 1976.

Human trichinosis is of importance in Spain because of the national gastronomic habits, such as the consumption of uncooked pork, ham, "chorizo" sausages, and other pork products, and because pork is one of the main sources of animal protein for a large portion of the population. The rate of human clinical trichinosis was reported to be decreasing in Spain in the 20-year period from 1948 to 1968 (Cordero del Campillo *et al.*, 1970). In 1948, 96 cases of human trichinosis were reported, and the number of cases reached a peak of 411 in 1953. However, in 1968, there were only 10 reported cases. The decrease in the number of cases has been attributed to veterinary inspection and a national network of packing plants with deep-freeze facilities. The 340 cases of human trichinosis recorded for the period 1971–1975 occurred in four different locales and were attirubted to the consumption of pork in two locales and wild boar in the remaining two (Martinez *et al.*, 1978). In 1975, 240 human cases were reported; in 1976, 63 cases; in 1977, 38 cases; and in 1978, 15 cases (Martinez-Gomez, 1978, 1979).

3.9. Portugal

Trichinosis has been extremely rare in Portugal. The infection has been reported in 30 of 1,645,916 pigs examined during the years 1900–1955 in Lisbon abattoirs (Kozar, 1970). At least 22 of the 30 infected pigs were brought from Spain. Although Fraga de Azevedo and Palmeiro (1970) also listed 42 pigs as having been infected between 1890 and 1966, most of them were believed to have been imported from Spain. The authors felt that only 2 infected pigs have been known to be definitely indigenous to Portugal. Among other animals, the infection has been recorded only in 1 fox (*V. vulpes*).

Of the few cases of human trichinosis on record, the majority occurred near the Spanish frontier. According to Fraga de Azevedo and Palmeiro (1970), the first human case of trichinosis in Portugal was described in 1867; however, it was not certain that the infection was indigenous to Portugal. They cited a report of 1967 in which they recorded the only human case of trichinosis indigenous to Portugal. According to Kozar (1970), there was evidently a mild epidemic in 1951 with sporadic cases. This particular epidemic and other isolated cases throughout the years have been cited by Fraga de Azevedo and Palmeiro (1970) to be of doubtful origin, i.e., not necessarily indigenous to Portugal.

3.10. Italy

Sylvatic trichinosis occurs mainly in foxes in the mountainous regions of the Alps and Apennines. It has been reported that the infection rate may be as high as 17.0% in the foxes from these regions (Kozar, 1970).

The infection in dogs, cats, and rodents has been reported to be virtually nonexistent in Sicily, although in one locality near Foggie, 17 of 71 dogs examined were found to be infected (Kozar, 1970).

Swine trichinosis is thought to be rare in Italy. Sporadic trichinoscopic examinations have detected only 15 animals that were infected (Kozar, 1970). In 1958, compulsory trichinoscopic examination was instituted on all pigs slaughtered in Italy. Since that time, no pig has been found to be infected in northern and central Italy, although 4 pigs from southern Italy were found to be infected (Bellani et al., 1978).

Human trichinosis is considered to be extremely rare in Italy. According to Bellani et al. (1978), only 9 outbreaks have been reported since 1900, and all of them have been in rural area: 4 in Sicily, 3 in central-southern Apennines, and 2 in the Alpine region. An interesting outbreak of human trichinosis occurred in northern Italy at Bagnolo, a town of 6000 inhabitants in the Po Valley. There were 89 suspected cases, but no deaths. All infected persons had eaten raw horse meat. *Trichinella* was detected in 3 cats that had been fed the same horse meat. The outbreak was attributed to the ingestion of the meat from an imported horse (Bellani et al., 1978).

3.11. Greece

Information on the prevalence of trichinosis in wildlife in Greece is sparse, but there is evidence that the infection is present. In a review of the status of human trichinosis in Greece, Himonas (1971) cited reports of the presence of the infection in foxes and wolves. The incidence of trichinosis in rats varied from 0 to 60% depending on the place of their capture. There was no case of trichinosis in domestic or wild animals in Greece during either the 1975–1976 period (Himonas, 1978) or the 1976–1978 period (Himonas, 1979).

There is more information regarding the prevalence of trichinosis in swine, since the law in Greece requires that swine muscle be routinely inspected by trichinoscopy in all slaughterhouses (Himonas, 1971, 1978, 1979). According to Himonas (1971), *T. spiralis* larvae were found in 117 of 15,704 pigs slaughtered and examined in Athens from 1952 to 1953. In Thessaloniki, of the 57,165 pigs slaughtered during a 7-year period (1952–1958), 71 (0.12%) were found to be infected. Also, 23 pigs of 1034 (2.2%) slaughtered in Piraeus within 1 month in 1967 because of a foot-and-mouth disease outbreak were found to be infected. It has been estimated that in Greece, no more than 15 cases of swine trichinosis are detected each year, and that the incidence of slaughtered animals is about 0.02%. More recent data indicated that there was no case of trichinosis in swine in Greece for the 1975–1976 period (Himonas, 1978) or the 1976–1978 period (Himonas, 1979).

The exact incidence of human trichinosis in Greece is not known. From the first recorded outbreak in 1946 to 1952, only 22 cases or suspected cases have been reported (Himonas, 1971). Since then, no case has been reported, except for an incidental finding of *T. spiralis* larvae in a case of laryngeal tumor in 1968. Although no epidemiological survey has been carried out, it has been assumed that 1 case of human trichinosis occurs every year in Greece. Since pork products and their consumption were believed to have increased significantly in Greece during the last few years, a study was undertaken to determine the prevalence of latent trichinosis in humans. Samples of diaphragms of 154 cadavers, 50 g each, were digested. The observed incidence of 0.65% suggested that the incidence of human subclinical trichinosis might be much higher than had been suspected (Himonas, 1971). More recent data show that there was no human trichinosis reported in Greece for 1975–1976 (Himonas, 1978) or for 1976–1978 (Himonas, 1979).

4. SCANDINAVIA

4.1. Norway

Limited information on trichinosis in Norway is available from reviews by Kozar (1970) and Steele and Schultz (1978). Among wildlife in Norway, the rate of trichinosis was reported to be 22.0%. The infection rate was reported to be 6.0% in some 95,000 foxes and 11.0% in some 2200 minks.

The infection rate in dogs has been reported to be 1.0% or less, while in cats it was 17.0%. Only a few cases have been reported in swine.

An epidemic of trichinosis occurred in 1940 among German soldiers in Norway. An isolated case was reported 10 years later involving a person who apparently had contracted the disease while abroad. No indigenous cases have occurred in Norway since 1940.

4.2. Sweden

Wild carnivores, especially red foxes, have been observed to be infected with *T. spiralis* in Sweden. Since foxes seem to be a potential source of infection for swine, and hence for man, the prevalence of the infection in foxes has been a concern in Sweden. In 1966, Ekstam (1966) reported that 14.22% of foxes and 2.02% of badgers were infected with *T. spiralis*. A total of 1151 foxes (*V. vulpes*), killed during the hunting season and representing all 24 counties of Sweden, were examined for *Trichinella* by trichinoscopy; the parasite was found in 19.6% (Rońeus and Christensson, 1979). Infected foxes were found in all counties, except for the isolated island of Gotland. The infection was more common in old foxes (40.0%) than in young foxes (11.0%). The number of *Trichinella* larvae varied between 0.05 and 200 per gram of muscle. *Trichinella* has been reported in other wildlife, such as the badger, polecat, ermine, marten, lynx, mink, and rat, as well as in farmed foxes and minks, and in the tiger, lion, polar bear, and wolf from zoological gardens (Rońeus and Christensson, 1979).

The infection has been reported in dogs and cats (Rońeus and Christensson, 1979). According to Steele and Schultz (1978), trichinosis is seldom seen in rats, mice, and other rodents in Sweden.

The highest incidence of trichinosis in the pig occurred in 1921 (0.007%) and the lowest in 1960 (0.0003%) according to Ekstam (1966). During the years 1970–1977, of 29.3 million swine slaughtered and inspected, *Trichinella* was observed in 52 (0.00018%) (Rońeus and Christensson, 1979).

Outbreaks of human trichinosis are rare in Sweden. Since 1917, 9 epidemics and a few sporadic cases have been reported (Odelram, 1973). Most of the epidemics up to 1961 had occurred in the western middle part of Sweden. In 1937, 50 cases were reported from Lindesberg, and in 1946 there were 35 cases in Boras as cited by Ringertz *et al.*, 1962. Ringertz and colleagues reported an outbreak of trichinosis that occurred in Karlskrona and the eastern part of the county of Blekinge on the southeastern coast of Sweden in July of 1961. There was a total of 338 cases, and the source of infection was smoked sausage containing 40% pork. The majority of the cases were found within the distribution area of the slaughterhouse producing the sausage. Odelram (1973) reported an outbreak of 15 cases of trichinosis that had occurred in 1969 in Vadstena with no fatalities. Despite the investigation by epidemiologists, the source of the epidemic was not ascertained. During 1970–1977, the annual occurrence of human trichinosis was 2.1 cases. Based on the population of 8 million during these years, the infection occurred in approximately 0.00003% of the population (Roñeus and Christensson, 1979).

4.3. Denmark

In contrast to the situation in most European countries, *T. spiralis* was not detected in Denmark, in sylvatic or domestic animals, for many years. According to Clausen and Henriksen (1976) and Clausen (1978), the parasite was last demonstrated in a pig in 1930 and in a cat in 1942. The parasite had never been found in Danish game animals even after examination of more than 1000 foxes. However, in 1973, the parasite was found among wild boars (*S. scrofa*) living in a 600-acre enclosure in the northwest of Jutland. The rate of infection among the boars was 4.0%. The stock had been built up in the 1960s mainly with imported animals. The infection was also found in 3 foxes (*V. vulpes*) that had entered the fenced area where the wild boars lived, and the number of larvae varied from 5 to 15 larvae per gram of tail muscle.

As a result of these findings, a survey was conducted to determine the extent of infection among foxes and other free-living carnivores in Denmark (Clausen and Henriksen, 1976). A total of 5084 foxes (*V. vulpes*), of which 4 were found to be infected, were examined by the combined digestion and Baermann technique (Clausen and Henriksen, 1976; Clausen, 1978). This was the first account of *T. spiralis* infection in free-roaming Danish game animals. The prevalence of trichinosis among Danish foxes was less than 0.1%, which was lower than in most European countries. All the other 293 small carnivores were found not to be infected.

Trichinosis has not been demonstrated either in domestic swine or in humans (Henriksen, 1978, 1979). According to Steele and Schultz (1978), the last case in man was in 1910 and in swine in 1929. The absence of the infection may be a reflection, at least in part, of the Danish meat-inspection regulations, which require compulsory examination of slaughter swine of more than 100 kg carcass weight and of boars and sows.

4.4. Finland

A recent report (Valtonen, 1979) showed that trichinosis was present in wildlife. In 1976, the infection was detected in 1 lynx, in 1977 in 2 bears, and in 1978 in 3 foxes. In 1976, the infection was detected in 2 polar bears, but they were in a zoo; it was also detected in 3 foxes, but they were farm animals. In the following year, another fox on a farm was found to be infected, and 4 more foxes from the farm were found to be infected in 1978. A mink from a farm was found to be infected in 1977. Tiainen (1966) had reported earlier that of 76 rats caught at the Helsinki Zoological Gardens, 9 (12.0%) were infected. He also reported that 3 polar bears that were slaughtered at the zoo several decades ago had been infected.

Of domestic swine, 2 were found to be infected in 1977 and 1 in 1978 (Valtonen, 1979). Prior to this, during 1954–1964, only 16 cases had been reported in swine (Mäkelä, 1970; Steele and Schultz, 1978).

Human trichinosis is an extremely rare infection in Finland. The rare occurrence of trichinosis in humans has been attributed to effective inspection of pork and to very rare consumption of raw pork by the population. According to Mäkelä (1970), only 3 cases of human trichinosis have been described, all from the 1890s. He reported the first case since then in which the infection was due to the consumption of meat from a captive wild pig killed at a zoological garden. The patient was a zoo car driver who had eaten the meat of the slaughtered wild pig. The definitive diagnosis was based on the demonstration of *T. spiralis* larvae in a biopsy several months later.

5. EASTERN EUROPE

5.1. Poland

Poland has had a serious trichinosis problem in man and animals, although the incidence has declined. Kozar stated that there was a rich sylvan reservoir of *Trichinella*, which was responsible for continued infection of pigs and humans (Steele, 1970). Relatively high infection rates have been encountered in Poland among forest animals, such as wolves (26.0%), foxes (7.3%), badgers (2.9%), martens (1.5%), polecats (1.3%), and boars (0.11%) (Kozar, 1970). The greatest frequency of trichinosis in the wild has been noted in the southern regions of the Carpathian Mountains, with diminishing incidence toward the northern part of the country.

Of a total of 5484 small rodents belonging to 16 species and 7 genera, from different districts of Poland, *T. spiralis* has been found in only 1 specimen, *Mus musculus*. The low infection rate does not diminish the role played by small rodents in the epidemiology of trichinosis (Gerwel and Pawlowski, 1975). In a study in which small mammals from 16 provinces were examined, only 2 species (*R. norvegicus* and *V. vulpes*) caught in the region of the Bialystok province were positive (Zukowski and Bitkowska, 1978). Examination of fur-animals and rats from different regions of Gdansk–Gdynia and surroundings revealed *T. spiralis* in 17 of 188 breeding foxes and 15 of 238 minks (Czarnowski and Przyborowski, 1970). The infection rate was 1.18% in rats from the suburbs of Gdynia, where there were numerous fur farms and small agricultural farms. A 10.1% infection rate was demonstrated in animals from the Warsaw and Olsztyn provinces (Gancarz *et al.*, 1968), with the highest rate in cats (9 of 17), followed by foxes (6 of 16), dogs (3 of 17), and rats (4 of 30).

Approximately 3000 pigs and about 320 synanthropic and wild animals were examined by trichinoscopy and artificial digestion, but *T. spiralis* was found only in pigs (Gancarz *et al.*, 1970). In an earlier study by Kozar *et al.* (1965), of 171 dogs from Wroclaw, 2.33% were infected, and of 210 dogs from Jelenia Gora, 2.38% were infected. The infection in cats (2.29%) was only slightly lower than in dogs. More recent findings (Gerwel and Pawlowski, 1975) showed that *T. spiralis* was found in 6 of 36 dogs, 10 of 42 cats, and 11 of 111 rats. These findings point out the reservoir of *T. spiralis* in these animals despite the successful eradication of the focus in pigs.

Trichinoscopic examination is compulsory in Poland for all pigs and wild boars slaughtered for human consumption. The incidence of swine trichinosis is the highest in the eastern and central regions and less common in the western region of the country. On the basis of official trichinoscopy of pigs, of a total of 126,206,350 pigs examined in Poland in 1947–1963, 26,652 (0.021%) were found to be infected (Kozar and Ogielski, 1965). This was half the rate of the prewar period, 1923–1936, in which the infection rate was 0.055%. For the period 1957–1963, the infection rate was reduced to 0.0146%. During 1958–1960, the pigs and wild boars from Wroclaw province, including those imported from other provinces and slaughtered at the meat plant in Wroclaw province, were examined for *Trichinella*. The results showed that cases of trichinosis in pigs were detected principally in those from districts bordering Czechoslovakia and those from central provinces (Ramisz and Swiech, 1962). In 1975, 370 cases (0.0019%) of pig trichinosis were reported (Ramisz and Jarzebski, 1979). In 1976, there were 317 (0.0019%) cases; however, in 1977, the number increased to 461 (0.0032%) and increased further in 1978 to 1004 (0.0055%). The overall increases were attributed to trichinosis on certain farms where large numbers of pigs were infected.

Examination of rats may at best be an index of the sanitary condition of a given slaughterhouse (Kozar and Ogielski, 1965), but Ramisz and Balicka-Laurans (1981) recently concluded that rats were responsible for spreading the infection among swine on fattening farms. During 1977–1979, 8 of 40 rats examined from five fattening farms in Krakow and Nowy Sacz provinces were found to be infected with *T. spiralis*. On the three farms that harbored the infected rats, heavily infected pigs were found.

Human trichinosis in Poland is still considered to be an important epidemiological and clinical problem. The most reliable data on the incidence of trichinosis in man can be obtained from postmortem examinations. Kozar and Kozar (1965) examined 3065 specimens from 15 different regions, using both compression and digestion methods, and found infection in 103 (3.4%). During 1946–1970, of 13,288 cases reported in Poland, more than 15% were from Bialystok Province in the northeast (Boron *et al.*, 1978). The highest incidence in this province was observed in 1952 (43.8%), and another increase was observed in 1967 (35.4%). The lowest incidence was observed in 1969 (16.0%) and also in 1973 (1 case). In 1960–1973, 61% of the cases came from the urban environment and 56% were in women. The highest percentage (69.0%) was observed in the 10- to 40-year-old group; in children up to 10 years of age, the percentage was 11%, and in the group above 40 years of age, 20%. The highest frequency in this province occurred between December and April, suggesting greater consumption of pork during the family holidays that fall in these months. The decrease in the percentage of infected swine has accompanied a marked decline of human incidence in the Bialystok Province during the last few years.

In 1960–1963, the reported number of cases of human trichinosis was 3954. Of these, 14 died and a large number of severe cases had to be hospitalized for a long time (Gerwel and Pawlowski, 1975). Most of the severe cases occurred on small farms. Large epidemics were also reported in towns each year; however, the clinical course of the disease was much milder. It appeared that trichinosis among rural populations was, as a rule, due to illicit swine slaughter, whereas in town the infection resulted from negligence in carcass inspection by the veterinary service. Human trichinosis in Poland is still an important epidemiological and clinical problem.

5.2. Czechoslovakia

In a rather extensive review of trichinosis in Czechoslovakia, Prokopič (1962) stated that the first evidence of trichinosis in wildlife was in 3 of 15 foxes examined by Weiser in 1948. Two of the infected foxes came from Radošov in the south Moravian district and the other from Lány near Rakovník in central Bohemia. Trichinosis had also been found in 2 bears examined at Bratislava in 1948. According to various investigators, the highest percentages of trichinosis in carnivorous animals were found in *L. lynx* (66.6%), *C. lupus* (33.3%), *V. vulpes* (27.02%), *F. silvestris* (15.2%), and *F. catus domestica* (1.28%). There were other reports of sporadic cases in wildlife from West-Slovakian districts, north Moravia, Luhačovice, and Brno. According to Prokopič (1962), the increase in the incidence of trichinosis in Slovakia could be attributed to the migration of carnivores from neighboring countries where trichinosis was widely distributed. These carnivores are believed to play an important role in the transmission of the infection in Czechoslovakia today.

After passage of a bill for compulsory trichinoscopy of hogs in Prague in 1936, 17 of 213,236 (0.008%) pigs examined were found to be infected, of which 16 were of foreign origin and only 1 from Slovakia (Prokopič, 1962). Surveys showed that trichinosis occurred more often in pigs from Slovakia than in those from other parts of the country, but the percentage of infected imported pigs was also higher.

Historical survey of human trichinosis in Czechoslovakia showed that about 1000 persons have been infected during the last 100 years, with 5% mortality (Prokopič, 1962). Mild outbreaks recurred every few years in the southern regions of Czechoslovakia and northern Moravia. More recently, the incidence in eastern Slovakia has increased. Between 1962 and 1974, six epidemics were recorded, with 89 cases but no fatalities (Hovorka, 1975). The infection was mild in the majority of cases. All the epidemics occurred in the eastern part of Slovakia, and the main source of the infection was boar meat. Only 2 cases were caused by raw or smoked domestic pork. The owners of the pigs lived in mountainous regions where pigs grazed in the woods and thus could have become infected by eating meat of wild animals infected with *Trichinella*. All the epidemics occurred during winter when hunters prepare homemade sausages of boar meat or pork and eat them smoked or even raw.

5.3. Hungary

Information on the prevalence of trichinosis among wildlife in Hungary is sparse. Infection in foxes has predominated. On the average, 5.0% of the foxes have been reported to be infected, with higher percentages in enzootic areas (Neméseri, 1970). Infection in wild hogs has amounted to approximately 0.5–1.0%. Infection rates among insectivores and rodents were reported to be extremely low.

Approximately 2.0% of dogs and cats have been found to be infected in the enzootic area of Hajdu-Bihar County (Nemeséri, 1970). Since 1962, when trichinoscopy of swine was made mandatory in abattoirs, only a few infections have been found each year. Since the pig that is slaughtered at home is not examined, and the practice is still very common, the main source of trichinosis infection is the home-slaughtered pig.

In man, most cases have resulted from consuming uncooked or smoked sausages made of meat from home-slaughtered pigs or wild hogs. In several cases, housewives became infected by tasting fresh, ground spiced meat while preparing it. Outbreaks tended to be familial and occurred mostly in villages. From the first recorded outbreak in 1891 to 1950, 114 cases with 9 deaths have been recorded (Nemeséri, 1970). In the past 20 years, however, the number of cases has increased to 422 cases with 9 deaths. The records, thus far, have shown that of those areas observed, there were 536 cases with 18 deaths. In the most severe outbreak, which occurred in 1964, 116 became infected and 3 died. The source of this outbreak was infected sow meat that was used for sausage. Large numbers of *Trichinella* (100–200 larvae/gram sausage) were found. On the basis of examinations of 1141 diaphragms of human cadavers by several investigators using artificial digestion, the infection rate proved to be 1.5%. Hence, it has been assumed that a latent infection is not uncommon in the general population of Hungary.

5.4. Romania

The major reservoir of trichinosis in Romania appears to be wildlife, particularly the carnivores. *Trichinella spiralis* was detected in 24 of 12,000 wild boars (*S. scrofa ferus*) examined during 1956 through 1967, as cited by Cironeanu (1974a). Another 7744 wild boars examined in 1968–1971 revealed 22 (0.284%) to be infected. Most of the infected wild boars came from the northern regions of Moldavia and Transylvania. Cironeanu (1974a) cited the findings of Lupascu and colleagues in 1970, which showed that of the 98 bears (*U. arctos*) examined between 1958 and 1967, 10 (10.2%) were infected. Another study of 306 bears shot in the Carpathians during 1968 and 1971 led to the detection of 20 that were infected. Examination of wild and domestic animals in northern Moldavia from 1956 to 1970 showed the following infection rates (Cironeanu, 1974a): wild boars (*S. scrofa ferus*), 2.08%; bears (*U. arctos*), 18.18%; wolves (*C. lupus*), 100% (2 of 2 animals examined); foxes (*V. vulpes*), 22.55%; martens (*M. martes*), 10.00%; wildcats (*F. silvestris*), 8.33%; polecats (*P. putorius*), 18.51%; dogs (*C. familiaris*),

8.17%; and cats (*F. domestica*), 14.03%. The prevalence of trichinosis in domestic dogs and cats examined since 1956 has shown a rate that was never higher than 3.4%.

In the main slaughterhouses in Romania during 1950–1974, 0.039% of pigs were found to be infected (Cironeanu, 1974b). Of pigs from Moldavia region during a similar period, 1956–1971, 0.076% were infected. There appeared to be a higher frequency of infection in Moldavia, Oltenia, and the midlands of Transylvania. The more recent reports by Cironeanu (1979, 1981) showed that swine trichinosis was found only on small, private farms and not on modern breeding farms where rigorous hygienic measures were maintained. In the last 15 years, no trichinosis has been detected in approximately 3–8 million pigs originating yearly from modern breeding and fattening farms (Cironeanu, 1981). Sporadic outbreaks were attributed to individually raised hogs, probably infected in summer and fall when left free to feed on pastures near forests, rivulets, and floodland, where they could have found carcass remnants of rats or domestic or wild carnivores. *Trichinella* infection within hog-breeding farms was attributed to rats (*R. norvegicus*) (Cironeanu, 1974a). In one outbreak that occurred on a hog-breeding farm, the extent and intensity of the infection were unusually high in both rats and pigs.

Human trichinosis in Romania was largely caused by the ingestion of infected pork, wild boar, or bear meat (Lupascu *et al.*, 1970). Since 1961, reporting of trichinosis has been officially required, which has resulted in a better record of the foci of the infection. Between 1964 and 1968, there were 71 foci involving 1569 cases, of which 423 were hospitalized and 3 died (Lupascu *et al.*, 1970). There were indications of a higher frequency in the northwest region of Romania and in the vicinity of the forests. The Danube plain and Dobroudgea regions had the lowest prevalence rate. During 1975–1980, some cases of human trichinosis resulted from the consumption of venison meat and pork from private farms, although there was not a single case involving meat from a slaughterhouse (Panaitescu *et al.*, 1980).

5.5. Yugoslavia

Trichinosis in wildlife in Yugoslavia has been reported to be widespread, especially in foxes. In 1963–1965, the following animals from several regions of Slovenia were reported to be infected (Brglez *et al.*, 1968): 7 (8.54%) of 82 foxes, 1 (10%) of 10 wild cats, 3 (14.29%) of 21 bears, and 1 (3.45%) of 29 wild boars. When the dry and stored skins were examined by artificial digestion, 1 (2.38%) beech marten, 3

(4.38%) polecats, 1 (8.33%) wildcat, and 156 (26.3%) foxes were found to be infected. The infection rate of foxes was comparable to the rates in other alpine countries, such as northern Italy and Switzerland. Rukavina *et al.* (1968) examined the remains of muscles on dry skins of 4513 foxes, 57 wolves, 56 dogs, 259 badgers, 21 martens, 6 bears, 16 wildcats, 3 lynxes, 6 wild swine, 33 polecats, 6 otters, and 110 bizam rats. In addition, 220 mice and 272 rats were examined. The animals represented various districts. Trichinosis was found in the following animals: foxes (14.06%), wolves (43.86%), dogs (7.13%), and badgers (5.1%). Additional data on wild animals were reported by Rukavina and Brglez (1970), which included infected jackals (25.0%), wildcats (4.58%), minks (1.4%), martens (2.38%), bears (7.04%), wild swine (1.14%), and skunks (1.46%). The infection rate in foxes has varied from 4.93 to 27.7%. The findings in other animals have varied even more. The infection, particularly in foxes, has been diffusely spread throughout the country.

Trichinella has been found in domestic animals, such as dogs (4.15%) and cats (1.23%), as cited by Kozar (1970).

According to Kozar (1970), the infection rate of pigs in Zagreb was only 0.0022% during 1932–1938. Examination of swine conducted between 1945 and 1960 failed to show a single case of swine trichinosis in Bosnia or Herzegowina. During 1957, only 36 cases of swine trichinosis were registered in the entire country as detected by trichinoscopy.

Information is not available on the prevalence of human trichinosis in Yugoslavia.

5.6. Bulgaria

Information on the prevalence of trichinosis in wildlife in Bulgaria is very limited. Stoimenov *et al.* (1966) reported that 12 of 60 (20%) adult foxes (*V. vulpes crucigera*) were found to be infected as determined by the compression method. In his review, Kozar (1970) reported that the infection rate in foxes was 35.3% and in wolves, 55.0%. More recently, Stoimenov and Gradinarski (1981) reported that in a small region, the infection rate among foxes was 47.3%. The infection was detected only twice among boars, within 1 year, in another small region.

Of the domestic animals, the infection rate in dogs was 6.0% and in cats, 7.5% (Kozar, 1970). According to Stoimenov and Gradinarksi (1981), the infection was detected only twice in dogs, within 1 year, in one small district.

The swine infection rate in Bulgaria has dropped from 0.266% in 1910 to 0.01% in 1959 (Kozar, 1970). In 1969, Kallab (1969) reported that of the pigs imported from Bulgaria, approximately 0.035% were infected. More recent reports showed 21 cases of swine trichinosis that were detected by trichinoscopy in three slaughterhouses (Pavlov, 1979). In one small district, the infection was detected 89 times among pigs within 1 year (Stoimenov and Gradinarski, 1981).

Earlier data on human trichinosis in Bulgaria were based on the examination of 632 human cadavers, which revealed only 6 to be infected (Kozar, 1970). More recent information involved 24 human cases in 1978 from a village in the region of Kustendil, a town in the western part of Bulgaria (Pavlov, 1979). These individuals had eaten meat of wild boar that had not been examined by veterinary authorities.

6. UNION OF SOVIET SOCIALIST REPUBLICS

There have been numerous reviews of the epizootiology and epidemiology of trichinosis in the U.S.S.R., most of them in Russian. However, Merkushev (1970) has given an account in English of the infection in the U.S.S.R. More recently, Bessonov (1974) has analyzed the data on the epizootic and epidemiological situation of trichinosis in the U.S.S.R.

Merkushev (1970) summarized the results of examination of wildlife up to 1966, covering all geographic areas of the country. Trichinosis was most frequent among wolves (*C. lupus*), 61.0%; lynx (*F. lynx*), 34.9%; badgers (*M. meles*), 21.7%; raccoon-dog (*Nyctereutes procyonoides*), 19.0%; foxes (*V. vulpes*), 17.7%; and bears (*U. arctos*), 15.0%. The rate of infection varied according to the geographic area and climatic zone. For example, the rate of infection among wolves in eastern Siberia was lower than in the European part of the country. The infection was also found in the jackal (*C. aureus*), polar fox (*A. lagopus*), wildcat (*F. silvestris*), tiger (*F. tigris*), marten (*M. martes*), sable (*M. zibellina*), Siberian ferret (*M. sibiricus*), mink (*M. lutreaola*), polecat (*M. putorius*), weasel (*M. nivalis*), ermine (*M. erminea*), glutton (*G. gulo*), wild boar (*S. scrofa*), white bear (*T. maritimus*), Pinnipedia, shrew (*Soricidae*), mole (*Talpidae*), hedgehog (*Erinaceus europaeus*), red squirrel (*S. vulgaris*), and mice from forests and steppes. According to Bessonov (1974), trichinosis has been reported in 57 species of wild and domestic animals, including 34 species of carnivores, 14 species of rodents, 5 species of insectivores, 2 species of sea mammals, and 2 species of artiodactyls. The rates of infection among the carnivores differed somewhat from those cited earlier by Merkushev (1970), although both reported the highest rate for wolves. Bessonov's analysis of the data gave the following infection rates: wolf (*C. lupus*), 51 ± 1.24%; jackal (*C. aureus*), 36.58 ± 4.34%; wildcat (*F. silvestris*), 36.26 ± 5.04%; stone marten (*M. foina*), 27.73 ± 4.28%; raccoon-dog (*N. procyonoides*), 23.7 ± 0.959%; and fox (*V. vulpes*), 18.4 ± 0.430%.

Lukashenko *et al.* (1971), in their review of trichinosis in animals in the northern region of Chukotka in 1960–1968, reported that *Trichinella* was detected in 16.4% of the animals. The highest rate of infection was in blue polar foxes (*A. alopex*) kept in cages, 44.8%, followed by white polar foxes (*A. lagopus*), 18.2%; common foxes (*V. vulpes*), 17.5%; silver black foxes kept in cages, 15.5%; and the domestic dog (*C. familiaris*), 12.1%. The high incidence of trichinosis among blue polar foxes and silver black foxes on fur-animal farms in Chukotka where the food fed was predominantly the flesh of marine animals, such as walruses and pinnipeds, suggested that the marine mammals may be one of the sources of infection for caged animals.

The distribution of the infection in the Soviet Arctic is very different, in that the infection is common in both terrestrial and marine mammals. Merkushev (1963) examined 7 species and was able to demonstrate the parasite in seals, polar bears, ermines, and polar foxes.

Until rather recently, Kazakhstan was considered to be free from trichinosis. Boev *et al.* (1970) reported finding *Trichinella* in 15 species of wildlife, with high infection rates in wolf (*C. lupus*), 41.0%; stone marten (*M. foina*), 29.0%; bear (*U. arctos*), 20.0%; and fox (*V. vulpes*), 11.6%.

In Georgia, the highest rates of infection by *Trichinella* were recorded for stone marten (40.0%) and the jackal (36.6%), followed by the mountain fox (22.2%) and the steppe fox (20.2%), as reported by Kurashvili *et al.* (1970).

In the Latvian S.S.R., as in many parts of the U.S.S.R., the highest rate of infection was found in wolves (37.8%) (Viksne, 1970). Reports from Byelorussia also showed a high infection rate in wolves (28.5%) and in foxes (34.1%) (Goregljad and Bogush, 1970).

Trichinosis has been reported for synanthropic animals, i.e., cats, dogs, rats, and mice (Merkushev, 1970). The frequency of infection has been reported as follows: 13.0% for cats (*F. catus domestica*), 2.7% for dogs (*C. familiaris*), 1.6% for gray and black rats (*R. norvegicus and R. rattus*), and 0.77% for mice. Bessonov (1974) quoted an infection rate of 2.67 ± 0.105% for domestic dogs and 7.67 ± 0.281% for domestic cats.

The distribution of trichinosis in swine is not uniform throughout the U.S.S.R. The chief focus of infection was reported to be in Byelorussia, where more than half of all infected animals were found

(Merkushev, 1970; Bessonov, 1974), followed by the Ukrainian S.S.R. and then the Russian S.F.S.R. In Byelorussia, the infection rate in swine was 0.15–0.20%. During recent years, the rate of swine trichinosis has been declining in a number of districts of the U.S.S.R. due to advances in animal husbandry and other social and cultural changes. Such improvements have lowered the infection rate in swine in Byelorussia from 0.18% in 1956 to 0.02% in 1967 (Goregljad and Bogush, 1970).

Human trichinosis in the U.S.S.R. was caused in most cases (92.4%) by consumption of pork from pigs slaughtered at home and rarely (2.9%) by consumption of meat of wildlife (Bessonov, 1974). The highest rate of infection in humans (82.9%) was reported from Byelorussia (Bessonov, 1974). For example, from 1946 to 1967, approximately 12,000 cases of clinical trichinosis in humans were registered in the U.S.S.R., of which more than 80.0% were from the Byelorussian S.S.R. (Bessonov, 1972). The high incidence in this area was attributed to the habit of eating raw, smoked, or salted sausages and ham, to the custom of allowing pigs to graze in forests, and to the practice of slaughtering pigs at home. Human infections have also been traced to the use of salt lard containing streaks of muscle that were consumed without cooking. In the Ukraine, it was determined that 33.0% of the cases were due to lard, 21.0% to inadequately roasted or boiled pork, and the rest to homemade sausages or ham (Merkushev, 1970).

According to the data from examination of human cadavers, the infection rate of the U.S.S.R. population was 1.5 ± 0.12% (Bessonov, 1972, 1974). As assessed by the compression method only, the infection rate decreased from 1.5% in 1952 to 1.145% ± 0.102% in 1969, a decrease of 23.7% (Bessonov, 1974). Bessonov and Kaportseva (1968) had shown earlier that this method could not detect mild or very mild infections. They examined in two Moscow hospitals 407 cadavers and detected only 0.98% with trichinoscopy, but 4.17% by artificial digestion.

Human trichinosis was reported from other regions, such as the Lithuanian S.S.R., where, from 1955 to 1967, 196 persons were hospitalized for trichinosis (Biziulevicius et al., 1970). The infection was diagnosed in 26 individuals in 1976, 103 in 1977, and 35 in 1978 (Biziulevicius and Vitkauskiene, 1979). Obligatory trichinoscopy of all swine and boar carcasses remains the main control measure against human trichinosis in Lithuania.

From 1963 to 1965, human trichinosis was reported in the Latvian S.S.R., involving 36 individuals of hunter families, of whom 19 were hospitalized (Viksne, 1970). The infection was attributed to the consumption of wild boar meat.

In the Kazakhstan region, two outbreaks of human trichinosis involved 34 cases, of which 4 (11.8%) died (Boev *et al.*, 1970). Three had eaten wild boar meat, while one had eaten bear meat.

With the steady decline of swine trichinosis in Byelorussia, the Ukraine, and the southern Russian S.F.S.R., particularly Lithuania, the incidence of human infection has decreased. However, isolated outbreaks of human trichinosis have occurred quite often in the last few years, due to the consumption of meat from wild boar, bear, badger, and other wildlife. In 1975, 96% of all cases in the R.S.F.S.R. were infected by consumption of meat of wild boar and bear, and in Lithuania, all cases of human trichinosis coincided with the hunting season (Bessonov, 1981).

7. ASIA

7.1. Middle East

Data on trichinosis in the Middle East are fragmentary at best. Yamashita (1970), in his review, reported the presence of the infection in the dog, lynx, fox, jackal, mongoose, and wild boar in Israel, although no human case of trichinosis had been reported in over 80 years. The absence of human infection can be attributed to religious customs or sanitary measures that prevent man from eating raw pork.

The incidence of human and animal trichinosis in Lebanon is unknown, although according to Steele and Schultz (1978), Lebanon has probably the greatest trichinosis problem in that area. They cited outbreaks that occurred in 1939 involving 500 cases. It was found that 30.0% of the pigs slaughtered in Beirut were infected. Later investigations showed swine infection rates of 15.0 and 25.0% and a rat infection rate of 36.0%. Matossian *et al.* (1974) reported a small outbreak of trichinosis in a small community in Mount Lebanon involving 50 individuals, of whom 37 required treatment. Consumption of raw pork, and mutton adulterated with infected pork in the form of "kubbeh nayyeh," was responsible for the outbreak.

In 1977, Merdivenci *et al.* (1977) reported infection in a wild pig that was hunted in the mountainous region of Kastamonu, transported to Istanbul, and slaughtered without being examined by a veterinarian. Of 13 individuals who ate this pork, all developed trichinosis, confirmed by muscle biopsy. This was the first account of human trichinosis in Turkey. These findings suggested that sylvatic trichinosis existed in Turkey.

The first report of the existence of trichinosis in Iran was that of Afshar and Jahfarzadeh (1967). Between 1961 and 1967, the examination of 4950 carcasses of wild boars (*S. scrofa*) that were hunted in the central northern area of Iran revealed the infection in 2. Trichinosis among wildlife in the Caspian Sea area of northern Iran was reported by Mobedi *et al.* (1973). Of 21,143 wild boars (*S. scrofa*) that were mainly from the eastern half of the Caspian region, 5 were found to be infected, and 1 brown bear (*U. arctos*) from the Nour Forest near the city of Amal was the only one infected of the 16 bears examined. Among the carnivores examined, 38 (60%) of 63 golden jackals (*C. aureus*) and 2 of 3 jungle cats (*F. chaus*) were found to be infected. The highest incidence in jackals was in those hunted in the Nour Forest near Amal. These findings indicated the presence of a sylvatic focus of trichinosis in the Caspian area.

In a study to determine the presence of *Trichinella* in carnivores and rodents in Central (Isfahan) Iran (Sadighian *et al.*, 1973), the following animals were found to be infected: 2 stray dogs, 10 jackals, 2 red foxes, 1 hyena, and 1 rodent (*Meriones persicus*). The finding of the infected rodent was of interest, since not a single rodent in the northern region was found to be infected (Mobedi *et al.*, 1973). A more recent report indicated that trichinosis was enzootic in Iran. Massoud (1978) found *Trichinella* in jackals (55.7%), foxes (8.3%), hyenas (2 of 2), dogs (4.2%), wild boars (25.0%), and brown bears (6.2%). The boars were from the southern region of Khuzestan; the jackals were from the northern (Caspian), central (Isfahan), and southern (Khuzestan) regions. According to Mobedi *et al.* (1973), the only human trichinosis on record in Iran is the single doubtful case reported in 1966 by Moin, who made the diagnosis on clinical symptoms, history of eating undercooked wild boar flesh, and the presence of low-titer circulating antibody.

The first account of trichinosis in Afghanistan was by Kullmann (1966), who found the infection in a lynx (*F. chaus*), wolf (*C. lupus*), jackal (*C. aureus*), and red fox (*V. vulpes*) that had been shot in Afghanistan. The jackal was most heavily infected. When a greater number of mammals from nearly all the provinces of the country was examined (Kullman, 1970), the mongoose (*H. auropunctatus*) and Afghan hedgehogs (*Hemiechinus megalotis*) were found to be infected. These findings showed that there was a natural focus of trichinosis in Afghanistan. However, abstinence from eating pork due to religious prohibition has been responsible for the absence of human infection.

Epidemiological data on trichinosis in India are sparse, except for some accounts earlier in this century. In 1942, Maplestone and Bhaduri

(1942) found 1 heavily infected cat after examining 100 pigs, 100 dogs, 100 rats, and 74 cats. This finding definitely established the presence of *T. spiralis* in India. Kalapesi and Rao (1954) also found *Trichinella* in a cat that died in the Zoological Gardens in Bombay. Later, a wild toddy cat (*Paradoxurus hermaphroditus*) captured in East Calcutta in an area widely separated from any possible exotic source of the parasite was found to be infected (Parmeter *et al.*, 1968). The third finding of *Trichinella* in Calcutta was reported by Schad and Chowdhury (1967) in a wild civet cat (*Viverricula indica bengalensis*). According to Kalapesi and Rao (1954), the infection has been found in a pig in northern India and in squirrels in Lucknow and probably exists in man despite the lack of reference to it in recent literature.

7.2. Southeast Asia

The only information available on trichinosis in Thailand is accounts of outbreaks of human trichinosis. During 1962–1964, three outbreaks were reported in northern Thailand (Dissamarn and Chai-Ananda, 1966). In the third outbreak in Mae Ngon district involving 258 cases and 15 deaths, the source of infection was a wild pig that had been hunted near the Burmese border. Examination of 50 pigs in the area as well as a few specimens of wild animals proved to be negative. In 1965, however, 11.43% of hilltribe pigs from three provinces (Chiengmai, Prae, and Nan) were infected. The level of infection was 7–5570 larvae/100 g muscle. In the province of Prae, 1 of 12 rats (*R. rattus*) was also positive. There was no human trichinosis among the people in this region, since they ate well-cooked meat. An epidemic of trichinosis that occurred in 1967 was reported by Doege *et al.* (1969). Of 20 hunters, 13 became acutely ill after shooting a Himalayan bear and eating the meat raw with chili peppers. They all had to be hospitalized. An outbreak of trichinosis that occurred in Chiang Mai Province in 1975 was attributed to raw meat in the form of "lahbor nahm," a favorite dish of northern Thailand (Khamboonruang *et al.*, 1978). To establish the epidemiology of the disease, particularly the role of rodents in the transmission cycle, 1070 rodents were examined, but all proved to be negative. Of the 7598 pig diaphragms examined by digestion, only one diaphragm harbored the parasite (42 larvae per gram). The epidemiology of trichinosis in Thailand is still unclear due to the rarity of the infection in urban rodents and the lack of extensive surveys in wildlife. However, the hilltribe pig has been shown to be the major reservoir host for human infections (Dissamarn *et al.*, 1980).

Recently, there was a report of an outbreak of human trichinosis in Laos (Sicard *et al.*, 1976). Fifty patients were hospitalized at Vientiane during 1975 after eating pork (*som-mou*, *lap mou*, and *lap leuat*).

Holz (1962) reported that pigs were infected in Indonesia. The infection rate ranged from 3.06% in 1930 to 1.66% in 1939. The incidence among dogs was 1.54% in 1932 and 0.56% in 1939. Much later, Holz (1979) confirmed the presence of trichinosis in swine in Indonesia and pointed out that the local custom of cooking meat extremely well has been responsible for the absence of human trichinosis in Indonesia.

Trichinosis has not been observed in domestic or wild animals in the Philippines. Tacal and Pabello (1965) did not detect the parasite in any of the muscle samples from 260 brown rats (*R. norvegicus*) trapped in Manila and its suburbs, using both the compression and digestion methods. Of 46 serum samples from pigs slaughtered at the Manila abattoir, all were negative for trichinosis using the latex-agglutination test (Arambulo *et al.*, 1970). The negative findings lend support to the accepted assumption that trichinosis has not been established in the Philippines, at least not in rats and pigs.

7.3. Far East

Trichinosis in Japan was first recorded in a dog in Hokkaido in 1957. According to Steele and Schultz (1978), the infection was also found in a zoo polar bear in Hokkaido, and was attributed to dog meat that was fed to the zoo animals.

Up to 1974, the presence of human trichinosis in Japan was not conclusively known. In 1974, however, in a small village in Aomori Prefecture, in northern Honshu, a group of hunters contracted trichinosis after eating raw bear meat (Yamaguchi, 1978). Before the outbreak, no wildlife infection that could serve as the reservoir for human infection had been known. In July of the same year, *T. spiralis* was detected in the muscle of a dog in the same village.

In China, the presence of *Trichinella* has been known since 1881, when Patrick Manson found the parasite in two of 225 samples of pork in Amoy (Yamashita, 1970). As recorded by the same author, there were numerous reports of *Trichinella* infection in China prior to World War II, with the prevalence being high in dogs in some areas (20.8% in South Manchuria) but being very low in man and in swine. The rarity of infection in man is assumed to be due to the custom of cutting the pork into very small pieces and cooking the meat thoroughly. Data on the present status of trichinosis in China are very sparse. In recent years two clinical outbreaks in mainland China have been reported, one attributed to ingesting raw bear meat and another to uncooked mutton (WHO, 1982). The first documented outbreak of trichinosis in Hong Kong Chinese also has been reported recently (Pun *et al.*, in press).

There is no information available on the prevalence of trichinosis in man or animals in Korea.

8. AFRICA

Following an unconfirmed outbreak of trichinosis in Egypt in 1975, a survey was done to determine the prevalence of *Trichinella* in pigs slaughtered at the Cairo abattoir. Of more than 40,000 carcasses examined, 4.5% were infected. This very high prevalence was attributed to unhygienic swine management, including the feeding of uncooked garbage (El-Nawawi, 1981).

Trichinosis in Africa has received a comprehensive review by Nelson (1970). In 1961, it was shown for the first time that trichinosis was enzootic in the wildlife of East Africa, but it is now evident that the parasite is probably present in most areas of Africa south of the Sahara.

When *Trichinella* was found in man in 1961 (see below), a search was made for the parasite in wildlife (Nelson *et al.*, 1961). Of 537 animals examined, most were negative. However, *Trichinella* larvae were found in a leopard (*Panthera pardus*) collected near Kerugoya on the lower slopes of Mount Kenya and in a hyena (*C. crocuta*) from the Masai plains more than 100 miles from Kerugoya. The following year, a striped jackal (*Canis adustus*) from Narok was found to be infected (Nelson and Forrester, 1962). By 1963, more than 2000 wild animals, representing more than 50 species, had been examined in the search for natural hosts of *T. spiralis* in East Africa (Nelson and Mukundi, 1963; Nelson *et al.*, 1963). *Trichinella spiralis* was found in the bush pig (*Potamocherus porcus*), lion (*Leo leo*), leopard (*P. pardus*), serval cat (*F. serval*), spotted hyena (*Crocuta crocuta*), striped hyena (*H. hyaena*), side-striped jackal (*C. adustus*), and wild dog (*Lycaon pictus*). Of 4 lions (*L. leo*) examined in Kenya, 1 from the Ngong hills, near Nairobi, was infected with 15 *Trichinella* larvae per gram of diaphragm (Nelson, 1970). Four leopards (*P. pardus*) were examined in Kenya, of which one from the lower slopes of Mount Kenya was found to be infected. One serval (*F. serval*) that had been shot on a poultry farm near Nairobi was infected; its diaphragm contained more than 50 larvae per gram of muscle.

Of 23 spotted hyenas (*C. crocuta*) from Kenya and Tanzania that were examined, 10 were found to be infected with larval densities ranging from 0.5 to 31 larvae per gram (Nelson *et al.*, 1963). Sachs and Taylor (1966) also found 1 of 3 spotted hyenas from Tanzania to be infected. The occurrence of *T. spiralis* had never been reported in Tanzania prior to this finding. Later, Sachs (1970) reported that the spotted hyena was more frequently infected than other carnivores and that it should be regarded as the main reservoir of trichinosis in Africa. The distribution of the striped hyena (*H. hyaena*) is limited in Africa. Of 2 from Kenya that were examined, 1 was found to be infected with a density of 9 larvae per gram in the diaphragm (Nelson, 1970). Two specimens of the side-striped jackal (*C. adustus*) were examined; one had 30 *T. spiralis* larvae per gram of leg muscle.

The domestic dog (*C. familiaris*) was the first nonhuman animal to be found infected with *T. spiralis* (Nelson *et al.*, 1961; Nelson and Forrester, 1962). Of 30 dogs examined, 2 were infected, having 5 and 7 larvae per gram of muscle (Nelson *et al.*, 1963). Both were known to have eaten the meat of bush pigs, which also proved to be the source of human infections. It is interesting to note that from the first discovery of trichinosis in Kenya, it has been emphasized that rodents play no part in the maintenance of the infection in Kenya (Nelson and Mukundi, 1963; Nelson *et al.*, 1963). *Trichinella spiralis* has not been recorded from domestic pigs in Africa south of the Sahara (Nelson and Forrester, 1962).

An outbreak among 9 Europeans in Dakar in 1966 was attributed to the flesh of the warthog (*Phacochoerus aethiopicus*), hunted in Boundoum, the Senegal Delta (Gretillat and Vassiliadès, 1968). These authors also reported finding the infection in a jackal (*C. adustus*). Trichinoscopic examination of the carcasses of the jackal and the warthog shot during several safaris in the Senegal Delta and Lac de Guiers region again implicated these species as reservoirs of *T. spiralis* in West Africa (Gretillat, 1970a,b).

The first reported cases of trichinosis in South Africa were in a lion (*L. leo krugeri*), spotted hyena (*C. crocuta*), black-backed jackal (*C. mesomelas mesomelas*), and multimammate rat [*Praomys (Mastomys) natalensis*] from the Kruger National Park (E. Young and Kruger, 1967).

Human trichinosis in East Africa was reported by Forrester *et al.* (1961). No previous record of trichinosis in man or animals had been reported from any African country south of the Sahara before this account. In 1959, 11 males from villages in the lower slopes of Mount Kenya were hospitalized with severe symptoms of trichinosis. All cases were confirmed by muscle biopsy with larval densities that averaged nearly 2000 larvae per gram of muscle. A 7-year-old patient who died had 3429 larvae per gram of muscle. Later, it was discovered that they had all eaten meat from the same bush pig (*P. porcus*) (Nelson and Forrester, 1962). A new focus of trichinosis was reported in Nakuru, which is 100 miles from Mt. Kenya. Laboratory studies confirmed an epidemiological suspicion that the Kenya strain isolated from man and wildlife had an exceptionally low infectivity for rodents and swine compared to the European strains (Nelson, 1970), and it has been suggested that the parasite represents a separate species (see Chapter 2). In 1972, there was a report of a family outbreak of trichinosis in the Kajiado District, Kenya (Hutcheon and Pamba, 1972). The infected children claimed to have eaten a "roasted pig." Recently, Kaminsky and Zimmermann (1977) reported a Kenyan case of lymphocytic lymphoma involving the periorbital connective tissue and extraocular muscles, with an incidental finding of an encapsulated *T. spiralis* within the extraocular muscle. An addendum to the report noted another case of trichinosis diagnosed incidentally in a biopsy taken from a suppurating back lesion. These findings raise questions as to the real incidence of human trichinosis in Kenya.

Human trichinosis in Tanzania was first reported by Bura and Willett (1977) in 11 members of the Iragw tribe from Mbulu district, not far from national game parks. Two of the cases were fatal. The source of the outbreak was probably meat of the warthog (*P. aethiopicus*). The authors suggested that the epidemiology of trichinosis in Tanzania was changing and the infection was becoming a potential public health problem. The people of that area have recently begun raising domestic pigs and selling them over a wide area, creating a potential for rapid dissemination of the infection.

9. AUSTRALIA, NEW ZEALAND, AND PACIFIC ISLANDS

The incidental historical accounts of human trichinosis in Australia have been reviewed by Alicata (1970), but there is no defnite evidence that *T. spiralis* has ever been endemic in Australia. Attempts to demonstrate the parasite in wildlife and swine have failed. All of 62 stray cats and 178 wild rats (*R. norvegicus*) caught in the Brisbane area and examined by the digestion method failed to reveal any *T. spiralis* larvae (Waddell, 1969).

New Zealand, like Australia, has reported incidental cases of human trichinosis over the years. Prompted by an indigenous human case in 1964, a survey was conducted to determine the prevalence of trichinosis in animals of the area, particularly in pigs (Cairns, 1966). The investigation showed that the following animals were infected: 4 of 8696 pigs, 5 of 1433 wild rats, and 2 of 28 cats. However, 10 years later, in 1975–1976, no cases of trichinosis were reported in wildlife, domestic animals, or humans (Mason, 1978).

Sixty serum samples from Western Samoa were tested for *Trichinella* antibodies by the Suessenguth–Kline flocculation test; only one sample was positive, at 1:20 dilution, and that was from a boy suffering from typhoid fever (Berman and Weinstein, 1970). Forty-nine samples from the Fiji Islands were negative. These findings support the assumption that trichinosis is absent in the South Pacific Islands.

The only area in the Pacific in which trichinosis has been reported to be indigenous is the Hawaiian Islands. The incidence in rodents varied from 0.01% in Maui to 2.7% in Hawaii (Alicata, 1970). Of the various species of rats examined from the island of Hawaii, the infection rates were 4.8% in *R. norvegicus*, 2.9% in *R. rattus*, 0.5% in *R. rattus alexandrinus*, and 0.2% in *R. exulans*. The mongoose (*H. javanicus auropunctatus*) from the island of Hawaii had an infection rate of 21.4% (15 of 70), and those from the island of Maui, 9.1% (2 of 22). Trichinosis in wild hogs has been found only on the island of Hawaii. Although this host is believed to be the main source of human infection in the Hawaiian Islands, trichinosis has been rare in domesticated pigs, probably due to hygienic swine-feeding.

The incidental cases of human trichinosis in Hawaii have been reviewed by Alicata (1970). In most cases, the source of the infection was attributed to improperly cooked flesh of wild pig. According to Alicata, examination of 133 autopsies showed 7.4% to contain *Trichinella* larvae (in these cases, the source of the infection could not be ascertained). More recently, an epidemic of trichinosis was reported in which 45% of the adults who ate roast wild pig at a barbecue in Hawaii became ill (Barrett-Conner *et al.*, 1976).

REFERENCES

Afshar, A., and Jahfarzadeh, Z., 1967, Trichinosis in Iran, *Ann. Trop. Med. Parasitol.* **61**:349–351.

Alicata, J., 1970, Trichinosis in the Pacific Islands and adjacent areas, in: *Trichinosis in Man and Animals* (S.E. Gould, ed.), Charles C. Thomas, Springfield, Illinois, pp. 465–472.

Alicata, J.E., and Amiel, D.K., 1971, On the absence of *Trichinella spiralis* in mongooses and rodents in Jamaica, West Indies, *J. Parasitol.* **57**:807.

Alvarez, V., Rivera, G., Neghme, A., and Schenone, H., 1970, Triquinosis en animales de Chile, *Bol. Chil. Parasitol.* **25**:83–86.

Arambulo, P.V., III, Hicarter, V.P., Coda, A.B., and Sarmiento, R.V., 1970, On the serologic screening for trichinosis of pigs slaughtered in the Manila Abattoir, *Philipp. J. Vet. Med.* **9**:104–107.

Artois, M., 1978, First results of an investigation on trichinosis in wildlife in France (1976–1977), *Ann. Parasitol. Hum. Comp.* **53**:533–537.

Babero, B.B., 1960, A survey of parasitism in skunks (*Mephitis mephitis*) in Louisiana, with observations on pathological damages due to helminthiasis, *J. Parasitol.* **46**(Suppl.):26–27.

Bair, R.D., and Etges, F.J., 1969, Trichiniasis in man and animals in Cincinnati, Ohio, *J. Parasitol.* **55**:369–371.

Barr, R., 1966, Human trichinosis, *Can. Med. Assoc. J.* **95**:912–917.

Barrett-Conner, E., Davis, C.F., Hamburger, R.N., and Kagan, I., 1976, An epidemic of trichinosis after ingestion of wild pig in Hawaii, *J. Infect. Dis.* **133**:473–477.

Barriga, O.O., 1966, Prevalence of some parasitic zoonosis in fat stock and its impact on our national economy, *Wiad. Parazytol.* **12**:677.

Beard, R.R., 1951, Incidence of *Trichinella* infections in San Francisco, *J. Am. Med. Assoc.* **146**:331–334.

Beck, J.W., 1953, Xenodiagnosis techniques as an aid to diagnosis of trichinosis, *Am. J. Trop. Med. Hyg.* **2**:97–101.

Beckett, J.V., and Gallicchio, V., 1967, A survey of helminths of the muskrat, *Ondrata z. zibethica* Miller, 1912, in Portage County, Ohio, *J. Parasitol.* **53**:1169–1172.

Bellani, L., Mantovani, A., Pampiglione, S., and Filippini, I., 1978, Observations on an outbreak of human trichinellosis in northern Italy, in: *Trichinellosis* (C.W. Kim and Z.S. Pawlowski, eds.), University Press of New England, Hanover, New Hampshire, pp. 535–539.

Berman, H., and Weinstein, L., 1970, Search for *Trichinella* infection in western Samoa and Fiji, *Med. J. Aust.* **2**:583–584.

Bessonov, A.S., 1972, *Epizootiology and Control of Trichinellosis*, "Mintis," Vilnius, pp. 295–302.

Bessonov, A.S., 1974, Epizoology and epidemiology of trichinellosis in the U.S.S.R.: Prospects for eradication of the infection, in: *Trichinellosis* (C.W. Kim, ed.), Intext, New York, pp. 557–562.

Bessonov, A.S., 1981, Changes in the epizootic and epidemic situation of trichinellosis in the USSR, in: *Trichinellosis* (C.W. Kim, E.J. Ruitenberg, and J.S. Teppema, eds.) Reedbooks, Chertsey, England, pp. 365–368.

Bessonov, A.S., and Kaportseva, G.K., 1968, Trichinellosis in the autopsy material of Moscow hospitals, *Wiad. Parazytol.* **14**:244.

Bilbao, G.S., 1965, Nuevos casos de triquinosis en Coronel Pringles, Pcia, Buenos Aires, *Wiad. Parazytol.* **12**:677.

Biziulevicius, S., and Vitkauskiene, J., 1979, Trichinellosis in the Lithuanian SSR, *Wiad. Parazytol.* **25**:595–596.

Biziulevicius, S., Burakauskas, A., Kairiukstis, J., Svabonas, E., and Simkuniene, B., 1970, Trichinellosis in Lithuania, *Wiad. Parazytol.* **16**:71–72.

Boev, S.N., Bondareva, V.I., Sokolova, I.B., and Tazieva, Z.H., 1970, A study on the distribution of trichinellosis in Kazakhstan, *Wiad. Parazytol.* **16**:74–75.

Boron, P., Kolloto-Szymajda, B., Jezyna, C., and Klimowicz, J., 1978, Epidemiology of trichinellosis in the Bialystok Province (Poland), 1946–1973, in: *Trichinellosis* (C.W. Kim and Z.S. Pawlowski, eds.), University Press of New England, Hanover, New Hampshire, pp. 529–534.

Bouree, P., Kouchner, G., Gascon, A., Fruchter, J., Passeron, J., and Bouvier, J.B., 1977, Trichinosis: Review of the epidemic in the south suburbs of Paris in January, 1976 (125 cases), *Ann. Med. Intern.* **128:**647–654.

Bouree, P., Bouvier, J.B., Passeron, J., Galanaud, P., and Dormont, J., 1979, Outbreak of trichinosis near Paris, *Br. Med. J.* **1:**1047–1049.

Bourns, T.K.R., 1952, The discovery of trichina cysts in the diaphragm of a six week-old child, *J. Parasitol.* **38:**367.

Bouvier, G., 1966, Geographic distribution of some diseases in game and wild animals in Switzerland, *Wiad. Parazytol.* **12:**679.

Bowmer, E.J., 1974, Trichinosis in British Columbia: Eight incidents traced to pork and bear meat, in: *Trichinellosis* (C.W. Kim, ed.), Intext, New York, pp. 531–538.

Brglez, J., Rakovec, R., and Valentinic, S., 1968, Trichinellosis in foxes and other wild animals in the SR of Slovenia, *Wiad. Parazytol.* **14:**244.

Bura, M.W., and Willett, W.C., 1977, An outbreak of trichinosis in Tanzania, *E. Afr. Med. J.* **54:**185–193.

Cairns, G.C., 1966, The occurrence of *Trichinella spiralis* in New Zealand pigs, rats and cats, *N. Z. Vet. J.* **14:**84–88.

Cameron, T.W.M., 1943, Studies on trichinosis. IV. Human incidence in Montreal, *Can. J. Res.* **21:**413–414.

Cameron, T.W.M., 1970, Trichinosis in Canada, in: *Trichinosis in Man and Animals* (S.E. Gould, ed.), Charles C. Thomas, Springfield, Illinois, pp. 374–377.

Centers for Disease Control, 1968, Trichinosis Surveillance, Annual Summary 1967.

Centers for Disease Control, 1976, Trichinosis Surveillance, Annual Summary 1975.

Centers for Disease Control, 1980, Trichinosis Surveillance, Annual Summary 1979.

Centers for Disease Control, 1981, Annual Summary 1980, *Morbid. Mortal. Weekly Rep.* **29**(54).

Centers for Disease Control, 1982, Annual Summary 1981, *Morbid. Mortal. Weekly Rep.* **30**(50–52).

Chicoine, L., Proulx, C., Lafleur, L., and Tanner, C.E., 1966, Trichinosis: An epidemiological study in children using five immunological methods, *Can. J. Public Health* **57:**357–365.

Cironeanu, I., 1974a, Trichinellosis in domestic and wild animals in Rumania, in: *Trichinellosis* (C.W. Kim, ed.), Intext, New York, pp. 549–555.

Cironeanu, I., 1974b, Achievements and prospects of trichinellosis control in Romania, *Wiad. Parazytol.* **20:**141–145.

Cironeanu, I., 1979, Trichinellosis in Romania, *Wiad. Parazytol.* **25:**597–598.

Cironeanu, I., 1981, The absence of *Trichinella spiralis* in modern farms of swine, in: *Trichinellosis* (C.W. Kim, E.J. Ruitenberg, and J.S. Teppema, eds.), Reedbooks, Chertsey, England, pp. 377–379.

Clark, P.S., Brownberger, K.M., Asalow, A.R., Kagan, I.G., Noble, C.R., and Maynard, J.E., 1972, Bear meat trichinosis: Epidemiologic, serologic and clinical observations from two Alaskan outbreaks, *Ann. Intern. Med.* **76:**951–956.

Clausen, B., 1978, Ecological factors in spreading *Trichinella spiralis* in Denmark, in: *Trichinellosis* (C.W. Kim and Z.S. Pawlowski, eds.), University Press of New England, Hanover, New Hampshire, pp. 541–544.

Clausen, B., and Henriksen, S.A., 1976, The prevalence of *Trichinella spiralis* in foxes (*Vulpes vulpes*) and other game species in Denmark, *Nord. Vet. Med.* **28**:265–270.

Coffey, J.E., and Wiglesworth, F.W., 1956, Trichinosis in Canadian Eskimos, *Can. Med. Assoc. J.* **75**:295–299.

Cordero del Campillo, M., Martinez Fernandez, A., and Aller Gancedo, B., 1970, Some facts concerning the epizootiology of trichinellosis in Spain, *Wiad. Parazytol.* **16**:100–108.

Corridan, J.P., and Gray, J.J., 1969, Trichinosis in south-west Ireland, *Br. Med. J.* **2**:727–730.

Corridan, J.P., and O'Meara, P.B., 1968, Trichinosis in Cork, *Ir. J. Med. Sci. 7th Ser.* **1**:109–113.

Corridan, J.P., O'Rourke, F.J., and Verling, M., 1969, *Trichinella spiralis* in the red fox (*Vulpes vulpes*) in Ireland, *Nature (London)* **222**:1191.

Czarnowski, A., and Przyborowski, T., 1970, Trichinellosis of rats and fur-animals in the surroundings of Gdansk and Gdynia, *Wiad. Parazytol.* **16**:119–120.

Davies, L.E.C., and Cameron, T.W.M., 1961, Trichinosis in the North West Territories, *Med. Serv. J. Can.* **17**:99–104.

DeGiusti, D.L., and Field, W., 1952, A survey of *Trichinella spiralis* in rats, dogs, and cats in Detroit, *J. Parasitol.* **38**(Suppl.):16.

Dissamarn, R., and Chai-Ananda, P., 1966, The present position of trichinosis in Thailand, *Wiad. Parazytol.* **12**:678.

Dissamarn, R., Chai-Anan, P., and Aranyakananda, P., 1980, Prevalence of trichinellosis in Thailand, Fifth International Conference on Trichinellosis (abstract), The Netherlands, p. 138.

Doege, T.C., Theinprasit, P., Headington, T., Pongprot, B., and Tarawanich, S., 1969, Trichinosis and raw bear meat in Thailand, *Lancet* **1**:459–461.

Dyer, W.G., 1970, Helminths of the striped skunk, *Mephitis mephitis* Schreber, in North Dakota, *Proc. Helminthol. Soc. Wash.* **37**:92–93.

Ekstam, M., 1966, Trichinellosis, *Wiad. Parazytol.* **12**:679–680.

El-Nawawi, F.A., 1981, Swine trichinellosis in Egypt, *Arch. Lebensmittelhyg.* **32**:156–158.

Emson, H.E., Baltzan, M.A., and Wiens, H.E., 1972, Trichinosis in Saskatchewan, *Can. Med. Assoc. J.* **106**:897–898.

Ernst, S., and Aguilar, H., 1978, Frequency of some parasitic zoonoses in slaughtered animals in the province of Valdivia (Chile) 1970–1976, *Bol. Chil. Parasitol.* **33**:66–69.

Evans, C.H., Jr., 1938, Trichinosis in Cleveland: Post-mortem examination of diaphragm and skeletal muscle from 100 consecutive autopsies, *J. Infect. Dis.* **63**:337–339.

Faubert, G.M., Péchère, J.C., Delisle, R., Smith, H.-C., and Brindle, Y., 1981, An outbreak of trichinellosis in Canada: The enzyme linked immunosorbent assay (ELISA) and clinical findings, in: *Trichinellosis* (C.W. Kim, E.J. Ruitenberg, and J.S. Teppema, eds.), Reedbooks, Chertsey, England, pp. 269–274.

Famerée, L., Cotteleer, C., Van den Abbeele, O., Mollaert, P., Engles, L., and Colin, G., 1981, Recherches épidémiologiques sur la trichinose sauvage en Belgique: Resultats préliminaires et incidence alimentaire, *Schweiz. Arch. Tierheilkd.* **123**:145–155.

Forrester, A.T.T., Nelson, G.S., and Sander, G., 1961, The first record of an outbreak of trichinosis in Africa, south of Sahara, *Trans. R. Soc. Trop. Med. Hyg.* **55**:503–513.

Fraga de Azevedo, J., and Palmeiro, J.M., 1970, Trichinellosis in Iberian peninsula, *Wiad. Parazytol.* **16**:91–99.

Fréchette, J.I., and Panisset, M., 1973, Contribution à l'étude de l'épizootiologie de la trichinose an Québec, *Can. J. Public Health* **64**:443–444.

Gancarz, Z., Wolfram, A., Adonajlo, A., Wilczyński, M., and Mikulsi, Z., 1968, Epidemiologic and epizootiologic studies in foci of epidemic trichinellosis in the Warsaw and Olszryn provinces, *Wiad. Parazytol.* **14**:243.

Gancarz, Z., Wolfram, A., Adonajlo, A., Wilczyński, M., and Mikulski, Z., 1970, Complex epidemiologic and epizootiologic studies in foci of trichinellosis, *Wiad. Parazytol.* **16**:117–118.

Geller, E.H., and Zaiman, H., 1965, Incidence of infection with *Trichinella spiralis* in dogs, *J. Am. Vet. Med. Assoc.* **147**:253–254.

Gerwel, C., and Pawlowski, Z.S., 1975, Studies on the epidemiology and biology of trichinellosis in Poland 1964–1974 (Proceedings of the International Commission on Trichinellosis), *Wiad. Parazytol.* **21**:513–540.

Goregljad, H.S., and Bogush, A.A., 1970, Results of the sanitation work in trichinellosis foci of Belorussia, *Wiad. Parzytol.* **16**:69–70.

Gretillat, S., 1970a, Epidemiology of trichinosis of wild animals in West Africa: Warthog receptivity of the West-African strain of *Trichinella spiralis, J. Parasitol. (Suppl.)* **56**:124.

Gretillat, S., 1970b, Epidemiology of trichinosis in Senegal, *Wiad. Parazytol.* **16**:109–110.

Gretillat, S., and Vassiliadès, G., 1968, The presence of *T. spiralis* in carnivores and suids in the delta region of River Senegal, *Wiad. Parazytol.* **14**:239–240.

Guilbride, P.D.L., 1953, Veterinary public health: The importance of animal disease to public health in the Caribbean with special reference to Jamaica. V. Parasitic infections, *West Indian Med. J.* **3**:205–223.

Harrell, G.T., and Johnston, C., 1939, The incidence of trichinosis in the middle South, *South. Med. J.* **32**:1091–1094.

Harvey, P.W., and Kershaw, W.E., 1964, Low incidence of latent trichinosis near Blackpool compared with incidence elsewhere in England and Wales, *Br. Med. J.* **2**:1632–1634.

Henriksen, S.A., 1978, Report on *Trichinella spiralis* in Denmark (1975–1976), *Wiad. Parazytol.* **24**:110–111.

Henriksen, S.A., 1979, Report on *Trichinella spiralis* in Denmark (1977–1978), *Wiad. Parazytol.* **25**:582–583.

Herman, C.M., and Goss, L.J., 1940, Trichinosis in an American badger, *Taxidea taxus taxus, J. Parasitol.* **26**:157.

Himonas, C.A., 1971, The present status of human trichinosis in Greece, *J. Parasitol.* **57**:1368–1369.

Himonas, C.A., 1978, Report on *Trichinella spiralis* status in Greece (1975–1976), *Wiad. Parazytol.* **24**:114.

Himonas, C.A., 1979, Report on *Trichinella spiralis* status in Greece, *Wiad. Parazytol.* **25**:596–597.

Hinaidy, H.K., 1970, *Trichinella spiralis* beim Rotfuchs (*Vulpes vulpes*) in Oesterreich, *Wien. Tieraerztl. Monastsschr.* **57**:157–158.

Hinaidy, H.K., 1978, Report of trichinellosis in Austria, *Wiad. Parazytol.* **24**:109–110.

Holgersen, P.B., 1961, Trikinose i Upernavik vinteren 1959–1960, *Nord. Med.* **66**:1089–1093.

Holz, J., 1962, Trichinellosis in Raume Indonesia, *Wiad. Parazytol.* **8**:29–30.

Holz, J., 1979, Trichinellosis in Indonesia, *Wiad. Parazytol.* **25**:597.

Hörning, B., 1977, Weitere Trichinenfunde in der Schweiz (1975–1976), *Schweiz. Arch. Tierheilkd.* **119**:337–339.

Hörning, B., 1978, Short report concerning *Trichinella* in Switzerland (1975–1976), *Wiad. Parzytol.* **24**:123–124.

Hovorka, J., 1975, Trichinellosis in Czechoslovakia (1962–1974), *Wiad. Parazytol.* **21**:541–544.

Hunt, G.R., 1967, *Trichinella spiralis* in dogs and cats, *J. Parasitol.* **53**:659.

Hutcheon, R.A., and Pamba, H.O., 1972, Report of a family outbreak of trichinosis in Kajiado District—Kenya, *East Afr. Med. J.* **49**:663–666.

Jefferies, J.C., Beal, V., Jr., Murtishaw, T.R., and Zimmermann, W.J., 1967, Trichinae in garbage-fed swine, *Proc. U.S. Livestock Sanit. Assoc.*, pp. 349–357.

Jeffery, G., and Oliver-González, J., 1948, Absence of *Trichinella spiralis* in rats in Puerto Rico, *J. Parasitol.* **34**:254.

Juranek, D.D., and Schultz, M.G., 1978, Trichinellosis in humans in the United States: Epidemiologic trends, in: *Trichinellosis* (C.W. Kim and Z.S. Pawlowski, eds.), University Press of New England, Hanover, New Hampshire, pp. 523–528.

Kalapesi, R.M., and Rao, S.R., 1954, *Trichinella spiralis* infection in a cat that died in the Zoological Gardens, Bombay, *Indian Med. Gaz.* **89**:578–580.

Kallab, K., 1969, Trichinenfunde bei Schweinen aus Bulgarien, *Wien. Tieraerztl. Monastsschr.* **56**:70.

Kaminsky, R.G., and Zimmermann, R.R., 1977, *Trichinella spiralis*: Incidental finding, *East Afr. Med. J.* **54**:643–646.

Kampelmacher, E.H., Ruitenberg, E.J., and Berkvens, J., 1968, Human trichinellosis in the Netherlands, *Wiad. Parazytol.* **14**:242.

Kershaw, W.E., St. Hill, C.A., Semple, A.B., and Meredith Davies, J.B., 1956, The distribution of the larvae of *Trichinella spiralis* in the muscles, viscera and central nervous system in cases of trichinosis at Liverpool in 1953, and the relation of the severity of the illness to the intensity of infection, *Ann. Trop. Med. Parasitol.* **50**:355–361.

Khamboonruang, C., Thitasut, P., and Pan-In, S., 1978, The role of pigs and rats in the transmission of trichinellosis in northern Thailand, in: *Trichinellosis* (C.W. Kim and Z.S. Pawlowski, eds.), University Press of New England, Hanover, New Hampshire, pp. 545–550.

King, J.J., Black, H.C., and Hewitt, O.H., 1960, Pathology, parasitology and hematology of the black bear in New York, *N. Y. Fish Game J.* **7**:99–111.

Kluge, J.P., 1967, Trichinosis and sarcosporidiosis in a puma, *Bull. Wildl. Dis. Assoc.* **3**:110–111.

Kozar, Z., 1970, Trichinosis in Europe, in: *Trichinosis in Man and Animals* (S.E. Gould, ed.), Charles C. Thomas, Springfield, Illinois, pp. 423–436.

Kozar, Z., and Kozar, M., 1965, Incidence of *Trichinella spiralis* in the Polish population on the basis of post-mortem examinations, *Wiad. Parazytol.* **11**:233–243.

Kozar, Z., and Ogielski, L., 1965, Trichinellosis of pigs in Poland in post-war period with particular reference to the years of 1960–1962, *Wiad. Parazytol.* **11**:282–283.

Kozar, Z., Ramisz, A., and Kozar, M., 1965, Incidence of *Trichinella spiralis* in some domestic and wild living animals in Poland, *Wiad. Parazytol.* **11**:285–298.

Kuitunen-Ekbaum, E., 1941, The incidence of trichinosis in humans in Toronto, *Can. J. Public Health* **32**:569–573.

Kullman, E., 1966, The first findings of *T. spiralis* in Afghanistan, *Wiad. Parazytol.* **12**:678.

Kullman, E., 1970, Trichinellosis in wild animals in Afghanistan, *Wiad. Parazytol.* **16**:111–116.

Kurashvili, B.E., Rodonaja, T.E., Matsaberidze, G.V., Gurchiani, K.R., Savateeva, I.A., Japaridze, Z.A., and Petrashvili, I.I., 1970, Trichinellosis of animals in Georgia, *Wiad. Parazytol.* **16**:76–77.

Lehmensick, R., 1970, Inspection of pork and control of trichinosis in Germany, in: *Trichinosis in Man and Animals* (S.E. Gould, ed.), Charles C. Thomas, Springfield, Illinois, pp. 437–447.

Letonja, T., and Ernst, S., 1974, Trichinosis in dogs from Santiago, Chile, *Bol. Chil. Parasitol.* **29**:51.

Lukashenko, N.P., Volfson, A.G., Istomin, V.A., and Chernov, V.Y., 1971, Trichinellosis of animals in Chukotka, USSR: A general review, *Int. J. Parasitol.* **1**:287–296.

Lupascu, G., Tantareanu, J., Solomon, P., and Smolinski, M., 1970, Trichinellosis in Roumania: Epidemiological aspects, *Wiad. Parazytol.* **16**:78.

Lyman, D.O., 1974, Trichinellosis in California: A 52-year review, in: *Trichinellosis* (C.W. Kim, ed.), Intext, New York, pp. 571–577.

Mäkelä, T., 1970: Trichinosis in a zoo employee, *Scand. J. Infect. Dis.* **2**:75–76.

Maplestone, P.A., and Bhaduri, N.Y., 1942, A record of *Trichinella spiralis* (Owen, 1835) in India, *Indian Med. Gaz.* **77**:193–195.

Margolis, H.S., Middaugh, J.P., and Burgess, R.D., 1979, Arctic trichinosis: Two Alaskan outbreaks from walrus meat, *J. Infect. Dis.* **139**:102–105.

Martin, R.J., Schnurrenberger, P.R., Anderson, F.L., and Hsu, C.K., 1968, Prevalence of *Trichinella spiralis* in wild animals on two Illinois swine farms, *J. Parasitol.* **54**:108–111.

Martinez, F., Calero, R., Hernandez, S., Becerra, C., and Dominguez de Tena, M., 1978, Epidemiology of trichinellosis in Cordoba (Spain), *Wiad. Parazytol.* **24**:23–28.

Martinez-Gomez, F., 1978, Short report concerning trichinellosis in Spain (1975–1976), *Wiad. Parazytol.* **24**:122.

Martinez-Gomez, F., 1979, Short report concerning trichinellosis in Spain (1977 and 1978), *Wiad. Parazytol.* **25**:592–595.

Mason, P.C., 1978, Report on *Trichinella* in New Zealand (1975–1976), *Wiad. Parazytol.* **24**:121.

Massoud, J., 1978, Trichinellosis in carnivores in Iran, in: *Trichinellosis* (C.W. Kim and Z.S. Pawlowski, eds.), University Press of New England, Hanover, New Hampshire, pp. 551–554.

Matossian, R.M., Rebeiz, J., and Stephan, E., 1974, Outbreak of trichinosis in Lebanon, 1970, *Leban. Med. J.* **27**:267–273.

Maynard, J.E., and Pauls, F.P., 1962, Trichinosis in Alaska: A review and report of two outbreaks due to bear meat, with observations on serodiagnosis and skin testing, *Am. J. Hyg.* **76**:252–261.

McNaught, J.B., and Anderson, E.V., 1936, The incidence of trichinosis in San Francisco, *J. Am. Med. Assoc.* **107**:1446–1448.

McNaught, J.B., and Zapata, E.M., 1940, Incidence of *Trichinella spiralis* in garbage-fed hogs in San Francisco, *Proc. Soc. Exp. Biol. Med.* **45**:701–704.

Merdivenci, A., Aleksanyan, V., Girisken, G., and Perk, M., 1977, A case of *Trichinella spiralis* infection in man and wild pig in Turkey, *J. Fac. Vet. Med. Univ. Istanbul* **3**:46–71.

Merkushev, A.V., 1963, Trichinelliasis in the Soviet Arctic, *Wiad. Parazytol.* **9**:493–495.

Merkushev, A.V., 1970, Trichinosis in the Union of Soviet Socialist Republics, in: *Trichinosis in Man and Animals* (S.E. Gould, ed.), Charles C. Thomas, Springfield, Illinois, pp. 449–456.

Mobedi, I., Arfaa, F., Madadi, H., and Movafagh, K., 1973, Sylvatic focus of trichiniasis in the Caspian region, northern Iran, *Am. J. Trop. Med. Hyg.* **22**:720–722.

Most, H., 1965, Trichinellosis in the United States: Changing epidemiology during past 25 years, *J. Am. Med. Assoc.* **193**:871–873.

Most, H., and Helpern, M., 1941, The incidence of trichinosis in New York City, *Am. J. Med. Sci.* **202**:251–257.

Moynihan, I.W., and Musfeldt, I.W., 1949, A study of the incidence of trichinosis in swine in British Columbia, *Can. J. Comp. Med.* **13**:224–227.

Neghme, A., 1979, Trichinellosis in Latin America: Report for 1976–1978, *Wiad. Parazytol.* **25**:586–588.

Neghme, A., and Schenone, H., 1970, Trichinosis in Latin America, in: *Trichinosis in Man and Animals* (S.E. Gould, ed.), Charles C. Thomas, Springfield, Illinois, pp. 407–422.

Nelson, G.S., 1970, Trichinosis in Africa, in: *Trichinosis in Man and Animals* (S.E. Gould, ed.), Charles C. Thomas, Springfield, Illinois, pp. 473–492.

Nelson, G.S., and Forrester, A.T.T., 1962, Trichinosis in Kenya, *Wiad. Parazytol.* **8**:17–28.

Nelson, G.S., and Mukundi, J., 1963, A strain of *Trichinella spiralis* from Kenya of low infectivity to rats and domestic pigs, *J. Helminthol.* **37**:329–338.

Nelson, G.S., Rickman, R., and Pester, F.R.N., 1961, Feral trichinosis in Africa, *Trans. R. Soc. Trop. Med. Hyg.* **55**:514–517.

Nelson, G.S., Guggisberg, C.W.A., and Mukundi, J., 1963, Animal hosts of *Trichinella spiralis* in East Africa, *Ann. Trop. Med. Parasitol.* **57**:332–346.

Neméséri, L., 1970, The importance of trichinellosis in Hungary, *Wiad. Parazytol.* **16**:80–83.

Odelram, H., 1973, A trichinosis epidemic, *Scand. J. Infect. Dis.* **5**:293–298.

Oldham, J.N., and Beresford-Jones, W.P., 1957, *Trichinella spiralis* in the wild red fox in England, *Br. Vet. J.* **113**:34–35.

Olsen, O.W., 1960, Sylvatic trichinosis in carnivorous mammals in the Rocky Mountain region of Colorado, *J. Parasitol.* **46**(Suppl.):22.

Ossola, A., Rubiolo, J., Castillo, R., and Carrizo, G., 1969, Epidemas de triquinosis in Mercedes, San Luis, Argentina, *Bol. Chil. Parazitol.* **24**:123–127.

Panaitescu, D., Constantinescu, G., and Capraru, T., 1980, Trichinosis: Epidemiological surveillance by serological tests, Fifth International Conference on Trichinellosis (abstract), The Netherlands, p. 140.

Parmeter, S.N., Schad, G.A., and Chowdhury, A.B., 1968, Another record of *Trichinella spiralis* in Calcutta, *Wiad. Parazytol.* **14**:239.

Pavlov, P., 1979, Trichinellosis in Bulgaria, *Wiad. Parazytol.* **25**:580.

Prokopič, J., 1962, Trichinellosis in Czechoslovakia, *Wiad. Parazytol.* **8**:31–46.

Pullen, M.M., Seymour, M.R., and Zimmermann, W.J., 1977, Trichinosis in sows slaughtered at a Kentucky abattoir, *J. Am. Vet. Med. Assoc.* **171**:1171–1172.

Pun, K.K., Wong, W.T., and Wong, P.H.C., The first documented outbreak of trichinellosis in Hong Kong Chinese, *Am. J. Trop. Med. Hyg.*, in press.

Ramisz, A., and Balicka-Laurans, A., 1981, Studies on the occurrence of *Trichinella spiralis* in rats at industrial fattening farms, in: *Trichinellosis* (C.W. Kim, E.J. Ruitenberg, and J.S. Teppema, eds.), Reedbooks, Chertsey, England, pp. 369–372.

Ramisz, A., and Jarzebski, Z., 1979, Report on trichinellosis in pigs in Poland, 1975–1978, *Wiad. Parazytol.* **25**:599–600.

Ramisz, A., and Swiech, S., 1962, Trichinellosis in pigs and wild boars on the terrain of the Wroclaw Province, Poland, in 1958–1960, *Wiad. Parazytol.* **8**:51–55.

Rausch, R.L., 1970, Trichinosis in the Arctic, in: *Trichinosis in Man and Animals* (S.E. Gould, ed.), Charles C. Thomas, Springfield, Illinois, pp. 348–373.

Rausch, R., Barber, B.B., Rausch, R.V., and Schiller, E.L., 1956, Studies on the helminthic fauna of Alaska. XXVII. The occurrence of larvae of *T. spiralis* in Alaskan mammals, *J. Parasitol.* **42**:259–271.

Riley, W.A., and Scheifley, C.H., 1934, Trichinosis of man a common infection, *J. Am. Med. Assoc.* **102**:1217–1218.

Ringertz, O., Landbäck, H., and Zetterberg, B., 1962, Trichinosis in Sweden in 1961, *Acta Pathol. Microbiol. Scand.* **54**:351.

Roñeus, O., and Christensson, D., 1979, Presence of *Trichinella spiralis* in free-living red foxes (*Vulpes vulpes*) in Sweden related to *Trichinella* infection in swine and man, *Acta Vet. Scand.* **20**:583–594.

Roselle, H.A., Schwartz, D.T., and Geer, F.G., 1965, Trichinosis from New England bear meat: Report of an epidemic, *N. Engl. J. Med.* **272**:304–305.

Roth, H., 1949, Trichinosis in arctic animals, *Nature (London)* **163**:805–806.

Rothrock, T.P., 1965, Trichinosis in an Iowa swine herd, *J. Am. Vet. Med. Assoc.* **146**:366–367.

Ruitenberg, E.J., 1974, Trichinellosis in the Netherlands, *Wiad. Parazytol.* **20**:137–139.

Ruitenberg, E.J., 1975, *Trichinella spiralis* studies in the Netherlands, *Wiad. Parazytol.* **21**:545–546.

Ruitenberg, E.J., 1979, Report concerning *Trichinella spiralis* studies in the Netherlands 1977–1978, *Wiad. Parazytol.* **25**:589–591.

Ruitenberg, E.J., and Sluiters, J.F., 1974, *Trichinella spiralis* infections in the Netherlands, in: *Trichinellosis* (C.W. Kim, ed.), Intext, New York, pp. 539–548.

Ruitenberg, E.J., and van Knapen, F., 1978, Report 1975–1976 concerning *Trichinella spiralis* studies in the Netherlands, *Wiad. Parazytol.* **24**:117–120.

Rukavina, J., and Brglez, J., 1970, Trichinellosis of some species of wild animals in Yugoslavia, *Wiad. Parazytol.* **16**:79.

Rukavina, J., Delic, S., Dzumurov, N., and Pavlovic, R., 1968, Trichinellosis of wild animals in some districts of Jugoslavia, *Wiad. Parazytol.* **14**:244.

Sachs, R., 1970, Zur Epidemiologie der Trichinellosis in Africa, *Z. Tropenmed. Parasitol.* **21**:117–126.

Sachs, R., and Taylor, A.S., 1966, Trichinosis in a spotted hyaena (*Crocuta crocuta*) of the Serengeti, *Vet. Rec.* **78**:704.

Sadighian, A., Arfaa, F., and Movafagh, K., 1973, *Trichinella spiralis* in carnivores and rodents in Isfahan, Iran, *J. Parasitol.* **59**:986.

Sapunar, J., and Székely, R., 1977, Análisis clínico de 76 pacientes con triquinosis, *Bol. Chil. Parasitol.* **32**:31–36.

Sawitz, W., 1939, *Trichinella spiralis*. I. Incidence of infection in man, dogs, and cats in the New Orleans area as determined in postmortem examination, *Arch. Pathol.* **28**:11–21.

Schad, G.A., and Chowdhury, A.B., 1967, *Trichinella spiralis* in India. I. Its history in India, rediscovery in Calcutta, and the ecology of its maintenance in nature, *Trans. R. Soc. Trop. Med. Hyg.* **61**:244–248.

Schantz, P.M., Juranek, D.D., and Schultz, M.G., 1977, Trichinosis in the United States, 1975: Increase in cases attributed to numerous common-source outbreaks, *J. Infect. Dis.* **136**:712–715.

Schenone, H., Jacob, C., Rojas, A., and Villarroel, F., 1967, *Trichinella spiralis* infection in *Rattus norvegicus* from the Municipal Abbattoir of Santiago, Chile, *Bol. Chil. Parasitol.* **22**:176.

Schenone, H., Cornejo, L., Rivera, G., Jara, H., D'Acuna, G., Soljan, N., and Knierim, F., 1968, Epidemic of trichinellosis in Antofagasta, *Wiad. Parazytol.* **14**:240–241.

Schenone, J., Reyes, H., and Rojas, A., 1969, Prevalencia actual de la triquinosis humana en Santiago, estudio en 1,000 cadáveres, *Bol. Chil. Parasitol.* **24**:152–153.

Schenone, H., Székely, R., and Ramirez, R., 1972, Aspectos epidemiológicos de la triquinosis humana en Chile, *Bol. Chil. Parasitol.* **27**:103–107.

Schmitt, N., Bowmer, E.J., Simon, P.C., Arneil, A.S., and Clark, D.A., 1972, Trichinosis from bear meat and adulterated pork products: A major outbreak in British Columbia, 1971, *Can. Med. Assoc. J.* **107:**1087–1091.

Schmitt, N., Saville, J.M., Friis, L., and Stovell, P.L., 1976, Trichinosis in British Columbia wildlife, *Can. J. Public Health* **67:**21–24.

Schmitt, N., Saville, J.M., Greenway, J.A., Stovell, P.L., Friis, L., and Hole, L., 1978, Sylvatic trichinosis in British Columbia: Potential threat to human health from an independent cycle, *Public Health Rep.* **93:**189–193.

Schultz, M.G., 1970, Reservoirs of *Trichinella spiralis* in nature and its routes of transmission to man, *J. Parasitol.* **56**(Suppl.)**:**309.

Schultz, M.G., and Juranek, D.D., 1974, Trichinellosis surveillance in the United States, in: *Trichinellosis* (C.W. Kim, ed.), Intext, New York, pp. 593–595.

Schwartz, B., 1953, Prevalence, transmission, prevention: Trichinae in swine, *Public Health Rep.* **68:**418.

Semple, A.B., Davies, J.B.M., Kershaw, W.E., and St. Hill, C.A., 1954, An outbreak of trichinosis in Liverpool in 1953, *Br. Med. J.* **1:**1002–1006.

Sheldon, J.H., 1941, An outbreak of trichiniasis in Wolverhampton and district, *Lancet* **1:**203–205.

Sicard, D., Fontan, R., Richard-Lenoble, D., and Gentilini, M., 1976, Trichinose humaine: Une épidémie récente a Vientiane (Laos), *Bull. Soc. Pathol. Exot.* **69:**521–525.

Smith, H.J., 1978, Status of trichinosis in bears in the Atlantic provinces of Canada 1971–1976, *Can. J. Comp. Med.* **42:**244–245.

Smith, H.J., Anzengruber, A., and DuPlessis, D.M., 1976, Current status of trichinosis in swine in the Atlantic provinces, *Can. Vet. J.* **17:**72–75.

Solomon, G.B., and Warner, G.S., 1969, *Trichinella spiralis* in mammals at Mountain Lake, Virginia, *J. Parasitol.* **55:**730–732.

Spindler, L.A., and Permenter, D.O., 1951, Natural infections of *Trichinella spiralis* in skunks, *J. Parasitol.* **37**(Suppl.)**:**19–20.

Steele, J.H., 1970, Epidemiology and control of trichinosis, in: *Trichinosis in Man and Animals* (S.E. Gould, ed.), Charles C. Thomas, Springfield, Illinois, pp. 493–512.

Steele, J.H., and Arambulo, P.V., III, 1975, Trichinosis: A world problem with extensive sylvatic reservoirs, *Int. J. Zool.* **2:**55–75.

Steele, J.H., and Schultz, M.G., 1978, Trichinellosis: A review of the current problem, in: *Trichinellosis* (C.W. Kim and Z.S. Pawlowski, eds.), University Press of New England, Hanover, New Hampshire, pp. 45–75.

Stoimenov, K., and Gradinarski, I.W., 1981, A study on the epizootiology of trichinellosis in Bulgaria, in: *Trichinellosis* (C.W. Kim, E.J. Ruitenberg, and J.S. Teppema, eds.), Reedbooks, Chertsey, England, pp. 373–377.

Stoimenov, K., Bratanov, V., and Trifonov, T., 1966, Studies on the helminthofauna of the fox in Bulgaria, *Wiad. Parazytol.* **12:**680.

Tacal, J.V., Jr., and Pabello, P.D., 1965, Absence of *Trichinella spiralis* in brown rats (*Rattus norvegicus*) in the Philippines, *J. Parasitol.* **51:**957.

Tailyour, J.M., and Hampton, M.J., 1954, A check on the incidence of trichinosis in swine in six piggeries in British Columbia, *Can. J. Comp. Med.* **18:**311–312.

Tailyour, J.M., and Steele, J.R., 1960, *Trichinella* infection in swine in the Vancouver area, *Can. J. Public Health* **51:**309.

Tanner, C.E., 1979, Report on trichinellosis in Canada, *Wiad. Parazytol.* **25:**585–586.

Thing, H., Clausen, B., and Henriksen, S.A., 1976, Finding of *Trichinella spiralis* in a walrus (*Odobenus rosmarus* L.) in the Thule district, Northwest Greenland, *Nord. Vet. Med.* **28:**59.

Thorborg, N.B., Tulinius, S., and Roth, H., 1948, Trichinosis in Greenland, *Acta Pathol. Microbiol. Scand.* **25:**788–794.

Tiainen, O.A., 1966, Occurrence of *T. spiralis* at the Helsinki City zoological gardens, *Wiad. Parazytol.* **12:**680.

Todd, J.W., 1979, Trichinosis letter, *Br. Med. J.* **1:**1355.

Valtonen, M., 1979, Trichinellosis in Finland, *Wiad. Parazytol.* **25:**591–592.

Van Someren, V.D., 1937, The occurrence of subclinical trichinosis in Britain: Results from 200 London necropsies, *Br. Med. J.* **2:**1162–1165.

Viens, P., and Auger, P., 1981, Clinical and epidemiological aspects of trichinosis in Montreal, in: *Trichinellosis* (C.W. Kim, E.J., Ruitenberg, and J.S. Teppema, eds.), Reedbooks, Chertsey, England, pp. 275–278.

Viksne, A.E., 1970, Epizootiological and epidemiological problems of trichinellosis in Latvian S.S.R., *Wiad. Parazytol.* **16:**73.

Waddell, A.H., 1969, The search for *Trichinella spiralis* in Austrialia, *Aust. Vet. J.* **45:**207.

Wilson, R., 1967, Bear meat trichinosis: Profound serum protein alterations, minor eosinophilia, and response to thiabendazole, *Ann. Intern. Med.* **66:**965–971.

Winters, J.B., 1969, Trichiniasis in Montana mountain lions, *Bull. Wildl. Dis. Assoc.* **5:**400.

World Health Organization, 1982, Abstracts of recent Chinese publications on helminthiases, WHO/HELM/82.5, p. 4.

Worley, D.E., Fox, J.C., and Winters, J.B., 1974, Prevalence and distribution of *Trichinella spiralis* in carnivorous mammals in the United States northern Rocky Mountain region, in: *Trichinellosis* (C.W. Kim, ed.) Intext, New York, pp. 597–602.

Wright, W.H., Kerr, K.B., and Jacobs, L., 1943, Studies on trichinosis. XV. Summary of the findings on *Trichinella spiralis* in a random sampling and other samplings of the population of the United States, *Public Health Rep.* **58:**1293–1313.

Wright, W.H., Jacobs, L., and Walton, A.C., 1944, Studies of trichinosis. XVI. Epidemiological considerations based on the examination for trichinae of 5,313 diaphragms from 189 hospitals in 37 states and the District of Columbia, *Public Health Rep.* **59:**669–681.

Yamaguchi, T., 1978, Report on trichinellosis in Japan, *Wiad. Parazytol.* **24:**114–117.

Yamashita, J., 1970, Trichinosis in Asia, in: *Trichinosis in Man an Animals* (S.E. Gould, ed.), Charles C. Thomas, Springfield, Illinois, pp. 457–464.

Young, M.R., 1947, The incidence of *Trichinella spiralis* at necropsies in England, *J. Helminthol.* **22:**49–60.

Young, E., and Kruger, S.P., 1967, *Trichinella spiralis* (Owen, 1835) Railliet, 1895 infestation of wild carnivores and rodents in South Africa, *J. South Afr. Vet. Med. Assoc.* **38:**441–443.

Zimmermann, W.J., 1967, The incidence of *Trichinella spiralis* in humans of Iowa, *Public Health Rep.* **82:**127–130.

Zimmermann, W.J., 1970a, Trichinosis in the United States, in: *Trichinosis in Man and Animals* (S.E. Gould, ed.), Charles C. Thomas, Springfield, Illinois, pp. 378–400.

Zimmermann, W.J., 1970b, The epizootiology of trichiniasis in wildlife, *J. Wildl. Dis.* **6:**329–334.

Zimmermann, W.J., 1970c, Reservoirs of *Trichinella spiralis* in nature and possible routes of transmission from one host to another, *J. Parasitol.* **56**(Suppl.):378.

Zimmermann, W.J., 1974, The current status of trichinellosis in the United States, in: *Trichinellosis* (C.W. Kim, ed.), Intext, New York, pp. 603–609.

Zimmermann, W.J., and Brandly, P.J., 1965, The current status of trichiniasis in U.S. swine, *Public Health Rep.* **80:**1061–1066.

Zimmermann, W.J., and Hubbard, E.D., 1969, Trichiniasis in wildlife of Iowa, *Am. J. Epidemiol.* **90:**84–92.

Zimmermann, W.J., and Schwarte, L.H., 1958, Trichiniasis in dogs and cats of Iowa, *J. Parasitol.* **44:**520–522.

Zimmermann, W.J., and Zinter, D.E., 1971, The prevalence of trichinosis in swine in the United States, 1966–70, *Health Serv. Mental Health Admin. Health Rep.* **86:**937–945.

Zimmermann, W.J., Hubbard, E.D., Schwarte, L.H., and Biester, H.E., 1962a, *Trichinella spiralis* in Iowa wildlife during the years 1953–1961, *J. Parasitol.* **48:**429–432.

Zimmermann, W.J., Hubbard, E.D., Schwarte, L.H., and Biester, H.E., 1962b, Trichiniasis in Iowa swine with further studies on modes of transmission, *Cornell Vet.* **52:**156–163.

Zimmermann, W.J., Steele, J.H., and Kagan, I.G., 1968, The changing status of trichiniasis in the U.S. population, *Public Health Rep.* **83:**957–966.

Zimmermann, W.J., Steele, J.H., and Kagan, I.G., 1973, Trichiniasis in the U.S. population, 1966–1970: Prevalence, Epidemiologic factors, *Health Serv. Rep.* **88:**606–623.

Zukowski, K., and Bitkowska, E., 1978, Extensiveness of trichinosis (*T. spiralis*) in small mammals in Poland, *Wiad. Parazytol.* **24:**103–108.

15

Control I

Public-Health Aspects (with Special Reference to the United States)

JACK C. LEIGHTY

1. INTRODUCTION

Prevention of human trichinosis presents a complex challenge to scientists and public-health officials throughout the world. Where the problem does not yet exist, it must not be allowed to develop as animal production, processing, and marketing practices change (Steele and Arambulo, 1975). In countries in which effective control measures have practically eradicated the infection from swine, the costly vigilance must be continued indefinitely lest reintroduction occur with tragic results. Where a country's control of commercially slaughtered swine has not also been adequate to prevent human infection resulting from the consumption of farm-slaughtered pork, the task that remains is difficult but obvious (Kozar, 1961). A heavy burden of responsibility also rests with those countries that are major producers of swine but have incomplete programs for trichinosis control (Cockrill, 1963). *Trichinella*-infected pork, imported from such countries into countries that have

JACK C. LEIGHTY • Dunkirk, Maryland 20754.

controlled the problem at great expense, offers a threat to the health of their citizens and the economics of their pork industry that is understandably unacceptable (Ruitenberg and Kamplemacher, 1970).

2. MECHANISMS OF CONTROL

Strategies for the control of trichinosis must be economically acceptable and must account for all significant sources of human and animal infection. In this world in which famine and malnutrition are commonplace, it is neither desirable nor possible to institute and maintain programs that waste human or domestic animal foods or raise their costs unnecessarily.

2.1. Prevention of Swine Infections

When considered on a worldwide basis, infected pork is still the greatest single source of human infection. Swine can acquire trichinosis by ingesting the tissues of other species of omnivorous or carnivorous feral or domesticated animals (Zimmerman *et al.*, 1962), feces containing gravid intestinal worms (Hill, 1968), and infected pork.

While all sources of swine infection are of importance, infected pork is the single greatest problem, as with humans. Infected pork is available to swine through caudophagy, swine carcasses that are carelessly or deliberately made available for consumption by swine, and in the form of pork scraps that are by-products of the meat industry or of food preparation in domestic or institutional kitchens. The latter source, garbage, has received a great deal of attention internationally because it can also contain the agents of other important infectious diseases of swine. As might be expected, where garbage feeding has occurred on a significant scale or has occurred otherwise under circumstances that have enabled recognition by regulatory officials, effective control has often been obtained either by outright prohibition of garbage feeding or by requiring cooking. Where garbage feeding has occurred under circumstances that make it less obvious to regulatory officials, control has sometimes been ineffective and human infections have been the result (Centers for Disease Control, 1980).

Prevention of swine infections that result from the consumption of animal carcasses, the tails of unfortunate penmates, feces, or from occasional garbage feeding requires mechanisms that are quite different from those that are used effectively against more formal garbage-feeding operations. Programs for post mortem identification of infected swine and for the education of producers may be the best approach in such situations.

2.2. Detection of Infected Swine

Unfortunately, swine infected by *Trichinella* cannot be detected by the usual postmortem examination. However, a number of indirect systems have been used for many years for the identification of swine that contain infective *Trichinella* larvae in their tissues. Two principal approaches have been made. One involves the actual visualization of the larvae and is reviewed in Chapter 16. The other attempts to detect an immunological response to the entry of the larvae into the host tissues and is reviewed in Chapter 17.

2.2.1. Test Characteristics Desirable for Use in Programs to Control Infection in Swine

Trichinosis testing systems for identifying *Trichinella*-infected swine may be used in public-health programs in a variety of situations with a number of possible objectives. When a human infection occurs, it may be desirable to test meat and live animals for the purpose of preventing further human infection, if swine have been implicated, and to identify and eliminate the source of infection of the swine. In epidemiologically based control programs, blood samples may be taken from live swine and examined individually, or as pools, to determine the continuing *Trichinella* status of swine on individual farms (Ruitenberg *et al.*, 1979). However, the most frequent use of testing systems is as an adjunct to routine postmortem inspection to determine the suitability of swine for human food.

The economics and technology of meat hygiene programs are tied closely to the changing nature of the meat industry. In some abattoirs in the United States, swine are slaughtered at rates that give 1000 carcasses an hour. Cryogenic chilling makes it possible to begin cutting up carcasses within a few hours of slaughter. Worldwide, huge numbers of swine are slaughtered annually. In 1980, international slaughter totaled approximately 462 million swine (Foreign Agriculture Service, 1981). In 1980, in the United States, 90 million swine were slaughtered (Food Safety and Quality Service, 1981). The efficiency of the pig in converting feedstuffs that are unsuitable for immediate human consumption into meat is well known and would seem to indicate that its importance as a major source of high-quality protein for mankind will continue to increase. It is obvious that if food hygiene programs are to remain viable, inspection techniques must be capable of examining large numbers of pigs in abattoirs having high slaughter rates. It follows, then, that a test to be used for the detection of *Trichinella*-infected swine in abattoirs must be applied with automated equipment that does not fail during operation.

The cost of inspecting such large numbers of animals can make effective postmortem inspection programs economically prohibitive unless ingenious ways can be found to keep costs low and expand benefits. Systems that have served well in the past may soon have to be replaced. Materials, equipment, and manpower costs for testing must be minimized, and test results must serve a number of socially significant purposes.

An important goal of all meat hygiene programs is to prevent the transmission of infectious or toxic disease to persons who handle or consume meat. Many such disease agents, in addition to *Trichinella*, are not detectable by gross organoleptic examination. As the prevalence of animal diseases such as brucellosis and tuberculosis declines, the abattoir becomes increasingly the point of choice for obtaining the epidemiological data needed for control and eradication programs. The benefits of trichinosis inspection are increased enormously when the testing system used is capable of detecting one or more additional diseases of importance to human or animal health. In countries in which low trichinosis prevalence in swine encourages the consumption of uncooked pork, public-health officials must be aware of the tragic results of congenital toxoplasmosis. Further, when a disease such as trichinosis is controlled almost to the point of eradication, testing often must be continued because other reservoirs of *Trichinella* infection are a continuing threat to the swine. The maintenance of costly inspection programs, useful only for detecting a virtually nonexistent disease, may be very unpopular with those who must pay the inspection bill.

Specificity is also an essential characteristic. Action generated by a positive finding, whether it results in the loss of the value of an animal or a costly disease control action, must be based on reliable findings.

Sensitivity is equally important. All affected swine must be found. If human disease results from consumption of a passed animal, the program quickly loses the confidence and support of the public and the meat industry. Finding all affected animals would enable control programs to proceed more rapidly, and thus more economically, to their goal.

At present, the enzyme immunoassay seems to best meet the aforestated requirements. It is fast, sensitive, and specific, costs little, and appears to be amenable to automation (Leighty, 1974) (see Chapter 17). An additional characteristic of great significance is the ability of the system to detect other infectious and toxic agents. Enzyme immunoassays are under development for the detection of antibiotics in serum (Standefer and Saunders, 1978; Humphreys and Ragland, 1981) and for swine brucellosis and mycobacteriosis. (Thoen *et al.*, 1979, 1980) The development of automated equipment for applying the test under abattoir conditions remains to be done. As progress is made in this area, we may expect to see the development of immunoassays, slightly different in principle, that are even more capable of serving these important human and animal health needs.

2.3. Rendering Infected Pork Noninfective

Unless reliable evidence is available to assure that pork is free of *Trichinella* larvae, it is prudent to consider that it is infected and treat it accordingly. The treatments currently available are cooking, freeze-drying, freezing, curing, and radiation.

2.3.1. Cooking

Cooking is one of the most common methods of assuring that any *Trichinella* present are destroyed. The results of early studies, using decapsulated larvae on a heated microscope stage and pieces of infected meat in test tubes that were heated in a water bath, indicated that the thermal death point of *Trichinella* was 131°F (Ransom and Schwartz, 1919; Otto and Abrams, 1939). Studies by Carlin *et al.* (1969) determined that the thermal death point of *Trichinella* occurs at a point slightly above 135°F (57°C). They concluded that 170°F (77°C), a temperature that also produces satisfactory pork roasts, is well above the thermal death point of the parasite and could be recommended for food preparation.

2.3.2. Freeze-Drying

Spindler *et al.* (1946) conducted freeze-drying studies on *Trichinella*-infected pork and found that pork frozen to 0°F and dehydrated at a temperature of 120°F to a moisture content of 9% or less contained no viable trichina. Lower drying temperatures with longer drying times failed to destroy all *Trichinella*. Alboiu and Popescu (1978) were unable to infect mice with larvae recovered by digestion from freeze-dried meat. Meat was frozen at $-70°C$ using carbon dioxide snow or in a freezer at $-12°C$ for 17 hr. Freeze-drying was accomplished with a condensation temperature of $-45°C$ and a final vacuum of 10^{-2} torr with heat not exceeding 30°C for 60 min.

2.3.3. Freezing

Freezing at appropriate temperatures for an appropriate time period destroys *Trichinella*. Ransom (1916) conducted a rather extensive study of the effect of freezing pork on the viability of *Trichinella* and recommended that meat be refrigerated at a temperature not higher than 5°F for not less than 20 days, to provide a margin of safety of about 10 days.

Considering that the use of lower temperatures for shorter periods of time might be advantageous, Gould and Kaasa (1948) studied "quick"-freezing effects. They reported that a temperature of $-27°C$ ($-16.6°F$) maintained for 36 hr, $-30°C$ ($-22°F$) for 24 hr, $-33°C$ ($-27.4°F$) for 10 hr, $-35°C$ ($-31°F$) for 40 min, or $-37°C$ ($-34.6°F$) for 2 min in the central portions of pork was effective in killing all *Trichinella* larvae. Rust and Zimmerman (1972) froze 110-g pork patties with liquid nitrogen and liquid carbon dioxide and concluded that if an equilibrated temperature of $-29°C$ was attained, the pork was immediately rendered *Trichinella*-free. Studies by Smith (1952) confirmed that a temperature of about $-30°C$ appears to be a critical point below which *Trichinella* die very quickly.

2.3.4. Curing

One of the oldest methods of meat preservation known to man, curing, is still one of the most popular. In the United States, in 1979, of 15,450 million pounds of pork produced, 4511 million pounds were reported as cured (Economics and Statistics Service, 1980). If the *Trichinella*-free status of the pork cannot be assured, the curing process should be one known to be capable of destroying any *Trichinella* that may be present. If the process cannot be depended on to destroy *Trichinella* larvae and if the pork may contain such larvae, the pork should be frozen to render it safe before curing. A number of different combinations of salt, moisture, aging, and heat have been studied and found to be lethal to *Trichinella* (Food Safety and Quality Service, 1973; Gammon *et al.*, 1968; Zimmerman, 1971; Allen and Goldberg, 1962).

2.3.5. Radiation

Since Tyzzer and Honeij (1916) reported the effects of radiation injury on *T. spiralis*, there has been interest in the possibility of employing X-rays or gamma rays to destroy the larvae in pork. However, no known commercial process has been established. Again, the installation of costly facilities directed toward the destruction of one species of organism that occurs infrequently in swine cannot be regarded as economically attractive. The application of such a system might be more attractive if additional benefits are sought. These might include the destruction of pathogenic bacteria such as *Salmonella, Yersina,* and *Campylobacter* species and of the organisms that reduce shelf life of meat and meat products. A dosage range of 20,000–30,000 rads is considered to be effective to control *Trichinella* in meat. At this level, deleterious changes do not occur in the meat. The effect is independent of the number of cysts per unit of meat (Gibbs *et al.*, 1961, 1964).

2.3.6. Microwave Cooking

W.J. Zimmermann (personal communication, 1981), cooked pork roasts and pork chops containing *T. spiralis* larvae in six household-type microwave ovens representing five brands. Cooking procedures were generally those recommended by the manufacturers. Infective *Trichinella* were found in 9 of 51 products after cooking. Subsequent studies have provided further evidence that due to the uneven heating that occurs, cooking with currently available microwave ovens is not a reliable way to destroy *Trichinella* in meat.

2.4. Game Foods

As trichinosis becomes less prevalent in swine, the relative importance of feral animals as sources of both human and swine infection increases (Bessonov, 1979). In the United States, in 1979, of 135 cases of human trichinosis reported, 28 cases were acquired from the meat of wild animals (Centers for Disease Control, 1980). At least 75 species of wild animals in various parts of the world have been reported as natural hosts (Schultz, 1970), and in some parts of the world the principal source of human infection may be wild animals (Nelson *et al.*, 1961) (see Chapters 13 and 14). Our current knowledge of this aspect of the trichinosis problem would seem to indicate that public-health programs should provide educational programs for hunters and consumers of game foods and offer diagnostic examination services for game animals.

3. MEASURES ADOPTED IN THE UNITED STATES

In the past, measures taken by other countries, principally those of Western Europe, Eastern Europe, and Scandinavia, have been viewed as impractical in the United States (Chapter 1). Both the trichinoscope and pooled-sample digestion tests, the systems that are currently employed in those countries, are rather expensive and capable of detecting only one disease. Their application to detect only *Trichinella* in 90 million hogs slaughtered in many hundreds of Federal and state plants would be very expensive (Food Safety and Quality Service, 1981). The time required to complete either test is incompatible with the rate at which hogs are converted to pork and moved to markets from high-volume plants. On the other end of the production scale are the very small plants that because of their low volume would also pose difficult problems in the use of those rather cumbersome inspection techniques.

A disease that produces clinical illness in fewer than 100 persons a year, and rarely causes a death, must be seen by those who allocate public-health funds as having a relatively low priority. On the other hand, animal-health officials have placed high priority on preventing the transmission of infectious diseases of swine through garbage. And in doing so, they have serendipitously reduced both the frequency and the severity of *T. spiralis* infection in swine. Added to the impact of garbage control is the effect of commercially processing pork in a manner that destroys any *Trichinella* that may be present before the pork gets to the consumer or the garbage can.

Studies by Zimmermann (Chapter 16) indicate that 68% of *Trichinella*-infected swine in the United States bear fewer than 1 cyst per gram of tissue. Tests that rely on the examination of "representative" tissue samples are less effective than would be desirable in detecting such swine.

The swine industry and the public have yet to advocate strongly an animal identification system that would enable Federal and state epidemiologists to use the intelligence produced by a trichinosis testing program for the eradication and continued exclusion of the disease from swine.

While *Trichinella* control in the United States has for the aforestated reasons differed from those of other countries, the approaches that have been used in this country may be of interest to those who have similar problems.

3.1. Control of Garbage

In the United States, Public Law 96-468, of October 17, 1980, prohibits the feeding of garbage to swine unless the garbage is treated to kill disease organisms. Enforcement is delegated to the individual states contingent on their having adequate laws and regulations and a program for enforcement. In January 1981, there were 10,122 garbage-feeding premises feeding 488,217 swine. (Animal and Plant Health Inspection Service, 1981). Since most such feeding operations are continuous, and most swine are marketed at 4–6 months of age, one might reasonably surmise that these formally identified feeders market about 996,000 swine annually—a small but significant contribution to the nation's food supply.

3.2. Regulation of Commercial Pork Products

The commercial processing of pork is controlled by state and Federal inspection programs (Food Safety and Inspection Service, United States Department of Agriculture) to assure that pork products that may be eaten without further cooking are processed in a manner capable of destroying *Trichinella*. Products such as raw unsmoked sausage that are customarily well cooked in residential or institutional kitchens may be sold without treatment.

3.2.1. Cooking

The heating process required in inspected establishments must assure that all parts of pork muscle tissue are heated to a temperature not lower than 137°F. Methods of assuring that the required temperatures are reached must be applied.

3.2.2. Freezing and Freeze-Drying

Certain products that may be eaten without cooking require pork that is not cooked or cured. These may be made trichina-free by freezing. The pork to be frozen must first be chilled to 40°F, or frozen, after which all parts must be subjected continuously to temperatures specified. The treatment required is based on the thickness of the meat or the inside dimensions of the container. Treatment may also consist of freezing to −30°F in the center of the meat or of freeze-drying. A 1977 study of the use of freezing to certify pork as trichina-free found that the actual industry costs vary from a low of $0.35 per 100 pounds (45 kg) to $3.15 per 100 pounds for those processors who certify on-site and from $2.25 to $3.40 per 100 pounds for those who certify off-site. These do not include inspection costs (Francke *et al.*, 1977).

3.2.3. Curing

Sausage to be cured may be stuffed into animal or hydrocellulose casings or into cloth bags. During any stage of the process, the coverings may not be coated with paraffin or a similar substance, and no sausage may be washed during any prescribed drying period.

Processors may utilize the five methods of sausage preparation published in the Federal Regulations or may make use of an alternative method if it can be demonstrated to render *Trichinella* noninfective.

Two methods are specified as acceptable dry-salt curing processes for hams and pork shoulder picnics, and three methods are permitted for curing boneless loins.

Positive controls, such as recording thermometers, are required to ensure that proper amounts of curing agents are employed and specified time and temperature requirements are followed.

3.3. Game Foods

These are a particular problem in the United States, since any carnivorous or omnivorous feral animal must be considered a possible source of infection. The Federal and state meat inspection acts do not apply to game animals. However, if they are to be served commercially, the Food, Drug and Cosmetic Act of 1962 is applicable. Under that act, game meat bearing *Trichinella* cysts would be considered "adulterated." However, no testing of such meat is required. As previously indicated, the relative number of human cases attributable to the consumption of the meat of wild animals, particularly bear meat, continues to increase as the prevalence of trichinosis in swine decreases. The number of infections would indicate that hunters are not generally aware of the hazard, and diagnostic services are not readily available.

3.4. Education

Consumer awareness of the trichinosis problem undoubtedly has played some part in the relatively low incidence of human infections reported in the United States. One of the more popular cookbooks, which is quite typical (Rombauer and Rombauer Becker, 1967), states: "Pork demands thorough cooking. Otherwise the very harmful trichinae or parasites which often exist in it may be transmitted to the eater." The book goes on to recommend cooking to an internal temperature of 185°F. Currently, cooking temperatures of 170°F are being recommended, and many publications are being revised accordingly.

The U.S. Department of Agriculture distributed 10,000 copies of a leaflet on trichinosis in 1979.

The past success of all control measures in the United States, including the education of the consumer to cook pork well, must be considered in terms of the results achieved. In the period 1966–1970, a statistically designed study of 8071 human diaphragm samples found that the risk of infection was much less at that time than for persons of comparable demographic characteristic 30 years earlier (Zimmermann *et al.*, 1973): "An estimated 1 to 2 million persons became infected with the parasite in 1940 in contrast to 150,000 to 300,000 in 1970." The authors pointed out that most infections are nonclinical, based on frequent findings of live trichina in human diaphragm tissue in numbers that are believed to be too small to cause clinical symptoms. Their recommendations for an eradication program included educating producers, eliminating garbage, and using an effective diagnostic program at slaughter.

3.5. The Future

While the prevalence of trichinosis in swine continues to decline, full control of the problem may require new initiatives. Automated testing procedures, capable of improving the effectiveness of postmortem inspection by specifically identifying more diseases that are of interest to human- and animal-health officials and meat producers, are now available. They also have the potential for reducing the current high costs of postmortem inspection. An essential element of such a program, a national animal identification program, may now be technically possible with advances in marking and automatic data processing.

The relative decline in *Trichinella*-infected swine has been incidental to other animal-disease control efforts. In the future, actual control may be incidental to improved inspection efforts directed largely at the control of other diseases of significance to human and animal health.

REFERENCES

Alboiu, M., Popescu, S., 1978, Investigations concerning the resistance to freeze–drying of *Trichinella spiralis* in pig meat, *Arch. Vet.* **13**:165–171.

Allen, R.W., and Goldberg, A., 1962, The effect of various salt concentrations on encysted *Trichinella spiralis* larvae, *Am. J. Vet. Res.* **23**:580–586.

Animal and Plant Health Inspection Service, 1981, National Status of Control of Garbage Feeding, USDA, Washington, D.C.

Bessonov, A., 1979, Short review on trichinellosis in the USSR (Proceedings of the International Commission on Trichinellosis), *Wiad. Parazytol.* **25:**578–579.

Carlin, F.A., Mott, C., Cash, D., and Zimmerman, W.J., 1969, Destruction of trichina in cooked pork roasts, *J. Food Sci.* **34:**210–212.

Centers for Disease Control, 1980, Trichinosis Surveillance Annual Summary 1979.

Cockrill, W.R., 1963, International problems and practices in meat hygiene, *Vet. Rec.* **75:**875–883.

Economics and Statistics Service, 1980, Agriculture Statistics, USDA, Washington, D.C., 313 pp.

Food Safety and Quality Service, 1973, Meat and Poultry Inspection Regulations, USDA, Washington, D.C., pp. 125–131.

Food Safety and Quality Service, 1981, Meat and Poultry Inspection, 1980, Report of the Secretary of Agriculture to the Committee on Agriculture, House of Representatives and Committee on Agriculture, Nutrition and Forestry, U.S. Senate, USDA, Washington, D.C.

Foreign Agriculture Service, 1981, Foreign Agriculture Circular, Livestock and Meat, USDA, Washington, D.C., p. 11.

Francke, D., Hanrahan, M., and Wissman, D., 1977, Costs associated with the use of freezing to certify pork as trichinae free, Development Planning and Research Associates, Manhattan, Kansas.

Gammon, D.L., Kemp, J.D., Edney, J.M., and Varney, W.Y., 1968, Salt, moisture and aging time effects on the viability of *Trichinella spiralis* in pork hams and shoulders, *J. Food Sci.* **33:**417–419.

Gibbs, H.C., Macqueen, K.F., and Pullin, J.W., 1961, The effects of cobalt 60 radiation on *Trichinella spiralis* in meat, *Can. J. Public Health* **52:**232–240.

Gibbs, H.C., Macqueen, K.F., and Pullin, J.W., 1964, Further studies of the effects of gamma radiation on pork infected with *Trichinella spiralis*, *Can. J. Public Health* **55:**191–194.

Gould, S.E., and Kaasa, L.J., 1948, Low temperature treatment of pork: Effect of certain low temperatures on viability of trichinae larvae, *Am. J. Hyg.* **49:**17–24.

Hill, C.H., 1968, Fecal transmission of *Trichinella spiralis* in penned hogs, *Am. J. Vet. Res.* **29:**1229–1234.

Hymphreys, G.K., and Ragland, W.L., 1981, Comparison of competitive and uncompetitive (excess reagent) enzyme immunoassay (EIA) for penicilloyl (Agp) quantitation, Federation of American Societies for Experimental Biology 65th Annual Meeting, (unpublished paper).

Kozar, Z., 1961, *Trichinella* free, *Med. Weter.* **17:**332–336.

Leighty, J.C., 1974, The role of meat inspection in preventing trichinosis in man, *J. Am. Vet. Med. Assoc.* **65:**994–995.

Nelson, G.S., Rickman, R., and Pester, F.R.N., 1961, Feral trichinosis in Africa, *Trans. R. Soc. Trop. Med. Hyg.* **55:**514517.

Otto, G.F., and Abrams, E., 1939, Quantitative studies on the effect of heat on trichinae (*Trichinella spiralis*) larvae, *Am. J. Hyg.* **29:**115–120.

Ransom, B.H., 1916, Effects of refrigeration upon the larvae of *Trichinella spiralis*, *J. Agric. Res.* **5:**819–853.

Ransom, B.H., and Schwartz, B., 1919, Effects of heat on trichinae, *J. Agric. Res.* **17:**201–221.

Rombauer, I.S., and Rombauer Becker, M., 1967, *Joy of Cooking*, Bobbs-Merrill, Indianapolis, Indiana.

Ruitenberg, E.J., and Kamplemacher, E.H., 1970, Diagnostiche Methoden zur Feststelling der Invasion mit *Trichinella spiralis*, *Fleischwirtschaft* **50**:42–47.

Ruitenberg, E.J., van Knapen, F., and Weiss, J.W., 1979, Foodborne parasitic infections—a review, *Vet. Parasitol.* **5**:1–10.

Rust, R.E., and Zimmerman, W.J., 1972, Low-temperature destruction of *Trichinella spiralis* using liquid nitrogen and liquid carbon dioxide, *J. Food Sci.* **37**:706–707.

Schultz, M.G., 1970, Reservoirs of *Trichinella spiralis* in nature and routes of transmission to man, *J Parasitol.* **56**:309–310.

Smith, H.J., 1975, An evaluation of low temperature sterilization of trichinae infected pork, *Can. J. Comp. Med.* **39**:316–320.

Spindler, L.A., Dunker, C.F., and Hawkins, O.G., 1946, Trichina killed by 120-deg. F. dehydration, *Food Ind.* **18**:342–344, 466–468.

Standefer, J.C., and Saunders, G.C., 1978, Enzyme immunoassay for gentamicin, *Clin. Chem.* **24**:1903–1907.

Steele, J.H., and Arambulo, P.V., 1975, Trichinosis, a world problem with extensive sylvatic reservoirs, *Int. J. Zoon.* **2**:55–75.

Thoen, C.O., Armburst, A.L., and Hopkins, M.P., 1979, Enzyme-linked immunosorbent assay for detecting antibodies in swine infected with *Mycobacterium avium*, *Am. J. Vet. Res.* **40**:1096–1099.

Thoen, C.O., Hopkins, M.P., Armbrust, A.L., Angus, R.D., and Pietz, D.E., 1980, Development of an enzyme-linked immunosorbent assay for detecting antibodies in sera of *Brucella suis*-infected swine, *Can. J. Comp. Med.* **44**:294–298.

Tyzzer, E.E., and Honeij, J.A., 1916, The effects of radiation on the development of *Trichinella spiralis* with respect to its application to the treatment of other parasitic diseases, *J. Parasitol.* **3**:43–56.

Visnjakow, J.I., and Georgieu, M., 1972, Swine caudophogy, a new epizootiological link of trichinellosis in the industrial swine farms, *Acta Parasitologica Poloniza* **20**:597–604.

Zimmermann, W.J., 1971, Salt cure and drying time and temperature effects on viability of *Trichinella spiralis* in dry cured hams, *J. Food Sci.* **36**:58–62.

Zimmermann, W.J., Hubbard, E.D., Schwarte, L.H., and Biester, H.E., 1962, Trichinosis in Iowa swine with further studies on modes of transmission, *Cornell Vet.* **52**:156–163.

Zimmermann, W.J., Steele, J.H., and Kagan, I.G., 1973, Trichiniasis in the U.S. population, 1966–70, *Health Serv. Rep.* **88**:606–623.

16

Control II

Surveillance in Swine and Other Animals by Muscle Examination

WILLIAM J. ZIMMERMANN

1. INTRODUCTION

1.1. General Methods and Uses

The demonstration of *Trichinella spiralis* larvae ("trichinae") in the musculature of man, swine, or other carnivorous animals is a positive determination of infection. Various methods of direct diagnosis have been used, including trichinoscopy (also known as the compression or microscopic method), digestion or mechanical disintegration of muscle tissue, biopsy and microscopic section of muscles, and xenodiagnosis. The desired method will vary with objectives and circumstances (such as whether examination is to be made on living or dead hosts), economics, especially when related to slaughterhouse examination of swine, degree of efficacy desired, amount of muscle sample available, stage of infection, and availability of equipment.

WILLIAM J. ZIMMERMANN • Veterinary Medical Research Institute, Iowa State University, Ames, Iowa 50011.

The major use of direct diagnostic methods, especially the trichinoscopic and digestion procedures, has been for postslaughter detection of *Trichinella* larvae in swine carcasses. The trichinoscopic method has been the primary means for control of the public-health aspects of trichinosis in many countries.

1.2. Criteria for Use

Any diagnostic method used for postslaughter examination of swine should meet certain criteria in regard to safety, cost, and adaptability to slaughterhouse use. A safe method must be able to detect *T. spiralis* as early as 17 days postinfection, when the larvae generally become infective to a new host, and to be effective throughout the lifespan of the swine. The method should be sensitive enough to detect concentrations of at least 1 larva per gram of muscle, since this is regarded as the level necessary to induce clinical trichinosis in man (Schwartz, 1962). Preferably, the sensitivity should be high enough to preclude even subclinical infection in man.

Cost of examination is also important when examination is mandatory. About 85,000,000 swine are slaughtered per year in the United States. An examination cost of 50 cents per animal would result in an expenditure of over $40,000,000 per year. Adaptability is also important, since the method utilized should not interfere with normal slaughter operations. The method should be rapid enough so that examination is completed before swine are cut into parts and identification of infected carcasses lost.

The various direct diagnostic methods will be discussed, stressing desired applications and the pros and cons of their usage.

2. TRICHINOSCOPIC METHOD

2.1. Use

The use of this method for postslaughter detection of *T. spiralis* in swine has served as the primary approach to controlling trichinosis in many parts of the world. It was introduced in Germany in 1863 and subsequently made mandatory in Prussia in 1877. The procedure was soon adopted for use in many other countries of Europe. Although some discontent has arisen concerning its safety and cost, it is still used as a basic diagnostic procedure in many countries.

2.2. Procedure for Swine Diagnosis

The basic procedure as applied in West Germany (Lehmensick, 1970) is as follows: 4–5 g of muscle is taken from the diaphragm or other prescribed sites. Fourteen small pieces about the size of a grain of wheat are cut from each sample and compressed between glass plates (Fig. 1). Examination is made with a trichinoscope or microscope. A trichinoscope (Fig. 2) is a specially designed projection microscope that eases eyestrain. A specially trained veterinary inspector is allowed to examine 60 swine per day with a trichinoscope or 36 per day using a microscope. After examination is complete, the carcass or meat cut is stamped either as trichina-free (no *Trichinella* larvae) or unfit (infected). Unfit meat must be destroyed. In addition to examination of swine in slaughterhouses, the German law also mandates examination of home-slaughtered swine and any carnivorous animal that is to be used for human consumption, including dogs, wild boars, bears, and foxes.

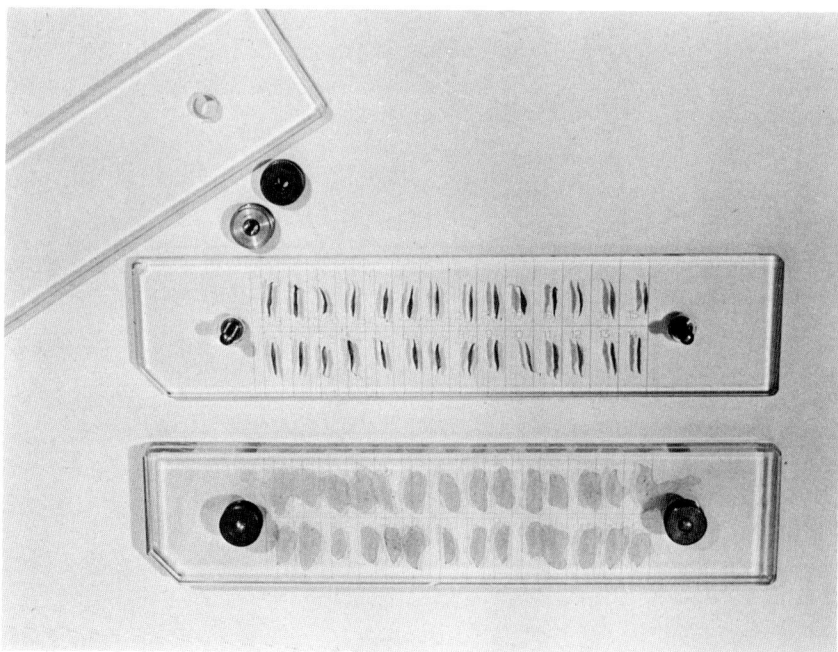

FIGURE 1. Trichinoscope slides. Unassembled slide contains groups of 14 snips from the crura of two pigs. Bottom slide is closed and ready for examination.

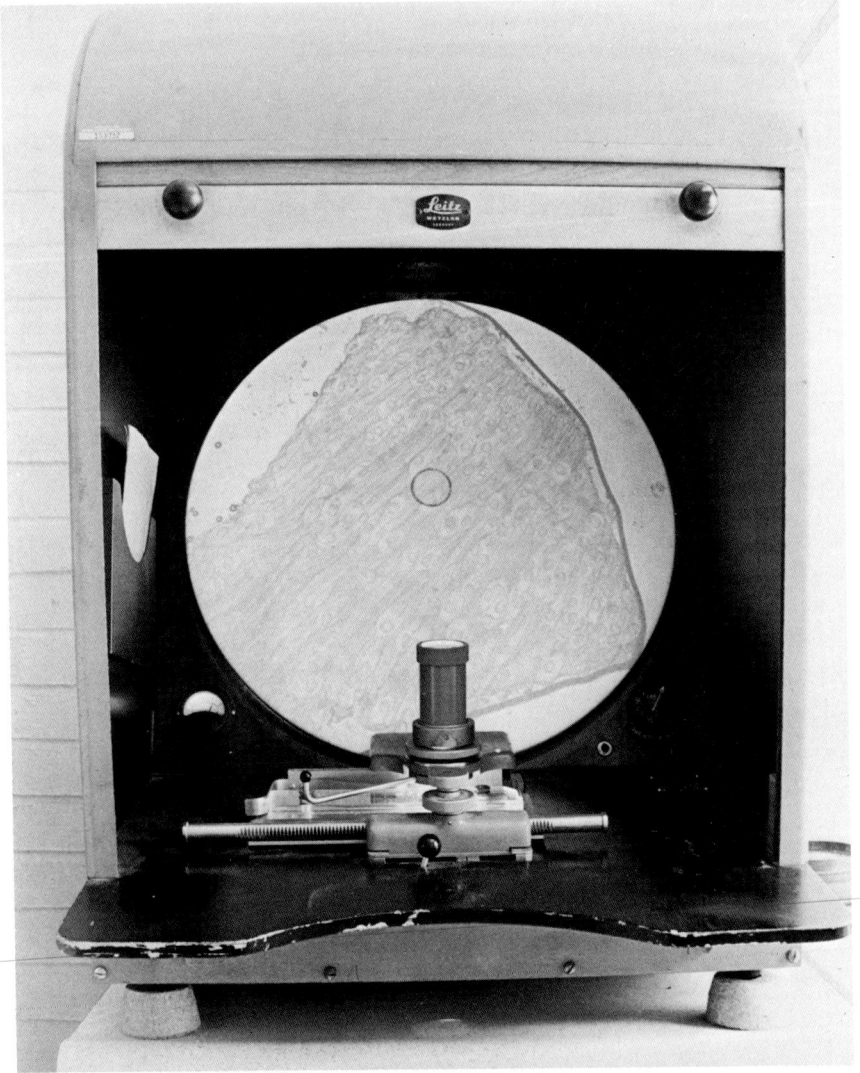

FIGURE 2. Trichinoscope in use for examination of slide from Fig. 1.

2.3. Drawbacks

Routine trichinoscopic examination is expensive, since the program requires specially trained veterinarians and there is a limitation on animals examined per day. Psychological problems may arise, since an inspector may spend his lifetime without finding a natural infection in countries such as West Germany, where the current infection rate is about 1 per 3,000,000 swine.

Sample size varies from 24 snips in the U.S.S.R. to only 3 snips in Chile. Many European countries use a 14-piece sample that is generally considered to weigh 1 g, although Thomsen (1976) stated that 0.5 g was the usual sample size. Ruitenberg and Sluiters (1974) consider the practical limit of sensitivity to be 3 trichinae per gram. Since 1 larva per gram of diaphragm is generally considered necessary to induce clinical infection in man (Schwartz, 1962), use of a 1-g sample should eliminate most clinical infections in man when the procedure is effectively applied. The destruction of infected carcasses also reduces the potential for transmitting the infection to other swine through pork scraps in garbage.

However, with use of a 1-g sample or less, light infections in swine will not be detected. W.J. Zimmermann and Zinter (1971) estimated that 68% of the infections in United States swine contain fewer than 1 larva per gram, and thus would likely be missed by the trichinoscopic method. Routine examination of swine by the trichinoscopic method in the Netherlands from 1926–1962 revealed no infected swine (Ruitenberg and Sluiters, 1974). However, studies in 1969–1971 using a digestion method with larger samples revealed a reservoir of low-grade infections in swine from throughout the country.

Another safety drawback of the trichinoscopic method is the difficulty in detection of nonencysted larvae. Clarity is often lacking, especially if larvae are not coiled. Since the wall of the cyst (nurse cell) does no become readily discernible until about 4 weeks after infection, there would be about a 10-day period when larvae are infective but not easily detected by low-power microscopic examination.

2.4. Other Uses

The trichinoscopic method has been used for human and animal prevalence studies. Results, again, may be influenced by sample size. In the United States, the trichinoscopic method has been used in conjunction with the digestion method for human prevalence studies. Calcified cysts and dead *T. spiralis* larvae may be detected by trichinoscopic examination but destroyed by digestion. In a national human prevalence study involving 335 positives in 8071 samples, W.J. Zimmermann *et al.* (1973) detected 39.4% of the infections by digestion only, 19.7% by the trichinoscopic method only, and 40.9% by both methods. The trichinoscopic method detected 191 infections with dead trichinae only, 5 with mixed live and dead, and 7 with live trichinae only. In this study, digestion did not markedly affect calcified cysts or dead trichinae, since 228 infections in this classification were detected by digestion.

3. BASIC DIGESTION METHOD

3.1. Basic Procedure

This procedure, first used by Thornbury (1897), applies the principles of gastric digestion. The muscle fibers and cysts are digested away, while live *T. spiralis* larvae, if present, will survive unless the digestion process is prolonged for much beyond 24 hr. The basic procedure currently used by the author is as follows: Muscle samples, generally from the diaphragm, are trimmed free of fat and fascia and finely ground with a mechanical food chopper. A sample of up to 100 g is placed in a 3-liter beaker to which is added 2.5 liters of digestive fluid containing 0.5% pepsin (NF 1:3000) and 0.7% hydrocholoric acid. The beaker is placed in a 43.3°C incubator, where the sample is digested for 17 hr with constant agitation provided by plastic paddles moving back and forth. After digestion, the solution is allowed to stand for 1 hr, after which the top two thirds of the supernate is siphoned off. The remaining fluid is poured into a 7-inch Baermann funnel with a 60-mesh sieve. Incubator-temperature water is added to cover the screen. After 1 hr settling, the clamp at the bottom of the funnel is released and the fluid is drawn into a 5-inch funnel. After an additional 1-hr settling period, a sample is drawn into a ruled Syracuse watch glass. The fluid in the dish is microscopically examined with a dissection microscope at 27×. Repeated examinations are made at 15-min intervals until two negative readings are obtained. If too many larvae are present to count, additional fluid is drawn into a beaker from which an aliquot is taken and examined.

3.2. Modifications

Various procedures have been used by other workers. Gould (1970) used a blender for tissue-grinding and a digestive fluid containing 1% pepsin and 1% hydrochloric acid. Digestion was carried out at 37°C for 16 hr with no agitation or in a water bath at 40°C for 3–4 hr with constant agitation. Some workers use intermittent manual stirring, while others produce agitation by magnetic stirrers, electric stirrers, or bubbling air. A repetitive settling–washing procedure may be substituted for the use of funnels, or concentration may be accomplished by centrifugation.

3.3. Advantages and Disadvantages

The primary advantage of the digestion procedure over the trichinoscopic method is that it allows increased sample size, up to 100 g or more as compared to 1 g or less. With the large samples, few infections will be missed, even when of minimal intensity. As cited earlier, dead larvae or calcified cysts may be destroyed by digestion. However, in the human study by W.J. Zimmermann *et al.* (1973), *Trichinella* infections were detected by the digestion method in 77% of 288 samples containing only dead *Trichinella*. A 20-mesh sieve in the Baermann funnel allowed passage of calcified cysts that had withstood digestion.

A disadvantage of the digestion method when used for individual samples is cost, primarily that of pepsin and of labor. Daily individual output would be about the same as that for trichinoscopic examination.

4. POOLED DIGESTION METHOD

4.1. Pooled-Sample Method: Procedure

The pork industry of the United States in 1966 requested increased research to develop an eradication program for trichinosis. The trichonoscopic method was deemed unsatisfactory as a diagnostic method due to questions of safety, as discussed earlier, and cost. Approximately 60,000 swine for export were examined with trichinoscopes in the United States during 1964 at a cost of about 70 cents per animal.

One of the options considered was the pooled-sample method (W.J. Zimmermann, 1967, 1974). This method is basically a modification of the previously described artificial digestion method as used by the author. The procedure is initiated by dividing the slaughtered swine into lots of 20–25 consecutive carcasses. A portion of the diaphragmatic crus is removed from each pig in each lot. Each sample is trimmed to 5–6 g for a 25-pig lot or 7–8 g for a 20-pig lot. The pooled sample is finely ground in a food chopper with 3-mm cutting-plate openings. Digestions are carried out for 4–6 hr at 43.4°C in a prewarmed digestive fluid containing 1% pepsin (NF 1:3000) and 1% hydrochloric acid. The remaining procedure is the same as that for the artificial digestion method described in Section 3.1.

The finding of a *Trichinella* larva indicates a positive lot. The carcasses comprising the lot are retained for further examination. A 50-g portion of the crus is collected from each pig and examined individually by the artificial digestion method. Any infected carcass in a lot is processed to kill trichinae by approved procedures (see Chapter 15). Negative carcasses in a lot are released for routine processing.

During a 32-week pilot study in an Iowa slaughter plant (Andrews *et al.*, 1969), 482,392 swine carcasses were examined, with 42 (0.0087%) being found infected. Of the infected carcasses, 24 contained fewer than 1 larva per gram, the theoretical limit of efficacy for the trichinoscope method. The procedure did not interfere with normal plant operation, even when the slaughter rate exceeded 500 swine per hour.

A 10-hr digestive period was used during the pilot study. Eight employees plus a veterinary supervisor were utilized: five employees on the day shift who collected samples and initiated digestion and three employees on the night shift who carried out concentration and examined samples. Had the trichinoscopic method been used, a crew of nearly 70 inspectors would have been necessary for a 4000-swine-per-day output. The cost per pig examined by the pooled-sample method during the pilot study was 9.35 cents.

4.2. Stomacher Method: Procedure

The development of the pooled-sample method stimulated interest in Europe. In contrast to the overnight cooling of carcasses before cutting into commercial cuts as used in the United States, carcasses are often cut warm in many European slaughterhouses, with subsequent identification of carcasses being lost. Therefore, attention was focused on the development of rapid digestion procedures. There was also hesitancy in using samples as large as the 5–8 g samples proposed for the pooled-sample method.

Thomsen (1976, 1977) developed the Stomacher method as an alternative. The Stomacher device was developed by Sharpe and Jackson (1972) to prepare bacterial suspensions from foods and other materials. The procedure by Thomsen involves use of a thermostatically controlled Stomacher laboratory blender (Fig. 3) in which digestion is activated by paddles pounding on plastic bags containing the pooled muscle samples and digestive fluid. A pool of 100, 1-g samples is used. The digestive fluid consists of 1.5 liters of water heated to 40–41°C, 25 ml 17.5% hydrochloric acid, and 6 g pepsin (NF 1 : 10,000). Digestion is carried out at 40–41°C for 25 min (recently revised from the original 10 min).

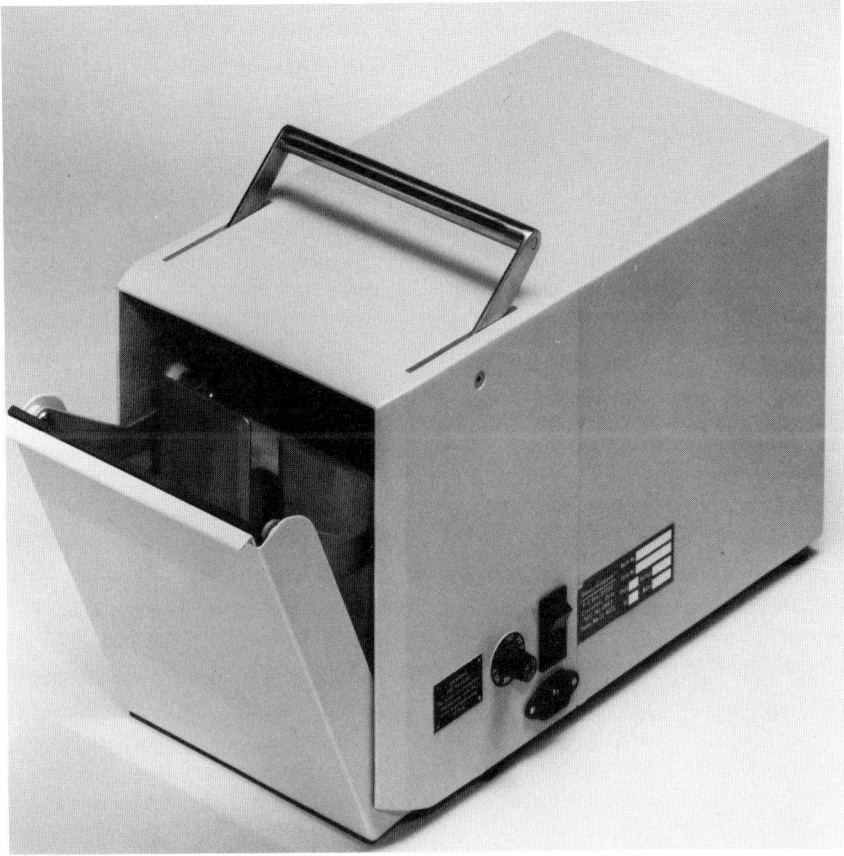

FIGURE 3. Stomacher. Plastic bag, containing sample and digestion fluid, is placed between paddles and door. Agitation is carried out by paddles pounding on bag. Courtesy of Tekmar Company, Cincinnati, Ohio.

The digestive fluid is then poured into a beaker to which flaked ice is added. After being chilled, the fluid is placed in a sedimentation funnel that is vibrated intermittently for 30 min. Then, 60–70 ml is quickly run off into a 100 ml cylinder. After 10 min settling, all but 15 ml is siphoned off. The remaining 15 ml is examined microscopically.

One person can examine about 200 pigs per hour by the Stomacher method, about 25 times the output of an inspector using a trichinoscope. This method has been approved in Denmark, Finland, Norway, Sweden, and Italy. It has also been accepted for examination of meat to be imported to West Germany.

4.3. Other Modifications

The pooled-digestion technique, with various modifications, has also been studied in other countries. Podhajecky (1974), in Czechoslovakia, using a digestive pool of 100 0.5-g samples, reduced the digestion–examination time to 1½ hr. Snobl and Kuklik (1976), also in Czechoslovakia, proposed a sample pool of 200 0.25-g samples, which involves smaller samples than most trichinoscopic methods. A procedure developed by Skovgaard (1975) in Denmark reduced the processing time to 6 hr for a pool of 100 1-g samples. Kohler (1977), in West Germany, reduced this period to 4 hr. Lotsch et al. (1979) reported that more than 4,000,000 swine slaughtered at 30 meat packing plants in West Germany have been examined by the group digestion method. Bessonov et al. (1978, 1981), in the U.S.S.R., developed an automated apparatus for recovery of Trichinella larvae (ART). Excluding time for mincing of samples, the total time for digestion and examination is 30–35 min. The procedure is used in nine U.S.S.R. slaughterhouses. The output per worker has increased 6-fold over that for the trichinoscopic method. Depending on the epizootiological situation in the area where the test was used, the sample pool varied from 20 5-g samples to 100 1-g samples. Forray and Szel (1975) and Simonffy et al. (1979) used both pepsin and papain in the digestive fluids. Many of the larvae remained encysted after digestion. Kohler (1979), using a magnetic stirrer, and Becker (1980), using an ultrasonic device, obtained highly efficient digestion and recovery of Trichinella larvae in minimal times. Kohler (1981) found little difference in efficacy of the magnetic stirrer method, the regular digestion method, and 25-min Stomacher digestion for detection of 40-week-old and 4-week-old infections of three intensity levels. A 12-min digestion with the Stomacher was only about 50% as effective as the other three methods. The trichinoscopic method was much less efficacious except for detection of heavy, 17-day infections, which were also detectable by the magnetic stirrer and digestion methods, but not by the Stomacher procedure. Modified procedures have also been used in Poland (Gerwel and Pawlowski, 1975), East Germany (G. Zimmermann, 1976), and Romania (Cristescu, 1973). Cristescu used a pool of 50 2-g samples. Henriksen (1978) developed a filtration staining technique to reduce the sedimentation period.

There is a direct relationship between safety and cost. Sample size, and therefore degree of safety for the consumer, must be determined by the extent of the problem, efficacy desired, and availability of funding. The 1-g samples proposed for use in most European countries should eliminate clinical infections in man. However, a reservoir of infection may remain in swine, since 68% of the infections in swine in the United States contain fewer than 1 larva per gram (Section 2.3).

5. OTHER DIRECT DIAGNOSTIC METHODS

5.1. Mechanical Disintegration Method

Since *Trichinella* larvae do not withstand digestion until approximately 17 days postinfection, 12 days after invasion of muscles, Levin (1941) developed a disintegration method (loosely termed "maceration method") to isolate young larvae from the musculature. Larvae are isolated from finely ground tissue by a series of mechanical agitations, washings, and filtrations. The procedure is recommended for examination of musculature 5–21 days postinfection.

5.2. Microscopic Section (Biopsy Method)

This method is occasionally used in an attempt to confirm clinical findings of trichinosis in humans. Sites recommended for biopsy include biceps, gastrocnemius, pectoral, gluteus maximus, and intercostals (Gould, 1970). Serial sections of the tissue should be examined to detect the parasite, cyst, or related inflammatory response. The biopsy method has drawbacks. If the infection is light, or recently acquired, *Trichinella* larvae may not be present in the tissues examined. Wright (1942) recommended that biopsy specimens not be taken before 21 days postinfection, since many larvae will not have reached the musculature before that time and those present may not have coiled, making the parasite difficult to detect. Parasites or cysts or both may also be present from older infections (McNaught, 1939). Therefore, the examiner should be familiar with pathological changes related to both old and new infections.

5.3. Xenodiagnosis

Occasionally, it is desirable to determine the presence or viability or both of larvae in the musculature of an animal or in pork products. This can be accomplished by feeding tissues to rats, mice, or other animals, then sacrificing the new host at 5 weeks postinfection to detect *Trichinella* larvae in musculature (Beck, 1953).

The author has extensively used the xenodiagnostic method, or a modification, to determine the viability of trichinae in meat-processing studies where the product has been heated, frozen, or cured for various periods of time. Often, instead of the meat being fed directly, the product is digested for 4 hr, the residue then being washed free of digestive fluid and injected orally into the stomachs of mice or rats. Microscopic examination of digestive residue often reveals larvae that appear coiled but somewhat abnormal in appearance. The xenodiagnostic method determines their viability.

6. SUMMARY

Each of the direct diagnostic methods has advantages and disadvantages that must be considered in selecting a method for a specific use. Although the trichinoscopic method has had widespread usage for routine surveillance of trichinosis in swine at slaughter, cost and efficacy considerations would make one of the pooled-digestion procedures preferable for this use. As experience is gained in Europe with use of the various modifications of the pooled-digestion procedure, additional improvements undoubtedly will be made.

The single-sample digestion method is preferred for prevalence studies in man, swine, and other animals, since the use of a relatively large sample makes it more efficacious than the trichinoscopic method. However, where dead or calcified trichinae may be encountered, as in human surveys, use of both methods may be advantageous.

The other methods, namely, mechanical disintegration, microscopic section, and xenodiagnosis, have more limitations, but there are specific applications for which these methods may be preferred.

REFERENCES

Andrews, J.S., Zinter, D.E., and Schulz, N.E., 1969, Evaluation of the trichinosis pilot project, Proceedings of the 73rd Annual Meeting, U.S. Animal Health Association, Milwaukee, October 12–17, 1969, pp. 332–353.

Beck, J.W., 1953, Xenodiagnostic technic as an aid in the diagnosis of trichinosis, *Am. J. Trop. Med. Hyg.* **2**:97–101.

Becker, H.-G., 1980, Beitrag zur Verkurzung der Inkubationszeit zum Trichinellennachweis bei Schlachtschweinen nach dem Digestionsverfahren, *Fleischwirtschaft* **60**:678–680.

Bessonov, A.S., Uspenskii, A.V., and Shekhovtsov, N.V., 1978, Group diagnosis of trichinellosis in pigs under conditions of meat-packing plants, in: *Trichinellosis* (C.W. Kim and F.S. Pawlowki, eds.), University Press of New England, Hanover, New Hampshire, pp. 519–522.

Bessonov, A.S., Upensky, A.V., and Shekhovtsov, N.V., 1981, Industrial trials of a method for mass diagnosis of pig trichinellosis in meat-packing plants, in: *Trichinellosis* (C.W. Kim, E.J. Ruitenberg, and J.S. Teppema, eds.), Reedbooks, Chertsey, Surrey, England, pp. 409–414.

Cristescu, M., 1973, Cu privire la diagnosticul trichinclozei porcine in abatoure de marc capacitate, *Rev. Zooteh. Med. Vet.*, pp. 81–88.

Forray, A., and Szel, G., 1975, Gyors emesztesi eljaras a sertes *Trichinella spiralis* okozta fertozottsegenetek megallapitasara, *Magy. Allatorv. Lapja.* **30**:187–189.

Gerwel, C., and Pawlowski, Z., 1975, Studies on the epidemiology and biology of trichinellosis in Poland (1964–1975). *Wiad. Parazytol.* **21**:513–540.

Gould, S.E., 1970, Clinical pathology: Diagnostic laboratory procedures, in: *Trichinosis in Man and Animals* (S.E. Gould, ed.), Charles C. Thomas, Springfield, Illinois, pp. 190–221.

Henriksen, S.A., 1978, A new technique for demonstration of *Trichinella spiralis* larva in suspensions of digested muscle tissue, *Acta Vet. Scand.* **19**:466–468.

Kohler, G., 1977, Zur Effektivät der Verdauungmethode beim Nachweis der Trichinellose des Schlachtschweines, *Fleischwirtschaft* **57**:421–423.

Kohler, G., 1979, Untersuchungen mit der Stomachermethode in Vergleich zu anderen Direktion verfahren beim Nachweis der Trichinellose des Schweines, *Fleischwirtschaft* **59**:1258–1261.

Kohler, G., 1981, Zur Nachweisbarkeit lang- und kurzfristiger *Trichinella spiralis*-infektionen beim Schlachtschweinen mittels direkter Verfahren, *Fleischwirtschaft* **61**:732–735.

Lehmensick, R., 1970, Inspection of pork and control of trichinosis in Germany, in: *Trichinosis in Man and Animals* (S.E. Gould, ed.), Charles C. Thomas, Springfield, Illinois, pp. 437–448.

Levin, A.J., 1941, Recovery of *Trichinella spiralis* larvae in early stages of infection, *J. Parasitol.* **27**:107–113.

Lotsch, R., Kubitz, K., and Heissinger, L., 1979, Wo steht die Trichinenuntersuchung Heute? Umfrage an deutsche EWG-Schlacht-Betriebe, *Fleischwirtschaft* **59**:1088–1092.

McNaught, J.B., 1939, The diagnosis of trichinosis, *Am. J. Trop. Med.* **19**:181–192.

Podhajecky, K., 1974, Orientacne vylucovacia metoda prehliadky masa osipanych na trichinely, *Veterinarstvi* **24**:303–304.

Ruitenberg, E.J., and Sluiters, J.F., 1974, *Trichinella spiralis* infections in the Netherlands, in: *Trichinellosis* (C.W. Kim, ed.), Intext, New York, pp. 539–548.

Schwartz, B., 1962, Trichinosis in the United States, in: *Trichinellosis*, Proceedings of the 1st International Conference on Trichinellosis, Warsaw, pp. 68–75.

Sharpe, A.N., and Jackson, A.K., 1972, Stomaching: A new concept in bacteriological sample preparation, *Appl. Microbiol.* **24**:175–178.

Simonffy, Z., Ando, P., Juhasz, J., Sari, G., and Takacs, J., 1979, Osszehasonlito vizsgalatok az emesztesi es a trichinoszkopos vizsgalat hatasfokara, *Magy. Allatorv. Lapja.* **34**:47–50.

Skovgaard, N., 1975, Fordøjelsesmetode til undersøgelse of samleprøver of 100 svin for trikiner, *Dansk. Vet. Tidsskr.* **58**:514–520.

Snobl, A., and Kuklik, K., 1976, Prohlidka veproveho masa na svalovce travici metodou ve velkprovoznich podminkach, *Veterinarstvi* **26**:272–273.

Thomsen, D.U., 1976, "Stomacher" trikinkontrol-metoden, *Dansk. Vet. Tidsskr.* **59**:481–490.

Thomsen, D.U., 1977, Den af Veterinaerdirektoratet godkendte version of Stomacher-trikinkontrolmetoden, *Dansk. Vet. Tiddskr.* **60**:337–341.

Thornbury, F.J., 1897, The pathology of trichinosis: Original observations, *Univ. Med. Mag.* **10**:64–79.

Wright, W.H., 1942, A consideration of the clinical and public health aspects of trichinosis, *J. Lancet.*, **62**:389–393.

Zimmermann, G., 1976, Vorschlag zur Einführung der Digestionsmethode als ein neues, verbessertes Untersuchungsverfahren in der gesetzlichen Trichenschau, *Schlacten Vermarkten* **9**:301–303.

Zimmermann, W.J., 1967, A pooled sample method for post slaughter detection of trichiniasis in swine, *Proc. 71st Annu. Meet. U.S. Livestock Sanit. Assoc.*, pp. 358–366.

Zimmermann, W.J., 1974, The modified pooled sample method for post-slaughter detection of trichinosis in swine, in: *Trichinellosis*, (C.W. Kim, ed.), Intext, New York, pp. 539–548.

Zimmermann, W.J., and Zinter, D.E., 1971, The prevalence of trichiniasis in swine in the United States, 1966–70, *HSMHA Health Rep.* **86**:937–945.

Zimmermann, W.J., Steele, J.H., and Kagan, I.G., 1973, Trichiniasis in the U.S. population, 1966–70: Prevalence, epidemiologic factors, *Health Serv. Rep.* **88**:606–623.

17

Control III

Surveillance in Swine by Immunodiagnostic Methods

E. JOOST RUITENBERG, FRANS VAN KNAPEN, and
ANNEKE ELGERSMA

1. INTRODUCTION

Tests for the detection of *Trichinella spiralis* infection in pigs at slaughter make use either of direct methods (trichinoscopy, digestion methods) by means of which the parasite itself can be demonstrated (see Chapter 16) or of indirect (serological or skin test) methods. With the latter, the presence of the parasite can be suggested by the demonstration of specific anti-*Trichinella* humoral or cell-mediated immunity. The reliability of these immunological methods depends largely on the quality of the reagents used. The presence of cell-mediated immunity can be assessed by a skin test, which has been employed only occasionally for *Trichinella* (Andrews *et al.*, 1976). Much more attention has been paid to the evaluation of a humoral response by a variety of serological techniques.

It should be realized that serological methods can be applied in two different ways: (1) clinical application, by which individuals are

E. JOOST RUITENBERG, FRANS VAN KNAPEN, and ANNEKE ELGERSMA • Rijks Instituut Voor de Volksgezondheid, 3720 BA Bilthoven, The Netherlands.

checked for the presence of the infectious agent by comparing antibody titers in paired sera; (2) for screening populations for the presence of a microorganism; in this case, the presence or absence of antibodies is used as a criterion.

In contrast to the first approach, in which at least two serum samples are needed to follow the kinetics of the antibody response, in the second approach, one serum sample is sufficient. However, screening should be carried out in a statistically valid sample of the population. In this chapter, we will discuss the possibilities of using serological methods for the surveillance of swine trichinosis.

2. SEROLOGICAL METHODS

2.1. Complement-Fixation Test

This universally applied method was first described by Frisch *et al.* (1947) for the diagnosis of human trichinosis, using soluble polysaccharide fractions of larval antigen. This relatively sensitive method, however, lacked sufficient specificity (Poggel, 1952), and since other serological methods became available, comparative studies in experimentally infected pigs and rabbits showed also that light infections were missed with the complement-fixation (CF) test (Kampelmacher and Streefkerk, 1965; Ruitenberg and Kampelmacher, 1970). Furthermore, routine application of this time-consuming method in the slaughterhouse was discouraged from the practical point of view.

2.2. Particle-Agglutination Methods

Various methods have been described that are based on the same principle; i.e., particles coated with *Trichinella* antigen may react with antibody-containing serum and form visible aggregations either on a glass surface or in glass tubes. In this respect, cholesterol crystals were used as early as 1944 (Suessenguth and Kline, 1944); later, cholesterol–lecithin, bentonite, and latex particles were introduced (reviewed in Ruitenberg and Kampelmacher, 1970). For practical field diagnosis, even a "card flocculation test" (Anderson *et al.*, 1963) allowing simpler interpretation (Schultz *et al.*, 1967) was developed. It should be emphasized here that these methods were introduced primarily for the diagnosis of human trichinosis and subsequently used for the screening of pigs at slaughter. The antigens used merely consisted of saline extracts of *T. spiralis* muscle larvae, which guaranteed sufficient specificity in man. In experiments with pigs, rats, and rabbits, however, all these tests proved to lack both sensitivity and specificity, which led to the conclusion that they could not be used to determine light infections in bacon pigs (Kampelmacher and Streefkerk, 1965; Sulzer and Chisholm, 1966; Scholtens *et al.*, 1966; Coats *et al.*, 1969).

2.3. Indirect Immunofluorescence Test

The indirect immunofluorescence (IF) test, which had already been used successfully for the diagnosis of other parasitic infections, was first described for *Trichinella* by Jackson (1959) and introduced for the diagnosis of human trichinosis by Sadun *et al.* (1962).

For the detection of specific *Trichinella* antibodies, muscle larvae are used as the antigen. Antibodies present in the serum react with the cuticle of the larvae. The antibody-coated cuticle is then incubated with antiporcine immunoglobulin labeled with a fluorochrome (fluorescein isothiocyanate) and visualized with ultraviolet light (Ruitenberg *et al.*, 1968; Scholtens *et al.*, 1966).

The advantages of this method over other methods are its specificity and sensitivity. Cross-reactions due to other commonly occurring infections in pigs (*Ascaris*) were not observed, and even slight infections of 100–200 larvae per pig at slaughter could be traced. The authors concluded that the test, which requires skill and the availability of a fluorescence microscope, can be performed only in central laboratories, rather than in the slaughterhouse. Therefore, this test was advocated as being suitable for keeping a permanent check on the presence or absence of antibodies against *T. spiralis* in a pig population.

The assay can be performed in various ways. First, the morphological structure of the parasite itself can be used. Only the muscle larvae and especially the antigenic properties of the cuticle have been evaluated by a number of authors. Variations of this approach included (1) the use of whole larvae in a so-called tube test, (2) cryostat sections of heavily infected musculature, and (3) isolated cuticles. Next, attempts to perform an indirect IF test using a crude soluble antigen of the muscle larvae have been described. In the latter case, an inert support has to be provided as antigen carrier. On this basis, the soluble-antigen/fluorescent antibody (SAFA) test has been developed. The enzyme immunoassays to be described below are based on the same principle.

2.3.1. Indirect IF Test with Whole Larvae in a Tube Test

This assay, originally developed for the diagnosis of human trichinosis (Sadun *et al.*, 1962), has been adapted for the serodiagnosis of porcine trichinosis (Ruitenberg *et al.*, 1968). The assay is based on the presence of specific antigens in the cuticle of muscle larvae. Positive reactions are assessed on the basis of specific fluorescence of the cuticle. Experimental studies in artificially infected slaughter pigs proved the technique to be both specific and sensitive. Early infections could be detected from day 17 after oral infection onward. This is a crucial finding, since larvae isolated from that postinfection time onward are able to resist digestion and are therefore potentially pathogenic for the consumer. Also, lightly infected animals could be detected, and no false-positive findings were reported. The efficacy of the assay under practical conditions can best be illustrated by citing the successful recognition of a very low incidence of *Trichinella* infection in The Netherlands after introduction of the assay in the surveillance of porcine trichinosis. Two years after its introduction, a *Trichinella* infection was reported in The Netherlands, a country always considered to be free of trichinosis (Ruitenberg and Sluiters, 1974).

2.3.2. Indirect IF Test Using Cryostat Sections

The technique was initially described for the diagnosis of human trichinosis (Ljungström, 1974) and was further evaluated for its application in porcine trichinosis by Henriksen *et al.* (1975). They reported that the method, using the cuticle fluorescence as criterion, yielded results similar to those of the tube test. However, when the fluorescence of the internal structures of the parasite was taken into account, the sensitivity was increased. This is in keeping with studies in experimentally infected mice (Ruitenberg *et al.*, 1975a).

2.3.3. Indirect IF Test Using Isolated Cuticles

Sulzer and Chisholm (1966) described the use of cuticles from muscle larvae as the antigen for an indirect IF assay. The aim of this approach was to make available a more stable antigenic preparation that would allow storage and facilitate distribution of the antigen to other laboratories.

2.3.4. Soluble-Antigen/Fluorescent-Antibody Test

The SAFA test was developed for the immunodiagnosis of trichinosis in man and experimental animals by Gore and Sadun (1968). Later, the assay was evaluated for swine trichinosis. Initial studies with crude saline extracts of muscle larvae proved the capriciousness of the technique (Ruitenberg and Berkvens, 1967, unpublished results). Clinard (1975) evaluated the technique in more detail. The author reported that only heavily infected pigs could be readily detected, as soon as 17 days after infection. Long-standing infections of both heavily and lightly infected animals were demonstrable for a period of 1 year. However, false-positive reactions were observed as well (Isenstein, 1974). In addition to the use of a crude antigen, the fluorometer technique available at that time was certainly responsible for the only partially satisfactory results obtained.

2.3.5. Comparative Studies with Indirect IF Assays

A number of authors have evaluated the applicability of the indirect IF technique. They include the groups of Kozar (Kozar and Kozar, 1969; Kozar et al., 1970), Belozyorov (1972, 1975), and Wikerhauser et al. (1980). Belozyorov (1975) stressed the unreliability of the test in the first 2 weeks after infection. Wikerhauser et al. (1980) observed both cases in which positive indirect IF results were combined with negative parasitological results and cases in which parasitologically positive animals did not have demonstrable antibodies. Köhler and Ruitenberg (1974) described the results of a comparative trial by five laboratories in Europe. The indirect IF test was compared with two conventional direct techniques: trichinoscopy and the digestion method. They concluded that the indirect IF test could be a useful tool for surveillance programs in various pig populations.

2.4. Enzyme Immunoassays

Enzyme immunoassays make use of a solid support for the antigen and an enzyme as amplifier for the specific antigen–antibody reaction. The enzyme is coupled to an antispecies immunoglobulin reacting with the original antigen–antibody complex. The amplification is based on the enzymatic reaction of a specific chromogenic substrate yielding a reaction product. This reaction product either precipitates on the solid phase or remains in solution. In both cases, the intensity of the color of the reaction product is related to the amount of antibodies in the body fluid tested. In porcine trichinosis, the enzyme immunoassay performed in polystyrene tubes or microtiter plates [the enzyme-linked immunosorbent assay (ELISA)] and the enzyme-labeled antibody (ELA) test have been described.

2.4.1. Enzyme-Linked Immunosorbent Assay

The assay can be performed both in polystyrene tubes (macroassay) (Ruitenberg *et al.*, 1974) and in microplates (microassay) (Ruitenberg *et al.*, 1975b; Saunders and Clinard, 1976). The principle of the technique is schematically presented in Fig. 1. Most reports describe the use of the enzyme horseradish peroxidase and the substrate 5-aminosalicylic acid. The antigen generally used is a crude saline extract of muscle larvae. As for all serological tests, the reliability of the technique depends largely on the quality of the reagents used. Adequate washing procedures are of particular importance (Ruitenberg *et al.*, 1976b). In contrast to most other serological assays, the interpretation of the test results is objective when a spectrophotometer is used. However, the test can also be read visually, as shown in Fig. 2.

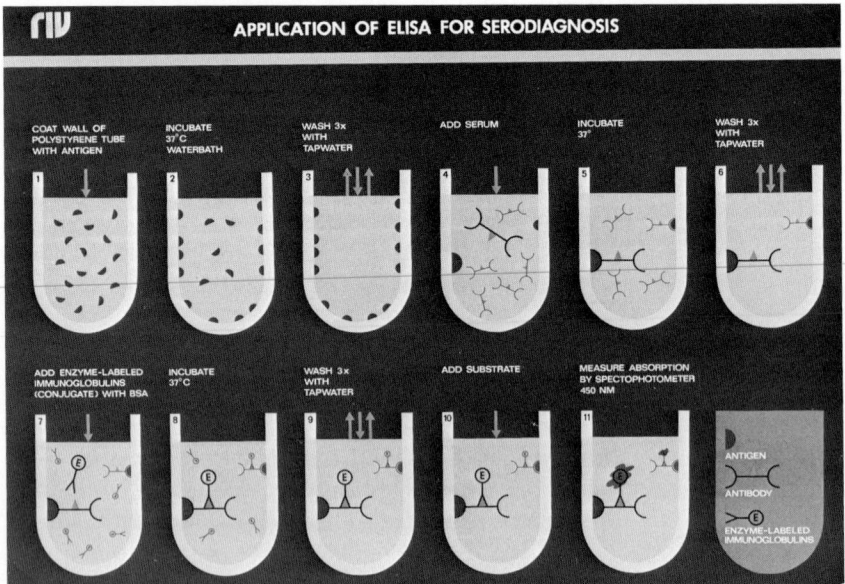

FIGURE 1. Schematic representation of the ELISA for the detection of serum antibodies.

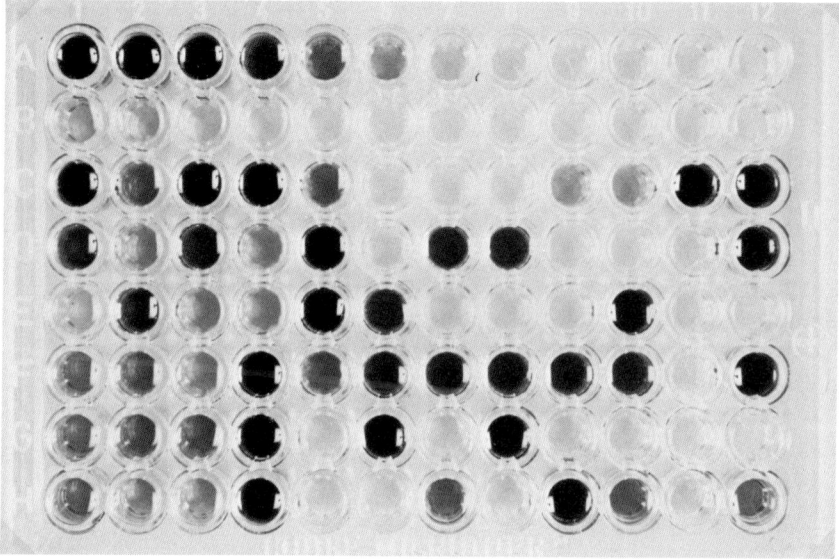

FIGURE 2. Micro-ELISA performed in a microplate. In the two top rows are serial dilutions of a positive reference serum (A) and a negative reference serum (B); all other cups contain single dilutions of individual sera.

2.4.2. ELISA in Tubes (Macroassay)

The original ELISA procedure was based on performance in polystyrene tubes (Ruitenberg *et al.*, 1976a). The tube wall is coated with the antigen without further pretreatment. It is unknown which part of the antigen solution adheres to the wall, since no detailed qualitative or quantitative analysis has been performed. Test results can be based on both serum titers and extinction values of a single dilution only. The test proved to be more sensitive than the indirect IF test, allowing the demonstration of the infection as early as at 4 days postinfection (Ruitenberg *et al.*, 1974). Long-standing infections, up to 40 weeks, can be diagnosed as well (van Knapen *et al.*, 1981). Of particular importance is the specificity of the assay. Based on results of experimentally infected pigs, possible cross-reactions with common porcine helminths such as *Ascaris suum* and *Trichuris suis* could be ruled out (Ruitenberg *et al.*, 1975c). The test is particularly suitable for large-scale screening using a single serum dilution only (see Section 6.1).

2.4.3. ELISA in Microplates (Microassay)

Soon after the introduction of the macro-ELISA, alternative meth-ods were studied to facilitate the handling of larger numbers of sera and to reduce the quantities of reagents used. The microplate test, in particular, met these criteria (Ruitenberg *et al.*, 1975b; Saunders and Clinard, 1976; Saunders *et al.*, 1977). Initially, some problems had to be overcome, since commercially available microplates were produced for handling liquids. Nothing was known about the adhesive properties of the polystyrene and the adequacy of the bottom for direct reading. As indicated in Fig. 2, visual interpretation is acceptable in some micro-ELISA applications, but for large-scale application and standardization, photometric reading is preferable. The mechanization aspects are discussed in Section 6.2. Here, we stress that the sensitivity and the specificity of the micro-ELISA for the serodiagnosis of porcine trichi-nosis are comparable with those of the macro-ELISA (van Knapen *et al.*, 1981).

2.4.4. Comparative Studies with Enzyme Immunoassays

In contrast to other serological methods, enzyme immunoassays offer the possibility of an objective assessment of the results based on the extinction values obtained with a single serum dilution. Evaluation of the test results is possible only on a relative basis, i.e., in comparison with a group of known negative reference sera. For application of the assay under slaughterhouse conditions, sera from conventionally raised pigs should be used as reference. A practical procedure is to determine the mean extinction value of a group of 100 reference sera. The cutoff point of the assay can be chosen arbitrarily on the basis of the mean and 3 times the standard deviation of the mean. This represents a 99% confidence limit (van Knapen *et al.*, 1980).

Various groups of authors evaluated the reliability of ELISA in both experimentally and naturally infected pigs. Ruitenberg *et al.* (1976b) reported that in 1 of 10 noninfected animals from The Netherlands, a false-positive ELISA result was obtained. With the use of the ELA test in populations of swine sent to packing houses for slaughter, positive rates of up to 15% were observed (Clinard *et al.*, 1978). Since the infection rate for swine in the United States is reported to be 0.12% for grain-fed animals and 0.5% for garbage-fed animals (Zimmerman and Zinter, 1971), these positives are believed to be largely false. Clinard (1979) tried unsuccessfully to further analyze the reason for these false-positive reactions. She concluded that there are at least two classes of immuno-globulins in the sera of *T. spiralis*-negative pigs that react with *T. spiralis* antigen and suggested that the specificity of the test could be improved by isolating an antigen fraction with greater specificity for *T. spiralis* IgG antibody than for false-positive IgG. Taylor *et al.* (1980) described the isolation of such a fraction that, when combined with some technical changes in the test procedure, both significantly reduced false-positive readings and simultaneously increased the sensitivity of the test. From Yugoslavia, Rapić (1980) reported the successful application of ELISA with crude saline extracts of muscle larvae under both experimental and field conditions. The reliability of ELISA results was proven by the demonstration of *T. spiralis* larvae at autopsy by trichinoscopy or the digestion method in all serologically positive animals and by the absence of larvae in all ELISA-negative animals. This confirms data by van Knapen *et al.* (1976) on the reliability of the ELISA in naturally infected Norwegian pigs. ELISA results agreed well with those obtained with the digestion of the diaphragm. In addition to high infection levels, ELISA was sensitive enough to detect extremely low *T. spiralis* infections in slaughter pigs as well.

Furthermore, comparative studies performed together with a number of European laboratories (using, however, material from pigs of Dutch origin) confirmed that the results of ELISA agreed with those of trichinoscopy, the digestion method, and the IF technique (van Knapen *et al.*, 1980, 1981). Material from pigs infected with 10,000, 5000, 500, 150, and 0 *T. spiralis* larvae was examined during a period from 17 days to 12 weeks postinfection. ELISA was more sensitive than IF during the onset of the infection in groups infected with higher numbers of larvae (1500, 5000, and 10,000 larvae). In general, however, results of ELISA and IF were comparable with regard to reliability. In pigs infected with a lower number of *T. spiralis* larvae, both serological assays were more sensitive than the direct methods (trichinoscopy and the digestion method). Figure 3 presents a schematic representation of the detection level of the various diagnostic methods for swine trichinosis based on these data.

2.5. Radioimmunoassay

Apart from the two more extensively studied serological methods using markers, i.e., the IF and enzyme immunoassays, some limited experience with the radioimmunoassay (RIA) has been reported. Movsessian (1971) and Biancifiori *et al.* (1980) reported a good sensitivity for the RIA when compared with the IF test. Also, the RIA results can

```
larvae        ┌─┐     techniques
per gram      │ │
              │ │
       3      ├─┤     trichinoscopy
              │ │
              │ │
       1      ├─┤     pooled-sample digestion methods (100 x 1 g)
              │ │
     0.1      ├─┤     IF test
    0.01      ├─┤     digestion method (5 x 20 g); ELISA
   <0.01      └─┘     ELISA
```

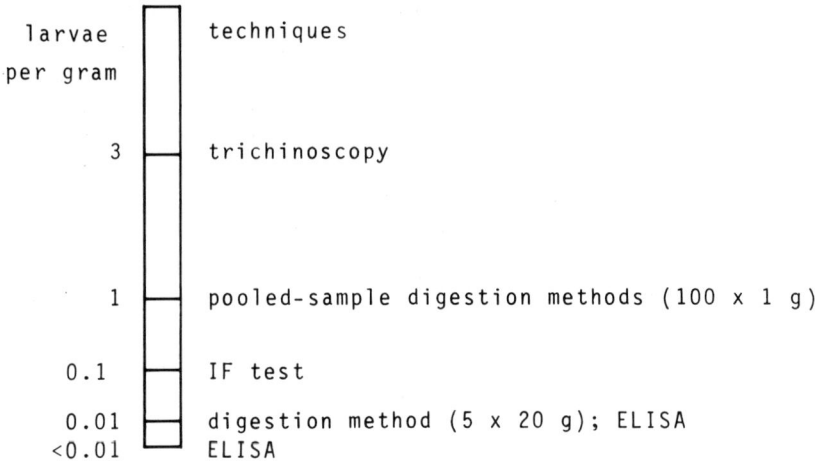

FIGURE 3. Schematic representation of the detection levels of various diagnostic methods for swine trichinosis.

be evaluated quantitatively. A drawback is, however, the use of radioactively labeled material in a slaughterhouse laboratory.

3. SENSITIVITY AND SPECIFICITY

The reliability of all serological tests depends on their sensitivity and specificity. These criteria are directly linked with the quality of the reagents, the standardization of the technique, and the availability of reference methods and materials. Only limited work has been performed to meet these standards for the serological methods used in porcine trichinosis (WHO, 1976). Particularly, when using the test in screening larger populations, a proper balance between the sensitivity and the specificity should be maintained to obtain reliable information. False-negative results, related to the sensitivity of the technique, and false-positive results, related to the specificity, should be kept within statistically valid confidence limits. For practical purposes, the 99% confidence limit chosen for ELISA (Ruitenberg and van Knapen, 1977) offers a good starting point to apply this technique for epidemiological surveys (see Section 2.4.4).

4. ANTIGEN PREPARATION AND PURIFICATION

The IF technique uses the morphological structures of the parasite as antigenic sites, but in all other serological techniques, antigens have to be prepared from the parasite. Consequently, one of the advantages of IF has always been that the whole larvae or sections could be employed directly as the antigen. It appeared that specific antigens were localized in both the cuticle and the internal structures of the muscle larvae. With the earlier-developed techniques, i.e., the Suessenguth–Kline test (Suessenguth and Kline, 1944; Suessenguth et al., 1965), the cholesterol–lecithin slide and charcoal card flocculation tests (Anderson et al., 1963), and the CF (Tompkins and Muraschi, 1955) and SAFA tests (Gore and Sadun, 1968), the problem of antigen isolation was recognized. However, with the introduction of the IF tube test and the cryostat methodology, the isolation and purification problem seemed to be temporarily overcome.

Nevertheless, with the successful introduction of the enzyme immunoassays, the problem of obtaining a reliable antigen reappeared. Previously, various techniques for isolating specific antigens had been employed, e.g., those based on the acid-soluble fraction of muscle larvae prepared according to Melcher (1943). Other publications dealing with antigen extraction and characterization include those of Wodehouse (1956), Labzoffsky et al. (1959), Tanner and Gregory (1961), Barriga and Segre (1972), Beltran-Hernandez et al. (1974), and Sukhdeo and Meerovitch (1979). These protein antigens were never carefully characterized, partly due to lack of reliable immunochemical techniques. In the enzyme immunoassays, a crude saline extract of muscle larvae has been employed (Ruitenberg et al., 1974). This antigenic material is then coated onto the solid phase at a pH of 9.8. Nothing is known about the quality or quantity of the specific antigenic components actually bound to the surface. Taylor et al. (1980) reported further fractionation of the crude protein antigen by gel filtration on a Sephadex G-200 column. The authors claim that with this purification of the antigen, the accuracy of the ELISA can be enhanced. This approach was also used by Despommier and Laccetti (1981). They demonstrated that the soluble protein (S_3) of a large-particle fraction derived from the muscle larvae is a rich source of antigens. The large majority of proteins thus isolated were glycoproteins with low isoelectric points. The antigenic portion of the S_3 fraction was identified with immunoelectrophoresis and counterimmunoelectrophoresis. Thus, the electrophoretic mobility of each of the 20 antigens in the S_3 fraction could be revealed. With a number of the antigens, also, protection against Trichinella in mice could be induced. Although not further analyzed, it is highly likely that a number of the antigens thus isolated may also be very useful as tools for diagnosis of porcine trichinosis. Preliminary experiments (van Knapen, 1980, unpublished data) with the ELISA method using the purified antigen prepared by Despommier indicated a high degree of discrimination between positive and negative sera and much lower background reactions. Further work should be performed to analyze and standardize the antigenic preparations. For an exhaustive review of this subject, see also Chapter 9.

5. EVALUATION OF SEROLOGICAL METHODS IN VARIOUS GEOGRAPHIC AREAS

Serological methods are indirect ways to suggest the presence of a disease agent. Examination of a large number of sera yields information on the infection in a certain area. Large-scale screening with serological methods has been conducted only with the IF and enzyme immunoassays. Absence or presence of specific antibodies was used as a criterion to suggest absence or presence of the infection. As with all serological techniques, the sensitivity of the test is based on a proper balance between "signal," the presence of antibodies, and "noise," i.e., background reaction. Apart from the possibility that other (disease) agents may influence the test due to possible shared antigens, the presence of unknown serum factors may give rise to variations in background reactions. For epidemiological surveys, it is therefore essential that comparisons be made with control sera from the same geographic area. Only then can the "signal"-to-"noise" ratio be properly evaluated. Various attempts have been made to study the differences in background reactions using predominantly the enzyme immunoassays in various geographic areas.

5.1. Evaluation of the Enzyme-Linked Immunosorbent Assay in the United States

As already mentioned in Section 2.4.4, Clinard *et al.* (1978) reported an unaccountably high (15%) level of presumably false-positive reactions in testing sera from packinghouse pigs. The authors reported that most of these reactions were due to the presence of a nonspecific serum factor that bound to components of the crude antigen preparation used. Attempts were made to remove this nonspecific reaction (Clinard, 1979). However, the ultimate answer to this source of false-positive results will certainly be the further purification of the antigen.

5.2. Evaluation of the Enzyme-Linked Immunosorbent Assay in European Countries

In preliminary examinations of porcine sera originating from The Netherlands, the United States, and Norway (van Knapen *et al.*, 1976;

unpublished data), marked differences in extinction values of parasitologically negative pigs were observed. Therefore, during comparative studies by the European Community Working Group on Trichinellosis to evaluate the reliability of ELISA, special attention was paid to the background reactions in different countries (van Knapen *et al.*, 1981). For this purpose, mean extinction values were calculated for sera from parasitologically *Trichinella*-free conventional slaughter pigs. On the basis of this mean value, a 99% confidence limit (detection level) was calculated. Detection levels for pig populations in 11 European countries were established simultaneously to avoid differences due to the test system itself. Again, remarkable differences were observed among the background extinction levels calculated from groups of 100 normal pig sera. Extinction values in the United Kingdom, two Scandinavian countries (Denmark and Sweden), and southern Poland (Krakow region) were low. High values were seen in western Germany (Berlin), Italy, eastern Poland (Bialystock region), and northern Ireland. Background reactions in the Republic of Ireland, The Netherlands, Belgium, and France were intermediate. The reason for this has still to be determined. However, some obvious reasons can be excluded, e.g., cross-reactions due to *Ascaris suum* (Ruitenberg *et al.*, 1975c). On the other hand, antigenic relationship between *Trichinella* and *Salmonella typhi* (Weiner and Neely, 1964) has to be reconsidered. Differences in background levels could also be caused by the difference in husbandry (Taylor and Kenny, 1978). It is interesting to note that in Poland, high background levels were observed in the eastern region, where *Trichinella* infections are endemic, whereas in the *Trichinella*-free southern region, low background levels were observed. This could possibly indicate that the background levels are at least partially due to contact with *Trichinella* antigen and therefore may be due to a specific immunological response. Careful absorption studies to clarify this point have, however, not been performed. In countries with a high background, the problem of false-negative reactions may exist. Low-level infections causing minor antibody response can readily be missed. Two ways to solve this problem can be suggested: (1) the use of a more specific antigen (see Section 4) and (2) the use of higher serum dilutions for routine screening, which might be a means of discriminating between positive and negative results in areas with a high background reaction.

6. MECHANIZATION

From the previous sections, it will be clear that of the serological methods, only the enzyme immunoassays are sufficiently specific and

sensitive to be suggested for routine application. The enzyme immunoassays share a relative ease of performance, using a solid phase to
which the biological reagents can be passively adsorbed and which can
also be used as antigen carrier during the test procedure. For the
enzyme immunoassay, polystyrene tubes (macro-ELISA) or microplates
(micro-ELISA) have been introduced to antigen carriers, serving also
as a liquid holder. These characteristics are of fundamental importance
when considering mechanization or automation. Since mechanization
of practically all steps of the assay is possible, on-line systems for both
macro-ELISA and micro-ELISA have been described (Ruitenberg and
Brosi, 1978).

6.1. Mechanized System for the Macro-Enzyme-Linked Immunosorbent Assay

The macro-ELISA system was based partially on specific commercially available equipment selected because it matched the ELISA
requirements most closely, particularly with regard to the multiple
dispensing and photometric system. The original system was modified
and extended in more detail as described elsewhere (Ruitenberg and
Brosi, 1978). The system includes:

1. Sample tubes (not made of polystyrene, to prevent undesired
   adhesion of biological material to the wall).
2. Working tubes (disposable polystyrene tubes with cuvette quality enabling direct measurement through the wall).
3. Sample blocks to be used both as carrier (tube holder) between
   sampling site and laboratory and as transport block in the on-
   line rail system.
4. Working blocks to be used both as transport blocks in the on-
   line rail system and as cuvette blocks in the photometer.
5. Identification device.
6. Dispenser for multiple samples.
7. Washing device for multiple samples.
8. Shaker.
9. Photometer and processor.
10. On-line rail system with carts and elevators for large-scale
    processing.

On the basis of this system, an on-line routing procedure was
developed that allowed the processing of a daily total of 4000 samples.
The test results are presented on a data sheet as a combination of the
sample identification number and the extinction value. Extinction values

can be presented as absolute figures, i.e., measured against the substrate controls as blank values, or as relative figures. In the latter situation, the optical density is first measured against the substrate control as blank value. Next, a preset confidence limit based on the extinction values of a number of known negative sera is subtracted from the absolute extinction value. In addition to the on-line system described in detail above, the macro-ELISA can be performed with commercially available equipment allowing dispensing and reading with a maximum daily workload of about 600 samples.

6.2. Mechanized System for the Micro-Enzyme-Linked Immunosorbent Assay

Successful attempts have been described to develop, as well, a mechanized system using conventional microplates. A particular problem to be solved was the direct reading of the plates. Although an adaptation of the macro-ELISA reader for measuring microplates has been developed (Ruitenberg *et al.*, 1976a) and successfully applied in a mechanized micro-ELISA system (Ruitenberg and Brosi, 1978), an essential breakthrough has been the development of a reader especially designed for microplates (Ruitenberg *et al.*, 1980). Together with a dispenser for multiple samples, based on the 12 × 8 cup figuration of conventional microplates and a microplate washer, a mechanized system was developed (Fig. 4). The essential elements of the system include:

1. Sample tubes.
2. Microplates (12 × 8 cups, flat-bottomed for optimal photometric reading).
3. Dispenser for multiple samples (based on a parallel transfer system of 96 syringes).
4. Microplate washer, consisting of a head with 96 outlets.

The reading and expression of test results can be done as mentioned for the macro-ELISA system (Section 6.1). In addition to the micro-ELISA system described in detail above, equipment for manual and mechanized processing is commercially available from various companies. The crucial element of the whole procedure remains the microplate. Originally, these plates were produced for handling liquids. Nothing was known about the adhesive properties of the polystyrene or polyethylene and the adequacy of the bottom for direct reading. The adhesive properties of the polystyrene are influenced by the speed of the polymerization process. This explains why batch-to-batch variations may occur. Some companies started with rigid quality control of

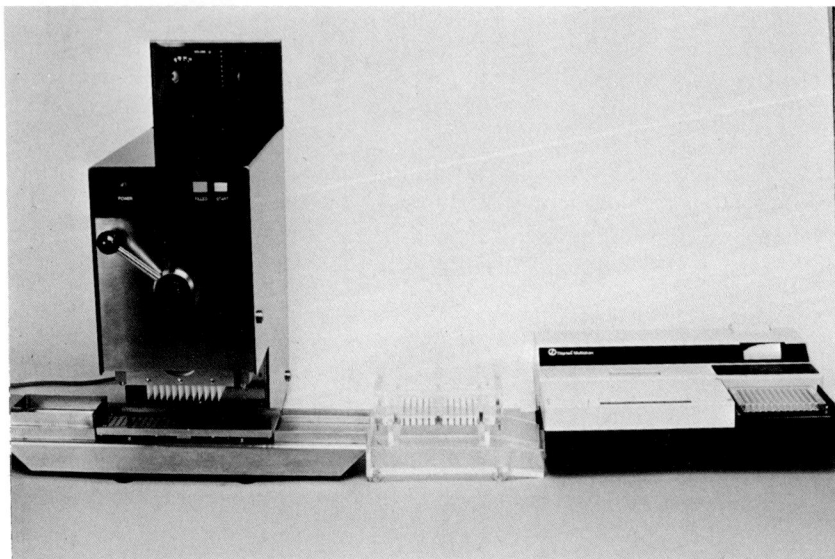

FIGURE 4. Mechanized system for micro-ELISA, showing (from left to right) dispenser, washing device, and photometer for vertical through-the-plate reading.

the adhesive properties of the microplates. It is clear that this is an essential prerequisite for standardization of the micro-ELISA. In general, however, reliable qualitative determinations can be achieved at present by both macro- and micro-ELISA. Although one of the advantages of the microplate assay in particular is the simplicity of performance without additional sophisticated equipment, both types of assays can be mechanized and thus be used for large-scale screening.

7. SURVEILLANCE BY SEROLOGICAL METHODS

Prevention of *Trichinella* infection in man by adequate meat control has been one of the stimuli to start organized meat inspection. The possibility of examining food products prior to human consumption depends on the availability of reliable and simple detection methods. In the case of trichinosis, these have been trichinoscopy and the digestion method, which allowed the direct visualization or isolation of the parasite. With the development of serological techniques, which are in general more sensitive than the direct methods, more reliable examination of slaughter pigs is feasible. It has been reported that the ELISA, as either a macro- or a micromethod, is a very sensitive technique to detect both early and long-standing infections in conventionally kept bacon pigs (van Knapen *et al.*, 1981). This is especially evident in low-grade infection. However, it should be realized that low-grade infections resulting in extremely low numbers of parasites in the musculature may give rise to serum antibodies without being a threat to public health. Furthermore, pigs may occasionally give a relatively poor antibody response, causing false-negative results (Ruitenberg and van Knapen, 1977). Consequently, before serological methods are suggested for surveillance purposes, the position and value of all serological methods in the framework of meat inspection should be further analyzed.

7.1. Inspection at the Slaughterhouse

In keeping with the statements made above, it is clear that when serological, i.e., indirect, methods are to be used for control in the slaughterhouse, a hierarchical model of examination, based on a two-step procedure, should be adopted. After serological screening, pigs can be divided into negative and positive categories (Ruitenberg *et al.*, 1979). With a negative serological result, the animal may be directly released. Since as yet insufficient data are available on the frequency of occurrence of low-responder animals, i.e., animals with a low antibody response, a certain risk should be taken into account. However, under field conditions, even extremely low infections were recognized with the ELISA (van Knapen *et al.*, 1976). In case of a positive serological finding, the animal has been exposed to the parasite. No conclusion, however, can be drawn as to the stage of infection, i.e., past exposure or present infection. Therefore, a reexamination with a direct method should be carried out. A negative result with the latter method would then indicate that the meat is safe for the consumer. Consequently, the serological method, e.g., the ELISA, is used to screen for the absence of infection, but the final confirmation of the infection and the assessment of the public-health relevance is based on the result of a direct method.

7.2. Inspection at the Farm

As interesting as the application of serological methods in the framework of preventive control is the potential of these methods, including ELISA, for screening animals at the farm. Seroepidemiological surveys can be carried out, permitting constant surveillance of the degree of infection in a certain area. Furthermore, serological results from individual animals can also be used for preventive control purposes. A positive result in an animal on the farm or in a herd would mean reexamination with a direct method at the slaughterhouse. With a negative test result, however, the farmer could receive a certificate for slaughter without further examination of the animal at the slaughterhouse.

7.3. Individual vs. Population Control

With the introduction of reliable serological methods, reassessment of control procedures becomes realistic. However, a distinction should be made between the situation in endemic and nonendemic areas. In endemic areas, i.e., areas with reported clinical trichinosis in man, individual control of all slaughter pigs remains essential. Thus, the procedure described in Section 7.1 may be adopted. Serological methods may be used for screening all pigs, and confirmation of positive findings should be done with direct methods.

In nonendemic areas, where neither animal nor human trichinosis has been noticed for many years, a different approach may be followed. Here, permanent surveillance programs based on sensitive detection methods and adequate administration can monitor the absence of infection in pigs and subsequently in man. Serological methods, including ELISA, are ideal for this type of epizootiological survey. In The Netherlands, the ELISA has been used on this basis as a routine screening method. Approximately 1% of all pigs presented for slaughter (14 million annually) are examined. Sera are collected weekly from 35 slaughterhouses distributed all over the country. Due to adequate individual identification of all pigs, a further survey at the farm of origin is possible whenever a positive finding suggests exposure to *Trichinella*.

7.4. Legislation

In a number of experiments, serological techniques, including IF and ELISA, were evaluated for the control of *Trichinella* infections in pigs by the Working Group on Trichinellosis from the European Communities (van Knapen *et al.*, 1980, 1981). In this Working Group, countries outside the European Economic Community (EEC) have actively participated. Comparisons were made with the trichinoscopy and digestion methods approved by the EEC. IF and ELISA proved to be suitable for epidemiological surveys, allowing screening for the absence of the infection. Although the EEC recognized the potential utility, not enough evidence is available as yet to suggest serological methods, including ELISA, as alternatives for control of individual animals in the slaughterhouse. Since there are differences in the various pig populations with regard to nonspecific background reactions, further research is needed. It is considered essential that screening programs, using serological techniques, should also be started in endemic areas to further evaluate the usefulness of these methods.

8. CONCLUDING REMARKS

Serological methods for the detection of antibodies to *Trichinella* in pigs have a relatively long history. With the introduction of marker assays such as immunofluorescence and enzyme immunoassays, the sensitivity has greatly improved. Consequently, they can now be regarded as competitive with direct methods such as trichinoscopy and digestion methods for application to meat inspection. The mechanization possibilities of ELISA give this assay in particular a potential for large-scale application. ELISA prompts a reorientation of the conventional slaughterhouse control. The assay offers the potential for screening all pigs presented for slaughter in a rapid and less laborious way. Positive findings should be confirmed by direct methods. Furthermore, ELISA can be used for epizootiological surveys in the framework of continuous surveillance programs.

REFERENCES

Anderson, R.I., Sadun, E.H., and Schoenbechler, M.J., 1963, Cholesterol–lecithin slide (TsSF) and charcoal card (TsCC) flocculation tests using an acid soluble fraction of *Trichinella spiralis* larvae, *J. Parasitol.* **49**:642–647.

Andrews, J.S., Hill, C.H., and Henson, L.A., 1976, Evaluation of a trichina-cyst antigen for the intradermal diagnosis of trichiniasis in live hogs, *Proc. Helminthol. Soc. Washington* **43**:81–84.

Barriga, O.O., and Segre, D., 1972, Dianosis of trichinellosis by hemagglutination with a purified larval antigen, in: *Trichinellosis* (C.W. Kim, ed.), Intext, New York, pp. 421–442.

Belozyorov, S.N., 1972, Comparative study of antigens in the indirect immunofluorescent tests used for diagnosing pig trichinelliasis, *Byull. Vses. Inst. Gel'mintol. K.I. Skryabina.* **9**:11–13.

Belozyorov, S.N., 1975, Vital diagnostics of pig trichinellosis, *Veterinariya* **6**:70–72.

Beltran-Hernandez, F., Gomez-Priego, A., and Figueroa-Villalva, V.E., 1974, Immunological characterization of antigenic fractions of *Trichinella spiralis* larvae, in: *Trichinellosis* (C.W. Kim, ed.), Intext, New York, pp. 175–187.

Biancifiori, F., Frescura, T., Gialletti, L., and Morozzi, A., 1980, Solid-phase micro-radio immunoassay for antibodies to *Trichinella spiralis*, *Arch. Vet. Ital.* **31:**44–47.

Clinard, E.H., 1975, Evaluation of soluble-antigen fluorescent antibody test for antibodies to *Trichinella spiralis* in experimentally infected swine, *Am. J. Vet. Res.* **36:**615–618.

Clinard, E.H., 1979, Identification and distribution of swine serum immunoglobulins that react with *Trichinella spiralis* antigens and may interefere with the enzyme-labeled antibody test for trichinosis, *Am. J. Vet. Res.* **40:**1558–1563.

Clinard, E.H., Saunders, G.C., and Leighty, J.C., 1978, Prospects for use of the ELA test in control of trichinellosis in swine, in: *Trichinellosis* (C.W. Kim and Z.S. Pawlowski, eds.), University Press of New England, Hanover, New Hampshire, pp. 501–507.

Coats, M.E., Leland, S.E., Jr., and Kelly, P.C., 1969, Evaluation of the charcoal test for trichinosis in swine, *J. Parasitol.* **55:**679.

Despommier, D.D., and Laccetti, A., 1981, *Trichinella spiralis*: Proteins and antigens isolated from a large-particle fraction derived from the muscle larva, *Exp. Parasitol.* **51:**279–295.

Frisch, A.W., Whims, C.B., and Oppenheim, J.M., 1947, Complement fixation and precipitation tests in trichinosis, *Am. J. Clin. Pathol.* **17:**24–28.

Gore, R.W., and Sadun, E.H., 1968, A soluble antigen fluorescent antibody (SAFA) test for the immunodiagnosis of trichinosis in man and experimental animals, *Exp. Parasitol.* **23:**287–293.

Henriksen, S.A., Buys, J., and Ruitenberg, E.J., 1975, Immunofluorescence technique in diagnosis of trichinellosis in swine. II. Comparative investigations with the tube test and the cryostat method, *Nord. Veterinaermed.* **27:**199–202.

Isenstein, R.S., 1974, The soluble antigen fluorescent antibody test in detecting trichinellosis in swine: Problems and recent progress, in: *Trichinellosis* (C.W. Kim, ed.), Intext, New York, pp. 385–388.

Jackson, G.J., 1959, Fluorescent antibody studies of *Trichinella spiralis* infection, *J. Infect. Dis.* **105:**97–117.

Kampelmacher, E.H., and Streefkerk, C.W., 1965, Experiments with a latex-slide test for the serodiagnosis of trichinosis, *Wiad. Parazytol.* **11:**317–326.

Köhler, G., and Ruitenberg, E.J., 1974, Comparison of three methods for the detection of *Trichinella spiralis* infections in pigs by five European laboratories, *Bull. W.H.O.* **50:**413–419.

Kozar, Z., and Kozar, M., 1969, Indirect fluorescence antibody test in diagnosis of trichinellosis, *Wiad. Parazytol.* **16:**7–13.

Kozar, Z., Kozar, M., and Staroniewicz, Z., 1970, An attempt of using some serologic methods in the diagnosis of trichinellosis in slaughter pigs, *Wiad. Parazytol.* **16:**41–44.

Labzoffsky, N.A., Kuitunen, E., Morrissey, L.P., and Hamros, J.J., 1959, Studies on the antigenic structure of *Trichinella spiralis*, *Can. J. Microbiol.* **5:**395–403.

Ljungström, I., 1974, Antibody response to *Trichinella spiralis*, in: *Trichinellosis* (C.W. Kim, ed.), Intext, New York, pp. 449–459.

Melcher, L., 1943, An antigenic analysis of *Trichinella spiralis*, *J. Infect. Dis.* **73:**31–40.

Movsessian, M., 1971, The use of the test of fluorescent and radioactive antibodies in helminthoses, *Tr. Vses. Inst. Gel'mintol, K.I. Skryabina* **17:**293–294.

Poggel, H., 1952, Die Komplementbindung zur Feststellung der Trichinose bei Tieren, insbesondere bei Schweinen, und über die Anwendbarkeit der Reaktion mit Schweineseren im allgemeinen, D.V.M. dissertation, University of Giessen.

Rapić, D., 1980, The enzyme linked immunosorbent assay (ELISA) in the serodiagnosis of *Trichinella spiralis* infections in experimentally and naturally infected pigs, *Acta Parasitol. Iugoslav.* **11**(1–2):49–57.

Ruitenberg, E.J., and Brosi, B.J.M., 1978, Automation in enzyme immunoassay, *Scand. J. Immunol.* **8**(7):63–72.

Ruitenberg, E.J., and Kampelmacher, E.H., 1970, Diagnostische Methoden zur Feststellung der Invasion mit *Trichinella spiralis, Fleischwirtschaft* **50**:41–44.

Ruitenberg, E.J., and Sluiters, J.F., 1974, *Trichinella spiralis* infections in the Netherlands, in: *Trichinellosis* (C.W. Kim, ed.), Intext, New York, pp. 539–548.

Ruitenberg, E.J., and van Knapen, F., 1977, The enzyme linked immunosorbent assay and its application to parasitic infections, *J. Infect. Dis.* **136**(Suppl.):267–273.

Ruitenberg, E.J., Kampelmacher, E.H., and Berkvens, J., 1968, The indirect fluorescent antibody technique in the serodiagnosis of pigs infected with *Trichinella spiralis, Neth. J. Vet. Sci.* **1**(2):143–153.

Ruitenberg, E.J., Steerenberg, P.A., Brosi, B.J.M., and Buys, J., 1974, Serodiagnosis of *Trichinella spiralis* infections in pigs by enzyme linked immunosorbent assays, *Bull. W.H.O.* **51**:108–109.

Ruitenberg, E.J., Ljungström, I., Steerenberg, P.A., and Buys, J., 1975a, Application of immunofluorescence and immunoenzyme methods in the serodiagnosis of *Trichinella spiralis* infection, *Ann. N. Y. Acad. Sci.* **254**:296–303.

Ruitenberg, E.J., Steerenberg, P.A., and Brosi, B.J.M., 1975b, Microsystem for the application of ELISA (enzyme linked immunosorbent assay) in the serodiagnosis of *Trichinella spiralis* infections, *Medikon Ned.* **4**(3):30–31.

Ruitenberg, E.J., Steerenberg, P.A., Brosi, B.J.M., and Buys, J., 1975c, ELISA (enzyme linked immunosorbent assay) as preventive and representive control method for the detection of *Trichinella spiralis* infections in slaughter pigs, *Wiad. Parazytol.* **21**(4–5):747–751.

Ruitenberg, E.J., Brosi, B.J.M., and Steerenberg, P.A., 1976a, Direct measurement of microplates and its application to enzyme-linked immunosorbent assay, *J. Clin. Microbiol.* **3**:541–542.

Ruitenberg, E.J., Steerenberg, P.A., Brosi, B.J.M., and Buys, J., 1976b, Reliability of the enzyme-linked immunosorbent assay (ELISA) for the serodiagnosis of *Trichinella spiralis* infections in conventionally raised pigs, *J. Immunol. Methods* **10**:67–83.

Ruitenberg, E.J., van Knapen, F., and Weiss, J.W., 1979, Food-borne parasitic infections— a review, *Vet. Parasitol.* **5**:1–10.

Ruitenberg, E.J., Sekhuis, V.M., and Brosi, B.J.M., 1980, Some characteristics of a new multiple-channel photometer through-the-plate reading of microplates to be used in enzyme linked immunosorbent assay, *J. Clin. Microbiol.* **11**(2):132–134.

Sadun, E.H., Anderson, R.I., and Williams, J.S., 1962, Fluorescent antibody test for the serological diagnosis of trichinosis, *Exp. Parasitol.* **12**:423–433.

Saunders, G.C., and Clinard, E.H., 1976, Rapid micromethod of screening for antibodies to disease agents using the indirect-enzyme labeled antibody test, *J. Clin. Microbiol.* **3**:604–608.

Saunders, G.C., Clinard, E.H., Bartlett, M.L., and Sanders, W.M., 1977, Application of the indirect enzyme-labeled antibody microtest to the detection and surveillance of animal diseases, *J. Infect. Dis.* **136**(Suppl.):258–266.

Scholtens, R.G., Kagan, I.G., Quist, K.D., and Norman, L.G., 1966, An evaluation of tests for the diagnosis of trichinosis in swine and associated quantitative epidemiologic observations, *Am. J. Epidemiol.* **83:**489–500.

Schultz, M.G., Kagan, I.G., an Warner, G.S., 1967, Card flocculation test in the field diagnosis of trichinosis, *Am. J. Clin. Pathol.* **47:**26–29.

Suessenguth, H., and Kline, B.S., 1944, A simple rapid flocculation slide test for trichinosis in man and swine, *Am. J. Clin. Pathol.* **14:**471–484.

Suessenguth, H., Schnurrenberger, P.R., Bauer, A.B.S., Wentworth, F.H., and Masterson, R.A., 1965, Swine trichinosis: Serologic reactivity in experimental infections with small numbers of *Trichinella* larvae, *Am. J. Vet. Res.* **26**(115):1298–1302.

Sukhdeo, M.V.K., and Meerovitch, E., 1979, A comparison of the antigenic characteristics of three geographical isolates of *Trichinella, Int. J. Parasitol.* **9:**571–576.

Sulzer, A.J., and Chisholm, E.S., 1966, Comparison of the IFA and other tests for *Trichinella spiralis* antibodies, *Public Health Rep.* **81:**729–734.

Tanner, C.E., and Gregory, J., 1961, Immunochemical studies on the antigens of *Trichinella spiralis*. I. Identification and enumeration of antigens, *Can. J. Microbiol.* **7:**473–481.

Taylor, S.M., and Kenny, J., 1978, The influence of concurrent infection with *œsophagostomum* species on the interpretation of the ELISA test for trichinosis in pigs, *Vet. Parasitol.* **4:**257–264.

Taylor, S.M., Kenny, J., Mallon, T., and Davidson, W.B., 1980, The micro-ELISA for antibodies to *Trichinella spiralis*: Elimination of false positive reactions by antigen fractionation and technical improvements, *Zentralbl. Veterinaermed. Reihe B* **27:**764–772.

Tompkins, V.N., and Muraschi, T.F., 1955, Complement-fixation test for trichinosis, *Am. J. Clin. Pathol.* **25:**206–213.

van Knapen, F., Framstad, K., and Ruitenberg, E.J., 1976, Reliability of ELISA (enzyme-linked immunosorbent assay) as control method for the detection of *Trichinella spiralis* infections in naturally infected slaughter pigs, *J. Parasitol.* **62**(2):232–233.

van Knapen, F., Franchimont, J.H., Ruitenberg, E.J., Baldelli, B., Bradley, J., Gibson, T.E., Gottal, C., Henriksen, S.A., Köhler, G., Skovgaard, N., Soulé, C., and Taylor, S.M., 1980, Comparison of the enzyme-linked immunosorbent assay (ELISA) with three other methods for the detection of *Trichinella spiralis* infections in pigs, *Vet. Parasitol.* **7:**109–121.

van Knapen, F., Franchimont, J.H., and Ruitenberg, E.J. (on behalf of the members of the EEC Working Group on Trichinellosis), 1981, The reliability of the enzyme linked immunosorbent assay (ELISA) for the detection of swine trichinellosis, in: *Trichinellosis* (C.W. Kim, E.J. Ruitenberg, and J.S. Teppema, eds.), Reedbooks, Chertsey, Surrey, England, pp. 399–404.

Weiner, L.M., and Neely, J., 1964, The nature of the antigenic relationship between *Trichinella spiralis* and *Salmonella typhi, J. Immunol.* **92:**908–911.

WHO, 1976, The enzyme-linked immunosorbent assay (ELISA), *Bull. W.H.O.* **54:**129–139.

Wikerhauser, T., Dzakula, N., Rapić, D., and Zuković, M., 1980, A comparison of the indirect fluorescence antibody test, trichinelloscopy and digestion method in the diagnosis of *Trichinella spiralis* infection in pigs, *Acta Parasitol. Iugoslav.* **11**(1–2):39–47.

Wodehouse, R.P., 1956, Antigen analysis and standardization of trichinella extracts by gel diffusion, *Ann. Allergy* **14:**128–138.

Zimmerman, W.J., and Zinter, D.E., 1971, The prevalence of trichiniasis in swine in the United States, 1966–70, *HSMHA Health Rep.* **86:**937–945.

Appendix 1

Synopsis of Morphology

DICKSON D. DESPOMMIER and
WILLIAM C. CAMPBELL

1. INTRODUCTION

A synopsis of the general morphology of *Trichinella spiralis* is presented herein. The material is designed to provide a concise source of information on the anatomical features referred to in the various chapters of this book. This summary is intended to complement those chapters and thus make possible a comprehensive understanding of the species.

Much additional morphological information, including ultrastructural detail and data on infraspecific variation, will be found in Chapters 2 and 3. The morphology of *T. pseudospiralis* is similar to that of *T. spiralis* except for differences noted in Chapter 2. The measurements given below are approximate.

2. MORPHOLOGY OF THE ADULT MALE

The colorless male measures 1.0–1.5 mm in length by 0.03 mm in width (Fig. 1A). Its cuticle is smooth, but exhibits pseudosegmentation

DICKSON D. DESPOMMIER • Division of Tropical Medicine, School of Public Health, Columbia University, New York, New York 10032.   WILLIAM C. CAMP-BELL • Merck Institute for Therapeutic Research, Rahway, New Jersey 07065.

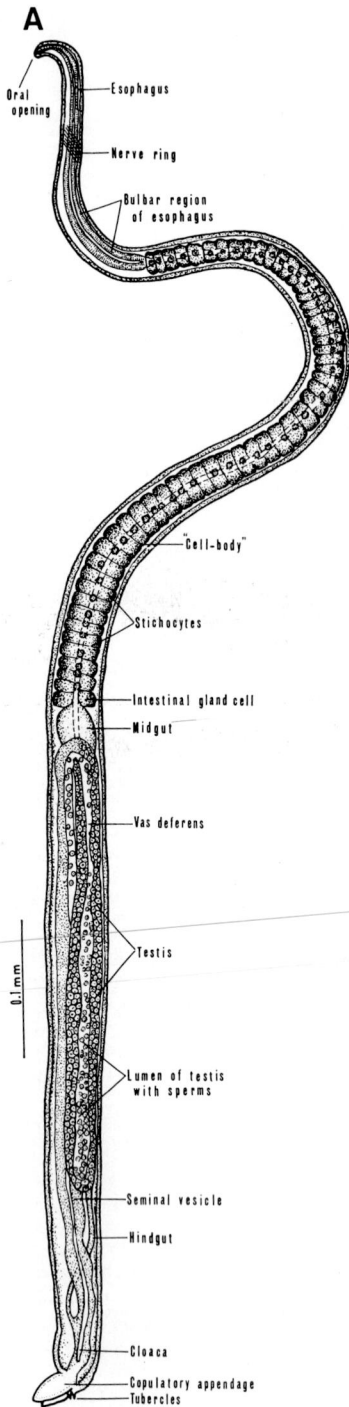

A

Oral opening

Esophagus

Nerve ring

Bulbar region of esophagus

"Cell-body"

Stichocytes

Intestinal gland cell

Midgut

Vas deferens

Testis

Lumen of testis with sperms

Seminal vesicle

Hindgut

Cloaca

Copulatory appendage
Tubercles

0.1mm

FIGURE 1. (A) Diagram of adult male *T. spiralis*. (B) Diagram of adult female *T. spiralis*. From Villella (1970).

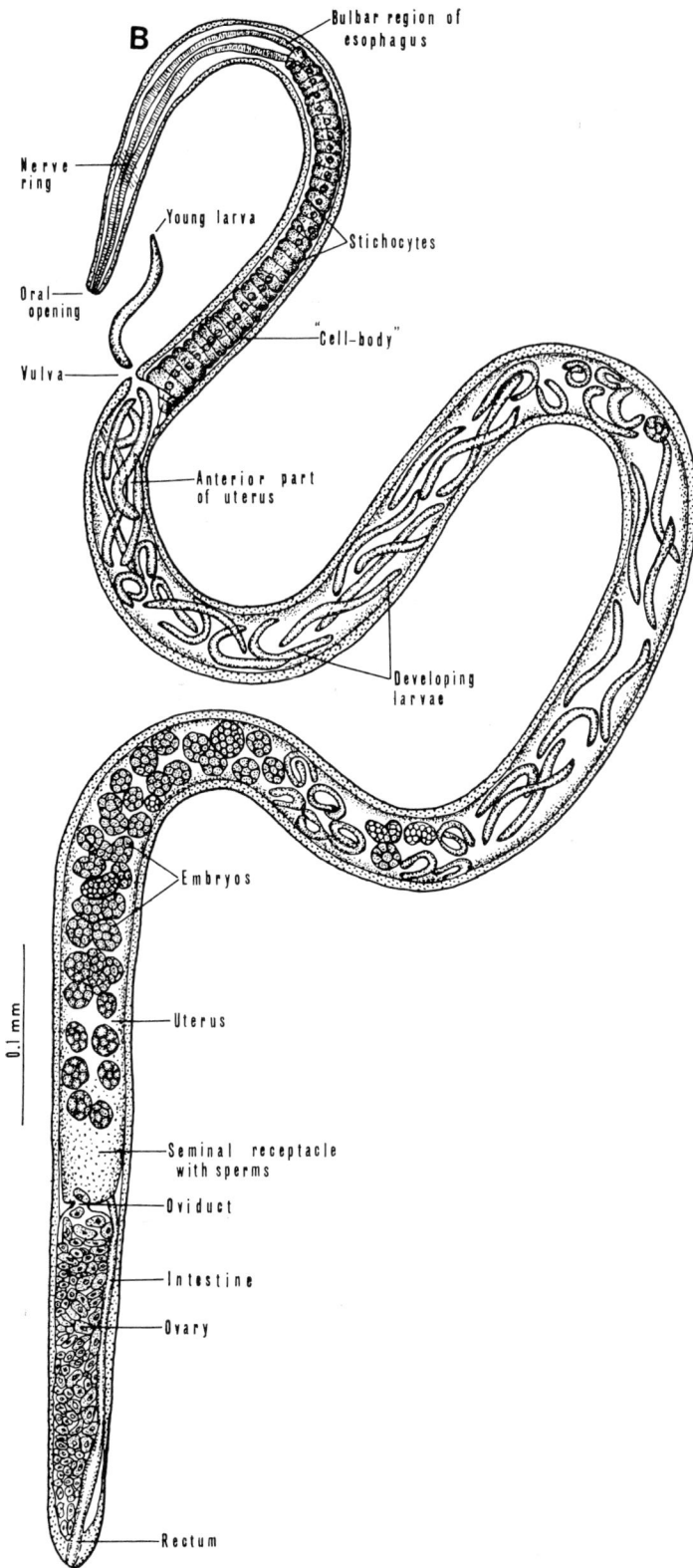

B

Bulbar region of esophagus

Nerve ring

Young larva

Oral opening

Stichocytes

"Cell-body"

Vulva

Anterior part of uterus

Developing larvae

Embryos

0.1 mm

Uterus

Seminal receptacle with sperms

Oviduct

Intestine

Ovary

Rectum

and is periodically interrupted by dorsal and ventral pairs of hypodermal gland cells (Chapter 3, Figs. 7 and 8). Its genital terminalia are distinctive, consisting of a pair of flattened copulatory appendages (Fig. 2D,E,G, and H, and Chapter 3, Fig. 16) and accessory papillae.

The alimentary tract consists of an oral cavity, capillary esophagus, midgut with brush border, and hind gut. The oral cavity is probably unarmed, although some authors have described a stylet. The eosphagus and hindgut are lined with cuticle, while the midgut is not. The stichosome, a collection of 45–55 specialized cells or stichocytes, lies in the anterior portion of the worm, with each cell emptying its products into the esophagus through individual ducts (Fig. 1 and Chapter 3, Figs. 28–30). The hind gut opens through the cloaca (Fig. 2G).

The morphology of muscle and nervous tissue is described in Chapter 3. The reproductive tract consists of a single testis, connected to the vas deferens, which in turn expands into a short seminal vessicle (Fig. 2). The copulatory bell (Fig. 2D and Chapter 3, Fig. 17) is a modified portion of cuticle that expands outward, giving the appearance of a bell.

3. MORPHOLOGY OF THE ADULT FEMALE

The nonpigmented female measures 2.5–3.5 mm in length by 0.05 mm in width (Fig. 1B). Externally, the cuticle possesses the same features as the male, with two exceptions: there are no copulatory appendages, and the vulva (birth pore) is evident at the posterior limit of the stichosome.

The alimentary tract closely resembles that of the male. The reproductive tract begins with a single ovary that leads to the oviduct, which in turn connects with the uterus (Figs. 1B and 3) Since living larvae are produced (see Chapter 3 for morphology of newborn larva), all stages of embryogenesis can be observed within the uterus. The

---

→

FIGURE 2. (A) Male reproductive system. (B) Hind body of enteric-stage male larva of *T. spiralis,* lateral view. First enteric-stage larva, approaching first molt. (C) Third enteric-stage larva of male with genital-junction cell between developing ejaculatory duct and rectum; outline of copulatory papilla and rectal tube in loose sheath. (D) Male, showing copulatory bell and copulatory muscle. (E) Male, showing posterior end with copulatory tube distended by sperm cells. (F) A portion of distal end of testis with sperms in lumen. (G) Male, ventral view of caudal end, showing copulatory appendages, papillae, and cloacal opening. (H) Male, showing posterior end with empty, folded copulatory tube and copulatory muscle. (A, D–H) From Wu (1955), by courtesy of the author and the editor. (B, C) From Ali Khan (1966), by courtesy of the author and the editor.

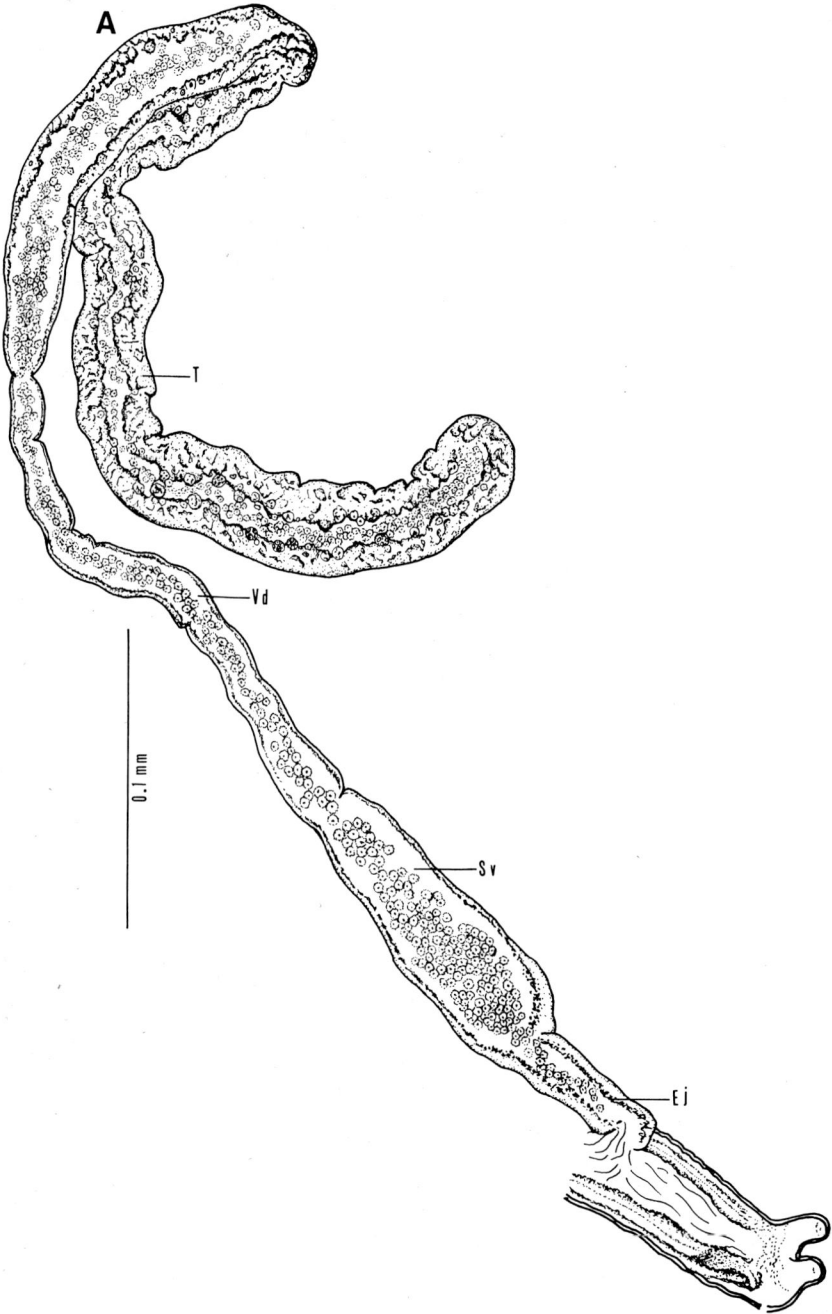

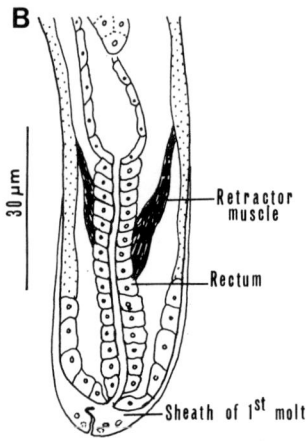

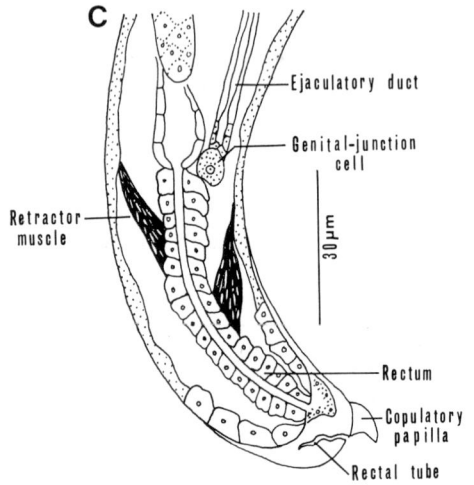

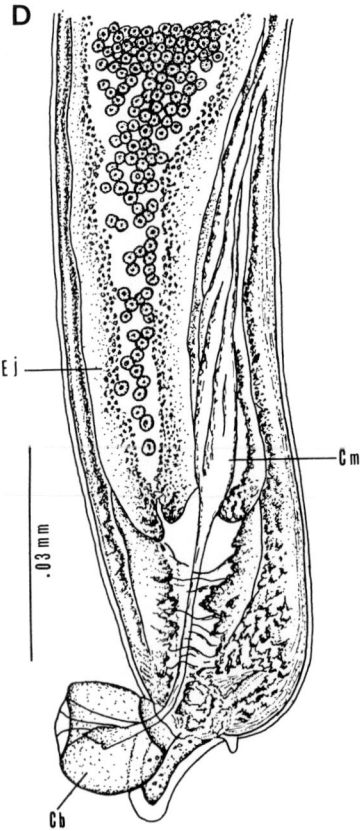

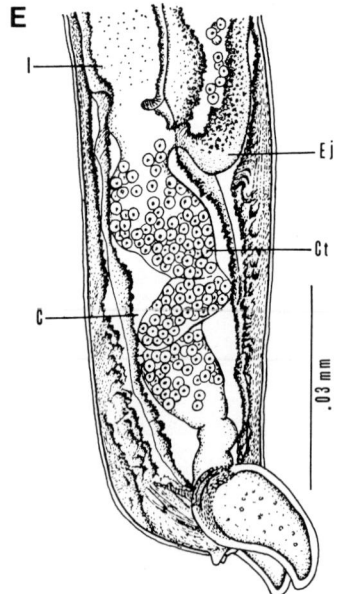

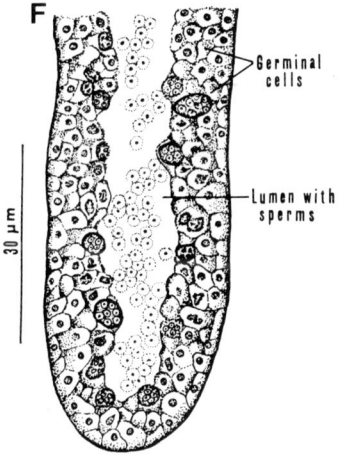

F

Germinal
cells

Lumen with
sperms

30 μm

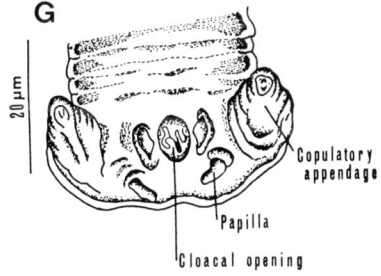

G

20 μm

Copulatory
appendage

Papilla

Cloacal opening

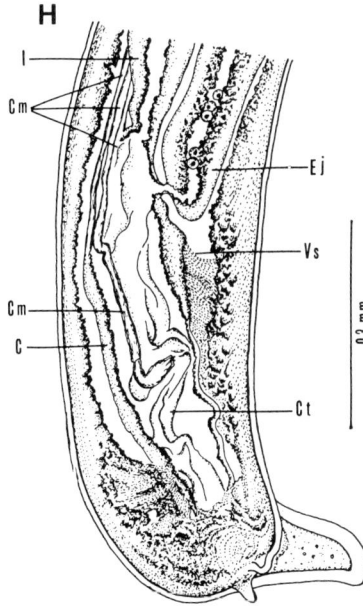

H

I

Cm

Ej

Vs

Cm

C

Ct

.03 mm

birth pore leads, through a thickened portion of cuticle, to the outside of the worm.

4. MORPHOLOGY OF THE INFECTIVE FIRST-STAGE LARVA

The encysted muscle-dwelling L_1 larva (Fig. 4) is faintly salmon-colored due to the hemoglobin in its pseudocelom. This feature is best observed when worms are seen *en masse*. This stage measures 1.0 mm in length by 0.03 mm in width. Its cuticle is smooth and exhibits pseudosegmentation, but hypodermal gland cells are not present. Each end is rounded, with no unusual projections or appendages.

The gut tract is complete (see Chapter 3). The reproductive system consists of an undifferentiated genital primordium, but the males can be distinguished anatomically from females (see Chapters 2 and 3). Some workers have observed a cluster of special cells or granules (Farre's granules) lying near the surface, about one fifth of the length of the larva from the posterior end, and perhaps representing the primordium of the seminal receptacle.

REFERENCES

Ali Khan, Z., 1966, The post-embryonic development of *Trichinella spiralis* with special reference to ecdysis, *J. Parasitol.* **52:**248–259.

Villella, J.B., 1970, Life cycle and morphology, in: *Trichinosis in Man and Animals* (S.E. Gould, ed.), Charles C. Thomas, Springfield, Illinois, pp. 19–60.

Wu, L.-Y., 1955, Studies on *Trichinella spiralis*, I. male and female reproductive systems, *J. Parasitol.* **41:**40–47.

⟶

FIGURE 3. Structures of enteric-stage larva of *T. spiralis* in lateral view. (A) Stichocytes, hypodermal cells of vaginal plate, and developing uterus of first enteric-stage larva. (B) Uterus of second enteric-stage larva, showing genital-junction cell touching vaginal plate. (C) Genital-junction cell touching pouched vaginal plate of third enteric-stage larva. (D) Ovary, oviduct, seminal receptacle, uterus, and nonpatent vagina with degenerating genital-junction cells, just before fourth molt. (E) Anterior portion of ovary, oviduct, seminal receptacle, and part of the uterus. (A–D) From Ali Khan (1966), by courtesy of the author and the editor. (E) From Wu (1955), by courtesy of the author and the editor.

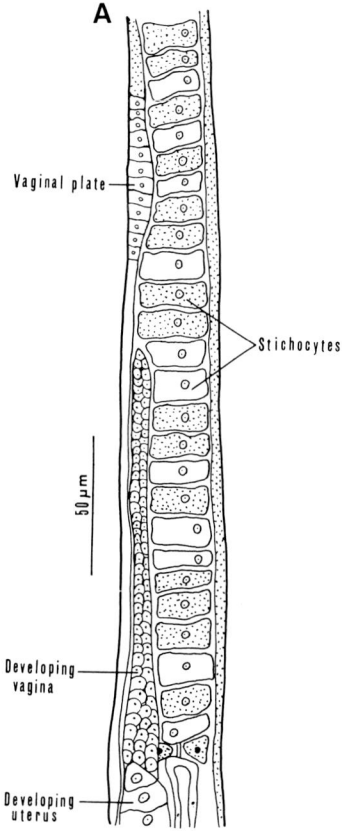

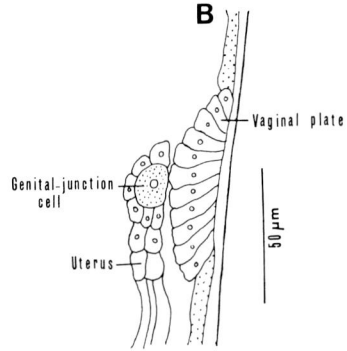

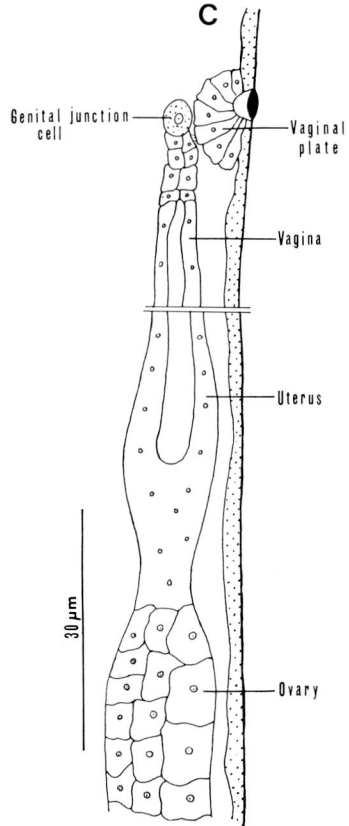

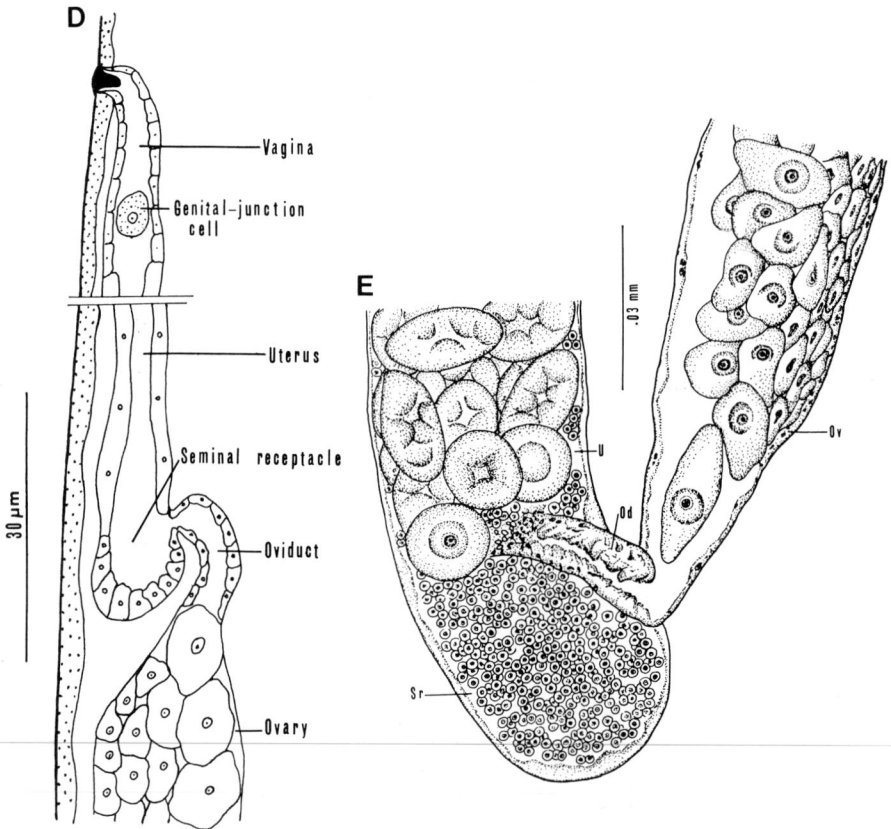

FIGURE 3 (*Continued*)

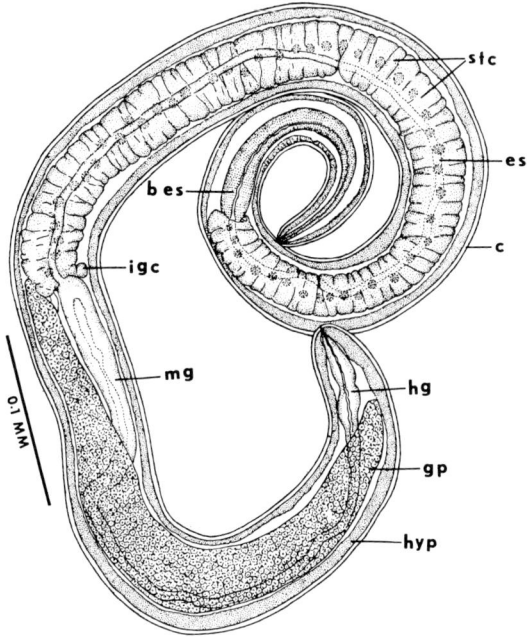

FIGURE 4. Drawing of infective muscle-dwelling larva (male). (c) Cuticle; (es) esophagus; (stc) stichocyte; (b es) bulb of esophagus; (igc) intestinal gland cell; (mg) midgut; (gp) genital primordium; (hyp) hypodermis; (hg) hindgut. From Villella (1970).

Appendix 2

Laboratory Techniques

LYNDIA SLAYTON BLAIR

METHODS

The use of *Trichinella spiralis* as a research tool usually involves maintaining the parasite in laboratory animals. Most experimental objectives require estimation of the number of worms present in individual animals at certain times postinoculation. Methods suitable for such work may be ferreted from the literature, but, for convenience, some basic techniques are outlined herein. They apply primarily to studies in mice and rats, the most commonly used hosts.

Recovering and Counting Adult Worms. The purpose is to determine the number of adults (enteral phase) in an individual host. Ordinarily, this would be done 4–7 days postinoculation. However, for studies on the immunological phenomenon of self-cure, other times may be chosen (see Chapter 8).

1. Kill the host animal and remove the entire small intestine. Because the worms migrate from the intestinal wall soon after host death, it is important to work quickly and process each mouse before proceeding to the next animal.

2. Open the intestine longitudinally. (Enterotome scissors with small blunt tips greatly aid in this task.)

3. Remove gut contents by dipping intestine gently into a beaker

LYNDIA SLAYTON BLAIR • Merck Institute for Therapeutic Research, Rahway, New Jersey 07065.

of saline once or twice. This step must be omitted if the host has been dead more than a couple of minutes. It must also be omitted if one wishes to count worms less than 2 days old.

4. Place gut in saline in 100 × 20 mm petri dish. Cut the gut into pieces 5–10 cm in length. This helps to prevent intertwining and may facilitate emergence of the worms.

6. Incubate the covered petri dish at 37°C for 4–5 hr. Not all worms emerge from the gut in less time. Longer incubation results in significant disintegration of the gut, which makes counting much more difficult.

7. Remove gut pieces and discard.

8. Count worms in petri dish under a dissecting microscope. To ensure that the entire dish is examined systematically, the dish may be set inside a petri dish lid on which parallel lines have been scored.

9. Differentiation of females from males is relatively easy on the basis of size and the absence of copulatory appendages (see Appendix 1).

Harvesting Adult Worms en Masse. The purpose is to obtain large numbers of adults when one is not concerned about collecting each and every worm.

1. Inoculate rats orally with 2000–10,000 larvae per rat.

2. Collect adults 5–7 days postinoculation, using a thermal migration chamber. The unit portrayed in Fig. 1 is Dr. John R. Egerton's modification of the chamber originally described by Despommier (1973). Add 37°C saline (0.85%) to a depth of about 2 cm over the screen (which has approximately 6.0-mm openings and has the center portion removed to form a ring; it is raised about 6 cm from the bottom of the dish by means of three or four rubber stoppers). Turn light bulb on and adjust the height so that it almost touches the bottom of the deep dish. The temperature in the center of the dish should not exceed 37°C. Peripheral temperatures will be lower.

3. Kill one of the infected rats and remove anterior half of the small intestine. Open longitudinally and rinse gently in saline. Drape intestine on the ring-screen so that it is submerged in the saline. Repeat for as many rats as desired; each 190-mm-diameter deep dish will accommodate up to 10 rat intestines.

4. Within an hour, small white clumps (the worms) begin to move toward the center of the chamber (or toward any other warmer areas). These may be lifted out in clean condition with a wide-mouth Pasteur pipette. If one is less concerned with obtaining clean worms, the screen and intestines can be gently lifted and removed after 1–2 hr and the remaining saline passed through a 200-mesh screen (pore size 74 μm).

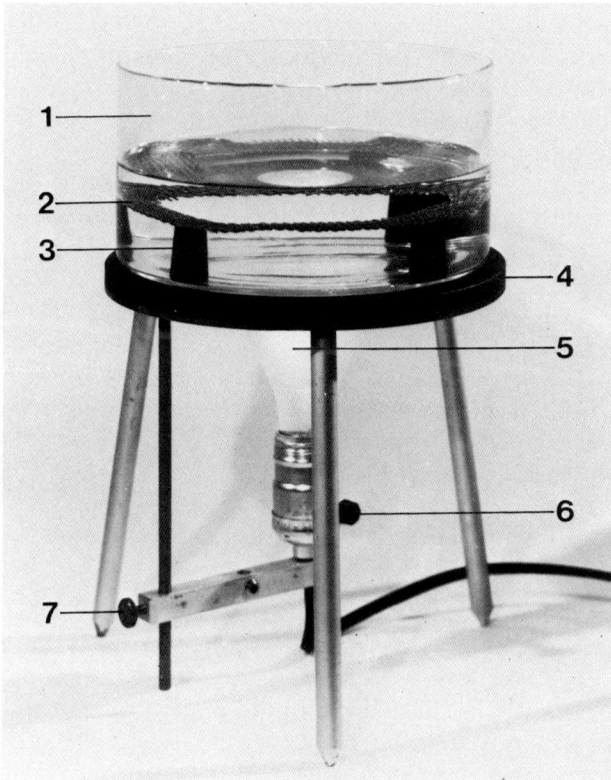

FIGURE 1. Thermal migration apparatus for collection of adult *Trichinella*. (1) Glass dish, 190 mm diameter; (2) ring of metal screen (pore size 6 mm × 6 mm square); (3) rubber stopper (or glass vial or other suitable object) as support; (4) disk of phenolic plastic, 0.13 cm thick, painted flat black on top and copper-colored underneath, with a 5 cm diameter circle removed from center; (5) light bulb, 60 W; (6) socket and switch for light bulb; (7) screw and arm for adjusting height of light bulb.

Adult worms remaining on the screen may then be gently backwashed with saline into a convenient container.

5. Allow collected worms to settle—15 min is usually sufficient. Aspirate the supernatant and resuspend the worms in any desired culture medium.

Harvesting Newborn Larvae

1. Incubate adult worms (obtained from mass collection described above) overnight at 37°C in Medium 199 with 29% calf serum and 1%

antibiotic–antimycotic solution [penicillin 10,000 U/ml, Fungizone 25 μg/ml, streptomycin 10,000 μg/ml (Dennis *et al.*, 1970)].

2. Use additional culture medium to wash contents of dish through a 500-mesh screen (pore size 25 μm). Adults will be retained on the screen, while newborn larvae will pass through and may then be collected in centrifuge tubes.

3. Concentrate newborn larvae by centrifugation for 2 min at 600*g*. Quickly aspirate supernatant and resuspend larvae in desired volume.

Estimating Fecundity

1. Incubate individual female *Trichinella* in small amount (1.0 ml) of maintenance medium in well (1.5-ml capacity) of multiple-well polystyrene plate. Repeat with as many worms as desired—a commonly used plate has 80 wells (Despommier *et al.*, 1977).

2. Cover entire plate with plastic and place in moist chamber at 37°C for 24 hr.

3. Count total number of newborn larvae in each well.

Harvesting and Counting Infective Larvae from Muscle. The purpose is to determine the number of larvae in a given carcass. In an infection less than 17 days old, larvae do not resist pepsin digestion but may be isolated from muscle by mechanical disintegration (see Chapter 16) or by tryptic digestion of minced muscle (0.25% trypsin at 37°C at pH 8.2). Our experience would suggest that for optimal recovery of larvae, it is better to wait (where the experimental objective permits) until at least 35 days postinoculation and to use the peptic digestion method described below.

1. Kill, skin, and eviscerate mouse. This operation is facilitated, without appreciable loss of larvae, by cutting off and discarding the feet and the tip of the snout.

2. Prepare digestive fluid. Add hydrochloric acid to warm tapwater (38–40°C) to give 1.0% concentration (vol./vol.). Add pepsin to give 1.0% concentration (wt./vol.) and stir gently until dissolved.

3. Place carcass in blender with about 100 ml digestive fluid. Blend *briefly*. (We blend for 10 sec at high speed followed by 5 sec at low speed, but individual blenders vary. The object is to obtain the smallest possible pieces of muscle without cutting and killing the muscle larvae.) A meat grinder may be used in place of a blender to mince the muscle.

4. Pour blended or ground carcass into 1- to 2-liter container with leak-proof lid. Rinse blender with additional digestive fluid and add this to container. Add enough additional fluid to give approximately

25 ml digestive fluid per gram of carcass. An excess does not harm the larvae. A volume of 400–600 ml is sufficient for a mouse carcass.

5. Place containers on incubated shaker at 37°C. The container chosen should be large enough to allow vigorous movement of the fluid. If an incubated shaker is not available, the digestion fluid may be agitated by means of a magnetic stirrer or bubbled air. Digestion can be accomplished (though not efficiently) by just shaking the sample periodically by hand and maintaining it at 37°C. Complete digestion requires 1–2 hr on the shaker, the use of other equipment may require additional time.

As an alternative to steps 3–5, the disintegration and digestion of muscle may be carried out by means of a Stomacher apparatus (see Chapter 16).

6. Pour the digested material through a layer of cheesecloth onto a 200-mesh screen (pore size 74 μm). Wash vigorously with water. (We use tapwater, but it is unsuitable in some areas.) Discard cheesecloth and its contents. If digestion is not complete, the cheesecloth and its contents may be returned to the container and digested further. Wash material (consisting almost entirely of larvae) from screen into suitable container. Adjust fluid content of each container to constant volume—typically 50 or 100 ml.

7. Estimate number of total larvae per mouse by aliquot sampling and extrapolation to the total volume. We base counts on 4–8 aliquots of 0.05 ml each, drawn from the same place while the material is magnetically stirred. If larvae are not seen in the aliquots, the material is removed from the stirrer and allowed to settle for at least 15 min, at which time most of the supernatant is remove by aspiration and the entire sediment is examined for larvae. A method for counting larvae electronically has been described (Velebny et al., 1979).

Live larvae can be distinguished by their motility, or, if cold, their tightly coiled appearance. Dead larvae assume the shape of the letter C or the number 6. Differentiation of males from females is possible (but not quickly accomplished with a dissecting microscope during routine counting procedures). For distinguishing criteria, see Chapter 3, Table IV.

As a rule, it is not practical to blend the carcasses of animals larger than mice. They may be treated in one of several ways. The whole carcass may be ground in a meat grinder and digested in its entirety. Another alternative would be to take a random sample of a given volume or weight of the ground carcass. It is also common to take all of a specific muscle (e.g., diaphragm) or, in the case of larger animals such as swine, a portion of one or more muscles. If only a portion of a given muscle is sampled for enumeration purposes, the entire muscle should be ground and randomly sampled. One should remember that "random sample" means that each sample has an equal chance of being selected.

Observation of Intact Capsules (Nurse Cells). Trichinella capsules may be observed by pressing a small bit of infected muscle between two glass slides and compressing tightly while examining under the microscope. The mouse diaphragm is ideal for this purpose. If larval viability is not a consideration, capsules may be isolated by digesting the muscle in a solution of sodium hypochlorite (Seagrave and Holm, 1974). It is convenient to blend 4–5 g muscle in 500 ml diluted household bleach (e.g., 2% Chlorox; Chlorox contains 5.25% sodium hypochlorite). The material is settled in copious amounts of water and finally screened on a 200-mesh screen (pore size 74 μm) and flushed into a container.

Inoculation of Host Animals. The parasite is usually maintained in mice and may conveniently be passaged at 6- to 9-month intervals. Strains of mice differ in their susceptibility, but most are adequate for laboratory maintenance. Relatively few mice are required for maintenance because 20,000–50,000 muscle larvae are commonly harvested from each mouse.

The inoculum size will depend on strain of host, strain of parasite, and purpose of the experiment. With common laboratory strains of parasite and host, a typical inoculum for mice might be 200 larvae per animal. Rats from which one wishes to recover muscle larvae might be given 500–2000 larvae each, while those from which one wishes to recover only adults might be given 5000–10,000 larvae. When inoculated with a laboratory strain of *T. spiralis,* domestic piglets have tolerated an inoculum of 10,000 larvae/kg body weight, but twice that number has caused severe or fatal disease.

To prepare the inoculum, infective larvae are harvested from muscle by peptic digestion as described above. They are suspended in 5% gelatin and stirred with a magnetic stirrer. The magnetic stirrer should be adjusted to the minimum speed for continuous agitation (higher speeds may throw the larvae to the periphery of the container). Aliquots are used to determine the concentration of larvae in the suspension. Additional quantities of larvae or gelatin are added until larvae in the desired number are contained in an appropriate inoculum volume. For a mouse, an appropriate volume would be 0.2–0.3 ml.

Inoculum volume may affect the linear distribution of adults in the small intestine (Sukhdeo and Croll, 1981).

For infection of laboratory animals, syringes fitted with ball-tipped gavage needles are used to inoculate infective larvae into the esophagus. Each inoculum is drawn from the same place while the larval suspension is being stirred. Typically, the first, last, and a middle inoculum are set aside to monitor any change in number or condition of the larva during the inoculation period.

In Vitro Culture. It is relatively easy to maintain all stages of *Trichinella* for short terms in a variety of media (e.g., Medium 199). Development of newborn larvae to adults has not been accomplished *in vitro*. Maturation of infective larvae to adults has been reported, but is not a routine exercise. For further information, see Chapter 3, Meerovitch (1970), and Denham (1967).

A Word of Caution. Larvae that have reached the acid-pepsin-resistant stage of development in host muscle are infective to man. Suspensions of such larvae should never be pipetted by mouth. Surplus larvae should be killed before they are dumped down the drain. Leftover carcasses should be incinerated.

The techniques described above represent selected ways of doing things—for the most part, the way they are currently done at the Merck Institute for Therapeutic Research. For simplicity and brevity, the presentation has been rather arbitrary and references minimized. Numerous variations (probably some of them better methods) exist. Personal experience will no doubt suggest modifications. We hope that these procedures will provide an adequate basis for beginning.

REFERENCES

Denham, D.A., 1967, Applications of the *in vitro* culture of nematodes, especially *Trichinella spiralis*, in: *Problems of in Vitro Culture* (A.E.R. Taylor, ed.), Blackwell, Oxford and Edinburgh, pp. 49–60.

Dennis, D.T., Despommier, D.D., and Davis, N., 1970, Infectivity of the newborn larva of *Trichinella spiralis* in the rat, *J. Parasitol.* **56**:974–977.

Despommier, D.D., 1973, A circular thermal migration device for the rapid collection of large numbers of intestinal helminths, *J. Parasitol.* **59**:933–935.

Despommier, D.D., Campbell, W.C., and Blair, L.S., 1977, The *in vivo* and *in vitro* analysis of immunity to *Trichinella spiralis* in mice and rats, *Parasitology* **74**:109–119.

Meerovitch, E., 1970, Cultivation of *Trichinella spiralis in vitro*, in: *Trichinosis in Man and Animals* (S.E. Gould, ed.), Charles C. Thomas, Springfield, Illinois, pp. 102–108.

Seagrave, J.D., and Holm, D.M., 1974, Physical methods for rapid on-line detection of *Trichinella* in pork, in: *Trichinellosis* (C.W. Kim, ed.), Intext, New York, pp. 579–592.

Sukhdeo, M.V.K., and Croll, N.A., 1981, The location of parasites within their hosts: Factors affecting longitudinal distribution of *Trichinella spiralis* in the small intestine, *Int. J. Parasitol.* **11:**163–168.

Velebny, S., Spaldonova, R., and Corba, J., 1979, Electronical counting of *Trichinella spiralis* larvae, *Helminthologia* **16:**199–206.

Index

This Index should be used in conjunction with the list of Contents. Words such as *rat, antigen,* and *eosinophilia,* which are apt to occur throughout the book, are listed in the Index to guide the reader to discussions of these subjects but not to identify every page on which the words appear.